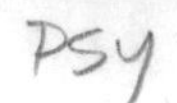

The Control of Eye Movements

The Symposium on the Control of Eye Movements was held under the auspices of the Smith-Kettlewell Institute of Visual Sciences of the Pacific Medical Center and the Department of Visual Sciences of the University of the Pacific Graduate School of Medical Sciences, San Francisco, California, November 10-11, 1969.

The Symposium was sponsored by DHEW, National Institutes of Health Grant Number 1 R 13 ET 00512-01A1.

Publication costs of this volume were defrayed in part by USPHS General Research Support Grant Number 5 SO1 FR 05566.

The Control of Eye Movements

EDITED BY **PAUL BACH-Y-RITA**
CARTER C. COLLINS

Smith-Kettlewell Institute of Visual Sciences
University of the Pacific Graduate School
of Medical Sciences
San Francisco, California

Associate editor
JANE E. HYDE

Smith-Kettlewell Institute of Visual Sciences
University of the Pacific Graduate School
of Medical Sciences
San Francisco, California

Academic Press
New York and London **1971**

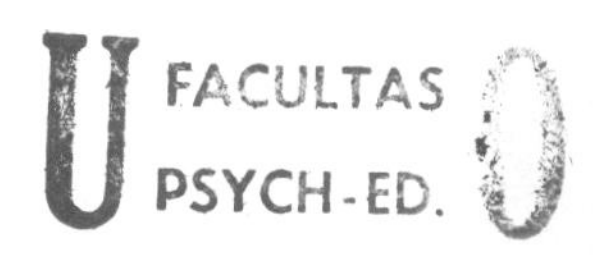

ACADEMIC PRESS, INC.
111 Fifth Avenue, New York, New York 10003

United Kingdom Edition published by
ACADEMIC PRESS, INC. (LONDON) LTD.
Berkeley Square House, London W1X 6BA

Library of Congress Catalog Card Number: 73-117101

PRINTED IN THE UNITED STATES OF AMERICA

CONTENTS

PART I. PHYSIOLOGICAL ASPECTS OF EYE MOVEMENT CONTROL

PART II. THE HUMAN EYE MOVEMENT CONTROL SYSTEM

CONTRIBUTORS

Paul Bach-y-Rita, Smith-Kettlewell Institute of Visual Sciences, University of the Pacific Graduate School of Medical Sciences, San Francisco, California

Malcolm B. Carpenter, Department of Anatomy, Columbia University, New York, New York

Bernard Cohen, Department of Neurology, Mt. Sinai School of Medicine, New York, New York

Carter C. Collins, Smith-Kettlewell Institute of Visual Sciences, University of the Pacific Graduate School of Medical Sciences, San Francisco, California

Robert B. Daroff, Neurology Service, Miami Veterans Administration Hospital, and Department of Neurology, University of Miami School of Medicine, Miami, Florida

Kenneth E. Eakins, Department of Ophthalmology, College of Physicians and Surgeons, Columbia University, New York, New York

Derek H. Fender, Booth Computing Center, California Institute of Technology, Pasadena, California

Leon Festinger, The New School of Social Research, New York, New York

Albert F. Fuchs, Department of Physiology and Biophysics and Regional Primate Research Center, University of Washington, Seattle, Washington

Ragnar Granit, Department of Physiology, Nobel Institute, Stockholm, Sweden

William F. Hoyt, Department of Ophthalmology and Neurosurgery, University of California Medical Center, San Francisco, California

G. Melvill Jones, Aviation Medical Research Unit, McGill University, Montreal, Canada

CONTRIBUTORS

Ronald Katz, Department of Ophthalmology, College of Physicians and Surgeons, Columbia University, New York, New York

Dietrich Lehmann, Smith-Kettlewell Institute of Visual Sciences, University of the Pacific Graduate School of Medical Sciences, San Francisco, California

Jacob L. Meiry, Department of Aeronautics and Astronautics, Massachusetts Institute of Technology, Cambridge, Massachusetts

George P. Moore, Department of Engineering and Physiology, University of Southern California, Los Angeles, California

Lee Peachey, Department of Biochemistry, University of Pennsylvania, Philadelphia, Pennsylvania

Cyril Rashbass, Maudsley Hospital, London, England

David A. Robinson, Department of Engineering, Johns Hopkins Medical School, Baltimore, Maryland

Alan B. Scott, Smith-Kettlewell Institute of Visual Sciences, University of the Pacific Graduate School of Medical Sciences, San Francisco, California

Lawrence Stark, Department of Optometry, University of California, Berkeley, California

Gerald Westheimer, Department of Physiology, University of California, Berkeley, California

Laurence R. Young, Department of Aeronautics and Astronautics, Massachusetts Institute of Technology, Cambridge, Massachusetts

Bert L. Zuber, Department of Information Engineering, College of Engineering, University of Illinois, Chicago, Illinois

PREFACE

Although a number of new contributions to the physiology of ocular kinetics have appeared in the literature, the publications have been scattered and seemingly unrelated. In 1962 a symposium on the oculomotor system was held at Mount Sinai Hospital in New York. The express purpose was assemblage of various scientists and clinicians to exchange their views on the known anatomy, physiology, and clinical applications of disorders of eye movement. Seven years later leading investigators were assembled in San Francisco for this second symposium on the control of eye movements. The twofold objectives were to provide current observations on physiological aspects and clinical correlations and to bring together a number of scientists who approach the analysis of eye movement control from the point of view of modeling.

A valuable aspect of this conference was the diversity of the participants: physiologists, pharmacologists, psychologists, biophysicists, biomedical engineers, "visual scientists," and clinicians. Such a meeting is apt to advance knowledge of functions of the oculomotor system and ultimately lead to better insight into the physiology of the total nervous system.

The first half of the volume is devoted to presentations of anatomical, physiological, pharmacological, psychological, and clinical correlations of eye movements. The material presented should provide a valuable reference source as well as increase our awareness of the need for further investigation of many aspects of the basic physiology of eye movements.

The second half of the volume presents a series of papers dealing with models of various parts of the oculomotor system. The modeling approach to control of eye movements is still in its infancy as witnessed by the fact that this work presents the first comprehensive survey of biophysical, mathematical, and engineering aspects of eye movement control. At such an early stage it is perhaps appropriate to point out some of the possible pitfalls of such an approach. For example, if a complete theory for sensory (visual, vestibular) and oculomotor system interactions is to be valid, it must be generally applicable for other sensori-motor integrations such as that involved in walking, talking, or head movement. It should also apply for all motor performances including a simple sensori-motor model. Doubtless, there are differences between limb movements which may be unilateral, individual, or partial and eye motions which are always binocular, coordinate, and limited in type. In the view of John Hughlings Jackson, the two eyes act as a unit, performing a single action such as ocular deviation or the act of convergence. Physiologically, the important common denominator for motor performance in each instance is laterality. One cerebral hemisphere exerts control over the contralateral limb and binocular movements to the contralateral side. The concept of total function of eye movement should always be borne in mind in studies of individual or patterns of ocular movements. There are investigators who emphasize the data on a single phase of an eye movement. Such information may be extremely important, but the findings must be correlated in a setting of total patterned activity. It is to be hoped that by making available in one volume the present thoughts regarding modeling systems, as well as pointing out the limitations of such models, stimulation for thought and experimentation has been provided.

Interdisciplinary meetings should include discussions on new techniques and instrumentation, description and recording of behavioral changes under varied conditions, comparative studies in animals and man, and theoretical considerations with evaluation of new data and introduction of new concepts. This symposium has achieved many of these goals.

Morris B. Bender
Henry P. and Georgette Goldschmidt
Professor of Neurology and
Chairman of The Department of Neurology
Mt. Sinai School of Medicine
of The City University of New York

PART I

PHYSIOLOGICAL ASPECTS OF EYE MOVEMENT CONTROL

THE PROBABLE ROLE OF MUSCLE SPINDLES AND TENDON ORGANS IN EYE MOVEMENT CONTROL

RAGNAR GRANIT

It is not possible in this context to cover the information we possess on the role of muscle spindles, the gamma-loop and the tendon organs in posture and locomotion. The author has reviewed our knowledge and hypotheses in a book in course of publication (Granit, 1970) entitled, *The Basis of Motor Control,* and to this the reader is referred for the evidence behind the brief statements to be given below.

Eye muscles provided with muscle spindles are regularly found only in primates and ungulates. For these species the extrinsic eye muscles are stated to be the spindle richest in the body competing in this respect with the neck muscles. They are innervated by fusimotor gamma fibres of the static type (definitely shown) and the dynamic type (suggested by indirect evidence). It is not known whether fusimotor alpha innervation is present. The slope of curves illustrating impulse frequency in the afferent nerve fibres from spindle primaries plotted against muscle length increases a great deal, up to sevenfold, under fusimotor gamma stimulation, implying that the static sensitivity to stretch increases under pull. Impulses have never been recorded from the afferents of spindle secondaries in eye muscles, but since these are provided with a static fusimotor innervation, their impulse frequency-length curves are likely to follow those of the primaries.

The statements to the effect that stretch reflexes are absent in extrinsic eye muscles need not be taken too seriously. Stretch reflexes are absent also in the skeletal musculature of normal subjects, unless the fusimotor neurons are specifically activated and the alpha motoneurons (of the extrafusal musculature) in an active state, i.e., sufficiently depolarized. Normally only the brief stretch reflexes known as "tendon jerks" can be elicited. Good stretch reflexes are obtained in normal subjects by activating muscle spindles by rapid vibrations applied at the tendons. All the evidence at present available shows that the stretch reflex is an adjunct to contraction and that alpha and gamma motoneurons are activated together in working muscles. This is the concept of alpha-gamma linkage. Thus, for instance, in respiration gamma activated spindles fire in the contraction phase of intercostal muscles; in volitional activation of muscles of the extremities the spindles likewise fire during contraction, as shown by recent successful attempts to record spindle impulses in man. Many other examples could be mentioned. Essentially, the gamma-activated spindle mechanism may be regarded as a governor of muscular performance both in tone and locomotion. As long as we do not possess as precise information of spindle and tendon organ functions in the normal operations of eye muscles as we have for muscles of the extremities and the ribs, the best one can do in order to understand the role of these organs in eye movements is to apply the principles derived from the other fields of study to the case in hand.

One of the best known tasks of the gamma-assisted stretch reflex is to provide a stable length-setting at any desirable length of the muscle. This is determined by the amount of gamma-bias applied. If the contracting muscle is stretched by a load, the spindles produce automatic *load compensation;* if it is contracted in excess of the applied gamma bias, the silent period *unloads* the spindles thereby preventing excitation of the muscle's alpha motoneurons. It seems more than probable that settings of the gaze are servo-assisted in this manner. The reason for this conclusion is that these two operations will all be automatic as soon as the spindles are under fusimotor influence.

Good evidence for feedback control of the eye muscles is provided by Dr. Carter Collins at this Symposium (Chapter 10). He and his co-workers have shown that in man the tension-extension curves of an extrinsic eye muscle in man are parallel at whatever angle of gaze stretching is begun. The experience from experimental work with the muscle-nerve preparation or with so-called alpha rigidities of cats tells us that in pure alpha activity stretch should produce a set of curves of different slopes depending on the number and firing rate of the alpha fibres. Parallel curves are a definite sign of proprioceptive control, probably executed jointly by spindles and tendon organs on the alpha motoneurons, the former excitatory, the latter inhibitory.

When two antagonist forces are active, as in non-reciprocal eye movements, the consequent variations of loading will automatically activate the muscle spindles and then fusimotor "settings" across the gamma-loop will determine the sensitivity of the muscle to changes of length. In reciprocal action the opposing force will be the elastic pull on bulbar tissue and this, too, will contribute to determining the static sensitivity in relation to angle of gaze.

Eyes without spindles can provide but a crude imitation of the mechanism of the gamma-controlled stretch reflex. This reflex at any one length (angle of gaze) lacks the automatic control that the gamma-spindle mechanism provides for this particular task.

The unvolitional saccadic movements in the eye of the cat are far less prominent and of much lower frequency than in man. Even though these movements are centrally induced and symmetrical in the two eyes, they are likely to make use of the built-in spindle control of the muscular acts which then would operate on binocular alpha-gamma linkage controlled from the same central station. The higher the sensitivity of the fusimotor setting, the greater would be the frequency of the saccades.

There has been no work specifically on muscle spindles in extrinsic eye muscles as involved in the actual process of controlling eye movements. But it is known from work on ungulates (goat) that the static sensitivity, also called the position sensitivity, may increase up to seven times under the influence of fusimotor gamma activity. A powerful augmentation of this order of magnitude can hardly be negligible for the motoneurons controlling the extrinsic muscles, unless the spindle input differs fundamentally from its central distribution elsewhere in the body where spindle projections go to the motoneurons of their own muscle. Regrettably we have no precise information on this important issue and the suggestions given above presuppose that spindle afferents project on the motoneurons of the eye muscles in which these organs are situated. They likewise presuppose that spindle primaries are excitatory and tendon organs inhibitory in the stretch reflex, as these organs are elsewhere in the body. As long as it has not been shown that in this respect these proprioceptors possess central projections differently organized from what they are elsewhere, it is necessary to assume that they are similar, that is, both mono- and polysynaptic.

Finally, it should be pointed out that dynamic fusimotor fibres sensitize the spindle primaries to velocity of stretch. As to the spindle secondaries, which only possess static sensitivity, some doubt may be entertained about their role in eye muscle control. These organs have been found to be excitatory on flexor muscles and inhibitory on extensor muscles. For this there is no obvious parallel in the organization of eye movements.

REFERENCE

GRANIT, R. (1970) *The Basis of Motor Control.* Academic Press, London.

NEUROPHYSIOLOGY OF EYE MOVEMENTS

PAUL BACH-Y-RITA

The oculomotor system has long attracted the attention of many physiologists. The study of this highly precise system offers both challenges and rewards to the basic scientist in addition to providing background essential to the clinical understanding of disorders of oculomotion. The extremely fine coordination of the oculorotary muscles of the two eyes, the variety of types and speeds of movements which are mediated by a very limited number of muscles, and the differences between cranial and spinal motor systems are only a few of the factors influencing some of us to devote our attention to the physiological analysis of the oculomotor system.

Neurophysiological studies of ocular motility present several unique problems to the investigator. The nerves leading to the eye muscles are short, completely embedded within the cranium, and without separate motor and sensory roots. In contrast, the long spinal nerves are surrounded by bone for only a small part of their course, and have dorsal roots conveying afferent information and ventral roots carrying efferent impulses. The three pairs of cranial nuclei providing motor innervation to the extraocular muscles (EOMs) are deeply buried in the brainstem, and are not readily accessible even with the use of stereotaxic techniques. The central connections, both afferent and efferent, have proven difficult to trace. Marked species differences exist with respect to the presence and distribution of sensory receptors in the EOMs. Finally, there is one extraocular muscle, the retractor bulbi, which is found only in some species; even in these its structure is not uniform.

In spite of the difficulties inherent in physiological analyses of ocular movements, this motor system appeared to offer solutions to a number of questions fundamental to an understanding of movement in general, as well as of movement of the eyes. What is the significance of ocular proprioception? i.e., what role is played by sensory receptors in oculorotary muscles? What can we determine of the fundamental physiological properties of the oculorotary muscles? What type of peripheral innervation supplies the EOMs so that they can move with the swiftness of a saccade or the slow smoothness of a following movement? To what extent can we correlate structure with function?

The present chapter represents a summary of efforts to date which

The research reported on in this paper was largely supported by Public Health Service Program Project Research Grant No. NB 06038 and Research Career Program Award No. K3-NB-14,094.

attempt to answer some of these questions. Inasmuch as the majority of studies from our laboratory have concentrated on the peripheral neuromuscular apparatus, the primary emphasis will be on afferent and efferent innervation of the EOMs. Results of studies of stretch receptors and their pathways, types of motor innervation, and muscle fiber types will be presented. A few pertinent aspects of CNS control will be included, although the subject of supranuclear control of eye movements has been extensively reviewed in other chapters of this volume (Cohen; Carpenter) as well as in earlier published summaries (Whitteridge, 1960; Bender, 1964).

AFFERENT MECHANISMS

Background

The importance of proprioceptive muscle afferents in the control of eye movements has been debated since the last century. The two principal opposing views were held by Helmholtz and Sherrington. Helmholtz (1962) suggested that proprioception from the eye muscles was unnecessary because of the presence of the retina (a highly efficient exteroceptor) and the ability of the central nervous system to monitor the efferent outflow from the brain stem. Sherrington (1918), on the other hand, minimized the importance of monitoring the efferent outflow, and strongly supported the concept of a perceptual role for EOM proprioception.

The confusion in regard to the presence or absence of eye muscle "proprioception" has been due in part to differences in definition (Christman and Kupfer, 1963). To some, proprioception means conscious position sense; to others it signifies subconscious nervous control of muscular contraction. The muscle spindle has been thought to be the principle afferent receptor of proprioception in somatic muscles. In the past both conscious and subconscious roles have been assigned to this receptor. Currently, however, the principal function of limb muscle spindles is believed to be in the subconscious nervous control of muscular contractions, rather than in conscious position sense (Matthews, 1964). This is consistent with recent evidence that there is no conscious perception of eye position (Brindley and Merton, 1960), although human eye muscles are richly endowed with muscle spindles.

The role of muscle afferents in the control of eye movements is further complicated by the fact that muscle spindles are present in the eye muscles of some species but not of others, and that the presence or absence of these organs does not appear to be related either to phylogeny or to discreteness of eye movements. Thus, spindles are present in the eye muscles of man, some monkeys, goats and cattle, but not in cat, dog, rat or certain of the monkeys (Cilimbaris, 1910; Cooper and Daniel, 1949; Cooper, Daniel and Whitteridge, 1955; Greene and Jampel, 1966; Cooper and Fillenz, 1955; Bach-y-Rita, 1959). Indeed the eye muscles of the squirrel monkey not only appear to lack spindles, but there is no evidence for any other type of stretch receptors (Ito and Bach-y-Rita, 1969).

Inasmuch as several thorough reviews of extraocular proprioception appeared between 1955 and 1961 (Cooper, Daniel and Whitteridge, 1955; Bach-y-Rita, 1959; Whitteridge, 1960; Hosakowa, 1961), the present paper will emphasize the principal findings of the past ten years, with a discussion of the possible role of proprioception in eye movements.

Stretch receptors

Encapsulated organs with several intrafusal fibers have been identified in the EOMs of several animal species as well as man. These muscle spindles differ from typical limb muscle spindles in size, motor innervation, thickness of capsule, distribution within the muscle, types of sensory endings, and morphology of the intrafusal muscle fibers.

In the eye muscles of man, the muscle spindles are small and have thin capsules; they are distributed in the proximal and distal thirds of the muscles. The intrafusal fibers are similar in diameter to the extrafusal fibers, and do not have distinct nuclear bag regions (Cooper and Daniel, 1957). The sensory endings are apparently not divided into primary and secondary terminals as they are in limb muscle spindles.

The properties of extraocular muscle spindles have been most thoroughly studied in the goat, by Cooper, Daniel and Whitteridge (1955). In the EOMs of this species the muscle spindles are relatively large and numerous; the afferent pathways are separate from the efferent (Winkler, 1937; Whitteridge, 1955).

In addition to muscle spindles and tendon organs, other morphologically distinct receptors have been identified in eye muscles (see previous reviews). Some structures earlier identified as sensory are now known to be motor, subserving the multi-innervated muscle fibers. A recent report on cat eye muscles has described the properties of stretch receptors which are neither muscle spindles nor tendon organs (Bach-y-Rita and Ito, 1966b). While these structures have not been identified histologically, the evidence suggesting that they may be a form of spiral ending is presented below.

In collaboration with Dr. Ito a study was made of the properties of 52 receptors in the inferior oblique muscles of 30 cats (Bach-y-Rita and Ito, 1966b). Between 10 and 28 receptors were noted in each, although it was possible to study only a few receptors in each muscle. Spontaneous discharge was recorded from only one receptor in each of four muscles. The conduction velocities of the afferent fibers from these four receptors ranged from 17-41 m/sec. In the remaining 26 muscles, the minimum stretch eliciting a response varied from 3 to 150 grams, with a peak at 10-20 g. Nineteen of the minimum threshold receptors were quick-adapting and 7 were slow-adapting. Conduction velocities of the corresponding afferent fibers ranged from 6.5 to 52 m/sec with a peak at 10-15 m/sec. (Fig. 1).

All of the receptors were in the muscle, none were in the tendon. It was possible to demonstrate that forty-seven receptors were in parallel, and two

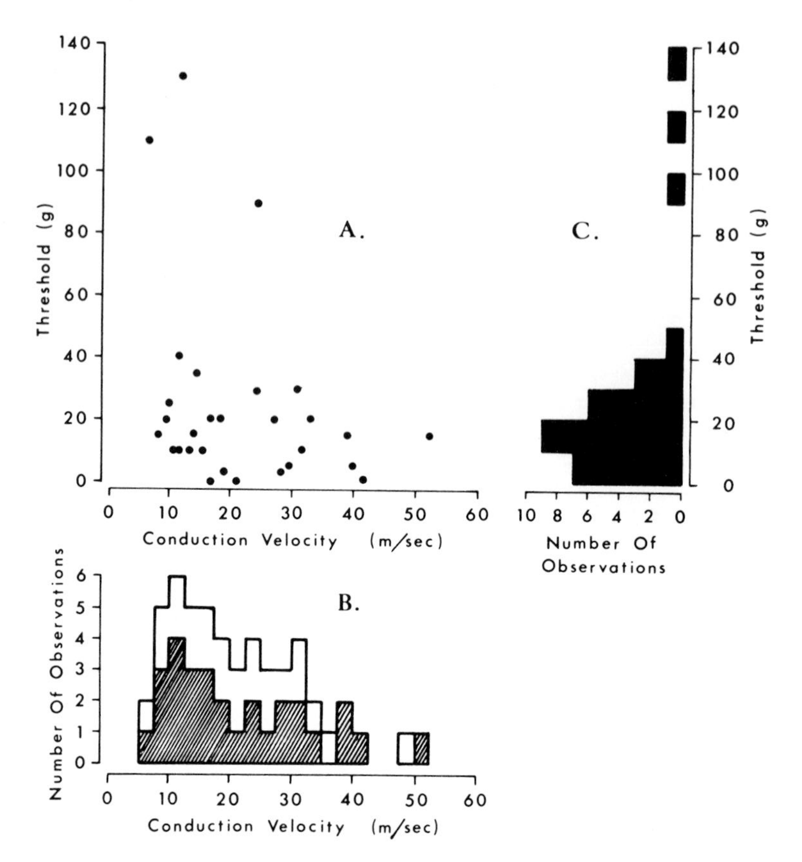

Fig. 1. A. Relation between the threshold value and the conduction velocity for the minimal threshold receptors in individual inferior oblique preparations. **B.** A histogram of the conduction velocities of the afferent fibers from the minimal threshold receptors represented in A (29 units in the hatched area), and for all receptors tested (fifty-two cases). **C.** A histogram of the threshold distribution for the minimal threshold receptors represented in A. (Reprinted by permission of *J. Physiol.* 1966, **186,** 663-668).

were in series with contractile elements (Fig. 2). The dynamic and static indices of all receptors were approximately equal; both increased on increasing initial length. Thus, there did not appear to be a region of reduced viscosity which could compare to that in the equatorial region of intrafusal fibers in limb muscle spindles.

Physiologically there appeared to be a single type of stretch receptor, with or without spontaneous discharge. For the four spontaneously discharging receptors, the minimum load which produced a change in frequency was 0.4 g. Fig. 3 illustrates an increase in discharge frequency of one of these

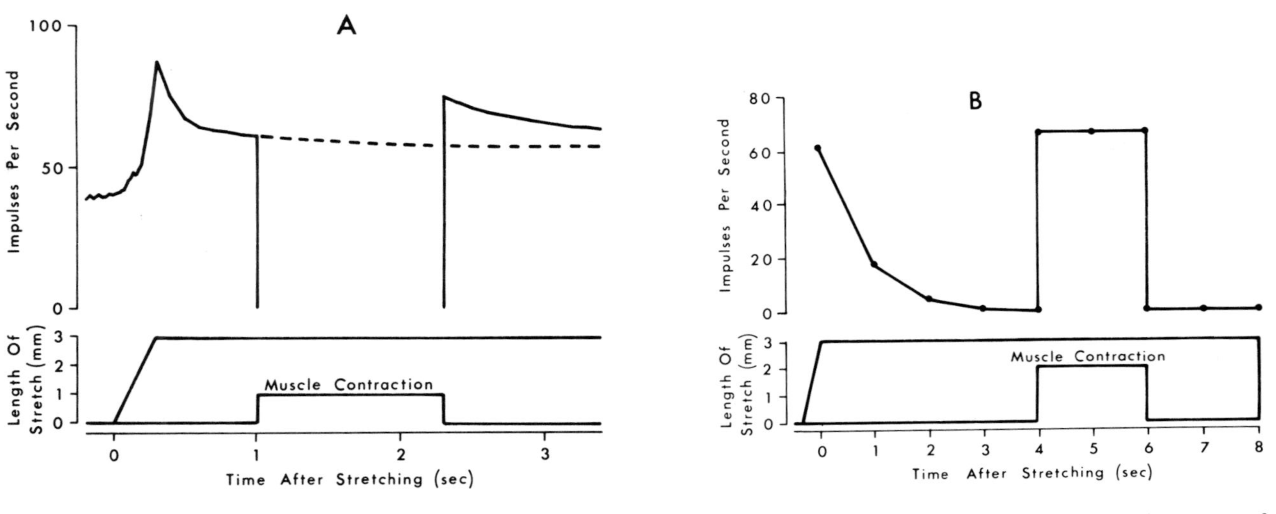

Fig. 2. Effect of tetanic contraction of the inferior oblique muscle on the responses of an in parallel receptor during muscle stretch. **A.** The response of a spontaneously discharging receptor (P-25) to stretching the muscle 3 mm at 10 mm/sec fell to zero frequency during tetanic contraction of the muscle induced by maximal nerve stimulation at 100 c/s (continuous line), in comparison with the control in the absence of nerve stimulation (interrupted line). The diagrammatic representations of the length scale and the muscle contraction are derived from the original records. **B.** Effect of tetanic contraction of the muscle on the responses of an in-series receptor during muscle stretch. The response of a rapidly adapting nonspontaneously discharging receptor (P-12) after 3 mm stretch from +7 mm initial length at 10 mm/sec increased during tetanic contraction of the muscle induced by maximal nerve stimulation at 100 c/sec. (Reprinted by permission of *J. Physiol.* 1966, **186**: 663-668.)

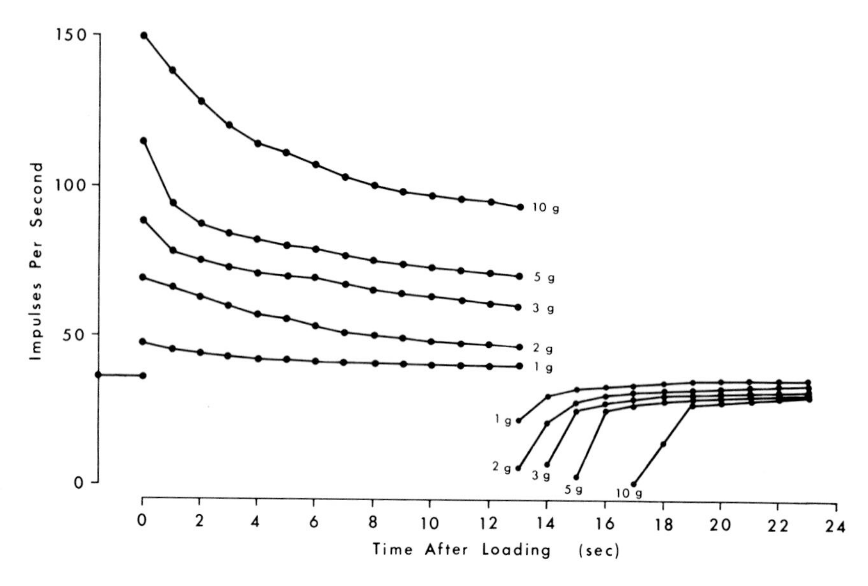

Fig. 3. Frequency of response of a spontaneously discharging receptor (preparation number P-25) after various loads were hung on and removed from the inferior oblique muscle. (Reprinted by permission of *J. Physiol.* 1966, **186**: 663-668).

receptors in response to loads of 1 g or more, and shows a temporary drop below the resting discharge frequency on removal of the loads.

In contrast to the responses from primary endings in de-efferented limb muscle spindles, no initial acceleration in the discharge frequency was noted at the beginning of stretch of the EOM. Increasing the velocity of stretch resulted in a greater maximum discharge frequency and a greater fall-off at the end of the dynamic period. During excessive stretch the receptor appeared to "slip". This, together with the other evidence presented above, suggested to us that the receptor was a type of spiral ending (Fig. 4). We could not be certain which type of muscle fiber was surrounded by these proposed spiral type endings in cats. However, Sas and Appletauer (1963) have shown that spiral endings in the middle third of human extraocular muscles are on the peripheral, thin muscle fibers. Cooper (1966) has shown that the fibers located in the outer layers are multi-innervated, and have characteristics similar to intrafusal fibers. Thus it is possible that the receptors which produced the responses in our study (Bach-y-Rita and Ito, 1966b) were in contact with small, peripheral multi-innervated muscle fibers.

A "silent period" in receptor discharge was noted on stimulation of motor nerve fiber bundles (Bach-y-Rita and Murata, 1964; Bach-y-Rita and Ito, 1966b). Granit (personal communication) has suggested that this "silent

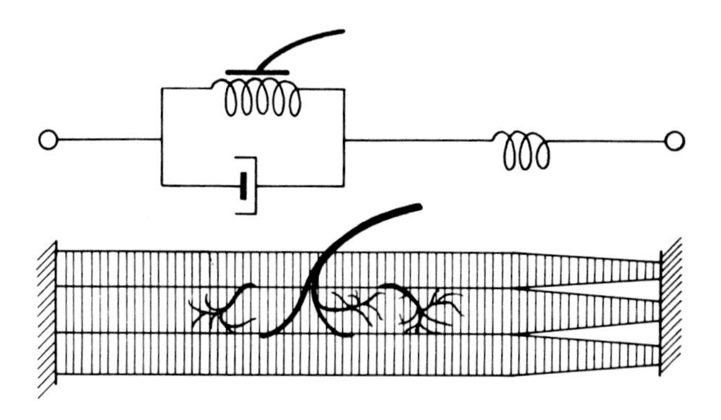

Fig. 4. Schematic diagram of an ending surrounding an extrafusal muscle fiber in the cat's extraocular muscle (lower figure of A) with its functional viscoelastic model (upper figure). (Reprinted by permission of *J. Physiol.* 1966, **186**: 663-668).

period" may have been due to the fact that the spiral afferent endings surround the slower twitch fibers, which may be briefly unloaded when the fast twitch fibers contract.

In the squirrel monkey, no evidence for true stretch receptors was uncovered by physiological studies of the inferior oblique and lateral rectus muscles (Ito and Bach-y-Rita, 1969). However, some receptors were noted which, while unresponsive to stretch, were highly sensitive to temperature, and were silenced by topically applied or intravenously administered adrenaline. The conduction velocities of the afferent fibers from these receptors ranged from 8.6-30 m/sec, with a peak at 15-20 m/sec. On the basis of the above evidence, we suggested that these might be blood vessel receptors (Ito and Bach-y-Rita, 1969). Sas and Appletauer (1963) have described a receptor in the vicinity of an arteriole in a human eye muscle, and Hosokawa (1961) mentions that terminal boutons have been described on EOM blood vessels. It is possible that some of our previous records from cat eye muscles (Bach-y-Rita and Murata, 1964; Bach-y-Rita and Ito, 1966b) may also have been from blood vessel receptors.

Peripheral pathways

Winkler (1937) and Cooper, Daniel and Whitteridge (1955) have shown in goats that the afferent fibers from EOMs travel intraorbitally to a branch of the V nerve, and enter the brainstem with it. The peripheral pathways are less clear in man and in other species (Hosokowa, 1961; Bach-y-Rita, 1959). For example, in the cat there is evidence that afferent fibers cross from the eye muscle nerves to the V nerve (Kumoi and Jampel, 1966; Manni, Bortolami and Desole, 1968; Cooper and Fillenz, 1955; and others). In contrast, in the cat Bach-y-Rita and Murata (1964) have recorded lateral rectus stretch receptor responses from the VI nerve immediately external to the brain stem. The latter observation demonstrates that in cats at least some of the afferents from the eye muscles do not cross over to the V nerve peripherally. In monkeys, Tozer and Sherrington (1910) demonstrated that the III, IV and VI nerves are mixed, carrying afferent impulses to the brain stem as well as motor impulses from the brain stem to the EOM. Taren (1964) on the other hand has demonstrated afferent fibers from EOMs in the IV, V and VI nerves in monkeys, and suggests that afferent fibers in the VI nerve pass through the VI nucleus on the way to the mesencephalic nucleus of the V nerve. Hogg (1964) has observed few, if any, afferents in the III nerves of man or of albino rats.

Ganglion cells

The cells of origin of the EOM stretch receptors have been postulated to have various locations. Some investigators have located these in the mesencephalic nucleus of the V; others propose cells along the course of the EOM nerves. Even the brainstem motor nuclei of the eye muscles have been implicated, but the investigators who suggested the latter location presumably were misled by believing either 1) that the motor endings of the multi-innervated fibers were sensory endings; or 2) that the presence of two distinct sizes of cells in the motor nuclei indicated that one type mediated proprioception.

Manni, Bortolami and DeSole (1968) have recorded numerous afferent responses in a cellular pool in the medial dorsolateral portion of the semilunar ganglion of the V nerve in sheep and pigs, but not in cat. However, as noted above, the fact that in the cat some afferent fibers enter the brain stem via the "motor" nerves to the EOMs (Bach-y-Rita and Murata, 1964) indicates that at least in this species some of the ganglion cells must be located in the brain stem, although the exact location remains unclear.

Central pathways

There has been little clarification of the central nervous system (CNS) pathways for afferent stretch impulses from EOMs since the classical study of Cooper, Daniel and Whitteridge (1953a&b). These authors recorded afferent impulses from EOM in the medial longitudinal fasciculus, central tegmental tract, reticular formation, superior colliculus, occipital lobe, cerebellar tracts and cerebellum.

In most cases the responses showed characteristics and latencies suggesting that the afferent impulses had crossed at least one synapse. Identifiable first order responses were recorded in the mesencephalic nucleus of the V nerve, and from varying sites in the fifth nerve complex in the brain stem (Cooper, Daniel and Whitteridge, 1953a). It was not always possible to be sure the polysynaptic responses were produced by stretch receptors; some could have been from periosteal pain receptors (Cooper, Daniel, Whitteridge, 1953b).

Recently Fuchs and Kornhuber (1969) have shown averaged evoked responses in the cerebellum on stretching eye muscles in the cat. The minimum latency was 4 msec but most of the responses occurred at 15 msec, and the responses were markedly affected by sodium pentobarbitone, indicating second order responses.

One significant advance in knowledge of CNS pathways is found in a recent study by Gernandt (1968) in cats. Gernandt noted that EOM afferent impulses interact in the brain stem with impulses traveling over the slower of the two routes from the vestibular system to the eye motor nuclei. The reticular formation route (the slower of the two routes) was greatly inhibited by preceding EOM stretch, whereas when vestibular stimulation preceded EOM stretch, there was little or no effect on the reticular formation neurons or on EOM motoneurons responding to strong muscle stretch.

Functional role

While the functional role of EOM stretch receptors remains almost as unclear today as when reviewed ten years ago (Bach-y-Rita, 1959), there have been some advances in recent years. Thus it is now evident that the EOM stretch receptors do not mediate conscious position sense (Brindley and Merton, 1960), and there is little evidence that messages from muscle spindles reach consciousness (Cooper, Daniel and Whitteridge, 1955). Matthews (1964), in a discussion of limb muscle spindles, suggested that the main function of muscle spindles was in relation to the subconscious nervous control of muscular contraction. Christman and Kupfer (1963) among others have pointed out that conscious position sense is mediated by capsular receptors in contact with the articulation between two bones, and these are absent in the oculomotor apparatus.

Various postulations on the functional role of EOM stretch receptors have been suggested. Thus Fuchs and Kornhuber (1969) propose that these receptors play a role in a cerebellum-mediated proprioceptive feedback loop for the control of eye movements, providing information to the cerebellum as to the magnitude or the end point of saccades. Christman and Kupfer (1963) offer the theory that the stretch receptors may have a role in fixation micronystagmus. Gernandt (1968) postulates that they may dampen and correct overshoot of eye movements and oscillation. Fender and Nye (1961) propose that EOM proprioception provides negative feedback, especially for small deviations from fixation, but propose further that this negative feedback becomes very slight with large deviations. Otherwise, heavy damping would prevent execution of rapid eye movements. Sasaki (1963) and Sears, Teasdale and Stone (1959) suggest that EOM stretch receptors inhibit motor neurons to the eye muscles. Sasaki (1963) noted that, in the cat, EOM stretch could produce hyperpolarization of motor neurons in the III nucleus. However, Whitteridge (1962) has evidence that the muscle spindles in goat EOMs do not influence the spontaneous discharges of motor neurons. Bach-y-Rita and Ito (1966) have postulated a possible "protective" function of the spiral endings in cat eye muscles to prevent overstretch, similar to the function of Golgi tendon organs in limb muscles. Hyde and Davis (1960) indicated, in cats, a possible role of EOM proprioception in the determination of the end point of movement of the eyes.

There are some species, such as the cat, in which the EOMs have no true muscle spindles, but do have stretch receptors in contact with muscle fibers. It is possible that these extrafusal fibers are playing a role similar to the intrafusal fibers found in other somatic muscles. The equivalent of a "gamma bias" may be mediated by the gamma range nerve fibers to the slow multi-innervated twitch fibers; the latter may have dual properties, whereby the individual fibers can contract both segmentally and with propagated impulses (see below). There are examples of such duality in other species. For example, Ginsborg (1960) has noted such fibers in avian muscles and Koketsu and Nishe (1957b) have suggested that they exist in frog muscle spindles. In frog tongue muscles, Siggins, Berman and McKinnon (1968) have observed fibers with multiple "en grappe" endings and resting potentials averaging -63 mv that produced propagated action potentials. Finally, rabbit limb muscle spindles have been shown to contain only one type of muscle fiber, with only primary sensory endings, but with both "en grappe" and "en plaque" endings on the same fiber. These fibers are capable of mediating all of the phenomena that utilize separate nuclear bag and chain fibers in other species (Edmonet-Denard, LaPorte and Pages, 1964). Granit (this symposium) has analyzed the data obtained from human EOMs by Collins (this symposium) and finds evidence for both muscle spindle (facilitation) and tendon organ (inhibition) type responses.

Thus it is evident that much attention has been lavished on the possible functional roles of the EOM stretch receptors. The role of neck muscle stretch receptors in control of eye position and posture has generally been considered to be minor. For example, Sherrington (1918) assigned the neck receptors a minor role in the control of posture in comparison to the three primary factors of retinal impulses, proprioception from EOMs and impulses from the otic labyrinth. However, several authors (de Kleyn, 1908; Cohen, 1961; Biemond and DeJong, 1969) have presented evidence that proprioceptive impulses from the neck may indeed be of considerable importance in eye movement control and spatial orientation, as well as posture.

EFFERENT MECHANISMS

Eye movement is produced by the 4 rectus and the 2 oblique muscles as well as the retractor bulbi muscle when present. Kennard and Smyth (1963) consider that the eye lid muscle is an EOM. They have demonstrated two types of lid movements, smooth tracking and rapid step-like saccadic adjustments of position, and have demonstrated interactions between blinks and vertical following movements. However, this presentation has been limited to an analysis of the neurophysiology of only those muscles (the 4 rectus, 2 oblique and the retractor bulbi) that move the globe.

Muscle fiber types and neuromuscular endings

The morphological aspects of EOMs have been described in detail by Peachey (this volume), who has presented evidence for 5 types of EOM fiber types. Two widely studied fiber types are a large singly innervated and a small multi-innervated type of fibers. However, fiber bundles in EOMs are tightly packed, which complicates the identification of multiply innervated fibers. Thus both Peachey and Alvarado (personal communications) have dissected out what appeared to be single fibers, only to find on electron microscopic examination that the "single fiber" was in reality a bundle containing several fibers.

Properties of EOM fibers

1. Electrical properties

Although some authors suggest, on the basis of electron microscopy, histological and histochemical evidence, that there are more than two types of fibers in the EOMs, the majority of investigators of the physiological properties of muscle fibers have not been able to clearly differentiate more than two types of fibers. Intracellular microelectrode studies of EOMs in rabbits by Matyushkin (1961) and Ozawa (1964) and in cats by Hess and Pilar (1963) have clearly established that the large singly innervated muscle fibers have high membrane potentials and respond to nerve stimulation with propagated action potentials. These authors, however, suggest that the second type of fiber (corresponding to the small, multi-innervated fibers) does not respond with propagated impulses but rather responds with slow junctional potentials, similar to amphibian slow fibers.

In collaborative studies with Dr. Ito (Bach-y-Rita and Ito, 1966a) we also found propagated impulses from the large singly innervated twitch fibers in cats. However, in contrast to the above, we were able to demonstrate that the multiply innervated fibers are also capable of producing propagated action potentials. Therefore we have labeled them "slow multi-innervated twitch" fibers. (Physiological evidence that these fibers are innervated by more than one nerve fiber is presented in a later section).

In anesthetized *in vivo* cat preparations, the inferior oblique (Fig. 5) and the superior rectus were studied (Bach-y-Rita and Ito, 1966a). The *in situ* superior rectus preparation preserved the insertion of the muscle in the globe and thus allowed intracellular microelectrode exploration of the two types of fibers in their normal anatomical relationship. We noted that the small multi-innervated twitch fibers were located predominantly in the outer (orbital) surface of the superior rectus (S.R.), in conformity with the histological evi-

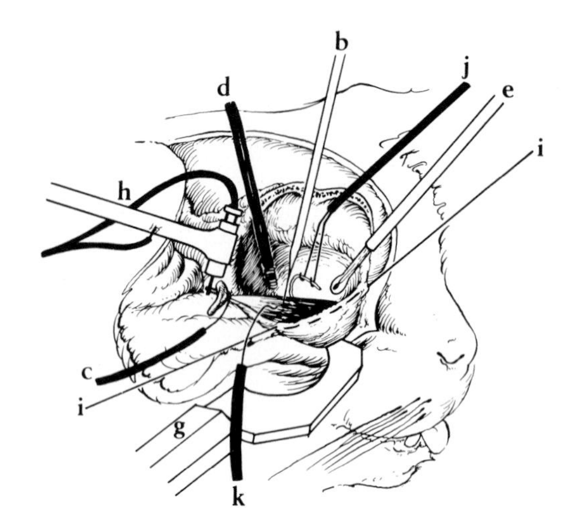

Fig. 5. An illustration of the preparation. The head of the anesthetized cat is held in the stereotaxic instrument. The inferior oblique preparation: (b) micropipette; (c) indifferent electrode; (d) heater; (e) thermistor; (g) part of the stereotaxic instrument; (h) RCA 5734 strain gauge tube and holder; (i) nictitating membrane held by a suture to form an oil pool; (j) platinum electrodes holding nerve to inferior oblique. (Reprinted by permission of *J. Gen. Physiol.* 1966, **49**: 1177-1198).

dence presented by Kato (1938) and Cooper and Fillenz (1955) on the layer organization of small and large fibers in EOMs.

Namba, Nakamura, Takahashi and Grob (1968) have also noted in rat EOMs that the small multi-innervated fibers are found in greater concentration on the orbital surface, away from the globe, in all muscles except for the superior oblique (S.O.). It would therefore seem possible that some of the differences in the results of Hess and Pilar (1963) and Pilar (1967), and those of Bach-y-Rita and Ito (1966) may be due to the fact that the detailed studies of Hess and Pilar (1963) and Pilar (1967) were undertaken on the S.O. which has a different fiber organization than other EOMs and contains a greater percentage of "slow" fibers (Hess and Pilar, 1963), whereas our own studies were on S.R. and inferior oblique (I.O.). Also, the *in vitro* studies of cat EOM by Hess and Pilar (1963) were performed at room temperature, which is far below the body temperature at which the muscles are normally maintained.

Cooling inhibits action potentials in mammalian (Nakanish & Norris, 1970) and frog muscle fibers (Ling & Woodbury, 1949). Indeed, this may be a natural mechanism for reducing energy consumption in cold blooded animals. For example, frogs are more sluggish in the cold, and physiologists have found differing results in studies on summer and winter frogs.

In our studies (Bach-y-Rita and Ito, 1966a) it was found that fast singly innervated and slow multi-innervated twitch fibers can be distinguished on

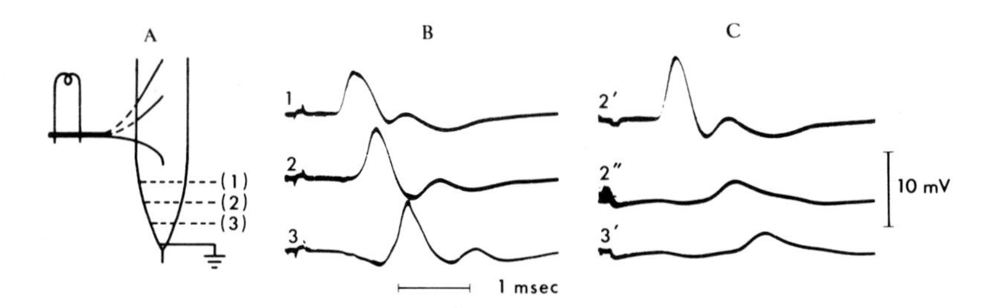

Fig. 6. Action potentials recorded externally from an inferior oblique muscle. **A.** The branch of the third cranial nerve to the inferior oblique has been cut at the level of the ciliary ganglion, and placed over stimulating electrodes. At its entrance into the muscle, the nerve divides into three branches; the proximal and central branches have been cut. The recording electrode has been placed on the muscle, and moved toward the distal end in 1 mm steps. The indifferent electrode is located at the distal end. **B.** Responses to maximal nerve stimulation (cathode excitation); Nos. 1, 2, and 3 correspond to the numbered recording sites on the muscle (in part A). **C.** 2" and 3' are the responses to anode block stimulation, recorded from points (2) and (3), in comparison with a response (part C-2') on maximal cathode stimulation. (Reprinted by permission of *J. Gen. Physiol.* 1966, **49**: 1177-1198).

the basis of impulse conduction velocities (Fig. 6); ranges of membrane potentials; amplitudes and frequencies of miniature end plate potentials; responses to the intravenous administration of succinylcholine (a depolarizing blocking agent); the frequency of stimulation required for fused tetanus; the rise and decay times of their twitch responses to nerve stimulation; and the velocities of conduction of the nerve fibers innervating each of the types of muscle fibers. The technique of anode block stimulation also differentiates the two types of fibers, by activating only the small multi-innervated twitch fibers, not the large fast singly innervated twitch fibers (Fig. 7).

Certain difficulties attend the study of EOM fibers with intracellular microelectrodes. For example, the small multi-innervated twitch fibers are more delicate and more easily injured than the large singly innervated fibers. In our study, action potentials were recorded only from those small fibers whose membrane potential exceeded 48mV. In four preparations, the average membrane potential of 88 fibers, known to be small twitch fibers on the basis of activation by anode block stimulation, was 59 mV. In contrast, the membrane potential of 875 large fast fibers recorded from four muscles ranged from 64-106 mV. In one muscle, of 153 small multi-innervated muscle fibers, only 39 produced propagated action potentials. We (Bach-y-Rita and Ito, 1966a) interpreted this to mean that the other multiply-innervated twitch fibers had decayed due to injury and thus were no longer able to produce action potentials. This was observed to occur on numerous occasions in our experiments (Fig. 8) and Ginsborg (1960) observed a similar phenomenon in avian muscle fibers. Also, in some cases when a hyperpolarizing current was passed through the same microelectrode (using a bridge circuit) into a decayed small fiber, we were again able to record action potentials.

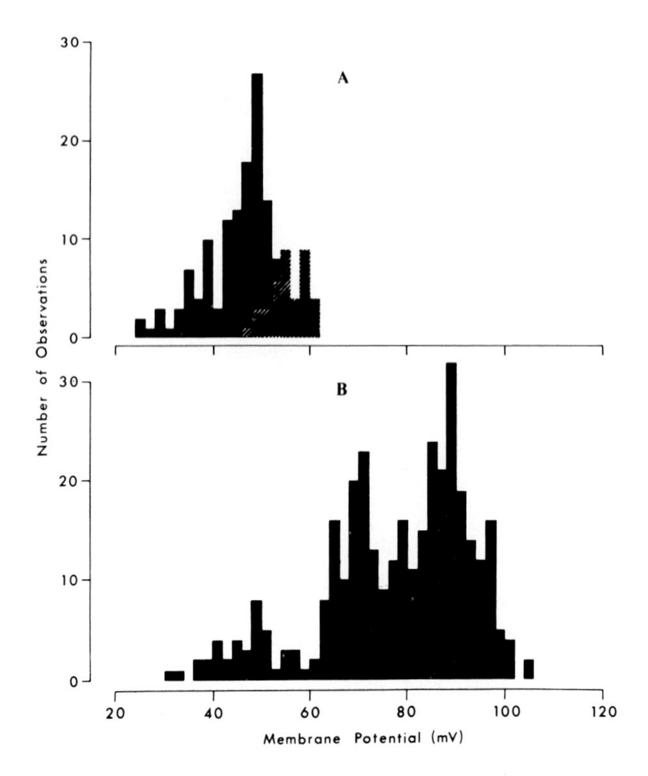

Fig. 7. Resting potentials of muscle fibers in an inferior oblique muscle. **A.** The potentials of fibers that responded to anode block stimulation of the nerve; fibers that responded with overshoot spikes are represented in crosshatching. **B.** Potentials of fibers that did not respond to anode block excitation. The fibers in the slow fiber range of membrane potentials fall between the arrows. (Reprinted by permission of *J. Gen. Physiol.* 1966, **49**: 1177-1198).

Similarly, Koketsu and Nishi (1957a&b) found that many of the multi-innervated intrafusal muscle fibers of frog limb muscles produce overshoot spike potentials, but others produce only junctional potentials. They considered the inability of these fibers to produce spike potentials to be due to membrane injury caused by insertion of the microelectrode, and the consequent loss of membrane potential. Ginsborg (1960) concurred in this opinion. Koketsu and Nishi (1957b) also noted (in frog intrafusal fibers) that spike discharges could be produced by hypopolarization even when none was produced by depolarization.

In addition to multi-innervated twitch fibers with properties similar to those described by Koketsu and Nishi (1957a&b) in frog intrafusal fibers, cat eye muscles may include fibers with properties similar to those of frog "tonus"

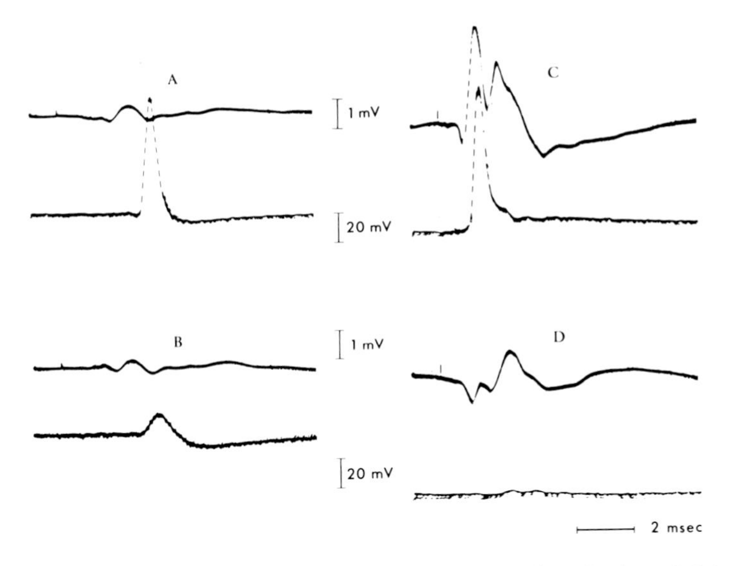

Fig. 8. Intercellular records of responses in slow (parts A, B bottom lines) and fast (parts C, D bottom lines) muscle fibers of an inferior oblique muscle, in comparison with the extracellular responses displayed on the zero volt reference line (top lines). **A.** Anode block excitation followed by a long latency overshoot spike when the membrane potential was 68 mv. **B.** A nonovershoot response when the membrane potential (same fiber as in part A) had decreased to 45 mv. **C.** A short latency overshoot spike response to maximal nerve stimulation (cathode excitation) in the fast fiber. **D.** No response to an anode block excitation in the same fiber as part C. Parts A and C have been retouched with dashed lines. (Reprinted by permission of *J. Gen. Physiol.* 1966, **49**: 1177-1198).

fibers which do not produce propagated action potentials. Peachey (this volume) has found a small percentage of this type of fiber in cat EOMs.

R. Adrian (personal communication) has suggested a possible reason for the loss of spike potentials by the small but not the large twitch fibers in the region of the recording electrode. When a micropipette is placed inside a fiber, there is a leakage around the tip of the pipette and thus a resistance shunt. If the specific resistance of the sarcoplasm and membrane do not change with fiber diameter, the input resistance of a fiber is inversely proportional to the 3/2 power of the fiber diameter. Thus, for the same shunt at the microelectrode, the reduction of the membrane potential in the region of the microelectrode will be greater in small fibers than in large fibers. This factor may produce the truncated action potentials, and the electrical events which look similar to slow junctional potentials, such as we (Bach-y-Rita and Ito, 1966a) and Koketsu and Nishi (1957a&b) note in many slow multiply-innervated twitch fibers (Fig. 8). In a large fiber, a comparable degree of fiber injury would not significantly affect the propagated action potential.

A further complicating factor in the analysis of certain electrical events recorded intracellularly from both fast and slow twitch fibers is the possibility of mechanical artifacts. The EOMs are capable of extremely rapid contraction, and have a twitch rise time of about 5 msec (see next section). Also, the conduction velocities of the motor nerve fibers (Yamanaka and Bach-y-Rita, 1968) are sufficiently rapid to allow the mechanical events to be initiated within a few msec of nerve stimulation in both types of fibers (Bach-y-Rita and Ito, 1966a). It therefore follows that the electrical events recorded after a few msec following nerve stimulation may be obscured by mechanical artifacts. Thus the late (more than 5 msec) electrical events observed by us and others (Matyushkin, 1961, 1964; Hess and Pilar, 1969; Pilar, 1967) cannot be adequately identified, since they are undoubtedly contaminated by movement of the muscle, even when this is held "isometrically."

Utilizing direct physiological-morphological correlations, we have recently demonstrated that small orbital-layer fibers with demonstrable multiple neuromuscular endings are capable of producing propagated action potentials (Alvarado, Adrian, Bach-y-Rita and Peachey; in preparation). This study employed the intracellular dye techniques of Thomas and Wilson (1966) in which a dye is driven out of the microelectrode by electrophoresis. This technique permits intracellular labelling of the individual muscle fibers that have been studied by physiological methods. The neuromuscular endings are demonstrated by histochemical techniques and the fine structure can be elucidated by electron microscopy. Ozawa and collaborators (Ozawa, *et al.*, 1969) had previously demonstrated by similar techniques that both singly and multiply-innervated rabbit EOM muscle fibers are capable of producing propagated action potentials.

2. Mechanical properties

The eye muscles exhibit the most rapid contraction of any mammalian muscles. The rise time of the twitch on nerve stimulation is 5 to 8 msec, with a half-decay time of approximately 7 msec (Cooper and Eccles, 1930; Brown and Harvey, 1941; Bach-y-Rita and Ito, 1966) (Fig. 9).

The twitch obtained on maximal stimulation of the nerve (Fig. 9A and B) includes two components: the fast fiber twitch (Fig. 9Ba) and the slow multiply-innervated twitch (Fig. 9, Bb). The slow component does not contribute to the peak of twitch tension, since its rise time is 20-27 msec while the fast component has a rise time of 5-7 msec; thus the maximum amplitude of the slow twitch occurs after the peak of twitch tension, when the fast twitch is almost fully decayed. The slow twitch component produces the long, late decay portion of the total muscle twitch, since the total duration of the slow twitch is about 200 msec (Bach-y-Rita and Ito, 1966a).

In the I.O. the maximum twitch tension recorded by Brown and Harvey (1941) was 1.6 grams. Bach-y-Rita and Ito (1966a) recorded a maximum twitch tension of 3 grams.

The maximum tetanic tension of the cat I.O. was 40 gr. (Bach-y-Rita and Ito, 1966a). The stimulus frequency necessary for a fused tetanus was reported to be 350 c/s by Cooper and Eccles (1936) and Brown and Harvey

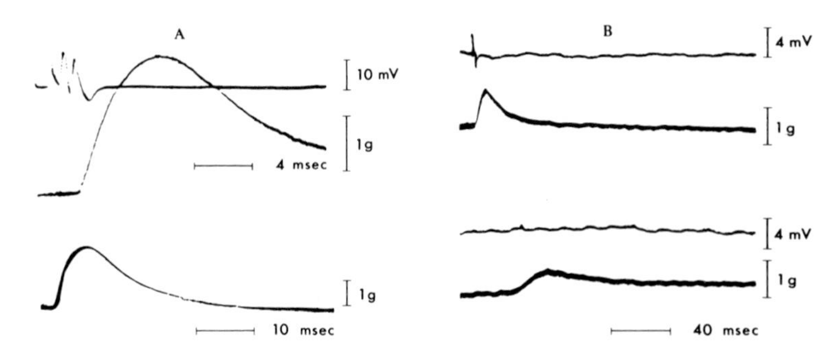

Fig. 9. Isometric twitches in response to nerve stimulation of the inferior oblique muscle. A. Time courses of maximal twitch responses to cathode excitation of a nerve in which none of the three branches had been cut; initial tension 2.6 g (a) a single twitch (lower trace) and the simultaneously recorded surface potential indicating both fast and slow fibers were activated (upper trace); (b) the total contraction time course of a single twitch. B. Single twitch response when the proximal and central branches of the innervating nerve had been cut. Initial tension 5.5 g (a) a single twitch of fast fibers selectively stimulated by a threshold cathode excitation to the nerve (lower trace) and a simultaneously recorded extracellular action potential showing only the fast fiber activation (upper trace). (b) a single twitch of slow fibers, selectively stimulated by anode block excitation (lower trace) and the simultaneously recorded extracellular action potential showing only the slow fiber activation (upper trace). (Reprinted by permission of *J. Gen. Physiol.* 1966, **49**: 1177-1198).

(1941), while we (Bach-y-Rita and Ito, 1966a) noted fusion frequencies up to 450 c/s (Fig. 10). It is possible that this discrepancy may merely be due to differences in recording techniques. For example, Buller and Lewis (1965) noted that higher amplification always results in higher fusion frequencies. Thus they have employed the term "apparent fusion frequency" for results obtained at typical amplification. In the case of cat muscles, the "apparent fusion frequency" is approximately 400 c/s.

In our studies the tetanic force in the I.O. approached a plateau approximately 40 msec after initiation of stimulation at 350 c/s (Fig. 10), but did not reach maximum until 125-150 msec. from initiation of stimulation (Bach-y-Rita and Ito, 1966a). This long late small rise in tension may be due to the slow component. In limb muscle, Buller and Lewis (1965) have shown that the slow twitch fibers (which in limb muscles are singly innervated) produce the slow, late, small rise in tension.

The EOMs exhibit a resting "tone" in the absence of movement. This appears as "motor unit discharges" when studied by means of electromyography (EMG) in human eye muscles (Bjork and Kugelberg, 1953). We (Yamanaka and Bach-y-Rita, 1966) have shown, in cats, that only the slow nerve fibers (to the slow multi-innervated muscle fibers) discharge spontaneously (see below). However, review of the literature failed to reveal any direct measurement of the mechanical force of the tone. Therefore experiments were performed (Bach-y-Rita, unpublished data) in the cat VI nerve-lateral rectus and IV nerve-superior oblique preparations to measure the difference in

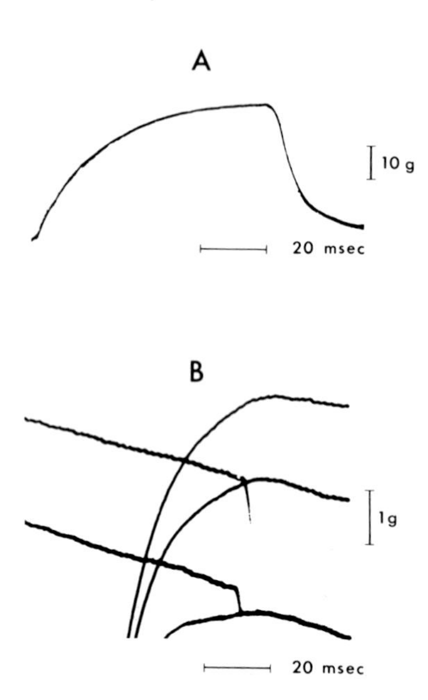

Fig. 10. Isometric tetanic contractions of the inferior oblique muscle in response to repetitive nerve stimulation. A. Maximal tetanic tension of an inferior oblique muscle preparation with all three branches intact; initial tension 3.8 g, stimulation frequency 350/sec. B. The same preparation as in part A with high gain amplification. Maximal intensity stimulation at (a) 400 and (b) 500/sec was followed by individual peaks of contraction; at 600/sec (c), the tetanic contraction was apparently fused. (Reprinted by permission of *J. Gen. Physiol.* 1966, **49**: 1177-1198).

resting tension in an anesthetized state (in which the tone is absent; Eliasson, Hyde and Bach-y-Rita, 1957) and when the cat was unanesthetized. The methods will be described briefly since the results are unpublished. The cats were anesthetized with fluothane, and a tracheal cannula inserted. The lateral rectus was freed from the globe, together with a portion of sclera. The globe was removed and the muscle tied to a strain gauge. The nerve was exposed and a suture was placed loosely around it. The initial tension was adjusted to 2 to 3 grams. The fluothane administration was suspended and as the cat approached a waking state a gradual increase in the tone was recorded. The tone reached up to 7 grams and usually stabilized, with some variations due to spontaneous movements. When a base line was obtained at this level of tension, the nerve was sectioned and the tension immediately dropped. Up to 5 grams of tone was noted in the lateral rectus, and up to 3.5 grams was recorded from the superior oblique. The tone is produced by muscle fibers which are innervated by small motor nerves (Yamanaka and Bach-y-Rita, 1968). Collins, Scott and O'Meara, (1969) have evidence that in human EOMs the tone may be as high as 15 grams.

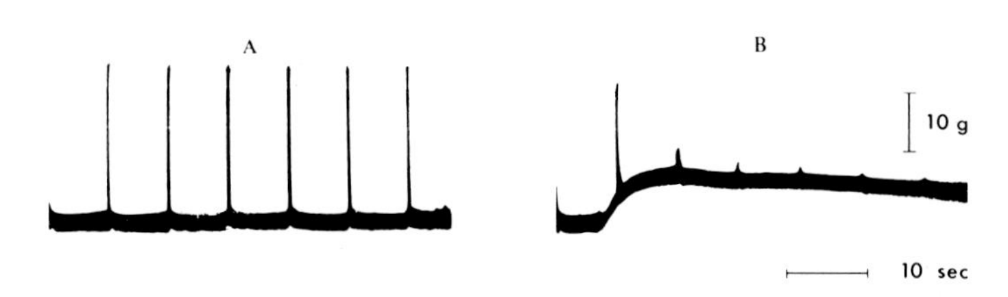

Fig. 11. Isometric contracture produced by succinylcholine, and the simultaneous decrease in the amplitude of the tetanic contraction of the inferior oblique muscle. Initial tension 2.6 g. **A.** Before the administration of succinycholine; maximal nerve stimulation at 350/sec for 150 msec which produced maximal tetanic tension, was delivered at the rate of 0.13/sec. **B.** After the administration of succinycholine; 250 μg in a 2.7 kg cat, injected in the femoral vein at the beginning of the trace (arrow). (Reprinted by permission of *J. Gen. Physiol.* 1966, **49**: 1177-1198).

3. Pharmacological properties

In addition to differences in electrical and mechanical properties between two types of EOM fibers, the large singly innervated and the small multi-innervated twitch fibers respond differently to depolarizing blocking agents such as succinylcholine (Ginsborg, 1960; Kern, 1965). While responses to these and other pharmacological agents will be presented in detail by Eakins and Katz in this symposium, certain pertinent studies on succinylcholine (Sch) will be presented here. In our studies (Bach-y-Rita and Ito, 1966a) we noted differences in the time course of Sch action on each fiber type (Fig. 11)and demonstrated that the Sch-induced contracture of the slow fibers could reach one-third of the maximum tetanic force of the muscle. The multiply innervated muscle fibers, in the outer layers of the muscles, produce the contracture (Kern, 1965).

The mechanism of action of Sch is apparently the same on each type of muscle fiber, maintained depolarization at the motor end plate. By means of multiple microelectrode penetrations along the length of single muscle fibers in *in vitro* frog muscles, Ito (1967) has demonstrated that Sch produced depolarization to approximately half the resting membrane potential in the region of the end plates. Thus, in multi-innervated fibers it is probable that most of the muscle fiber is depolarized, inasmuch as neuromuscular endings occur along the length of the fiber. Muscle shortening accompanies the depolarization at multiple foci. This would appear to explain why the multi-innervated fibers show marked contracture while the singly innervated fibers do not. The end plate region of singly innervated fibers occupies a very small part of the muscle fiber length, and thus a contracture here is obscured in mechanical recordings of the total muscle (Fig. 12).

In EOMs (and also in the stapedius and tensor tympani muscle of the ear, [Bach-y-Rita, unpublished observations]) the dominant picture following Sch administration is contracture. When the depolarization in any fiber is sufficiently rapid, action potentials are produced in that fiber by a post-

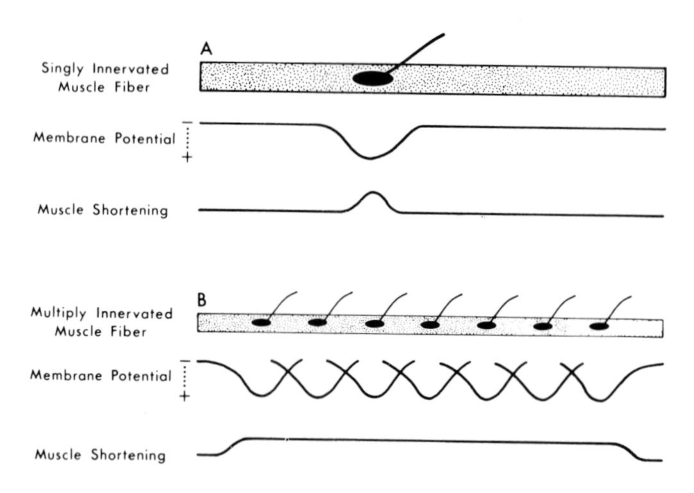

Fig. 12. Schematic representation of the responses of muscle fibers to succinylcholine, which produces muscle fiber deplorization in the region of the neuromuscular junction. **A.** A singly-innervated fiber is depolarized only in the region of the end plate. Only a small portion of the muscle is contracted, and thus tension recordings from muscles that have only singly-innervated fibers (e.g. the retractor bulbi) do not reveal a tension increase. **B.** A multiply-innervated fiber is depolarized along the entire length, and tension recordings reveal muscle shortening.

synaptic effect of the drug (Ito, 1967), thus accounting for the initial fibrillation observed clinically on administration of Sch.

Sch also produces antidromic responses along motor nerves in cats (Bach-y-Rita, Murata and Mulach, 1963) and in frogs (Ito, 1967). This is apparently due either to a presynaptic action or, as Ito (1967) suggests, to a direct effect on the motor nerve fiber. Ito (1967) noted that the threshold concentration for producing muscle membrane depolarization was higher than that for the antidromic activation of motor fibers.

Nerve fibers

1. Fiber spectrum

The nerves to the extraocular muscles contain large numbers of small, gamma range motor fibers (such as innervate muscle spindles in the limbs). Such small fibers are found even in those species, including the cat, which have no muscle spindles in the EOMs. O'Leary, Heinbacker and Bishop (1934) earlier noted that the nerves to EOMs in the cat contain up to 40% of these small fibers. Similar results have been found by other authors (Bjorkman and Wohlfart, 1936; Rexed, 1944; Donaldson, 1960; Pilar and Hess, 1966; Steinacker and Bach-y-Rita, 1968). However, in our recent studies (Steinacker and Bach-y-Rita, 1968) we have observed a greater number of large fibers than were observed in some earlier studies, possibly due to

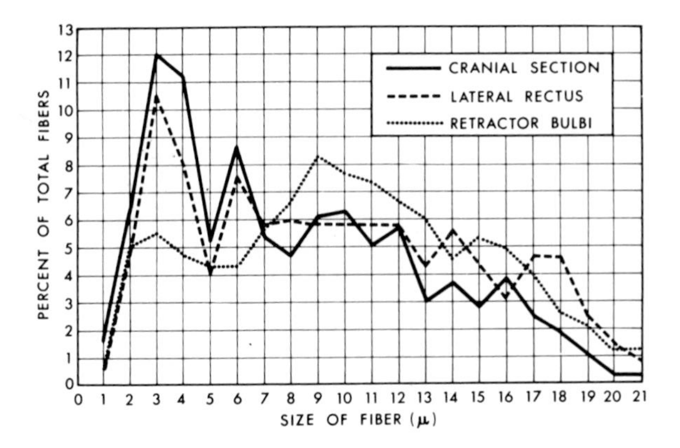

Fig. 13. Fiber diameter in 1 μ size increments plotted as % of total number of fibers in the VI nerve. Each value is the average of measurements at that diameter in 4 nerves. Average range of variability at any fiber size was 4.89% for the retractor bulbi, 5.68% for the lateral rectus, and 2.18% for the cranial sections. Statistical evaluation courtesy of Dr. J. Harrison. (Reprinted by permission of *Experientia (Basel)*, 1968, **24**: 1254-1255).

improved fixation methods that reduce shrinkage. Thus, although the largest fibers found in the cat VI nerve by Bjorkman and Wohlfart (1936) were 13 μ in diameter, we (Steinacker and Bach-y-Rita, 1968) found approximately 17% of the fibers were in the 13-21 μ range.

In our studies (Steinacker and Bach-y-Rita, 1968) the fiber spectrum of the cat VI nerve was explored at three levels: 1) at the emergence from the brain; 2) at the periphery, close to the entrance to the lateral rectus (LR), and 3) at the branch to the retractor bulbi (RB) muscle. The first two spectra showed peaks at 3-4μ and 6μ. The branch to the retractor bulbi, a muscle with a uniform population of singly innervated fast fibers (described below) exhibited a single peak between 6 and 14μ (Fig. 13). The measurements of fiber diameters included the myelin sheaths. The total number of nerve fibers increased approximately 30% between the cranial section and the peripheral sections. This is consistant with the findings of Eccles and Sherrington (1930) on fiber branching in the nerves to limb muscles. We also noted that approximately seven times as many fibers innervate the LR than the RB, although the latter probably contains more muscle fibers.

2. Innervation ratio

It is not possible at this time to specifically determine the ratios of motor nerves to muscle fibers in the EOMs for two reasons: 1) The number of afferent and autonomic fibers is not known since these are mixed with the motor nerves. For example, we (Bach-y-Rita and Murata, 1964) demonstrated that at least some of the afferent fibers from stretch receptors in the LR of the cat enter the brain via the VI nerve, but we were unable to estimate the number of such fibers in each nerve. It is not known how many, if any, of the muscle fibers in the EOMs extend from end to end of the muscle. Brown and Harvey (1941) stated that all do, but gave no evidence for this. Thus, the innervation ratio figures mentioned in the literature (1:3 to 1:7; Duke-Elder, 1961) may be inaccurate.

In the cat retractor bulbi Alvarado (in preparation) presents data from electron microscopic studies that indicate the fibers do not extend from end to end. This muscle, which has a uniform population of fibers, cannot be compared directly with the other EOMs. However, it should be noted that in the retractor bulbi we (Steinacker and Bach-y-Rita, 1968) have estimated a ratio of approximately one nerve fiber to 50 muscle fibers, assuming that the mid-muscle section (Alvarado, in preparation) includes most of the fibers.

3. Innervation of muscle fibers

In the cat EOMs, the small (gamma range) motor neurons supply multiply innervated muscle fibers, as shown by intracellular, mechanical and surface potential studies (Bach-y-Rita and Ito, 1966a) (described above). The larger motor fibers innervate the fast, singly innervated twitch fibers. Sas and Schab (1952) have shown in cats that the branch of the nerve to the distal third of the inferior oblique is made up largely of small nerve fibers. In contrast, the branch supplying the middle third of the muscle, where the "innervation band" of the singly innervated twitch fiber is located includes both small and large nerve fibers. In species that have muscle spindles in the EOM's, some of the small fibers may innervate intrafusal fibers.

The ranges of conduction velocities of both small and large motor fibers in cat EOMs were determined to be 6-40 m/sec for the slow group of motor fibers, and 41-83 m/sec for the fast fibers (Yamanaka and Bach-y-Rita, 1968; Ito, Bach-y-Rita and Yamanaka, 1969). A correlation of these conduction velocities with functional roles of the fast, and of the slow multiply innervated twitch fibers will be discussed below.

4. Polyneuronal innervation

Some of the muscle fibers of the EOMs are each apparently supplied by several motor nerve fibers. Strong evidence that they are polyneuronally innervated has been provided by the following three studies from our laboratory:

a) In the first study, (Bach-y-Rita and Ito, 1966) the proximal and middle branches of the nerve to the inferior oblique were sectioned as noted in Fig. 6. The section eliminated approximately 75% of the motor input to the muscle since the one remaining branch was the smallest in diameter. Stimulation of this remaining branch produced a response in 75% of the slow fibers studied, rather than in 25% as would be expected if the fibers were not polyneuronally innervated.

b) In six cats the nerve to the inferior oblique was divided and each section was placed on stimulating electrodes. In this study (Bach-y-Rita, unpublished data) a comparison was made of the mechanical responses to stimulation of each branch separately and of both simultaneously. The total amplitude of the twitches produced by stimulation of each portion was approximately 95% of the amplitude of the twitch produced by simultaneous stimulation of both branches. This resulted from the fact that the peak tension of the twitch is produced by fast, singly innervated fibers (see above). In contrast, however, the amplitude of the tetanic response to simultaneous stimulation of both portions of the nerve was only 65% of the sum of the amplitudes of the responses to tetanic stimulation of each portion separately. The tetanic response is produced by both fast and slow twitch fibers.

c) With the nerve to the I.O. separated into two portions (as in the study described above), we (Alvarado, Bach-y-Rita and Ito, in preparation) have obtained intracellular recordings from fibers that respond with action potentials to stimulation of each branch, indicating dual innervation.

On the basis of these observations it would appear appropriate to consider these fibers polyneuronally innervated.

Retractor bulbi muscle

In addition to the four rectus and two oblique muscles, species that have a nictitating membrane also have another extraocular muscle, the retractor bulbi (RB). The functional role of the RB is protective: it retracts the globe, forcing the intraorbital fat against the base of the nictitating membrane and causing the latter to sweep across the globe (Motais, 1885).

The RB is inserted in the globe proximal to the rectus and oblique muscles. It has differing forms in the various species in which it is found (Motais, 1885). In the cat, the muscle is composed of four slips, and is innervated by a branch of the VI nerve (Hopkins, 1916; Bach-y-Rita and Murata, 1964; Steinacker and Bach-y-Rita, 1968).

The RB has been shown to differ physiologically (Bach-y-Rita and Ito, 1966), histologically (Alvarado, Steinacker and Bach-y-Rita, 1967) and pharmacologically (Bach-y-Rita, Levy and Steinacker, 1967) from the other 6 EOMs. For example, it does not exhibit contracture on the administration of Sch either in the *in vivo* (Bach-y-Rita and Ito, 1965) or the *in vitro* preparations (Bach-y-Rita, Levy and Steinacker, 1967).

Further, the RB lacks slow, multi-innervated twitch fibers. Rather it has a uniform population of fast twitch fibers (Alvarado, Steinacker, and Bach-y-Rita, 1967; Alvarado and Peachey, in preparation) with single motor end plates (Namba, Nakamura, Takahashi and Grob, 1968). The fibers apparently do not extend from end to end of the muscle. Alvarado (in preparation) has sectioned a slip of the RB at three levels and found 3118 fibers at the midpoint, 2449 at the proximal third, and 1790 fibers at the distal third.

In our studies (Bach-y-Rita and Ito, 1966; Steinacker and Bach-y-Rita,

1968) we have found the electrical and mechanical properties of the RB to be intermediate between the fast and the slow, multi-innervated twitch fibers of the I.O. The RB has a mean twitch rise time of 13 msec, a contraction duration of 60 msec, a maximum twitch tension of 0.79 for each slip, a tetanic rise time of 150 msec and a fusion frequency of 175/sec. The mean maximum tension was 10.5 gm per slip (approximately 40 gm for the total RB). The mean membrane potential of the fibers is 71 mV. The fibers produce action potentials (mean -93 mV) with a mean latency of 2.6 msec on stimulation of the VI nerve nucleus.

Some functional localization of the RB within the VI nucleus has been noted: stimulation of the upper portion of the nucleus produced contractions of the superior slips, stimulation of the lower portion produced contraction of the lower slips, and stimulation of the mid portion produced contraction of all four slips (Bach-y-Rita and Ito, 1965).

The RB apparently does not have tonic properties nor is it capable of producing finely graded movements. The RB muscle is an ideal muscle for control studies on EOMs since it has a uniform muscle fiber population and a motor nerve fiber spectrum with a single peak, and since the physiological, pharmacological, histological and mechanical properties differ from those of the other EOMs.

CENTRAL MECHANISMS

The central mechanisms controlling eye movements are complex and incompletely understood. However, it is clear that cortical areas play important roles: the frontal cortex apparently is related to saccadic movements and to the liberation of the eye movements from reflex control, allowing initiation of voluntary movements (Smith, 1949); the occipital cortex is more related to following movements. However, the functional divisions between the cortical areas are not clearly established, nor are the pathways from the cortex to the EOM motor nuclei known with certainty; the pathways are not direct, but rather appear to synapse in the reticular formation (Carpenter, this symposium).

Some additional central structures involved in EOM control include: cerebellum, vestibular system, superior colliculi, lateral geniculate nuclei, motor nuclei of the EOMs and the reticular formation. All of these are discussed in other chapters of this symposium, and have been reviewed previously (Whitteridge, 1966; Bender, 1964). In this section discussion will be limited to a brief presentation of selected studies on the EOM motor nerves and the reticular formation in vertebrates, together with a short description of the possibilities for further work in invertebrate preparations.

EOM motor nuclei

The motor nuclei of the EOMs, III, IV and VI, contain the cell bodies of the final common pathway to the EOMs. It has been known for a long time that cells of different sizes are located in the nuclei. Tsuchida (1906) found three sizes, the smallest of which were 1/3 the size of the largest. In the rabbit, Fukuda (1964) found that of the 5400 cells in the III nucleus, 2300 were small (20 to 25 by 15 to 20μ), and the rest large (40 to 50 by 30 to 38μ). Cells of both types were mixed, but many of the smaller cells were located in the periphery of the nucleus.

It has only recently become apparent that several different functional systems are present in eye muscles, and that these are reflected in distinct firing patterns of the motor neurons (Schaefer, 1965; Schubert and Bornschein, 1962; Yamanaka and Bach-y-Rita, 1968). From recordings of spontaneous activity in the cat oculomotor nucleus, Schubert and Bornschein (1962) postulated the presence of tonic and phasic neurons. Further, Schaefer (1965) differentiated tonic and phasic activity in the rabbit VI nucleus on the basis of microelectrode recordings of spike amplitudes and discharge patterns. Approximately 1/3 of the nerve fibers to EOM are small, gamma range fibers (discussed above), with conduction velocities of 6 to 40 m/sec (Yamanaka and Bach-y-Rita, 1968); these supply the slow multiply innervated twitch fibers (Bach-y-Rita and Ito, 1966) and possibly originate in the small motor neurons described above.

Sasaki (1963) has analyzed the spontaneous discharges of the motor neurons in the cat III nerve nucleus and the responses to orthodromic and antidromic stimuli. His results and those of Baker, Mano and Shimazu (1969), agree with previous studies (Cajal, 1952; Lorente de No, 1933; Baldesera and Broggi, 1968) demonstrating that recurrent collaterals (Renshaw cells) do not exist in this system. Sasaki (1963) has also studied the interneurons, identified by a lack of antidromic responses to stimulation of the III nerve. The interneurons did, however, respond following stimulation of other structures, such as the VIII nerve.

It would appear (Carpenter, this symposium) that the motor nuclei of the EOM have few demonstrable direct connections to the cortical oculomotor areas or to the superior colliculi. Additionally it would seem that other cellular groups in the region of the oculomotor complex (such as the interstitial nucleus of Cajal) do not contribute fibers to the nerves leading to the EOM.

The pattern of anatomical connections, as well as the results of physiological studies, suggest that highly complex relations exist between afferent impulses, central structures such as the cortex, and integrating areas. The motor neurons and their axons are but the final pathway to the muscles that produce the extremely fine and highly coordinated eye movements; the patterns of nerve impulses that travel along these nerves have been determined in oculomotor integrating areas.

Reticular formation and oculomotor integration

The phylogenetically old reticular formation is an area of many synapses; it is extremely sensitive to anesthetic agents (French, Verzeano and Magoun,

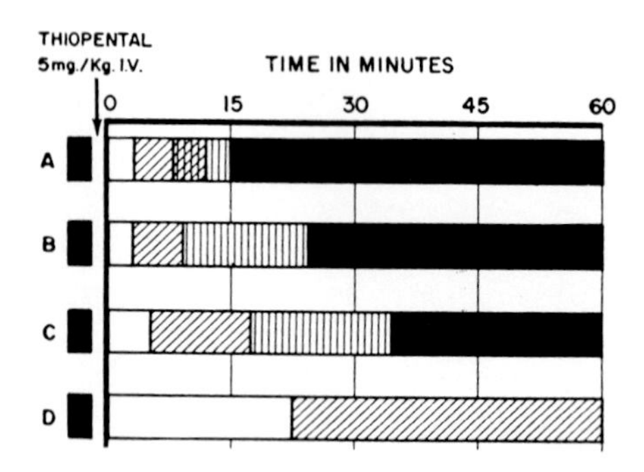

Fig. 14. Relative sequence of evoked eye movements after thiopental, 5 mg/kg i.v. A. Average of 10 sites in tegmentum of medulla (control response to stimulation: ipsilateral conjugate deviation). B. Average of 4 sites in dorsal midbrain tegmentum (control response: contralateral conjugate deviation). C. Average of 4 sites in ventral midbrain tegmentum (control response: ipsilateral deviation). D. Average of 7 cortical sites (control response: contralateral deviation). Black: conjugate deviation evoked. White: no response to stimulation. Diagonal cross-hatch: midpositioning evoked. Vertical cross-hatch: partial conjugate movement. (Reprinted by permission of *Amer. J. Physiol.* 1957, **191**: 203-208).

1953) and has multiple connections to other central structures (Carpenter, this symposium; Cohen, this symposium). Most of the individual reticular neurons are highly convergent, receiving inputs from many sources (for references *cf.* Bach-y-Rita, 1964). For these reasons, it has been difficult to assess the role of the reticular formation in any particular system, such as that of oculomotion. However, its importance in the control of eye movements is well documented.

As early as 1933 Lorente de No (1933) described some of the connections between the reticular formation and other central structures involved in the control of eye movements. Hyde and Eliasson (1957) stimulated 8,500 sites, extending from posterior diencephalon to medulla, and up to 3.5 mm from the midline in the cat brainstem. They noted that half of the stimulus sites produced eye movements, although under chloralose anesthesia only 30% produced eye movements. However, anesthesia markedly changes the character of these movements. Eliasson, Hyde and Bach-y-Rita (1957) noted that as little as 5 mg/kg of thiopental (approximately 1/6 of the anesthetic dose) produced marked effects on both spontaneous and brainstem evoked eye movements in encéphale isolé cats (Fig. 14). The simultaneously recorded electromyogram showed a gradual decrease in tonic discharges following intravenous administration of the drug. These two studies demonstrated that the multisynaptic oculomotor integrating areas of the reticular formation are highly sensitive to anesthetic agents, and thus "lightly anesthetized" preparations (commonly used in many experimental laboratories) may produce unphysiological results. Cooper, Daniel and Whitteridge (1953) acknowledged that anesthetic agents may have had an important effect on the distribution and latencies encountered in their studies of CNS responses to

EOM stretch. From their results these investigators postulated the existence of a brainstem "neuronal pool to which messages are delivered by a multiple of parallel pathways. Such a pool would integrate the messages and would play on the final motorneurons to initiate eye movements under suitable conditions." A review of the evidence in 1956 (Bach-y-Rita, 1956) and studies since that time strongly suggest that such an oculomotor integrating area or "pool" exists in the brainstem.

Invertebrate preparations

The complexities of neural systems in vertebrates have prompted a number of investigators to take advantage of the relative simplicity of neural systems in invertebrate preparations for an approach to the study of basic neural mechanisms. For example, the decapod Crustacea offer features admirably suited to such an analysis of the central mechanisms controlling eye movements.

The eye of the decapod, *Carcinus,* has been shown to be capable of three reflex movements and four small amplitude movements which require no visual movement stimulus. The reflex movements are 1) an optokinetic nystagmus in the horizontal plane, 2) statocyst (vestibular) controlled movements to maintain an absolute position of the eye in space, and 3) withdrawal movements of the eye into the socket in response to mechanical stimulation. The small amplitude movements comprise (1) a tremor of 2-5 cps and 0.05°-0.2° amplitude, (2) a flick or saccade of 0.05°-0.2° amplitude with an initial fast phase and a slow return phase, (3) scanning movements of 0.5°-1.0° amplitude and (4) a slow drift in the absence of light or visual contrast. These movements involve the coordination of slow and fast muscle fiber systems and have been shown not to involve proprioceptive control in their execution (Burrows and Horridge, 1968).

The directionally-sensitive movement detector units of the retina, which are a source of phasic sensory input to the oculomotor system, have been investigated in several decapods (Wiersma, 1967, Wiersma and Yamaguchi, 1967). These movement detector units may drive the oculomotor neurons to execute following movements. With the exception of the withdrawal reflex (Sandeman, 1969) few studies of the CNS in relation to eye movements have been undertaken on invertebrate preparations. Work is currently in progress (Steinacker, personal communication) utilizing a decapod preparation, to begin a study of the central mechanisms of the oculomotor system.

FUNCTIONAL CORRELATIONS

The principal function of the oculomotor system is to quickly acquire foveal localization of a target, and then to follow it during movement relative to the environment (Walls, 1962). The substrates (muscle fibers, sensory receptors, neurons, central nuclei, nerve fibers and integrating areas) of this function have been discussed in this presentation and elsewhere in this

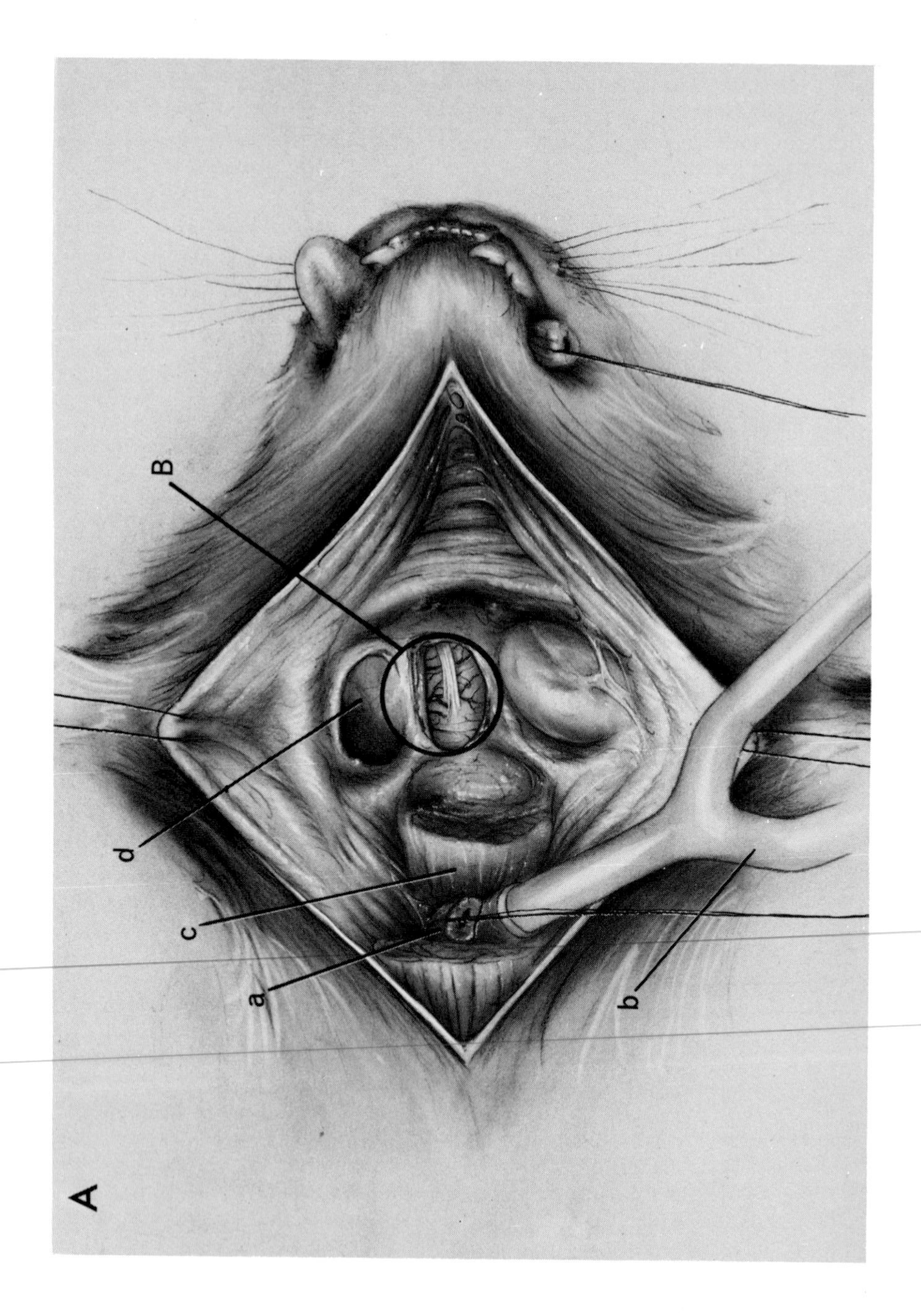
A
B
a
b
c
d

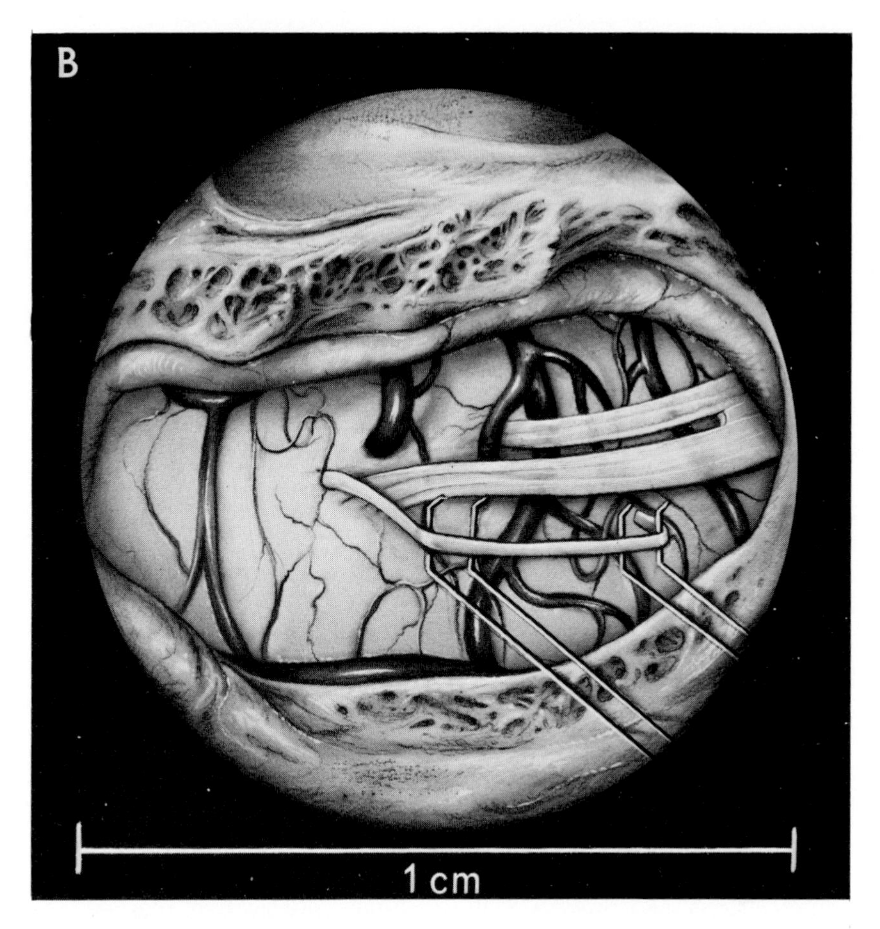

Fig. 15. An illustration of the VI nerve preparation. **A.** A view of the ventral exposure of the VI nerve emerging from the pons. (a) Esophagus; (b) endotracheal tube; (c) neck muscles retracted; (d) tympanic bulla opened. **B.** A detailed view of the circled area of A, showing the emergence of the VI nerve with the arrangement of the two pairs of recording electrodes. (Reprinted by permission of *Exp. Neurol.* 1968, **20**: 143-155).

symposium as have studies designed to determine functional roles for some of these substrates. The present section will be largely restricted to certain studies of muscle and nerve fiber types in which attempts were made to correlate structure with function in different types of eye movements.

In encéphale isolé cat preparations we (Yamanaka and Bach-y-Rita, 1968) correlated the activity of each of the two principal populations of nerve fibers in the VI nerve with the slow and fast movements of vestibular nystagmus. Small bundles of nerve fibers teased from the VI nerve at its

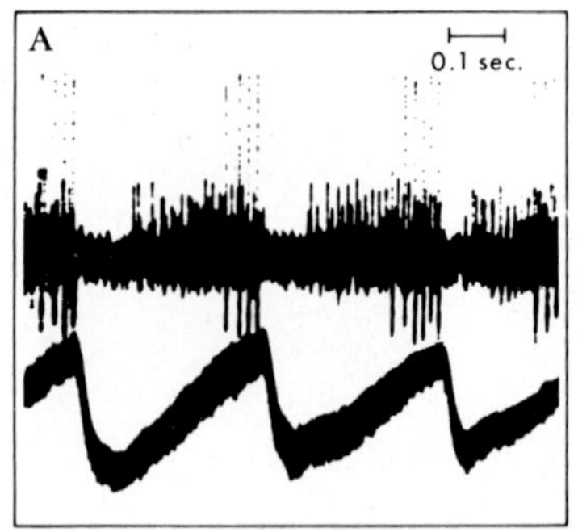

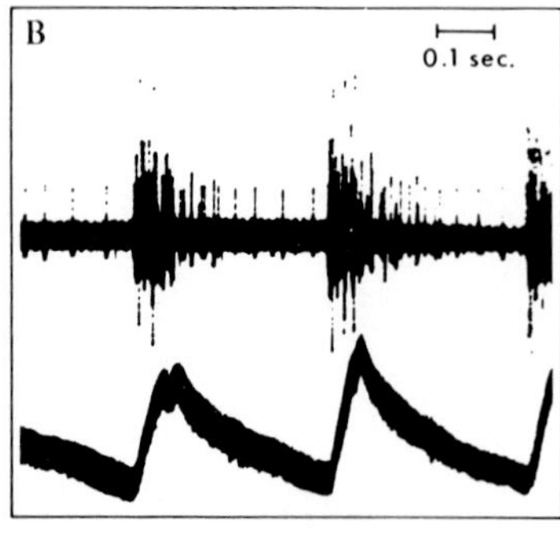

Fig. 16. Responses during vestibular nystagmus. The upper channel presents activity recorded from the VI nerve; the lower channel records lateral rectus muscle tension. **A.** From the nerve on the same side as the slow phase of nystagmus. Small spikes, representing a slow fiber (CV 25 m/sec) revealed a gradually increasing discharge frequency during the slow phase, with cessation of activity during the fast phase. Large spikes, from a fast fiber (CV 50 m/sec) appeared only during the last half of the slow phase. (The upper portions of the large spikes in A and B have been retouched). The CV of the fiber with very low-amplitude spikes, discharging almost simultaneously with the slow fiber, was not measured. **B.** From the nerve on the side opposite to the slow phase of nystagmus. Recordings were made from the same nerve fibers as in A, but the direction of nystagmus was reversed. The slow fibers showed a high-frequency burst during the fast (lateral) phase, with a gradual decrease in frequency during the slow phase of nystagmus to the opposite side. The fast fiber (large spikes) was silent during the contralateral slow phase and appeared as a high-frequency burst during the homolateral fast phase. (Reprinted by permission of *Exp. Neurol.* 1968, **20**: 143-155).

emergence from the pons were placed over two pairs of electrodes (Fig. 15) in order to determine the conduction velocities of the fibers active in the absence of movement (tonic control of eye muscles) and in each phase of vestibular nystagmus. Touching the exposed lateral semicircular canal with a wick of cotton induced nystagmus; removal of the wick reversed the direction of the nystagmus (Fig. 16). The conduction velocities (CV) of VI nerve fibers were found to be distributed in two groups: slow, 6-40 m/sec, and fast, 41-83 m/sec. Slow fibers were active in the absence of movement, in both phases of nystagmus, and during slow spontaneous eye deviations. Fast fibers were active during the fast phase and towards the latter portion of the slow phase of nystagmus. Fast fibers were never seen to discharge in the absence of movement.

In collaboration with Dr. Ito (Bach-y-Rita and Ito, 1966a) it was previously shown that the slow range of nerve fibers innervated the slow multi-innervated twitch fibers, and the fast nerve fibers innervated the fast, singly innervated twitch fibers. Therefore by extrapolation it appears that the slow nerve fibers and the slow twitch fibers of the EOMs are active principally during tonic movements, and the fast nerve fibers and large singly innervated twitch fibers are active principally during phasic movements, although each type of fiber contributes to some portion of each type of eye movement.

From the observation that spontaneous resting discharge was recorded only from the slow nerve fibers, one might be justified in concluding that the spontaneous electromyographic (EMG) activity that is recorded from human EOMs at rest (Bjork and Kugelberg, 1953) is a reflection of the slow nerve system to the slow multi-innervated twitch fibers. The extracellular EMG needle could only record unit spikes if they were produced by fibers with propagated action potentials.

Based on a mathematical analysis of the actions of individual extraocular muscles in the mechanics of eye movements, Boeder (1962) determined that muscle extension is just as important, from a mechanical point of view, as contraction. When we (Yamanaka and Bach-y-Rita, 1968) recorded from a fiber bundle contralateral to the direction of the slow phase of nystagmus, a decreasing rate of nerve discharge was noted (e.g., Fig. 16B). This may represent a graded muscle extension. This activity could only be recorded from slow nerve fibers, which suggests that the graded extension may be mediated by the multi-innervated muscle fibers supplied by these small nerve fibers.

Yellin (1969) has shown by histochemical techniques that several different types of muscle fibers are found in EOMs, possibly with different types of motor innervation. One type of fiber may have dual innervation. He suggests that this duality may signify differences in the functional capabilities of a muscle fiber during differential as well as simultaneous activation by its efferents. Our studies on anesthetized cats (Ito, Bach-y-Rita and Yamanaka, 1969) have differentiated three types of twitch fiber responses to semicircular canal stimulation. Intracellular microelectrode studies of each of the fiber types revealed differences in the latency and frequency of action potentials. The fibers with the largest membrane potentials, above 95 mV, revealed the lowest frequency and the longest latencies. In fibers with membrane potentials between 65 and 90 mv, the shortest latencies and highest frequencies (up to 83/sec) were noted. The fibers with the lowest range of membrane potentials (50-65 mv) showed frequencies of action potentials up to 60/sec (Fig. 17), and were also characterized by the occasional appearance of small potential deflections similar to end-plate potentials or to abortive spikes (Fig. 18). It is likely that this type of fiber is multiply innervated. A synchronous excitation of many neuromuscular endings may be necessary for initiation of a propagated impulse, since the amount of acetylcholine released by each nerve impulse should be less than at the larger endings of the other fiber types. This type of fiber may have a dual role: it may be able to contract segmentally during slow, finely graded movements such as following movements; it may also be able to contract with a propagated impulse and contribute to a saccade, as our studies (Yamanaka and Bach-y-Rita, 1968) suggest (Fig. 16).

Studies of the eye muscle slow multi-innervated twitch fibers revealed similarities with the multi-innervated frog limb intrafusal fibers studied by Koketsu and Nishi (1957a&b). Both, in addition to their small size and

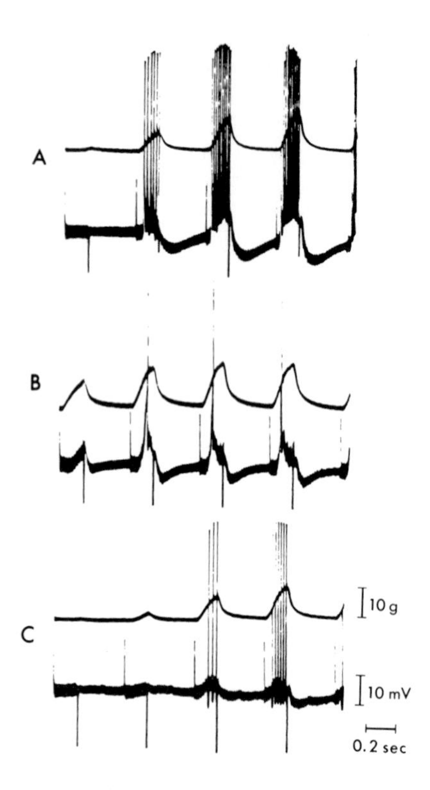

Fig. 17. Simultaneous records of tension (upper traces) and intracellular action potentials (lower traces) of a lateral rectus muscle at +4-mm initial length during 150-msec bursts of 0.1-msec pulses delivered to the contralateral semicircular canal at 1.5-sec intervals and at a frequency of 300 cycle/sec. The action potentials are from muscle fibers having resting potentials of 66 mv (A), 95 mv (B), and 65 mv (C). (Reprinted by permission of *Exp. Neurol.* 1969, **24**: 438-449).

multiple innervation, are capable of producing propagated spikes but lose this ability following a degree of local membrane injury that would not inhibit the spikes of fast twitch fibers (discussed above). Both, however, apparently can respond to stimulation with only local non-propagated responses, even in the absence of membrane injury. Koketsu and Nishi (1957b) have suggested that local muscle constraction can be produced in frog intrafusal fibers even when no spikes are initiated. They note that the role of intrafusal fibers is the production of afferent impulses from tension receptors in the muscle spindles, and that in this role the muscle fibers must maintain a long lasting contraction by the activation of efferent impulses. In cat EOMs, the slow multi-innervated fibers may play a similar role in afferent mechanisms, as well as their role in the production of slow and fast eye movements.

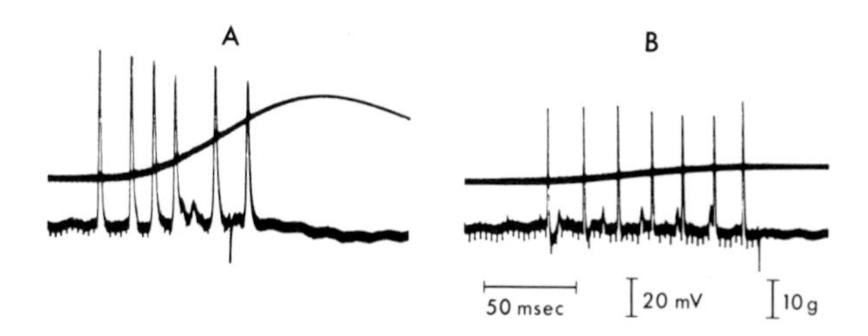

Fig. 18. Intracellular action potentials and end plate or abortive potentials (lower traces) of two muscle fibers, having resting potentials of 55 mv (A) and 52 mv (B), recorded simultaneously with the tension of the respective lateral rectus muscles (upper traces). Records were made during the third burst of 0.1-msec pulses delivered for 150 msec to the contralateral semicircular canal at a frequency of 300 cycle/sec and 1.5-sec interval between bursts. (Reprinted by permission of *Exp. Neurol.* 1969, **24**: 438-449).

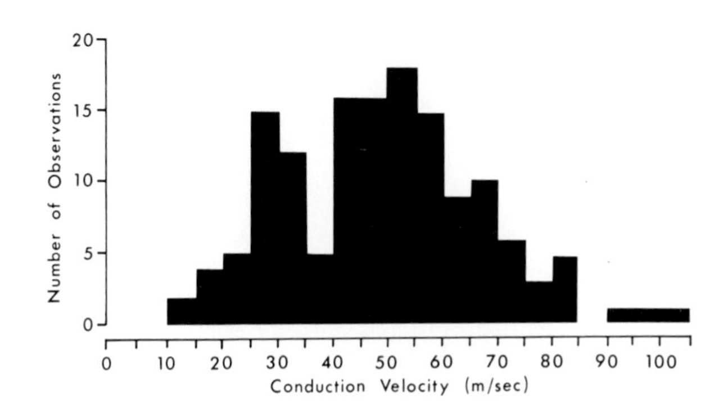

Fig. 19. A histogram of the velocities at which efferent impulses are conducted along the VI nerve in cats. Measurements were made from impulses recorded from small bundles teased from the nerve; 150-msec burst of 0.1-msec pulses delivered to the contralateral semicircular canal at a frequency of 300 cycle/sec and a 1.5-sec interval constituted the stimulus. (Reprinted by permission of *Exp. Neurol.* 1969, **24**: 438-449).

The classification proposed at this symposium by Peachey includes five fiber types. It is not possible at this time to correlate our physiological findings with Peachey's morphological classification.

An additional point on functional correlation is found in our observation (Ito, Bach-y-Rita and Yamanaka, 1969) that increases in muscle length reduced the latencies of the action potentials to vestibular stimulation. Analysis of the conduction velocities (Fig. 19) and the temporal distribution of the efferent fibers in the VI nerve during the "slow" movements following electrical vestibular stimulation revealed a lack of temporal distribution. A

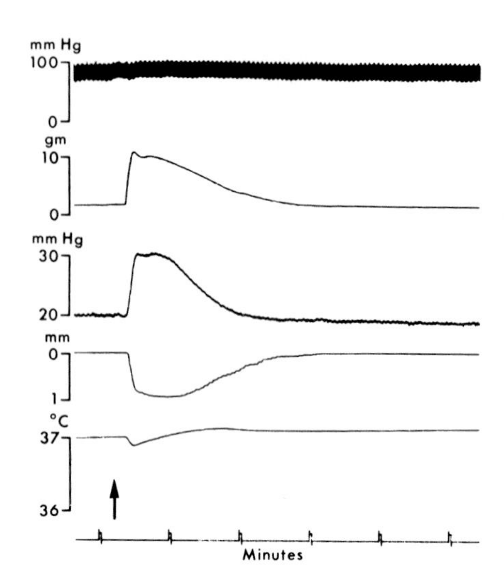

Fig. 20. Response to succinylcholine (30 μ g/kv, iv at arrow) in a cat. **A**: (top) arterial pressure. **B**: lateral rectus muscle tension. **C**: intraocular pressure rise. **D**: enophthalmos (downward). **E**: muscle surface temperature. (Reprinted by permission of *Amer. J. Physiol.* 1967, **213**: 1039-1043).

temporal distribution (e.g., during the initial portion of the slow phase contraction only slow nerve fibers discharge, as shown in Fig. 16) had previously been noted in vestibular nystagmus in nonanesthetized cats (Yamanaka and Bach-y-Rita, 1968). Therefore the contractions produced by electrical stimulation of the semicircular canal in anesthetized preparations cannot be considered the equivalent of the slow phase of nystagmus.

Finally, in addition to moving the eyes, the EOMs may have several other roles. For example, we have shown (Collins, Bach-y-Rita and Loeb, 1962) that changes in EOM tension can produce changes in intraocular pressure (Fig. 20). Muscle contractions produce a creasing of the globe, resulting in an uneven application of forces to the globe, as shown by an intraocular pressure - extraocular tension curve that is non-linear (Fig. 21).

EOM contraction can also affect the position of the globe in the orbit. Szentagothai and Schab (1956) have shown that stimulation of brainstem inhibitory areas in the cat produces an inhibition of muscle tone and exophthalmus. Tengroth (1960) has reported that in human subjects elimination of EOM tone produces as much as 3 mm of exophthalmus. In a further study on the globe deformation produced by an EOM tension increase, we (Bach-y-Rita, Collins and Tengroth, 1966) noted that a small dose (50μg/kg) of Sch produced axial length shortening and marked enophthalmus in cats. There were also concomitant hyperopic refractive changes of up to two diopters even without the participation of the intraocular muscles. It is tempting,

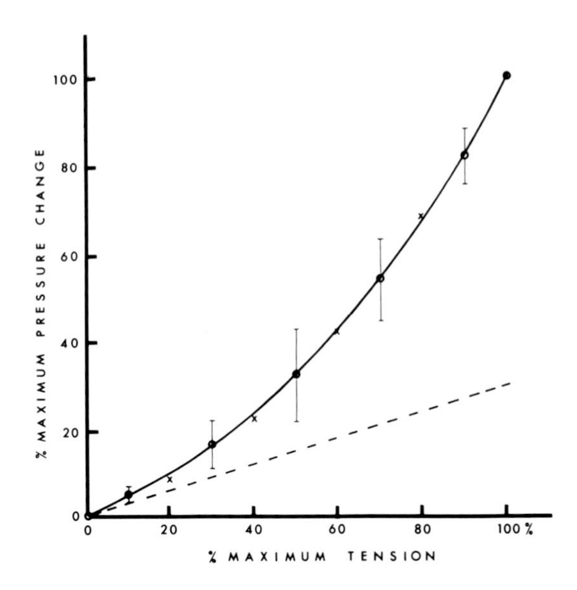

Fig. 21. Intraocular pressure change plotted as a function of oculorotary muscle tension. *Abscissa:* muscle tension as percent of maximum observed. *Ordinate:* intraocular pressure change as percent of maximal change. Open circles: mean intraocular pressure changes plotted as a function of lateral rectus tension following succinylcholine injections (averaged from 5 cats and 5 rabbits; SE indicated by vertical bars). Crosses: intraocular pressure plotted as a function of tension on a string bearing against 60° of the cornea; from one of five similar animals. Dashed line: intraocular pressure plotted as a function of force applied to a large scleral contact lens to simulate piston-like action of distributed muscle tension producing enophthalmos (average of four animals). (Reprinted by permission of *Amer. J. Physiol.* 1967, **213**: 1039-1043).

but inappropriate at this time, to speculate on the possible role that the EOMs may play in the development of refractive errors.

ACKNOWLEDGEMENT

I wish to acknowledge the invaluable aid of the Vision Information Center, a unit of the National Information network of the National Institute of Neurological Diseases and Stroke and of the National Eye Institute.

REFERENCES

Alvarado, J., Steinacker, A. and Bach-y-Rita, P. (1967). The ultrastructure of the retractor bulbi muscles of the cat. *Invest. Ophthal.* **6**, 548.
Bach-y-Rita, P. (1956). El sistema internuncial óculomotor. *Acta neurol. Latinoamer.* **2**, 65-71.
Bach-y-Rita, P. (1959). Extraocular proprioception. *Acta neurol. Latinoamer.* **5**, 17-39.
Bach-y-Rita, P. (1964). Convergent and long latency unit responses in the reticular formation of the cat. *Exp. Neurol.* **9**, 327-344.
Bach-y-Rita, P. (1964). Convergent and long latency unit responses in the reticular formation of the cat. *Exp. Neurol.* **9**, 327-344.
Bach-y-Rita, P., Collins, C. and Tengroth, B. (1968). Influence of extraocular muscle contructure on globe length. *Amer. J. Opthal.* **66**, 906-908.
Bach-y-Rita, P. and Ito, F. (1965). In vivo microelectrode studies of the cat retractor bulbi fibers. *Invest. Opthal.* **4**, 338-342.
Bach-y-Rita, P. and Ito, F. (1966a). In vivo studies on fast and slow muscle fibers in cat extraocular muscles. *J. gen. Physiol.* **49**, 1177-1198.
Bach-y-Rita, P. and Ito, F. (1966b). Properties of stretch receptors in cat extraocular muscles. *J. Physiol.* **186**, 663-688.
Bach-y-Rita, P., Levy, J. V. and Steinacker, A. (1967). The effect of succinylcholine on the isolated retractor bulbi muscle of the cat. *J. Pharm. Pharmacol.* **19**, 180-181.
Bach-y-Rita, P. and Murata, K. (1964). Extraocular proprioceptive responses in the VI nerve of the cat. *Quart. J. exp. Physiol.* **49**, 408-415.
Bach-y-Rita, P., Murata, K. and Mulach, V. B. (1963). Proprioceptive und antidrome Entladungen in den Augenmuskelnerven bei Muskeldehnung und nach Succinylcholin. *Pflüg. Arch. ges. Physiol.* **278**, 71-72.
Baker, R. G., Mano, N. and Shimazu, H. (1969). Postsynaptic potentials in abducens motoneurons induced by vestibular stimulation. *Brain Res.* **15**, 577-580.
Baldissera, F. and Broggi, G. (1968). Analysis of a trigemino-abducens reflex in the cat. *Brain Res.* **7**, 313-316.
Bender, M. B. (1964). *The Oculomotor System.* New York, Harper & Row.
Biemond, A. and DeJong, J. M. B. V. (1969). On cervical nystagmus and related disorders. *Brain.* **92**, 437-458.
Bjork, A. and Kugelberg, E. (1953). The electrical activity of the muscles of the eye and eyelids in various positions and during movement. *Electroenceph. clin. Neurophysiol.* **5**, 595-602.
Björkman, A. and Wohlfart, G. (1936). Faseranalyse der Nn. oculomotorius trochlearis und abducens des Menschen und des N. abducens verschiedener Tiere. *Zeitschr. mikr.-anat. Forsch.* **39**, 631-641.
Boeder, P. (1962). Cooperative action of extraocular muscles. *Brit. J. Ophthal.* **46**, 397-403.
Brindley, G. and Merton, P. (1960). The absence of position sense in the human eye. *J. Physiol.* **153**, 127-130.
Brown, G. L. and Harvey, A. M. (1941). Neuro-muscular transmission in the extrinsic muscles of the eye. *J. Physiol.* **99**, 379-399.
Buller, A. J. and Lewis, D. M. (1965). The rate of tension development in isometric tetanic contractions of mammalian fast and slow skeletal muscle. *J. Physiol.* **176**, 337-354.
Burrows, M. and Horridge, G. A. (1968). The action of the eyecup muscles of the crab, *Carcinus*, during optokinetic movement. *J. Exp. Biol.* **49**, 223-250.
Cajal, S. and Ramon y. (1952). *Histologie du Systeme Nerveaux de l'Homme et des Vertebres.* vol. I, p. 856. Madrid Consejo Superior de Investigaciones Cientificas, Instituto Ramon y Cajal.
Christman, E. and Kupfer, C. (1963). Proprioceptors in extraocular muscle. *Arch. Ophthal.* **69**, 824-829.
Cilimbaris, P. A. (1910). Histologische Untersuchungen uber die Muskelspindeln der Augenmuskeln. *Arch. mikr. Anat.* **75**, 692-747.
Cohen, L. (1961). Role of eye and neck proprioceptive mechanisms in body orientation and motor coordination. *J. Neurophysiol.* **24**, 1-11.
Collins, C. C., Bach-y-Rita, P. and Loeb, D. R. (1967). Intraocular pressure variation with oculorotary muscle tension. *Amer. J. Physiol.* **213**, 1039-1043.
Collins, C. C., Scott, A. B. and O'Meara, D. (1969). Elements of the peripheral oculomotor apparatus. *Amer. J. Optom.* **46**, 510-515.
Cooper, S. (1966). The small motor nerves to muscle spindles and to extrinsic eye muscles in man. *J. Physiol.* **186**, 28p-29p.
Cooper, S. and Daniel, P. (1949). Muscle spindles in human extrinsic eye muscles. *Brain.* **72**, 1-24.

Cooper, S. and Daniel, P. (1957). Responses from the stretch receptors of the goat's extrinsic eye muscles with an intact motor innervation. *Quart. J. Exp. Physiol.* **42**, 222-231.

Cooper, S., Daniel, P. and Whitteridge, D. (1951). Afferent impulses in the oculomotor nerve from the extrinsic eye muscles. *J. Physiol.* **120**, 471-490.

Cooper, S., Daniel, P. and Whitteridge, D. (1953a). Nerve impulses in the brainstem of the goat. Short latency responses obtained by stretching the extrinsic eye muscles and the jaw muscles. *J. Physiol.* **120**, 471-490.

Cooper, S., Daniel, P. and Whitteridge, D. (1953b). Nerve impulses in the brainstem of the goat. Responses with long latencies obtained by stretching the extrinsic eye muscles. *J. Physiol.* **120**, 491-513.

Cooper, S., Daniel, P. M. and Whitteridge, D. (1955). Muscle spindles and other sensory endings in the extrinsic eye muscles; the physiology and anatomy of these receptors and of their connections with the brainstem. *Brain.* **78**, 564-583.

Cooper, S. and Eccles, J. C. (1930). The isometric responses of mammalian muscles. *J. Physiol.* **69**, 377-385.

Cooper, S. and Fillenz, M. (1955). Afferent discharges in response to stretch from the extraocular muscles of the cat and monkey and the innervation of these muscles. *J. Physiol.* **127**, 400-413.

Donaldson, G. W. K. (1960). The diameter of the nerve fibers to the extrinsic eye muscles of the goat. *Quart. J. of exp. Physiol.* **45**, 25-34.

Duke-Elder, S. (1961). *System of Ophthalmology.* vol. II, p. 435. St. Louis, C. V. Mosby.

Eccles, J. C. and Sherrington, C. S. (1930). Numbers and contraction-values of individual motor-units examined in some muscles of the limb. *Proc. roy. Soc. B.* **106**, 326-357.

Edmonet-Dénand, F., Laporte, Y. and Pagés, B. (1964). Mise en évidence de fibres fusimotrices statiques chez le lapin. *C. R. Acad. Sci.*, Paris. **259**, 2690-2693.

Eliasson, S., Hyde, J. and Bach-y-Rita, P. (1957). Effects of intravenous thiopental on spontaneous and evoked eye movements in cats. *Amer. J. Physiol.* **191**, 203-208.

Fender, D. H. and Nye, P. W. (1961). An investigation of the mechanisms of eye movement control. *Kybernetik.* **1**, 81-88.

French, J., Verzeano, M. and Magoun, H. (1953). A neural basis of the anesthetic state. *Arch. Neurol. Psychiat.* **69**, 519-599.

Fuchs, A. F. and Kornhuber, H. (1969). Extraocular muscle afferents to the cerebellum of the cat. *J. Physiol.* **200**, 713-722.

Fukuda, M. (1964). Histological studies on the oculomotor nucleus of the rabbit. *Jap. J. Ophthal.* **8**, 59-67.

Ginsborg, B. L. (1960). Some properties of avian skeletal muscle fibers with multiple neuromuscular junctions. *J. Physiol.* **154**, 581-598.

Gernandt, B. E. (1968). Interactions between extraocular myotatic and ascending vestibular influences. *Exp. Neurol.* **20**, 120-134.

Greene, T. and Jampel, R. S. (1966). Muscle spindles in the extraocular muscles of the macaque. *J. comp. Neurol.* **126**, 547-550.

Helmholtz, H. von (1962). *Helmholtz's Treatise on Physiological Optics.* New York, Dover. vol. III, pp. 243-246.

Hess, A. and Pilar, G. (1963). Slow fibers in the extraocular muscles of the cat. *J. Physiol.* **169**, 780-798.

Hogg, I. D. (1964). Observations on the development of the peripheral portion of the oculomotor nerve in man and the albino rat. *J. comp. Neurol.* **122**, 91-112.

Hopkins, G. S. (1916). The innervation of the muscle retractor oculi. *Anat. Rec.* **11**, 199-206.

Hosokawa, H. (1961). Proprioceptive innervation of striated muscles in the territory of cranial nerves. *Tex. Rep. Biol. Med.* **19**, 405-464.

Hyde, J. and Davis, L. (1960). Extraocular proprioception in electrically induced eye movements. *Amer. J. Physiol.* **198**, 945-948.

Hyde, J. E. and Eliason, S. G. (1957). Brainstem induced eye movements in cats. *J. comp. Neurol.* **108**, 139-172.

Ito, F. (1967). The effects of succinylcholine on frog slow muscle fibers. *Jap. J. Pharmacol.* **17**, 550-556.

Ito, F. and Bach-y-Rita, P. (1969). Afferent discharges from extraocular muscle in the squirrel monkey. *Amer. J. Physiol.* **217**, 332-335.

Ito, F., Bach-y-Rita, P. and Yamanaka, Y. (1969). Extraocular muscle intracellular and motor nerve responses to semicircular canal stimulation. *Exp. Neurol.* **24**, 438-449.

Kato, T. (1938). Uber histologische Untersuchungen der Augenmuskeln von Menschen und Saugetieren *Okajimas Folia anat. Jap.* **16**, 131-145.

Kennard, D. W. and Smyth G. L. (1963). Interaction of mechanisms causing eye and eyelid movement. *Nature* (Lond.). **297**, 50-52.
Kern, R. (1965). A comparative pharmacologic-histologic study of slow and twitch fibers in the superior rectus muscle of the rabbit. *Invest. Ophthal.* **4**, 901-910.
DeKlejn, A. (1918). Actions reflexes du labyrinthe et du cou sur les muscles de l'oeil. *Arch. Neerland. Physiol.* **2**, 644-649.
Koketsu, K. and Nishi, S. (1957a). Action potentials of single intrafusal muscle fibers of frogs. *J. Physiol.* **137**, 193-209.
Koketsu, K. and Nishi, S. (1957b). An analysis of junctional potentials of intrafusal muscle fibers in frogs. *J. Physiol.* **139**, 15-26.
Kumoi, T. and Jampel, R. S. (1966). Influence of lateral rectus muscle contractions on the abducens nerve discharge evoked by vestibular nerve stimulation. *Exp. Neurol.* **15**, 180-191.
Ling, G. and Woodbury, J. W. (1949). Effect of temperature on membrane potential of frog muscle fibers. *J. cell. comp. Neurol.* **34**, 407-412.
Lorente de Nó, R. (1933). Vestibulo-ocular reflex arc. *Arch. Neurol. Psychiat.* **30**, 245-291.
Manni, E. Bortolami and Desole, C. (1968). Peripheral pathway of eye muscle proprioception. *Exp. Neurol.* **22**, 1-12.
Matthews, P. B. C. (1964). Muscle spindles and their motor control. *Physiol. Rev.* **44**, 219-288.
Matyushkin, D. P. (1961). Phasic and tonic neuromotor units in the oculomotor apparatus of the rabbit. *Sechenov physiol. J. U. S. S. R.* **47**, 65-69.
Matyushkin, D. P. (1964). Varieties of tonic muscle fibers in the oculomotor apparatus of the rabbit. *Bull. exp. Biol. Med.* **55**, 235-288.
Motais, E. (1885). Recherches sur L'Anatomie Humaine et l'anatomie comparee de l'appareil moteur de l'oeil (Part 3). *Arch D'Ophthal.* (Paris). **5**, 143-158.
Nakanishi, T. and Norris, F. H. (1970). Effect of local temperature on the resting membrane potential in rat muscle. *Electroenceph. clin. Neurophysiol.* (In press).
Namba, T., Nakamura, T., Takahashi, A., and Grob, D. Motor nerve endings in extraocular muscles. *Comp. Neurol.* **134**, 385-396.
O'Leary, J., Heinbecker, P. and Bishop, G. (1934). Analysis of function of a nerve to muscle. *Amer. J. Physiol.* **110**, 636-658.
Ozawa, T. (1964). Some electrophysiological properties of rabbit extraocular muscle recorded in vivo with intracellular electrode. *Jap. J. Ophthal.* **8**, 47-52.
Ozawa. T., Cheng-Minoda, K., Davidowitz, J., and Breinin, G. M. (1969). Correlation of potential and fiber type in extraocular muscle. *Documenta Ophthal.*, **26**, 192-201.
Pilar, G. and Hess, A. (1966). Differences in internal structure and nerve terminals of the slow and twitch muscle fibers in the cat superior oblique. *Anat. Rec.* **154**, 243-252.
Pilar, G. (1967). Further study of the electrical and mechanical responses of slow fibers in cat extraocular muscles. *J. Gen. Physiol.* **50**, 2289-2300.
Rexed, G. (1944). Contributions to knowledge of postnatal development of peripheral nervous system in man: study of bases and scope of systematic investigations into fiber size in peripheral nerves. *Acta psychiat. et. neurol.* Supp. 33, p. 1-206.
Sandeman, D. C. (1969). The site of synaptic activity and impulse initiation in an identified motoneuron in the crab brain. *J. Exp. Biol.* **50**, 771-784.
Sas, J. and Schab, R. (1952). Die sogenannten "Palisaden-Erdigungen" der Augenmuskeln. *Acta morph. Acad. Sci. hung.* **2**, 259-266.
Sas, J. and Appeltauer, C. (1963). Atypical muscle spindles in the extrinsic eye muscles of man. *Acta anat.* **55**, 311-322.
Sasaki, K. (1963). Electrophysiological studies on oculomotor neurons of the cat. *Jap. J. Physiol.* **13**, 287-302.
Schaefer, K. (1965). Die Erregungsmuster einzelner Neurone des Abducens-Kernes beim Kaninchen, *Arch Ges. Physiol.* **284**, 31-52.
Schubert, G. and Bornschein, H. (1962). Einzelfaseraktivität im N. oculomotorius bei vestibulärer Reizung. *Arch. Ges. Physiol.* **275**, 107-116.
Sears, M. L., Teasdall, R. D. and Stone, H. H. (1959). Stretch effects in human extraocular muscle: An electromyographic study. *Bull. Johns Hopk. Hosp.* **104**, 174-178.
Sherrington, C. D. (1918). Observations on the sensual role of the proprioceptive nerve supply of the extrinsic eye muscles. *Brain.* **41**, 332-343.
Siggins, G., Berman, H. and McKinnon, E. (1968). Striated muscle with unusual properties in the tongue of the frog. *Fed. Proc.* **27**, 236.

Smith, W. (1949). The frontal eye fields. *The Precentral Motor Cortex,* 2nd. ed. Bucy, P. (Ed.). Chicago, Ill. Press.

Steinacker, A. and Bach-y-Rita, P. (1968a). A mechanical study of the cat retractor bulbi muscle. *Experientia* (Basel) **24,** 1138-1139.

Steinacker, A. and Bach-y-Rita, P. (1968b). The fiber spectrum of the cat VI nerve to the lateral rectus and retractor bulbi muscles. *Experientia* (Basel) **24,** 1254-1255.

Szentágothai, J. and Schab, R. (1956). A midbrain inhibitory mechanism of oculomotor activity. *Acta. Physiol.* (Hung) **9,** 89-98.

Taren, J. A. (1964). An anatomic demonstration of afferent fibers in the IV, V, and VI cranial nerves of the macaca mulatta. *Amer. J. Opthal.* **58,** 408-412.

Tengroth, B. (1960). The influence of the extraocular muscles on the position of the eye. *Acta Ophthal.* **38,** 698-700.

Thomas, R. C. and Wilson, V. J. (1966). Marking single neurons by staining with intracellular recording microelectrodes. *Science.* **151,** 1538-1539.

Tozer, F. and Sherrington, C. (1910). Receptors and afferents of the III, IV and VI cranial nerves. *Proc. Roy. Soc. B.* **82,** 450-457.

Tsuchida, U. (1906). Uber die Ursprungskerne der augenbewegungs-nerven und uber die mit diesen in beziehung stehenden bahnen in mittel-und zwischenhirn. Normal-anatomische embryologische, patholgisch-anatomische und vergleicheld-anatomische Untersuchungen. *Arb. Hirnanat. Inst. Zur.* **2,** 1-205.

Walls, G. L. (1962). The evolutionary history of eye movements. *Vision Res.* **2,** 69-80.

Whitteridge, D. (1955). A separate afferent nerve supply from the extraocular muscles of goats. *Quart. J. Exp. Physiol.* **40,** 331-336.

Whitteridge, D. (1960). Central control of eye movements. *Handbook of Physiology-Neurophysiology.* vol. II. Amer. Physiol. Soc., Washington, D. C.

Whitteridge, D. (1962). Afferent mechanisms in the initiation and control of eye movements. Symposium XI, Optic and Vestibular Factors in Motor Co-ordination. *Proc. Internat. Union Physiol. Sci.,* Leiden Exerpta Medical Foundation, Amsterdam.

Wiersma, C. A. G. (1967). Visual central processing in crustaceans. *Invertebrate Nevous Systems.* C. A. G. Wiersma (Ed.). Chicago, Univ. of Chicago Press.

Wiersma, C. A. G. and Yamaguchi, T. (1967). Integration of visual stimuli by the crayfish central nervous system. *J. Exp. Biol.* **47,** 409-431.

Winkler, G. (1937). L'innervation sensitive et motrice des muscles extrinseques de l'oeil chez quelques ongules. *Arch. Anat. Strassbourg.* **23,** 219-234.

Yamanaka, Y. and Bach-y-Rita, P. (1968). Conduction velocities in the abducens nerve correlated with vestibular nystagmus in cats. *Exp. Neurol.* **20,** 143-155.

Yellin, H. (1969). Unique intrafusal and extraocular muscle fibers exhibiting dual actomyosin ATPase activity. *Exp. Neurol.* **25,** 153-163.

THE STRUCTURE OF THE EXTRAOCULAR MUSCLE FIBERS OF MAMMALS

LEE PEACHEY

All the muscles of the extraocular group with the exception of the retractor bulbi (when present) contain a mixture of muscle fibers of different types. These different types can be recognized by histological appearance, fine structure as seen in the electron microscope, innervation pattern, and histochemistry, as well as by various physiological properties such as electrical activity or speed of contraction. Ultimately we would like to understand how each of these fiber types contributes to eye movements. Attainment of this goal would clearly be facilitated by precise and correlated knowledge of the structural and functional properties of each muscle fiber type. Integration of this information with knowledge of the eye movements themselves, the mechanics of the orbit, and the activities of the central nervous system would give a complete picture of eye movements. However, for the present, we are faced with an incomplete and somewhat confused array of morphological and physiological parameters, unable to know with certainty the properties of any particular type of muscle fiber.

Dr. Bach-y-Rita already has reviewed the physiology of these muscles. I have been asked to review our knowledge of the structure of the extraocular muscles and to bring this together insofar as possible into an overall scheme. The main force of my presentation will be directed toward the presence in these muscles of fibers of different structural types. Obviously this is only one part of the general question of 'slow' vs. 'fast' muscle fibers in all muscles, a subject badly in need of careful consideration. However, the ambition to write a comprehensive review on this subject has eluded me for several years now, and I welcome this chance to address myself to the more restricted area defined by the fascinating muscles of the extraocular group. I will confine my review to mammals and to the extrafusal fibers of the six muscles within the orbit, excluding the retractor bulbi. I will start by discussing the histological arrangement of fibers in the muscles. Second, I will consider histochemical and ultrastructural aspects of the various fiber types, which will lead to a classification system including five different types of fibers. Third, and finally, I will discuss some problems of relating structure to function, and briefly discuss the motor nerve endings in these muscles.

HISTOLOGY

When I started preparing this review, I thought I should begin with a brief statement about the arrangement of muscle fibers and tendons in the extraocular muscles, at the histological level. However, I was surprised to find relatively little information on this beyond the common textbook statement (e.g. Wolff, 1964) that the fibers are unusually small in diameter, that they run parallel to the long axis of the muscle, that the muscles contain an unusually large amount of elastic tissue, and that the distal tendons glisten. The last point seems to be of rather dubious importance, at least in the present context. The more important point concerning whether any or all of the fibers run the whole length of the muscle, or whether some are shorter than others and end within the muscle away from either or both tendons, seems to have received little attention.

In 1931, Hines reported that in rabbits the one-third of the muscle near its origin is characterized by larger diameter fibers, whereas smaller diameter fibers are more common in the two-thirds of the muscle near its insertion on the eyeball. Many of the larger fibers were said to end abruptly in the middle third of the muscle, while many smaller fibers tapered before also ending within the middle third of the muscle. The picture was further complicated by the observation of branching of muscle fibers, either toward the origin end or toward the insertion end of the muscle. Lockhart and Brandt in 1938 cited previous reports in the literature of fibers terminating and arising in tapering cones in the course of the length of an extraocular muscle, but these workers could find no such tapered ends and concluded that 'In adult eye muscles the fibers ran all the way.' In contrast to Hines' finding of predominantly large fibers proximally and smaller ones distally, Cooper and Daniel (1949) reported that the proximal end of the inferior rectus of man contains a majority of small diameter fibers, as small as 10 μ. Only a few large, up to 50 μ diameter fibers, are found in this part of the muscle. Further distally the peripheral fibers remain small, but the central fibers, according to Cooper and Daniel 'appear to be increasing in diameter.' In the middle third of the muscle, the fibers 'become smaller in diameter again,' and some of the peripheral fibers end on the most proximal portion of the distal tendon of insertion. The structural arrangement of all the extraocular muscles of man was said by Cooper and Daniel to be essentially similar.

Apparently, in agreement with Lockhart and Brandt (1938), Cooper and Daniel (1949) wished us to believe that all the fibers run the whole length of the muscle, changing their diameters as they go. In fact, Cooper and Daniel found this 'variation in diameter of the extrafusal muscle fibers as they pass along the muscle' an 'interesting feature of eye muscles.' In a later paper, however, Cooper *et al.* (1955) were more uncertain about this particular point that the large diameter fibers in the core of the muscle stretch the whole length of the muscle and taper at their ends. Certainly if this is the case, we have a rather unacceptable situation from a physiological point of view. If the fibers do taper and have more fibril cross-section centrally, then the thicker central parts would produce more tension than the thinner ends. This would lead to an unstable mechanical situation during contraction if all the fibrils contracted equally. Alternatively, we could believe that the large fibers seen in the belly of the muscle terminate short of both ends of the muscle, as reported for the distal end by Hines (1931). If this is true, then we are left with a difficult problem in interpreting information based on cross-sections of unspecified regions in the muscle. There is no question that this needs to be resolved before we can fully evaluate the question of numbers of fibers of various types, since only in transverse sections can we hope to look at every fiber in the muscle, and even this can be complicated if some of the fibers end in the body of the muscle. However, for the present, and with these problems in mind, I should like now to proceed to a tentative consideration of the problem of fiber types and numbers in the extraocular muscles.

FIBER COUNTS

One of the more complete studies on the histology of the extraocular muscles was published by Kato in 1938 (Fig. 1). Kato concerned himself primarily with study of fiber size and number in transverse sections. Like earlier authors, he noted the fine diameter of the fibers, relative to other skeletal muscles, and their parallel arrangement. In an adult man, there were from 20-35,000 fibers in each rectus, and about 15,000 in each oblique. There was a tendency for the smaller fibers to be located peripherally, around an axial core of larger fibers. Incidentally, this peripheral location of small fibers is one histological point I have never seen challenged. Among the largest and the smallest fibers found by Kato in man were those of the inferior rectus. The superior rectus also contained relatively large fibers. In the newborn, most of the muscle fibers are of thin variety.

In a monkey, the results were similar to those in the adult man, except the muscles contained about one-third as many fibers, and these had a wider distribution of sizes, from about one-quarter the size of the smallest fibers up to over twice the size of the largest fibers in man.

In the lemur, the fibers tended to be larger than in man or in the monkey, and the distinction in fiber size between axial and peripheral portions of the muscle was not so striking.

The dog, according to Kato, has more prominent connective tissue septae, dividing the muscles into distinct fiber bundles. As in man and the monkey, axial and peripheral fibers differed appreciably in size in the dog. The border between the regions was not particularly sharp, there being considerable mixing of fiber sizes in the transition region. The cat gave results very similar to those of the dog, although the fibers generally were bigger. In the dog, cat, and rabbit, the muscle fibers within a bundle were more tightly bunched together than in the other species, at least in Kato's fixed preparations. The rabbit showed the clearest separation between peripheral small and axial large fibers of all the species studied, except for man and monkey.

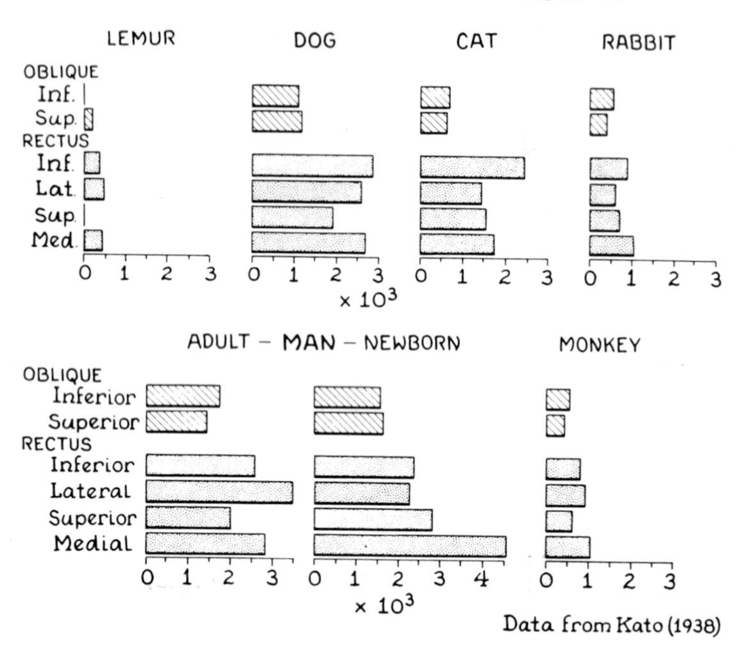

Fig. 1. Number of muscle fibers in extraocular muscles of various species, according to histological studies of Kato (1938). No values are given for two of the muscles in the lemur.

Figure 1 shows fiber numbers in the individual muscles of various species studied by Kato. No consistent pattern is apparent, except that the recti contain more fibers than the obliques.

Unfortunately Kato's description of segregation of fibers by size into regions or layers in the muscle largely has been ignored in physiological studies, with the notable exceptions of the papers by Kern (1965) and by Bach-y-Rita and Ito (1966). In trying to achieve our goal of correlating fiber structure with function, such regional information is very useful as it helps us toward associating a physiological response with a particular histological fiber type on the basis of location within the muscle. In this review, I will try to emphasize the fiber location while discussing morphological fiber types.

FIBER TYPES

Early in the histological literature, we find a suggestion of more than one type of muscle fiber in extraocular muscles. These are distinguished not only by fiber diameter, as already discussed, but by content of sarcoplasm, size of nuclei and 'fibrillae', and the presence or absence of hypolemmal rings

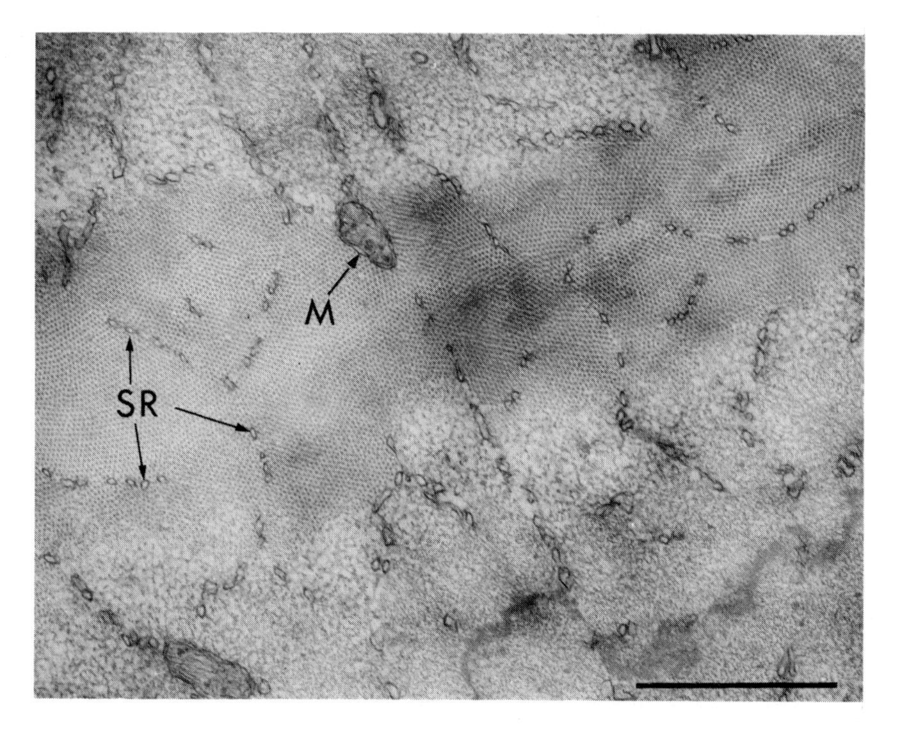

Fig. 2. Transverse section of a slow muscle fiber of a frog iliofibularis muscle. Fibrils are large and indistinct, only partially separated by a scant sarcoplasmic reticulum (SR) X 30,000. Line represents 1μ.

or bands. For example, Cilimbaris (1910) reported finding clear fibers with little sarcoplasm and few nuclei, and dark fibers, rich in sarcoplasm and with many nuclei, as well as intermediate types. Thulin (1914) reported three types, two of which were similar to the ones described by Cilimbaris. Thulin's third type contained peripheral fibrils oriented transversely or circularly around the fiber, not parallel to the axis of the fiber. These 'ring-fibrils' are relatively rare and may be associated with age or pathology (Voth and Rohen, 1962), so I think a discussion of them goes beyond the scope of this review.

Since more modern techniques of histochemistry and electron microscopy are so much better suited to studies of this kind than are the classic histological methods, I choose at this point to break off this very incomplete histological review and proceed to the studies of the last eight years.

The first person to examine extraocular muscles by electron microscopy was Arthur Hess (1961), whose results clearly established the presence of two morphological fiber types, one of which was reminiscent of fibers in

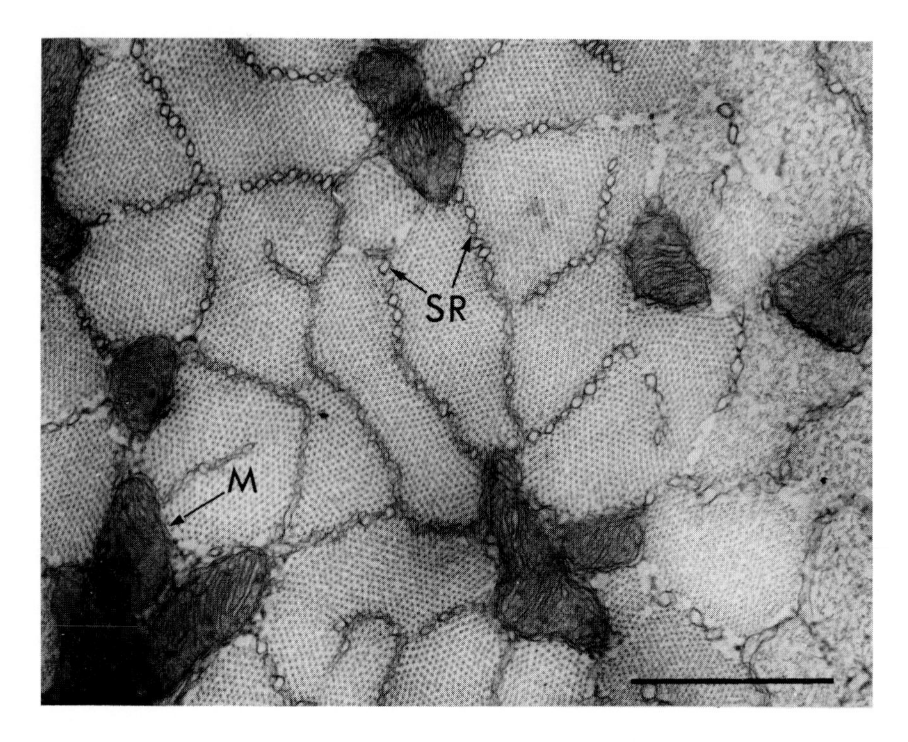

Fig. 3. Transverse section of a twitch or fast muscle fiber of a frog iliofibularis muscle. Fibrils are smaller and more distinctly separated by SR. More and larger mitochondria (M) are present. X 30,000. Line represents 1μ.

other vertebrates (birds, amphibians) where certain technical advantages had allowed the fibers to be shown to be physiologically slow. These pioneering and important morphological studies were done on guinea pig extraocular muscles, and two years later were extended to the cat, where they were combined with physiological studies confirming the presence of two different forms of contractile activity in extraocular muscles (Hess and Pilar, 1963). From this time on, no one has questioned the presence in extraocular muscles of at least two different types of fibers, distinguishable by morphological and physiological means. Many papers since that time have extended Hess' original observations, adding new species and new techniques, especially histochemical techniques, and have contributed considerable new information and even some confusion. Certainly no clear, consistent picture has emerged with regard to three critical questions. First, are there merely two fiber types, or are there more?: up to five have been proposed. Second, what are the morphological characteristics of these fiber types? And, third, which morphological fiber types are correlated with which particular physiological parameters observed in these muscles?

Before trying to answer these questions, I should like briefly to discuss some of the structural parameters available for fiber classification. Most of these can be illustrated by comparison between the fast and slow skeletal muscle fibers of amphibians, whose morphological and physiological properties are reasonably well established. Several of the limb muscles of frogs, for example, contain a majority of fast, twitch fibers and a minor population of distinct fibers that properly can be called slow fibers.

The physiology of these two fiber types has been reviewed (Peachey, 1961), and I will present this only very briefly. The fast fibers are singly innervated, and conduct propagated action potentials, each of which is followed by a brief twitch. The slow fibers, however, have multiple endings, and can give slower, graded contractions in the absence of action potentials. Presumably their dense, multiple innervation leads to depolarization of the whole fiber membrane and a spatial summation of local junctional potentials and contractions. In this way, the whole fiber is activated even without a propagated electrical response.

Morphologically, the two types of frog fibers are distinct and quite easily recognized (Peachey and Huxley, 1962; Page, 1965). A precise correlation between functional type and structure was obtained by Peachey and Huxley (1962), who dissected single fibers, tested them physiologically, and then examined them microscopically. Figures 2 and 3 are electron micrographs of transverse sections of frog slow and fast muscle fibers, shown for comparison to the published figures of extraocular muscles discussed later. These micrographs are taken from a bundle of fibers, but the two types are easily identified once the correlation with physiological type had been established on isolated fibers. An obvious difference between the two types is the size and form of the myofibrils. In the fast fiber, the fibrils are quite distinct and are almost completely separated by elements of sarcoplasmic reticulum (SR) and mitochondria. Fibrils of slow fibers, on the other hand, are irregular and indistinct, being poorly delineated by SR. The total amount of SR differs in the two types, there being more in the fast fiber. Mitochondria are also more prominent in the fast fiber, although this difference is more dramatic between red (many mitochondria) and white (fewer mitochondria) fibers of mammals (see Gauthier, 1969).

It is now widely accepted that the turning on and off of contraction in the living fiber results from the release and subsequent reaccumulation of calcium by the SR. The signal for this release is believed to be a depolarization spreading radially into the fiber from the surface along the transverse tubular system (Fig. 4), which associates with the SR in specialized structures called triads (in vertebrates: in invertebrates the equivalent structures are somewhat different and are called dyads. For reviews on this subject, see Sandow, 1965; Peachey, 1965, 1966; Ebashi and Endo, 1968). Suffice it to say for the present that a rapid cycle of contraction and relaxation depends

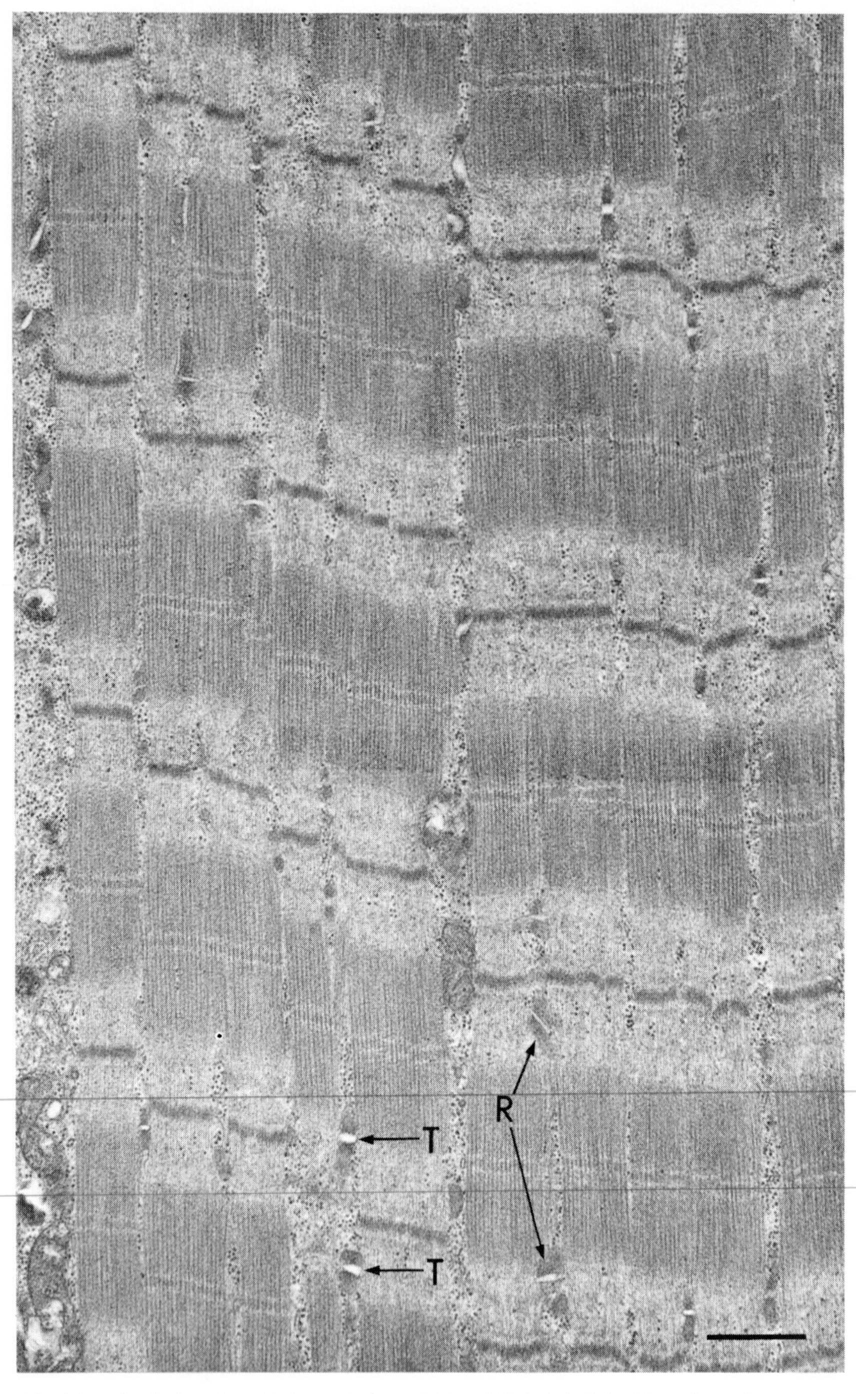

Fig. 4. Longitudinal section of a human leg muscle fiber. Triads (R) of the SR are located between the myofibrils near the ends of the dark A-bands. The central element of each triad is a transverse tubule (T). X 15,000. Line represents 1μ.

at least in part on the efficient functioning of the SR and transverse tubules. It follows from this to expect extensive development of these membrane systems in fast contracting muscles, and to expect slowly contracting fibers to have less of these systems. Obviously this agrees with the results on the frog, already discussed, where we have precise correlation between structural type and functional type, i.e., fast vs. slow. The important point here is that we can with some justification look at fibers in extraocular muscles with regard to their content of SR and triads as a clue to their possible functional type, but we must not forget that this is an extrapolation from information obtained from other types of muscles.

Another morphological parameter that varies considerably among various muscle fiber types, and that is fairly easily studied either histochemically or in the light or electron microscope, is mitochondrial content. So-called 'red' fibers contain many or large (or both) mitochondria, whereas 'white' fibers have a lower mitochondrial content. These mitochondria contain cytochromes, and these contribute part of the red color of some muscles. It is common to equate 'redness' with 'slowness' and 'whiteness' with 'rapidity' of contraction, and while this relationship holds most of the time, it is not absolute. This has been discussed elsewhere (e.g., Peachey, 1970), and I will merely advise caution here and suggest that redness and mitochondrial content relates to oxidative metabolism of the fiber, which in turn relates to demands on the fiber for long duration work. Nevertheless, mitochondrial content is an important and useful criterion for establishing fiber types, and we will use it extensively here.

Other morphological criteria we can use in describing muscle fibers are related to the appearance of the striations of the myofibrils (Z-lines and M-lines especially, see Fig. 4), content of lipid and glycogen (related to metabolism of the fiber, but also probably to nutritional state of the animal), activity of various enzymes as detected histochemically, and, very importantly, number and form of myoneural junctions on the muscle fiber. With these points in mind, I will now procede to an attempt to classify the fiber types in mammalian extraocular muscles.

The major recent histochemical and microscopic studies of extraocular muscles are those of Hess (1961, 1967), Hess and Pilar (1963), Kern (1965), Cheng and Breinin (1966), Miller (1967), and Mayr (unpublished). For the moment, I will exclude studies of endplate regions in order to concentrate on the muscle fibers themselves. These authors claim to have identified various numbers of differing fiber types, ranging from two to five in number. The trick here is to relate the fiber types of one author to those of another and this is not at all easy. However, one can make some sense of it all by first concentrating on the three papers giving the most complete detail: Cheng and Breinin (1966), Miller (1967), and Mayr (unpublished). I will key these papers as (CB, Mi, Ma) respectively. The animals used were the rhesus monkey (CB, Mi) and the rat (Ma).

Orbital layer

Miller and Mayr describe two fiber types that are concentrated on the orbital surface of the muscle and extend around its edges, so that these fibers form a sort of 'C' in transverse sections with the open side of the 'C' facing the globe. Cheng and Breinin describe no fiber whose structure fits very well with these fibers, so the following description of fibers from this orbital layer is based entirely on the work of Miller and of Mayr.

1. On the orbital surface of the muscle (Mi, Ma) and irregularly on the global surface (Mi), there is a layer of small diameter cells. These fibers are of two types. Most (Mi; 80% Ma) have a diameter of 5-20μ (Ma). They show a characteristic light microscopic staining pattern (Gomari's trichrome, Mi: Sudan black, Ma), revealing large groups of globular mitochondria in columns throughout the fiber and in even larger subsarcolemmal accumulations. These mitochondria contain many densely-packed cristae. Fibrils are indistinct and irregularly shaped in these fibers, the fibrils being only poorly separated by the sparse SR in the A-band region (Mi, Ma). Prominent Z-lines (Mi) are thin and straight (Ma), and no M-line is present (Mi, Ma). The SR is moderately well-developed in the I-band, is very sparse in the A-band, and has triads at the A/I junction (Mi, Ma). Lipid and glycogen content is high (Mi, Ma), and there is a strong reaction for succinic dehydrogenase (SD) and phosphorylase (Pase), and a weak alpha-glycerophosphate dehydrogenase (GPD) reaction (Mi). The innervation of these fibers is single, with large end plates with numerous post-junctional folds (Ma).

2. The less common fiber (Mi, 20% Ma) on the orbital surface is even smaller (Mi), measuring only 5-10 μ in diameter (Ma). Mitochondria are not particularly few in number, but are small, so their total amount is not large (Ma). They are arranged in narrow columns throughout the fiber, and are cylindrically elongated (Mi, Ma). Subsarcolemmal accumulations of mitochondria are reduced in comparison to the first type (Mi, Ma). Fibrils are again indistinct (especially in A-bands) (Mi) but smaller (Ma) than in the first fiber type, and again an M-line is lacking (Mi, Ma). In this case, well-defined Z-lines (Mi) are said to be thicker and more irregular than in the first type (Ma). SR is again moderately well-developed and found largely in the I-band (Mi), with triads at the A/I junction (Mi, Ma) and also elsewhere (Ma). Glycogen is moderate (Ma), and lipid droplets are absent (Mi, Ma). The reaction for SD and Pase is less than in the first type, and GPD activity is again weak (Mi). Nerve endings are found at all positions in the muscle, so it is presumed that these fibers are multiply-innervated (Ma). Short post-junctional folds are present in these endings, which are larger than the endings of the multiply-innervated fibers in the central portion of the muscle (Ma).

Central and global layers

In the central core of the muscle, and reaching to the global surface, where surface-type, small fibers may mix in, we have a population including medium and large-diameter muscle fibers (Mi, Ma). The fibers described by Cheng and Breinin apparently come from this part of the muscle. Cheng and Breinin classify the large fibers in two groups, 'large red' and 'large white'. They also describe a smaller fiber, which will be discussed later. Miller describes 3 types of large fibers in this region of the muscle: the first of these in the order he presents them seems to correspond to 'large red' and the third to 'large white'. The other large type of Miller will be discussed later. Mayr's description of fibers in this region provides for a medium-diameter fiber type and three groups of large fibers ranging from 'dark' (presumably red), through 'intermediate' to 'pale' (presumably white). In these large fibers, we seem to have a suggestion of a continuum of fiber types, but for the present I will describe the extreme thirds of Mayr's populations as separate types and leave the central third as possible intermediates.

3. The 'large red' fibers of Cheng and Breinin and the first large fiber described by Miller are similar to each other, and also similar in gross appearance to the small, dark fibers of the orbital layer (type 1) although larger in diameter (25-50μ,CB). Mayr's dark and intermediate fibers of this region are also similar, except smaller (10-30μ). However, it seems to be characteristic of these fibers that their diameter varies in different regions of the muscle, so these all may be one type. Like the surface fibers of a similar type, these fibers have broad columns and subsarcolemmal accumulations (CB, Mi) of large mitochondria with many cristae (Ma). A characteristic feature of these fibers is their small, distinct fibrils, compared to the larger, indistinct fibrils of all the fibers of the orbital surface (CB, Mi, Ma). Description of the Z-line varies (straight, CB; irregular, Ma), but authors agree on the absence of an M-line (CB, Mi, Ma). The SR is highly developed, with numerous triads at the A/I junctions (CB, Mi, Ma). Lipid is present in moderate to large amounts (CB, Mi, Ma) and glycogen in moderate amounts (Mi, Ma). Succinic dehydrogenase is the highest of any fiber type in the muscle, phosphorylases are moderately high, and α-glycerophasphate dehydrogenase is low (Mi). The innervation is single, endplates are large, and post-junctional folds are frequent (Ma).

4. The other large diameter fiber type in the central core of the muscle is the 'large white' fiber of Cheng and Breinin and the pale fiber of Mayr, whose descriptions are very similar to each other. The third large fiber described by Miller is similar except with regard to the description of mitochondria.

These fibers are 25-50μ in diameter (CB; 30-40μ, Ma), and have few mitochondria (CB, Mi, Ma), these being small and evenly distributed (CB, Ma) among the fibrils, particularly in the vicinity of the Z-lines (CB) and having relatively few cristae (Ma). (Miller's apparently corresponding type shows a few scattered, somewhat larger mitochondria). Myofibrils in this type are small (Ma) and well delineated by SR (CB, Mi). Z-lines are thin and straight (CB, Ma), and an M-line is distinctly seen (CB, Mi, Ma). A well formed SR with triads at the A/I junction (CB, Mi, Ma) and a moderate amount of glycogen (Mi, Ma) is present, but lipid droplets are rare (CB, Ma). Succinic dehydrogenase and phosphorylases are low to intermediate, corresponding to the small mitochondrial content, but α-glycerophasphate dehydrogenase is moderate to high (Mi). The innervation of these fibers is similar to that of the large, red fibers, i.e., single with large endplates with many post-junctional folds (Ma).

At this point, I must mention again the intermediate fiber type discussed by Mayr. It is said to have an intermediate level of granularity and staining intensity with Sudan black, and therefore presumably has an intermediate mitochondrial and lipid content. Its fibrils are small and distinct, like the pale and dark fibers of this group. No statement is made about the M-line of these intermediate fibers, but recall that the pale fibers have a distinct M-line while the dark fibers have none. What is intermediate between having an M-line and not having one?

5. The final fiber type to be described has many characteristics we would tend to attribute to a slow fiber, being rather similar to the small diameter slow fibers of the frog. These fibers are large (Mi) to medium diameter (8-15μ, CB; 18μ, Ma). They have small mitochondria, often transversely-elongated to form bracelets around the fibrils, which are large and indistinct, with a poorly-developed M-line (CB, Mi, Ma). Z-lines are broad (CB, Ma) and sometimes irregular (CB). Little SR is present, with few triads (CB, Mi, Ma). Glycogen content is moderate (Mi, Ma). Both succinic dehydrogenase and phosphorylase activity are minimal, while α-glycerophosphate dehydrogenase is low to moderate (Mi). Innervation, like that of frog slow fibers, is multiple, with small endings, generally with no post-junctional folds (Ma).

I now have described five classes or types of fibers based on these three papers. These are summarized in Table I. The five types described by Miller and by Mayr seem to have fallen rather well into the five groups, with the additional, intermediate type of Mayr falling in the third group or somewhere between the third and fourth type. All three of these papers can be brought into essential agreement, a task that seemed impossible to me only a few weeks ago, by assuming that Cheng and Breinin for some reason missed all the small diameter fibers on the orbital surfaces of the muscles. Looking at their Materials and Methods section, this seems entirely possible. Following a common procedure designed to aid penetration of fixative into the tissue, they cut the muscles into small pieces in the first fixation, and subsequently they could either intentionally or unintentionally have selected only pieces from the central portion of the muscle to carry through to microscopic examination. This is entirely consistent with their micrographs in comparison to those of Mayr, and with the descriptions given in the text, in that the three fiber types presented by Cheng and Breinin fit rather closely with the three types found both by Miller and by Mayr to be located centrally and toward the global surface.

TABLE I

FIBER TYPES IN EXTRAOCULAR MUSCLES

	TYPE 1	TYPE 2	TYPE 3	TYPE 4	TYPE 5
Location:	--------surface---------		--------------------interior-----------------		
Diameter:	5-20μ (small)	5-10μ	10-50μ (large)	25-50μ	18μ (medium)
Mitoch./Lipid/SD:	high	low	high	low	low (mitoch. elong. trans.)
Fibrils:	larger (indistinct) smaller		-------small,distinct----		large, indistinct
Z-line:	thin,straight	irregular	(descr. varies)	thin,straight	broad
M-line:	-------absent-----------		absent	present	weak or absent
Sarcopl. retic.:	moderate amount,mostly I, triads A/I		--much, triads A/I--------		little, few triads
GPD:	---------weak-----------		low	mod. high	low to mod.
Innervation	single, folds	mult.,short folds	------single, folds-------		mult.,no folds

Comments

What then remains to be done? First, I think we should try to see if the five classes can be reduced in number by combining them in some way. However, while I see many similarities between certain classes, especially between my class 1 (orbital, dark) and my class 3 (global, dark) I also recognize significant differences in the myofibrils of these types. Frankly, I see no advantage at the present time in trying to combine these or any other classes simply to reduce the number of fiber types. Of course, as additional evidence accumulates, this may turn out to be desirable.

Second, we might try to follow Mayr's lead, and consider the large diameter fibers in the central and global part of the muscle as a continuous spectrum. One type is red, with many mitochondria, and the other is white, with fewer mitochondria. While this color classification often has been overextended to imply physiological properties related to speed of contraction, it does indicate underlying biochemical differences, and is a useful distinction (see Gauthier, 1968). Also there seems to be an absolute difference between these classes in that one type of fiber has a prominent M-line, and the other has none. Unless one can show gradations of M-line presence in fibers of intermediate types, this would seem to speak against consideration here of a continuous spectrum of fiber types. However, the M-line has shown itself recently to be a rather labile part of the fibril (Knappeis and Carlsen, 1968; Stromer *et al.*, 1969). We must therefore be prepared to consider the possibility of differential extraction of the M-line substance during preparation for electron microscopy, leading to a false absence of this structure from particular fibers which in fact do have an M-line in the living state. Overall, I would argue here against consideration of a continuum of fiber types until we have observed gradations of all these properties or have demonstrated transformation from one type to another.

Another goal we might set for ourselves would be to try to fit some of the other morphological reports in the literature into the general scheme that I have presented. I think this may be a worthwhile effort, and I propose to use some of my remaining time in this direction.

Hess and Pilar (1963) in their study of cat extraocular muscles described two fiber types. In their highly-commendable and successful attempt to do electron microscopy on the very same fibers that had been used for cholinesterase studies, they were forced to use preparation methods that gave rather less than ideal preservation of fine structure. Therefore their early paper is somewhat incomplete at the fine structural level, but is neatly supplemented by a later report (Hess, 1967). The large (30-45μ diameter) fibers described by Hess and Pilar clearly fall into my classifications 3 or 4, simply on the basis of size. They also have the small, distinct myofibrils, extensive SR, and single endings characteristic of these types. On the basis of their relatively low mitochondrial content, they seem to fit better in class 4 than in class 3. Unfortunately the other, smaller (10-15μ diameter) fibers, with their multiple nerve endings could be either type 2 or type 5, and I can't decide between these two. This is unfortunate because this knowledge would help us in relating the physiological work of Hess and Pilar (1963) to that of Bach-y-Rita and Ito (1966). Also, this fiber is reported to have an M-line, but I am inclined to neglect this apparent inconsistency for reasons already stated.

Cheng-Minoda *et al.* (1968) used an approach similar to that of Hess and Pilar but with improved preservation of fine structure. This time the work was on rabbits. They distinguished 2 classes of fibers, selected by single versus multiple innervation. They noted that the two types of innervation were found both on the surface of the muscle, and in its interior, in agreement with work I have already discussed. Their description of the single innervated fibers, like that of Hess and Pilar fits well with my type 4 fibers, but again their class of multiply-innervated fibers could be type 2 or 5. It may have included both types, depending on whether the individual fibers studied came from the surface or the interior of the muscle. Their report makes a special point of the absence of an M-line from these multiply-innervated fibers.

Kern (1965) has done histological and pharmacological studies on rabbit lateral rectus, making ingenious use of the distinct layers in the rabbit, as described earlier by Kato (1938), by separating these layers for pharmacological experiments. Kern agrees with earlier authors in showing a superficial layer of small fibers and a deeper, large diameter fiber layer. He classifies the small fibers as Felderstruktur and the deeper fibers as Fibrillenstruktur, using the terminology of Krüger (1952), a classification I must take exception to in this case. Krüger's Fibrillen- and Felderstruktur refer to characteristic patterns seen in transverse sections particularly after fixation in Susa's fluid and staining with hematoxylin and eosin. Fixation in this case is poor, by modern standards. But while the pattern obtained is a shrinkage artifact in the fibrils, it must represent an underlying difference in fibril structure and therefore is useful. These patterns were demonstrated by Krüger and others (Peachey and Huxley, 1962) in frog muscles, and it has been shown, using isolated single fibers, that the Felderstruktur fibers are the slow fibers discussed earlier. However, I find Krüger's evidence for Felderstruktur in mammalian skeletal muscles very unconvincing and, likewise, I do not believe that Kern makes a good case for Felderstruktur in surface fibers of rabbit extraocular muscles. His pictures suggest to me Fibrillenstruktur in both regions of the muscle, with the superficial fibers merely having larger fibrils than those of the deeper fibers. I have no time to document my opinion here, but I must register my objection to any inference that superficial fibers in extraocular muscles have any necessary physiological relationship to frog slow fibers on the basis of an unconvincing appearance of Felderstruktur. If you have read much of the literature on extraocular muscle structure, you will recall the rather widespread use of this comparison with frog muscles to support the presence of 'slow fibers' in extraocular muscles.

Returning to Kern's paper, his pharmacological studies clearly show a greater sensitivity to acetylcholine (producing a long-duration contraction) in superficial fibers, so in this respect at least some of the fibers in this layer do resemble frog slow fibers. However, lacking further evidence, I would say that the comparison should end here, at least for the present.

NERVE ENDINGS

Time prevents me from presenting a comprehensive coverage of the nerve endings in extraocular muscles, but I would like to discuss two points that are of particular importance with regard to recent physiological studies already discussed by Dr. Bach-y-Rita.

Two types of motor nerve endings have been seen in a wide variety of vertebrate species. First there is the end-plate, or 'en-plaque' type of ending. This ending is the more common of the two, it usually is the only ending on the fiber, although there sometimes may be two. Considerable evidence has suggested that this type of ending is characteristic of twitch type muscle fibers, that is, fibers that conduct action potentials and respond to a single stimulus with a brief twitch.

The other type of ending was first described by Retzius (1892) and subsequently has become known as an 'en grappe' ending, for its resemblance to a bunch of grapes. These endings are smaller than the end plate endings, and in some cases have been shown to be present on multiply-innervated fibers, such as the slow fibers of the frog. These muscle fibers are generally considered not to conduct action potentials (Kuffler and Vaughan Williams, 1953), although apparently they can when denervated (Stefani and Steinbach, 1968). Nevertheless, it is clear that these frog slow fibers can respond to a series of impulses with a build-up of junctional potentials but no action potential in the muscle fiber membrane leading to a slow, graded type of contraction. The multiple innervation, spaced over the whole length of the fiber, presumably assures that the whole fiber is activated in spite of the absence of a conducted electrical response.

There has been a tendency to extrapolate these results from the frog directly into the extraocular muscles of mammals, following the observation of multiple innervation with 'en grappe' type endings in some fibers of these muscles (Hess and Pilar, 1963), but I think it may be time to look at this point more closely.

Hess and Pilar (1963) were quite cautious on this point and stated that 'Although this type of ending in cat extraocular muscles does not have a grape-like appearance, it is probably analogous to the 'en grappe' terminal in other species.' Many later authors, however, abandon this caution and state that extraocular fibers with these endings are physiologically equivalent to frog slow fibers.

More recently, it has been re-emphasized that the multiple endings in extraocular muscles do differ from classic 'en grappe' endings (Zenker and Anzenbacher, 1964; Teräväinen, 1968) in that post-synaptic folds are often seen in the former endings. Teräväinen (1968) divides multiply-innervated fibers in rat extraocular muscles into two groups. His type 2 multiple innervation consists of a large number (20-30) of endings along the muscle fiber, without subneural lamellae. These were not located in depressions, and in these respects do resemble the innervation of frog slow fibers (Page, 1965). The type 1 multiple innervation consisted of larger endings, approximately 1/3 the size of motor end plates in the same muscle, and usually only 2-5 such endings were found on one muscle fiber. Subneural lamellae were present, though difficult to demonstrate. This type 1 multiple innervation differs from the multiple innervation of frog slow fibers. Of particular interest is the number of endings per fiber, 2-5. This seems inadequate for full activation of contraction along the whole fiber if no action potential is conducted. Even if the fibers are only 5 mm. long (a guess) and there are 5 evenly-spaced endings, each ending would have to serve 1 mm. of fiber length. Again guessing, taking the surface resistance (R_m) of the fiber as 2000 ohm-cm^2, the interval resistivity (R_i) as 200 ohm-cm, and a diameter of 20μ, we calculate an electrical length constant ($\lambda = aR_m/2R_i$) of only 0.7 mm. This would seem to be marginal for activation of the whole length of the fiber in the absence of the propogated response, and we are left to consider seriously the possibility that this class of fibers with Teräväinen's type 1 multiple innervation may in fact, under certain conditions at least, conduct action potentials.

Combining this information with the descriptions of fiber types as I have already presented them, it seems likely that the type 1 multiple innervation occurs on the multiply-innervated fibers of the peripheral portions of the muscle, my class 2 fibers. It is interesting to note that this is precisely where Bach-y-Rita and Ito (1966) report finding their multiply-innervated twitch fibers, adding additional credence to the idea that Teräväinen's type 1 fibers can conduct.

An additional relevant point on innervation of these muscles is the statement by Teräväinen (1968) that both small (type 2) and larger (type 1) multiple endings can occur on the same fiber. Earlier, Hines (1931) reported an apparently different but possibly similar situation in which a single fiber in an extraocular muscle carried an end plate type ending, and a small 'accessory ending' as well. The 'accessory ending' was said to arise from a non-medullated axonal branch either from the same nerve fiber giving rise to the end plate or from another nerve fiber. It seems that we should be on the lookout for evidence of polyneuronal innervation of individual fibers in extraocular muscles, as well as multiple endings. The physiological possibilities this presents are extensive, but one perhaps deserves mention here. If two separate nerve fibers innervate the same muscle fiber at nearby points on the membrane, then the response of the fiber could depend on the temporal relationship between impulses arriving from the two nerve fibers. It is even possible that temporally separated impulses in the two nerves would give rise only to local responses, whereas two sufficiently close impulses could summate to exceed threshold for an action potential. If this could even be demonstrated it would be the first example, to my knowledge of a single vertebrate muscle fiber with two modes of response under central nervous control.

You may have detected throughout my presentation a careful avoidance of the application of terms such as twitch or slow to the fibers whose morphology I have been discussing, with the exception of reference to the frog. This compulsive avoidance is not, you may also recognize, shared by all my colleagues, and perhaps I should be asked at this point to justify my aberrant behavior. It seems clear to me that our information at this time is incomplete. Hess and Pilar (1963), and Bach-y-Rita and Ito (1966) as well, each recognize two types of fibers physiologically, but disagree on the properties of the slower fiber. Their differences of opinion could be explained simply by saying that they are looking at two different types of 'slow' fibers, although other explanations of the discrepancy of results are possible and there is no particular reason for favoring this one. However, even if we do accept this possibility, it provides us with only three physiological fiber types. In contrast, the morphology I have discussed today allows for at least 5 fiber classes. It may be that two or more morphological types of fibers could have indistinguishable physiological properties, but somehow this seems unlikely. Even if this is true, however, it needs to be shown to be true experimentally.

Therefore, I am going to take the position that we cannot safely relate morphological and physiological fiber types in extraocular muscles at the present time, except in a tentative way. This may seem a defeatist attitude, but I would hope that it could be called merely cautious. Also, I see it as a challenge; a challenge that we work until we have accomplished the precise understanding we desire. It seems clear that the approach that will eventually lead us to this level of understanding must include a real effort by morphologists and physiologists to work together and to do each other's thing. The physiologist must tell us where in the muscle he found a particular response, and from what size of fiber, and hopefully even get the fiber out for morphological examination. The morphologist, on the other hand, can help by providing precise, quantitative information whenever possible in place of the somewhat imprecise language so commonly used in structural papers.

I must emphasize in conclusion, in case this is not already apparent,that the grouping together of fiber types described by various authors is entirely my own doing. I have carefully read each paper, and have formed the best grouping I can, but I must admit that there was some difficulty in doing this. I suppose that if this presentation has any value at all, it is that I have saved you the work of doing this yourself. However, we must keep in mind that the grouping may not be legitimate, perhaps because no one author gives all the information we would like to have, because of differences in methods used, because of inadvertant selection or omission in the publications, because of species differences, or simply because I have not done my job very well.

I hope I have not been too critical; I have not meant to be unkind. I strongly feel that a sound morphological base is needed on which to build physiological experiments and interpretations, and a careful review of the literature has been, at least for me, a useful effort.

Dr. Robert Mayr (II. Anatomische Lehrkanzel der Universitat Wien, Wahringerstrasse 13, Wien, Austria) has kindly supplied me with an early draft of the introduction, methods, and results sections of a manuscript he is currently preparing for publication, and has generously consented to allow me to show some of his figures at this Symposium. I am extremely grateful to Dr. Mayr, since without the benefit of this excellent manuscript, this review would have been considerably more difficult to prepare, and the result would have been considerably less comprehensive.

REFERENCES

Bach-y-Rita, P. and Ito, F. (1966). In vivo studies on fast and slow muscle fibers in cat extraocular muscles. *J. Gen. Physiol.* **49,** 1177-1198.

Cheng, K. and Breinin, G. M. (1966). A comparison of the fine structure of extraocular and interosseus muscles in the monkey. *Invest. Ophth.* **5,** 535-549.

Cheng-Minoda, K., Davidowitz, J., Liebowitz, A. and Breinin, G. M. (1968). Fine structure of extraocular muscle in rabbit. *J. Cell Biol.* **39,** 193-197.

Cilimbaris, P. A. (1910). Histologische Untersuchungen uber die Muskelspindeln den Augenmuskeln. *Arch. f. mikr. Anat.* **75,** 692.

Cooper, S., and Daniel, P. M. (1949). Muscle spindles in human extrinsic eye muscles. *Brain.* **72,** 1-24.

Cooper, S., Daniel, P. M. and Whitteridge, D. (1955). Muscle spindles and other sensory endings in the extrinsic eye muscles; the physiology and anatomy of the receptors and of their connexions with the brain-stem. *Brain.* **78,** 564-583.

Ebashi, S. and Enda, M. (1966). Calcium ion and muscle contraction. *Progr. Biophys. Mol. Biol.* **18.**

Gauthier, G. F. (1969). On the relationship of ultrastructural and cytochemical features to color in mammalian skeletal muscle. *Z. Zellforsch.* **95,** 462-482.

Hess, A. (1961). The structure of slow and fast extrafusal muscle fibers in the extraocular muscles and their nerve endings in guinea pigs. *J. Cell. Comp. Physiol.* **58,** 63-79.

Hess, A. (1967). The structure of vertebrate slow and twitch muscle fibers. *Invest. Ophth.* **6,** 217-228.

Hess, A. and Pilar, G. (1963). Slow fibers in the extraocular muscles of the cat. *J. Physiol.* **169,** 780-798.

Hines, M. (1931). Studies on the innervation of skeletal muscle. III. Innervation of the extrinsic eye muscles of the rabbit. *Am. J. Anat.* **47,** 1-53.

Kato, T. (1938). Über histologische Untersuchungen der Augenmuskeln von Menschen und Säugetieren. *Okajunas Folia Anatomica Japonica.* **16,** 131-145.

Kern, R. (1965). A comparative pharmacologic-histologic study of slow and twitch fibers in the superior rectus muscle of the rabbit. *Invest. Ophth.* **4,** 901-910.

Knappeis, G. G. and Carlsen, F. (1968). The ultrastructure of the M-line in skeletal muscle. *J. Cell Biol.* **38,** 202-211.

Krüger, P. (1952). *Tetanus and Tonus der quergestreiften Skelettmuskel der Wirbeltiere und des Menschen,* Leipzig, Acad. Verlag, Geest and Portig.

Kuffler, S. W. and Vaughan-Williams, E. M. (1953). *J. Physiol.* **121,** 289.

Lockhart, R. D. and Brandt, W. (1938). Length of striated muscle fibers. *J. Anat.* **72,** 470.

Miller, J. E. (1967). Cellular organization of Rhesus extraocular muscle. *Invest. Ophth.* **6,** 18-39.

Page, S. (1965). A comparison of the fine structure of frog slow and twitch muscle fibers. *J. Cell. Biol.* **26,** 477-497.

Peachey, L. D. (1961). Structure and function of slow striated muscle. In: *Biophysics of Physiological and Pharmacological Actions,* A. M. Shaves, ed., A.A.A.S., Washington, 391-411.

Peachey, L. D. (1965). Transverse tubules in excitation-contraction coupling. *Fed. Proc.* **24,** 1124-1134.

Peachey, L. D. (1966). The role of transverse tubules in excitation-contraction coupling in striated muscles. *Ann. N. Y. Acad. Sci.* **137,** 1025-1037.

Peachey, L. D. (1970). Form of the sarcoplasmic reticulum and T-system of striated muscle. In: *The Physiology and Biochemistry of Muscle as a Food, III.* E. J. Briskey and R. G. Cassens, eds., U. Wisc. Press, Madison, pp. 273-310.

Peachey, L. D. and Huxley, A. F. (1962). Structural identification of twitch and slow striated muscle fibers of the frog. *J. Cell Biol.* **13**, 177-180.
Retzius, G. (1892). Zur Kenntniss der motorischen Nervenendigungen. *Biol. Untersuch. (n.F.)* **3**, 41-52.
Sandow, A. (1965). Excitation-contraction coupling in skeletal muscle. *Pharmacol. Rev.* **17**, 265-320.
Stefani, E. and Steinbach, A. B. (1968). Action potentials in denervated 'slow' muscle fibers of the frog. *J. Physiol.* **197**, 4-5 P.
Stromer, M. H., Hartshorne, D. J., Mueller, H. and Rice, R. V. (1969). The effect of various protein fractions on Z- and M-line reconstitution. *J. Cell Biol.* **40**, 167-178.
Teräväinen, H. (1968). Electron microscopic and histochemical observations on different types of nerve endings in the extraocular muscles of the rat. *A. Zellfarsch.* **90**, 372-388.
Thulin, I. (1914). Contribution a l'histologie des muscles oculaires chez l'homme et chez les singes. *Compt. Rend. Acad. Sce.* **76**, 490-493.
Voth, D. and Rohen, J. (1962). Experimentelle und histochemische Untersuchungen uber die Ringbinden der abguergestreiften Muskulatur. *Anat. Anz.* **111**, 165-174.
Wolff, E. (1955). *The Anatomy of the Eye and Orbit.* McGraw-Hill, New York, Fourth Edition.
Zenker, W. and Anzenbacher, H. (1964). On the different forms of myo-neural junction in two types of muscle fiber from the external ocular muscles of the Rhesus monkey. *J. Cell. Comp. Physiol.* **63**, 273-285.

CENTRAL OCULOMOTOR PATHWAYS

MALCOLM B. CARPENTER

The nuclei of the extraocular muscles belong to the group of cranial nerves functionally classified as general somatic efferent cranial nerves. In comparison with the branchiomeric cranial nerves and those nerves conveying impulses concerned with special sensory modalities, these cranial nerves are regarded as relatively simple. The nuclei of the general somatic efferent cranial nerves form an interrupted cell column which extends from the lower medulla to the rostral mesencephalon and includes the XII, VI, IV and the III cranial nerves. The nuclei of the extraocular muscles share common features, in that all: (1) are located near the median raphe ventral to the cerebral aqueduct or the fourth ventricle, (2) are exclusively efferent, and (3) innervate striate muscle derived from the preotic somites. Distinctive features concern the intraaxial course of the root fibers, the innervation of specific extraocular muscles, and the presence of visceral nuclei in the oculomotor complex.

NUCLEI OF THE EXTRAOCULAR MUSCLES

The abducens nucleus, consisting of typical multipolar motor neurons, is located beneath the floor of the fourth ventricle within the complex loop of the internal genu of the facial nerve. These structures produce an eminence in the floor of the fourth ventricle, referred to as the facial colliculus. Root fibers of the abducens nerve emerge from the ventromedial border of the nucleus, traverse the pontine tegmentum, the medial lemniscus and pass lateral to the corticospinal tract to emerge from the ventral surface of the brain at the junction of pons and medulla. Fibers of the abducens nerve course upward and forward in the subarachnoid space between the pons and basisphenoid. Near the upper border of the petrous pyramid, the fibers pierce the dura, enter the medial wall of the cavernous sinus, and course along the lateral side of the internal carotid artery. The abducens nerve is said to have the longest intracranial course and lesions of this nerve are said to be the most common. Because of its long intracranial course, an isolated lesion of the abducens nerve has no neurological localizing value. Lesions of the abducens nerve produce paralysis of the ipsilateral rectus muscle which is expressed by horizontal diplopia, maximal on attempted lateral gaze to the side

Supported by a research grant (NS-01538-12) from the National Institute of Neurological Diseases and Stroke.

of the lesion. The affected eye usually is adducted because the medial rectus muscle on that side is unopposed.

The abducens cranial nerve is unique in that it is the only cranial nerve in which lesions in the nucleus produce phenomena different from those associated with lesions in the root fibers. Unilateral lesions in the abducens nucleus produce a paralysis of lateral gaze to the side of the lesion. In paralysis of lateral gaze neither eye can be directed horizontally to the side of the lesion. Thus, the syndrome consists of: (1) paralysis of the ipsilateral lateral rectus muscle, and (2) paresis of contralateral ocular adduction on attempted gaze to the side of the lesion. Convergence generally is not impaired. While discrete lesions in the abducens nucleus are rare, they do occur (Garel, 1882; Bennet and Savill, 1889; Blocq and Giunon, 1891; Benvenuti, 1901; D'Espine and Démole, 1917). Large lesions in the dorsal pontine tegmentum involving the abducens nucleus and a variety of surrounding structures also produce this syndrome (Wernicke, 1877; Freeman, 1922; Froment, Dechaume and Colrat, 1930). Experimental studies of discrete lesions in the abducens nucleus in the monkey have led to some interesting conclusions (Carpenter, McMasters and Hanna, 1963). Discrete unilateral lesions in the abducens nucleus in the monkey produce enduring paralysis of ipsilateral conjugate horizontal gaze (Fig. 1, **A** and **B**). Following such lesions conjugate horizontal gaze has never been seen to the side of the lesion in animals observed for over one year. After lesions are inflicted in the abducens nucleus: (1) both eyes are forcefully and persistently directed to the side opposite the lesion, (2) there is a mild head tilt to the opposite side, (3) ocular convergence is unimpaired and (4) some, but not all, animals exhibit monocular horizontal nystagmus in the contralateral abducted eye. Gaze straight ahead is infrequent and fleeting.

Anatomical data indicates that complete destruction of the abducens nucleus is not required to produce this syndrome, but involvement of ventral portions of the nucleus seems critical. The production of this syndrome is not dependent upon concomitant destruction of fibers of the medial longitudinal fasciculus (MLF), though fibers of this bundle are invariably degenerated. Lesions limited to cells of the medial eminence (eminentia teres) do not produce the syndrome. Degeneration resulting from discrete lesions of the abducens nucleus virtually is confined to the root fibers of the nucleus and medial longitudinal fasciculi. Degeneration in the MLF is bilateral, but predominantly contralateral, and is distributed to all of the nuclei of the extraocular muscles (Fig. 1, **C**). Degeneration ascending in the contralateral MLF is distributed preferentially to the ventral nucleus of the oculomotor complex (Fig. 1, **D**), a cell group which innervates the medial rectus muscle on that side (Carpenter, McMasters and Hanna, 1963). These data suggest that the syndrome of lateral gaze paralysis resulting from lesions in the abducens nucleus probably consists of two elements: (1) an ipsilateral lower motor neuron lesion due to destruction of motor neurons of the abducens nucleus, responsible for the paralysis of the lateral rectus muscle, and (2) a paresis of

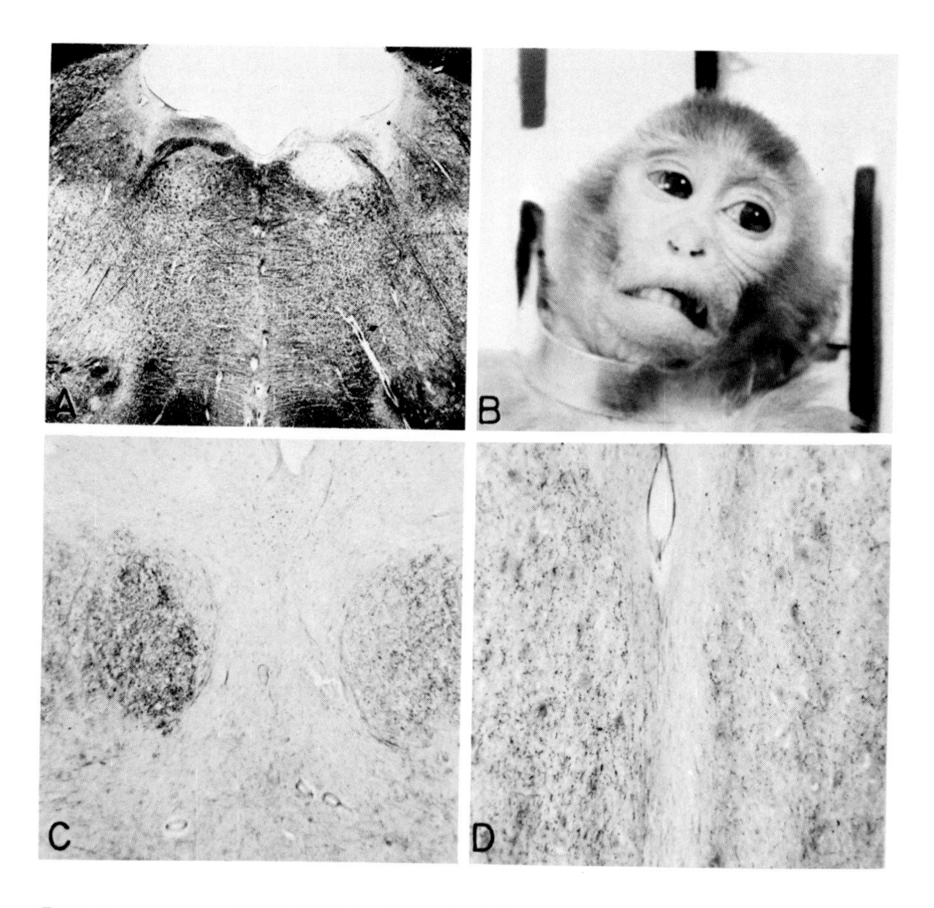

Fig. 1. **A** and **B.** Rhesus C-611. **A.** Photomicrograph of a localized lesion in the right abducens nucleus. Weil stain, X 8. **B.** Photograph showing forced gaze to the left and moderate head tilt to the left, occurring in association with paralysis of ipsilateral (right) conjugate horizontal gaze. **C.** Rhesus C-612. Ascending degeneration, predominantly in the left MLF, resulting from a discrete lesion in the right abducens nucleus, Nauta-Gygax stain, X 25. **D.** Rhesus C-622. Terminal degeneration projecting preferentially to the left ventral nucleus of the oculomotor complex following a lesion of the right abducens nucleus, not involving the MLF. Nauta-Gygax stain, X 160.

the contralateral medial rectus muscle due to interruption of ascending fibers which traverse the abducens nucleus, cross to the opposite side and project via the MLF preferentially to the ventral nucleus of the oculomotor complex. The precise origin of the ascending fibers destined for the contralateral ventral nucleus of the oculomotor complex is unknown. The so-called pontine center for lateral gaze has been referred to as the parabducens nucleus (Strong and Elwyn, 1943). While the so-called parabducens nucleus has never been described as an anatomical entity, the theoretical existence of this nucleus is acknowledged widely (Crosby, 1950, 1953; Cogan, 1956; Peele, 1961). This so-called nucleus is thought to be in the immediate vicinity of the abducens nucleus (Riley, 1930), and certain authors have postulated that the abducens nucleus and the "center for lateral gaze may constitute a single entity on the basis of lesions restricted to the abducens nucleus" (Bennet and Savill, 1889; d'Espine and Démole, 1917). Following section of the abducens nerve virtually all cells of the nucleus are reported to undergo chromatolysis (Van Gehuchten, 1898, 1904; Holmes, 1921; Warwick, 1953), so it seems unlikely that cells of the so-called parabducens are intermingled with those of the abducens nucleus. It has been postulated that fibers concerned with lateral gaze mechanisms could arise from the reticular formation or from the vestibular nuclei and merely traverse the abducens nucleus *en route* to the oculomotor complex. Secondary vestibular fibers from the medial and lateral vestibular nuclei follow this course, but there is no evidence that lesions restricted to these nuclei produce dissociated eye movements (McMasters, Weiss and Carpenter, 1966). It seems likely that cell groups in the reticular formation may give rise to fibers which pass through the abducens nucleus, enter the contralateral MLF and terminate upon cells of the opposite ventral nucleus of the oculomotor complex, but reticular neurons giving rise to fibers following this course have not been identified. Experimental studies of lesions in the brain stem reticular formation indicate that few, if any, fibers which ascend in the MLF are distributed to the nuclei of the extraocular muscles (Papez, 1926; Nauta and Kuypers, 1958). Most of the ascending fibers in the MLF rostral to the abducens nuclei are secondary vestibular fibers (McMasters, Weiss and Carpenter, 1966).

The trochlear nucleus is a small compact cell group ventral to the periaqueductal gray at the inferior collicular level which indents the dorsal surface of the MLF. This nucleus appears as a homogenous caudal appendage to the oculomotor complex. Root fibers from the nucleus arch dorsolaterally and caudally near the margin of the central gray and decussate completely in the superior medullary velum. Peripherally the nerve follows the lateral surface of the mid-brain, passes through the cavernous sinus, and ultimately innervates the superior oblique muscle. The superior oblique muscle serves to intort the abducted eye and to depress the eye when it is adducted. Isolated lesions of the trochlear nerve produce vertical diplopia which is maximal on downward gaze to the opposite side. Head tilt to the side opposite the lesion is seen in children. This is a mechanism that compensates for the impairment of ocular intortion of the affected eye.

The oculomotor nuclear complex is a collection of cell columns and discrete nuclei which: (1) innervate the inferior oblique and the superior, medial and inferior recti muscles, (2) the levator palpebrae muscle, and (3) provide preganglionic parasympathetic fibers to the ciliary ganglion. This complex lies ventral to the central gray of the midbrain in a "V" shaped trough formed by the obliquely diverging fibers of the MLF. The complex consists of paired lateral somatic cell columns, midline and dorsal visceral nuclei, and a discrete

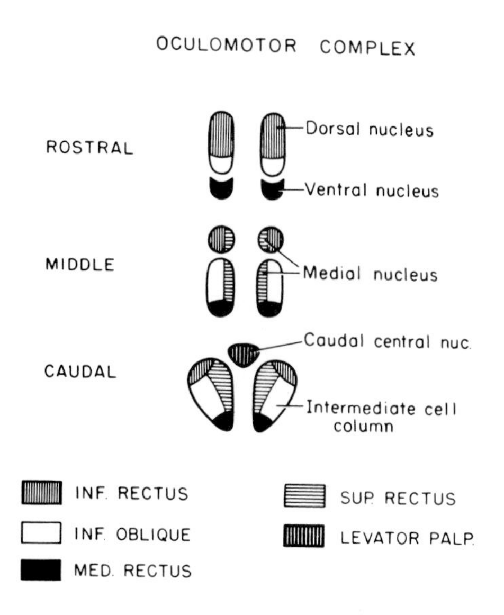

Fig. 2. Schematic diagram of the nuclear subdivisions of the oculomotor complex in the monkey (Warwick, 1953a). The visceral nuclei and the rostral pole of the complex are not shown. Root fibers innervating the inferior oblique and the inferior and medial rectus muscles are uncrossed, while fibers from the medial nucleus supply crossed fibers to the superior rectus muscle. Cells of the caudal central nucleus provide crossed and uncrossed fibers to the levator palpebrae muscle.

midline dorsal cell group, called the caudal central nucleus (Fig. 2). The lateral somatic cell columns innervate the extraocular muscles. The dorsal cell column (or nucleus) innervates the inferior rectus muscle, the intermediate cell column innervates the inferior oblique muscle, and the ventral cell column provides innervation for the medial rectus muscle (Warwick, 1953a). Root fibers arising from these cell columns are uncrossed. A cell column medial to the dorsal and intermediate cell columns, and unnamed by Warwick, provides crossed fibers that innervate the superior rectus muscle. This column of cells has been referred to as the medial nucleus (Carpenter and Strominger, 1964). The remaining somatic nucleus of the oculomotor complex, the caudal central nucleus, gives rise to crossed and uncrossed fibers that innervate the levator palpebrae muscle (Warwick, 1953a).

The visceral nuclei of the oculomotor complex consists of two distinct parts which rostrally are in continuity. The Edinger-Westphal nucleus consists of two slender columns of small multipolar cells dorsal to the rostral three-fifths of the oculomotor complex. In sections through the middle third of the complex each of these paired cell columns divides into two smaller cell columns which taper and gradually disappear. Rostrally the cell columns of the Edinger-Westphal nucleus merge in the midline dorsally and become

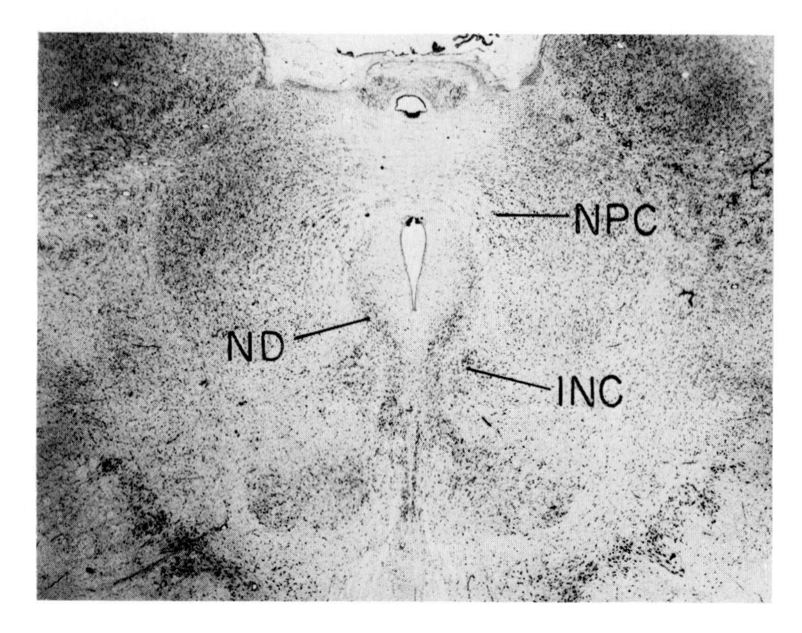

Fig. 3. Photomicrograph of a transverse section of the brain stem at the level of the posterior commissure showing the position of the nuclei of the posterior commissure (NPC), the nucleus of Darkschewitsch (ND), and the interstitial nucleus of Cajal (INC). Cresyl violet stain, X 8.

confluent with the visceral cells of the anterior median nucleus. Cells of the anterior median nucleus lie in the median raphe between the rostral portions of the lateral somatic cell columns (principally the dorsal cell column at this location). Cells of the anterior median nucleus are cytologically similar to those of the Edinger-Westphal nucleus and both of these nuclei give rise to uncrossed preganglionic parasympathetic fibers (Warwick, 1954).

In addition to the principal nuclei of the oculomotor complex there are certain accessory nuclei related to this complex which appear to play an important role with respect to oculomotor function. These nuclei are the interstitial nucleus of Cajal, the nucleus of Darkschewitsch and the nuclei of the posterior commissure (Fig. 3). There has been considerable confusion in the identification of, and in the nomenclature used to designate, these nuclei. Papers by Ingram and Ranson (1935) and Pompeiano and Walberg (1957) have helped to clarify this situation and the terminology used by these authors is employed here.

The interstitial nucleus (Cajal, 1908) is a small collection of neurons, multipolar in shape and smaller than somatic oculomotor cells, located among, and lateral to, the fibers of the MLF in the rostral midbrain. In the monkey this nucleus extends slightly beyond the rostral pole of the oculomotor complex and is present as an identifiable nucleus only in sections through the rostral half of the oculomotor complex. None of the cells of this nucleus contribute fibers to the oculomotor nerve (Warwick, 1954), but descending fibers passing in the MLF project to certain brain stem nuclei (Pompeiano and Walberg, 1957) and to spinal segments as far caudal as the lumbosacral region (Nyberg-Hansen, 1966).

The nucleus of Darkschewitsch (1889), formed by small cells, lies just inside the ventrolateral border of the central gray, dorsal and lateral to the somatic cell columns of the oculomotor complex. Rostrally the nucleus begins in the periventricular gray near the site where the fasciculus retroflexus traverses the red nucleus. This nucleus, difficult to distinguish from other cells of the central gray, is elliptical in shape, lies dorsal to the interstitial nucleus and the MLF and does not extend as far caudally as the interstitial nucleus. This nucleus does not give rise to any descending fibers that enter the MLF (Pompeiano and Walberg, 1957).

The nucleus of the posterior commissure, like the interstitial nucleus of Cajal, lies outside of the central gray. It is intimately associated with fibers of the posterior commissure and some cells extend across the midline. In spite of the assumptions of many authors, no fibers arising from the nucleus of the posterior commissure descend in the MLF.

One other frequently referred to nucleus of the oculomotor complex is deserving of comment mainly because of dogmatic statements in textbooks concerning its existence and function. This is the so-called central nucleus of Perlia. Since the reports of Knies (1891) and Brouwer (1918) most subsequent authors have regarded the nucleus of Perlia as a midline cell group concerned with convergence. According to Warwick (1955) this cell group was well developed in the midbrains of only 9 of 100 monkeys and was absent in 77 of this number. This same author usually was able to identify the nucleus of Perlia in the human and chimpanzee midbrains, but Tsuchida (1906) reported its absence in about 20 percent of human brains. Clark (1926) considered the so-called nucleus of Perlia to be absent or ill-defined in the tarsius and in monkeys despite their binocular vision, although a well developed central nucleus was found in the squirrel and tree shrew, animals not having binocular vision. According to Warwick (1956) cells of the central nucleus, when present in the monkey, were found to supply portions of the superior rectus muscle. Thus, both the existence and function of the so-called central nucleus of Perlia remain in doubt.

AFFERENT PATHWAYS TO THE NUCLEI OF THE EXTRAOCULAR MUSCLES

Afferent impulses to the nuclei of the extraocular muscles are thought to be conveyed directly or indirectly from the cerebral cortex, the cerebellum, and from certain nuclear masses and structures of the brain stem. Most of these pathways are poorly understood and it seems likely that important details are lacking even in those regarded as established.

Corticofugal fiber systems

A system of corticofugal fibers projecting to the motor nuclei of the cranial nerves is a long established concept in neurology. Fibers of this system are referred to as corticobulbar, but it is obvious in the light of recent developments that such fibers constitute a rather specialized group of corticofugal fibers (Truex and Carpenter, 1969). These fibers arise primarily from the precentral gyrus, descend in the internal capsule and basal portions of the brain stem, and constitute part of the upper motor neuron for certain motor cranial nerve nuclei. Most of the fibers regarded as "corticobulbar" in this restricted sense are distributed to cells of the brain stem reticular formation which in turn are thought to convey impulses to the motor cranial nerve nuclei. In the cat and rat it has not been possible to trace any corticofugal fibers to direct terminations in motor cranial nerve nuclei (Walberg, 1957; Kuypers, 1958; Zimmerman, Chambers and Liu, 1964). In man and primates this indirect system is supplemented by a relatively small number of direct corticobulbar fibers that terminate upon cells of the trigeminal, facial, hypoglossal, and supraspinal nuclei (Kuyper, 1958a). These observations suggest that cortical impulses to the nuclei of the extraocular muscles in rodents, carnivores, primates and man are conveyed by a phylogenetically old indirect system in which relays occur in the reticular formation. This hypothesis is supported by Golgi studies of the intrinsic organization of the reticular formation (Scheibel and Scheibel, 1958), which indicate that reticular neurons in the brain stem give rise to abundant collaterals projecting to both motor and sensory cranial nerve nuclei.

The fact that regions of the frontal and occipital cortex exert tonic effects upon conjugate deviation of the eyes has long suggested that cortical regions other than the motor cortex play an important role in conjugate eye movements. The so-called frontal eye field in man lies in the caudal part of the middle frontal gyrus (corresponding to parts of Brodmann's area 8) and extends into contiguous portions of the inferior frontal gyrus. The entire frontal eye field does not lie within a single recognized cytoarchitectonic area. Electrical stimulation of the frontal eye field in man produces strong conjugate deviation of the eyes, usually to the opposite side. The frontal fields are thought to be concerned with voluntary eye movements which are not dependent upon visual stimuli. The conjugate eye movements are commonly called "movements of command" since they can be elicited by instructing the subject to look to the right or left (Cogan, 1956). Studies in man and primates suggest a double representation of specific eye movements in each frontal eye field (Crosby, 1953; Lemmen, Davis and Radnor, 1959; Crosby, Humphrey and Lauer, 1962). These authors divide the frontal eye field into upper (frontal eye field I) and lower (frontal eye field II) parts which have a mirror image arrangement.

The concept of an occipital center for conjugate deviation of the eye is based upon the fact that stimulation of occipital cortex produces conjugate eye movements to the opposite side, and lesions of the occipital cortex are associated with transient deviation of the eyes to the side of the lesion. Unlike the frontal eye field, the occipital center for conjugate eye movements is not localized to a small part of this lobe, and eye responses can be obtained from a wide area. In the monkey the lowest threshold was found in area 17 about the calcarine sulcus (Walker and Weaver, 1940), but responses could be obtained from the parastriate (area 18) and the peristriate (area 19) cortex. The occipital centers for conjugate eye movements are assumed to subserve movements of the eyes induced by visual stimuli, such as following a moving object (Cogan, 1956). These pursuit movements of the eyes are considered to be largely involuntary, though they are not present in the young infant. The occipital eye centers, unlike the frontal eye fields, are interconnected on the two sides by fibers passing in the corpus callosum. Further, the threshold for excitation is higher in the occipital lobe than in the frontal eye field; the latency of the eye responses is longer, and eye movements tend to be smooth and less brisk.

The pathways by which responses from the frontal and occipital eye fields are mediated are not known, but it seems likely the superior colliculus is involved since both of these cortical areas give rise to particularly profuse projections to that structure. In a recent systematic study of cortical projections to the brain stem in the monkey, Kuypers and Lawrence (1967) described a particularly abundant projection to the superior colliculus and pretectum from a cortical lesion rostral to, and within, the concavity of the arcuate sulci (i.e., his monkey 1c; areas FDΔ and FDτ). The area ablated in this animal corresponded closely with area 8 according to the Brodmann nomenclature (1905). In the superior colliculus degenerated fibers terminated in the stratum griseum profundum, the stratum album intermedium and, especially, in the stratum griseum intermedium; fibers reached these layers via a transtegmental course. Fewer fibers were seen in the superior colliculus following other ablations of the frontal lobe. Lesions involving portions of the precentral and postcentral gyri produced little or no degeneration in the superior colliculus. Cortical areas, other than area 8, described as projecting a significant number of fibers to the superior colliculus, were in the temporal, occipital and caudal portions of the parietal lobes.

The most substantial and highly organized projection to the superior colliculus arises from the visual cortex (Altman, 1962; Garey, Jones and Powell, 1968). Fibers from the visual cortex reach the superior colliculus via the pretectum and brachium of the superior colliculus, mainly enter the stratum opticum, and pass into the ventral part of the stratum griseum superficiale and into the stratum griseum intermedium. Thus corticotectal fibers enter the superior colliculus by the same route as fibers from the retina and appear to terminate in the same layers. Whether these different afferent fibers terminate upon the same or different cells has not been determined, but the laminar distribution indicates a very close relationship (Garey, Jones and Powell, 1968). Although retinal and visual cortical projections to the superior colliculus are similar, these projections show certain important differences.

The retinal projection is bilateral and is greatest contralaterally; the cortical projection is strictly unilateral. Fibers from these two sources course through different levels within the stratum opticum; retinal fibers are superficial to cortical fibers. Small lesions suggest that at least areas 17 and 18 have independent projections to the superior colliculus. Observations in the cat (Garey, Jones and Powell, 1968) suggest that parts of the visual cortex and superior colliculus related to a particular region of the retina are interconnected. This relationship indicates that superior portions of the retina are represented anteriorly in the visual cortex and laterally in the superior colliculus, while inferior portions of the retina are represented posteriorly in the visual cortex and medially in the superior colliculus. Data have not been reported for lesions restricted to area 19, but it seems likely that this area also has an independent projection to the superior colliculus. These observations indicate that essentially the same cells of the superior colliculus receive two distinct but related inputs, one from the ganglion cells of the retina, and another of a more complex nature from the cortical cells of the visual cortex. Thus at one brain stem level there is the possibility of a potent interaction and integration of peripheral sensory impulses with the output from the complex activities of the visual cortex. Further there is evidence that the superior colliculus may receive peripheral and cortical impulses related to other sensory systems (Kuypers and Lawrence, 1967).

Superior Colliculus

The precise pathways by which impulses from the superior colliculus are conveyed to the nuclei of the extraocular muscles are unknown. Experimental studies based upon lesions restricted to the superior colliculus indicate that no efferent fibers from this structure project directly into the oculomotor complex or to the trochlear or abducens nuclei (Papez and Freeman, 1930; Rasmussen, 1936; Marburg and Warner, 1947; Szentágothai, 1950; Altman and Carpenter, 1961). Available data suggest that connections between the superior colliculus and the nuclei of the extraocular muscles probably are indirect and involve accessory oculomotor nuclei and/or the brain stem reticular formation. Lesions restricted to the superior colliculus produce bilateral degeneration in the nuclei of Darkschewitsch and the interstitial nucleus of Cajal (Altman and Carpenter, 1961), a finding which suggests that impulses from the superior colliculus may reach the oculomotor complex via these accessory nuclei. Fibers projecting to these nuclei on the opposite side appear to cross in the commissure of the superior colliculus (Fig. 4).

In addition the superior colliculus gives rise to an extensive system of tectoreticular fibers which in the mesencephalon are distributed bilaterally, but with homolateral preponderance. These fibers arise from deep layers of the superior colliculus and are distributed predominantly in dorsal regions of the reticular formation. In the pons and medulla tectoreticular fibers are exclusively crossed, pass caudally in the tectobulbar tract (predorsal bundle),

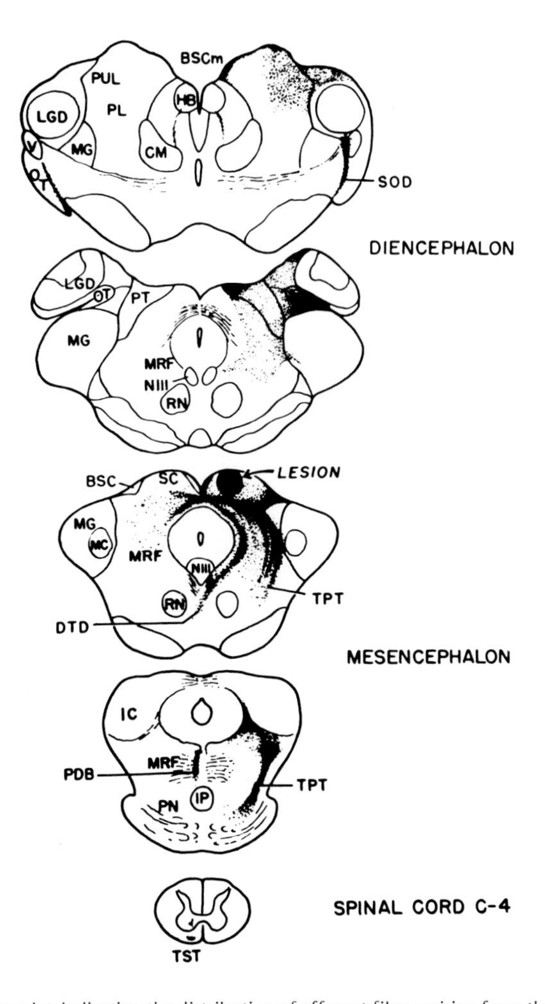

Fig. 4. Schematic drawing indicating the distribution of efferent fibers arising from the superior colliculus in the cat. The black area indicates the lesion and stippling indicates degenerated fibers. Abbreviations are: BSC, *brachium of the superior colliculus;* DTD, *dorsal tegmental decussation;* HB, *habenular nucleus;* IC, *inferior colliculus;* IP, *interpeduncular nucleus;* LGD, *lateral geniculate, dorsal part;* LGV, *lateral geniculate, ventral part;* MG, *medial geniculate;* MGMC, *medial geniculate, magnocellular part;* MRF, *midbrain reticular formation;* NIII, *nucleus of third nerve;* OT, *optic tract,* PDB, *predorsal bundle;* PL, *posterolateral nucleus;* PN, *pontine nuclei;* PT, *pretectum;* PUL, *pulvinar;* RN, *red nucleus;* SC, *superior colliculus;* SOD, *supraoptic decussation;* TPT, *tectopontine tract;* TST, *tectospinal tract.*

and give rise to modest terminations about reticular neurons in a paramedian location. It has been postulated (Jefferson, 1958) that tectoreticular fibers distributed to mesencephalic regions are involved in activation of broad areas of the cerebral cortex in response to visual stimuli. It also seems likely that neurons in the midbrain reticular formation may convey impulses to parts of the oculomotor complex. Golgi studies by the Scheibels (1958) indicate that reticular neurons project abundant collaterals to cranial nerve nuclei.

Cerebello-oculomotor fibers

In the older anatomical literature there are descriptions of cerebello-oculomotor fibers (Klimoff, 1896, 1899; Van Gehuchten, 1905; Wallenberg, 1905; Allen, 1924; Winkler, 1927; Sachs and Fincher, 1927; Gerebtzoff, 1936; 1941; Clark, 1936), which have been regarded as somewhat of a curiosity because few, if any cerebellar efferent fibers have been demonstrated to project directly to lower motor neurons. However, physiological studies have shown that electrical stimulation of certain regions of the cerebellum, especially the vermis, may produce conjugate deviation of the eyes toward the side stimulated. While it was recognized that these phenomena may involve primarily cerebellar efferent fiber systems projecting to the vestibular nuclei, it seemed worthwhile to explore the possibility of a direct cerebello-oculomotor system. A systematic study of cerebello-oculomotor fibers done several years ago in the rhesus monkey produced interesting findings (Carpenter and Strominger, 1964). This study confirmed the observations of earlier investigators, who used the Marchi method, that some cerebellar efferent fibers project to the contralateral somatic cell columns of the oculomotor complex. In the monkey cerebello-oculomotor fibers arise from the dentate nucleus, particularly ventral parts of this nucleus. These fibers enter ventral parts of the superior cerebellar peduncle, cross the midline in the caudal mesencephalon, and project to two distinctive subdivisions of the contralateral somatic cell columns of the oculomotor nucleus (Fig. 5). Fibers from both dorsal and ventral parts of the dentate nucleus project to the rostrolateral part of the dorsal nucleus of the oculomotor complex, a cell column which gives rise to uncrossed root fibers that innervate the inferior rectus muscle (Warwick, 1953a). The restricted oral part of the dorsal nucleus where these fibers end appears rostral to locations where most secondary vestibular fibers ascending in the MLF terminate. Cerebello-oculomotor fibers arising almost exclusively from ventral parts of the dentate nucleus, project to the medial nucleus of the oculomotor complex, a cell column which gives rise to root fibers that cross and innervate the contralateral superior rectus muscle. There is no evidence that efferent fibers from the fastigial or interposed nuclei project directly to the oculomotor nuclear complex.

Observations reported above suggest that certain cerebellar efferent fibers are organized to convey impulses directly to selected portions of the oculomotor complex. Anatomical evidence indicates that direct cerebellar influences upon eye movements may be confined to cell groups that innervate extraocular muscles whose prime functions involve eye movements in a vertical plane. Although most physiological studies (Hoshino, 1921; Mussen, 1927; Magoun, Hare and Ranson, 1937; Dow and Moruzzi, 1958) relate cerebellar stimulation to conjugate horizontal deviation of the eyes, Hare,

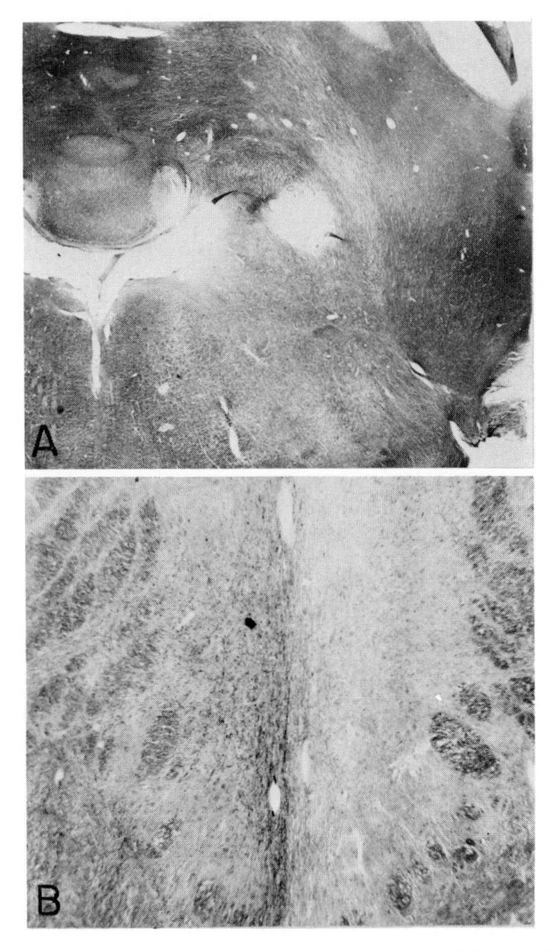

Fig. 5. Rhesus C-681. Photomicrographs of a lesion in the ventral part of the superior cerebellar peduncle (A) which produced degeneration in the contralateral medial nucleus of the oculomotor complex (B). Nauta-Gygax stain, X7, X32.

Magoun and Ranson (1937) commented that "the eyes have by far the most widespread representation in the hemisphere of the cerebellum of any part of the body." It seems probable that direct stimulation of the cerebellum excites or inhibits multiple neuronal pathways, so that resulting effects represent only a summation of complex effects. The fact that cerebello-oculomotor fibers appear to represent the only cerebellar projection which terminates directly upon cells of a lower motor neuron suggests that this unique pathway is one of major importance in the regulation of eye movements.

Vestibulo-oculomotor projections

Quantitatively the most important brain stem projections to the nuclei of the extraocular muscles arise from the vestibular nuclei. The labyrinths, the vestibular nuclei and secondary vestibular pathways projecting to the nuclei of the extraocular muscles play a major role in the control of conjugate eye movements. Physiological studies (Szentágothai, 1952; Fluur, 1959; Cohen, Suzuki and Bender, 1964) provide clear evidence of a precise functional correlation between particular semicircular canals and eye movements in specific directions. The investigations of Szentágothai (1950a) leave little doubt that the most important impulses mediating ocular movements in response to stimulation of the semicircular canals ascend in the medial longitudinal fasciculus (MLF). These results suggest that impulses from the individual semicircular canals ultimately must be transmitted differentially to all nuclei of the extraocular muscles, including specific subdivisions of the oculomotor complex.

A systematic study of secondary vestibular projections to the nuclei of the extraocular muscles was made recently in the rhesus monkey (McMasters, Weiss and Carpenter, 1966). Stereotaxic lesions were produced in individual vestibular nuclei and degeneration was studied in sections stained by the Nauta-Gygax (1954) technic. Lesions in the medial, inferior and superior vestibular nuclei were selective, but lesions in the lateral vestibular nuclei invariably involved portions of either the superior or inferior vestibular nuclei. Efferent fibers from the superior vestibular nucleus ascend exclusively in the lateral process of the ipsilateral MLF and project only to ipsilateral nuclei of the extraocular muscles. The major projections of the superior vestibular nucleus are to: (1) the trochlear nucleus, and (2) the dorsal nucleus of the oculomotor complex (Fig. 6). A relatively small number of fibers pass to the intermediate cell column of the oculomotor complex. These observations suggest that ascending fibers from the superior vestibular nucleus provide controlling influences for extraocular muscles involved primarily in vertical and rotatory eye movements. Physiological observations by Cohen, Suzuki and Bender (1964) suggest that secondary vestibular fibers arising from the superior vestibular nucleus may be concerned exclusively with inhibitory activities, since no excitatory influences were observed in the ipsilateral inferior oblique or the contralateral superior oblique muscles following stimulation of any of the semicircular canals. The superior vestibular nucleus is the only nucleus of the vestibular complex which gives rise to secondary vestibular fibers distributed in this manner.

Ascending secondary vestibular fibers from the medial vestibular nucleus project via the MLF bilaterally, asymmetrically and differentially to all nuclei of the extraocular muscles (Fig. 7). Particularly prominent among these projections are fibers to: (1) the contralateral trochlear nucleus, (2) the contralateral intermediate cell column of the oculomotor complex and (3) the ipsilateral ventral nucleus of the oculomotor complex. Fibers from this nucleus projecting to the abducens nucleus were distributed asymmetrically but were quantitatively similar.

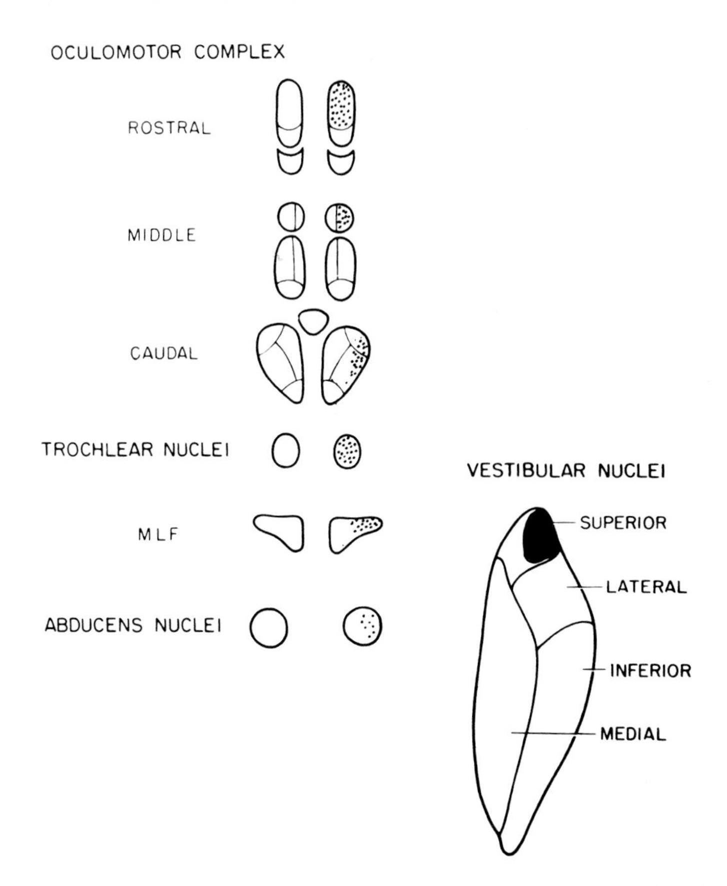

Fig. 6. Schematic diagram of degeneration in the nuclei of the extraocular muscles resulting from a lesion in the superior vestibular nucleus.

Ascending secondary vestibular fibers from the inferior vestibular nucleus appeared less numerous than those from other vestibular nuclei, arose mainly from the rostral third of the nucleus, and projected bilaterally to the abducens and oculomotor nuclei and to the contralateral trochlear nucleus. These findings suggested that the inferior vestibular nucleus and its ascending projections probably play a relatively minor role in the control of extraocular eye movements.

The lateral vestibular nucleus gives rise to ascending fibers in the MLF which are distributed primarily to: (1) the contralateral abducens and trochlear nuclei, and (2) asymmetrically to specific portions of the oculomotor complex bilaterally (Fig. 8). These secondary vestibular fibers arise only from ventral portions of the lateral vestibular nucleus, which receive primary vestibular fibers. The projection in the oculomotor complex is to: (1) the

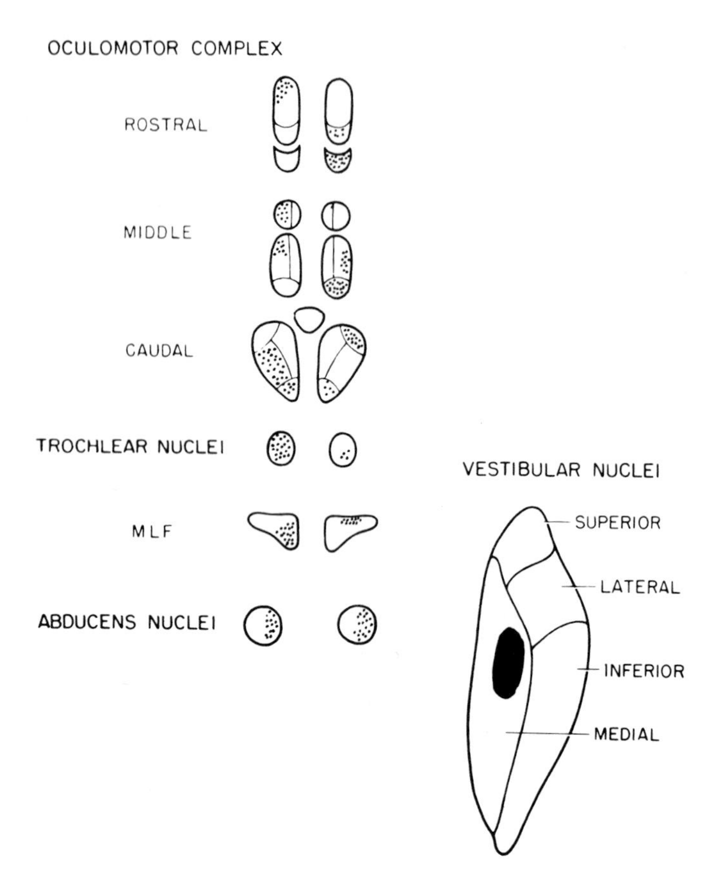

Fig. 7. Schematic diagram of degeneration in the nuclei of the extraocular muscles resulting from a lesion in the medial vestibular nucleus.

ipsilateral ventral and dorsal nuclei, and (2) the contralateral intermediate, medial and dorsal cell columns. The lateral vestibular nucleus appears unique in that it alone projects fibers to the medial cell column, a cell group which innervates the contralateral superior rectus muscle. The above pattern of degeneration within the nuclei of the extraocular muscles suggests that considerable overlap may exist in the projections of the medial and lateral vestibular nuclei. Part of this overlap conceivably might be due to concomitant interruption of efferent fibers from the lateral vestibular nucleus that traverse portions of the medial vestibular nucleus, but our observations indicate that most of the fibers from the lateral vestibular nucleus pass medially along the ventral border of the medial vestibular nucleus, an area not infringed upon by lesions in the medial vestibular nucleus. The second finding that mitigates against this possibility is the distinctive distribution of secondary vestibular

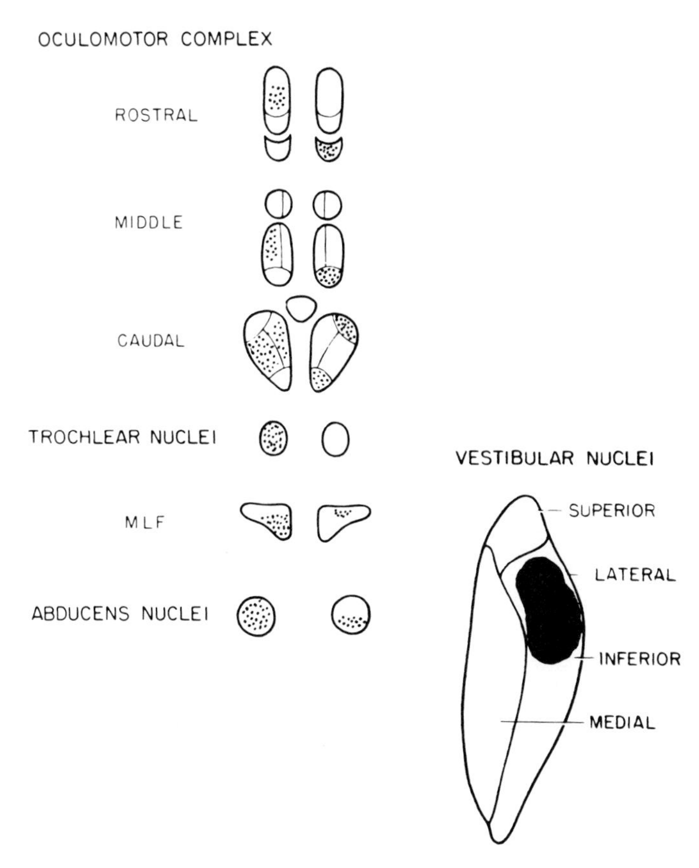

Fig. 8. Schematic diagram of degeneration in the nuclei of the extraocular muscles resulting from a lesion in the lateral vestibular nucleus that involved a small rostral part of the inferior vestibular nucleus.

fibers in the abducens and trochlear nuclei and in the medial cell column of the oculomotor complex.

Secondary vestibular fibers from the medial, lateral and superior vestibular nuclei also project fibers to the interstitial nucleus of Cajal; fibers to this nucleus from the medial and lateral vestibular nuclei are predominantly crossed, while those from the superior vestibular nucleus are uncrossed. It is of interest that no secondary vestibular fibers from any of the vestibular nuclei project to the caudal central nucleus, the visceral nuclei or to the ipsilateral medial nucleus of the oculomotor complex.

Vestibulo-oculomotor fibers arising from the medial and lateral vestibular nuclei appear capable of mediating most patterned eye movements obtained by stimulating the individual semicircular canals (Szentágothai, 1952), or the ampullary nerves (Cohen, Suzuki and Bender, 1964). In order to avoid overinterpretation of these data, only primary actions of the extraocular muscles will be considered. Since stimulation of the ampullary nerve from one horizontal canal produces conjugate horizontal deviation of the eyes to the opposite side, secondary vestibular fibers conveying excitatory impulses must reach the contralateral abducens nucleus and the ipsilateral ventral nucleus of the oculomotor complex. The only secondary vestibular fibers distributed in this manner arise from the medial and lateral vestibular nuclei.

Because stimulation of the ampullary nerve from the right posterior canal produces primary contractions in the right superior oblique and the left inferior rectus muscles, excitatory impulses must reach the contralateral trochlear nucleus, and dorsal nucleus of the oculomotor complex. Only secondary vestibular fibers arising from the medial and lateral vestibular nuclei are distributed to these contralateral nuclei.

Since stimulation of the ampullary nerve from the right anterior canal produces primary contractions of the right superior rectus muscle and the left inferior oblique muscle, excitatory impulses must reach the medial nucleus and the intermediate cell column on the left. Secondary vestibular fibers that could mediate these responses appear to originate only from the medial and lateral vestibular nuclei. Secondary vestibular fibers projecting to the contralateral intermediate cell column arise from both the medial and lateral vestibular nuclei, but only the lateral vestibular nucleus projects to the contralateral medial nucleus. While it seems likely that ascending fibers from secondary rostral portions of the inferior vestibular nucleus may be involved in some of the primary responses discussed above, the relative paucity of demonstrated fibers from this source makes it impossible to draw definite conclusions. Review of the presented findings suggests that secondary vestibular fibers from the medial and lateral vestibular nuclei to the nuclei of the extraocular muscles are most abundant to those nuclei innervating muscles whose primary functions concern horizontal and rotatory movements of the eyes.

Medial longitudinal fasciculus

The fact that lesions in the MLF produce dissociated horizontal eye movements (i.e., anterior internuclear ophthalmoplegia) suggests that ascending secondary vestibular fibers might play their most important role in mechanisms of conjugate horizontal gaze. Although this syndrome has been the subject of considerable study, both basic and clinical, many important questions remain unanswered. Experimental studies of discrete lesions of the MLF in the monkey (Carpenter and McMasters, 1963; Carpenter and Strominger, 1965) have revealed certain important findings. The syndrome of anterior internuclear ophthalmoplegia results from lesions in the MLF rostral to the abducens nuclei. It may also occur with lesions which interrupt the most medial fibers of the MLF at the level of the abducens nucleus

(Fig. 10, a and b), but it does not result from lesions of the MLF in the vicinity of the trochlear nucleus. Unilateral lesions of the MLF rostral to the abducens nucleus produce: (1) paresis of ipsilateral ocular adduction on attempted lateral gaze to the opposite side, and (2) monocular horizontal nystagmus in the abducting eye (Fig. 9, a and b). Convergence is not impaired, but bilateral transient vertical or rotatory nystagmus may occur. Paresis of ocular adduction resulting from lesions in the MLF in the monkey is enduring and is invariably associated with ascending degeneration in the MLF,

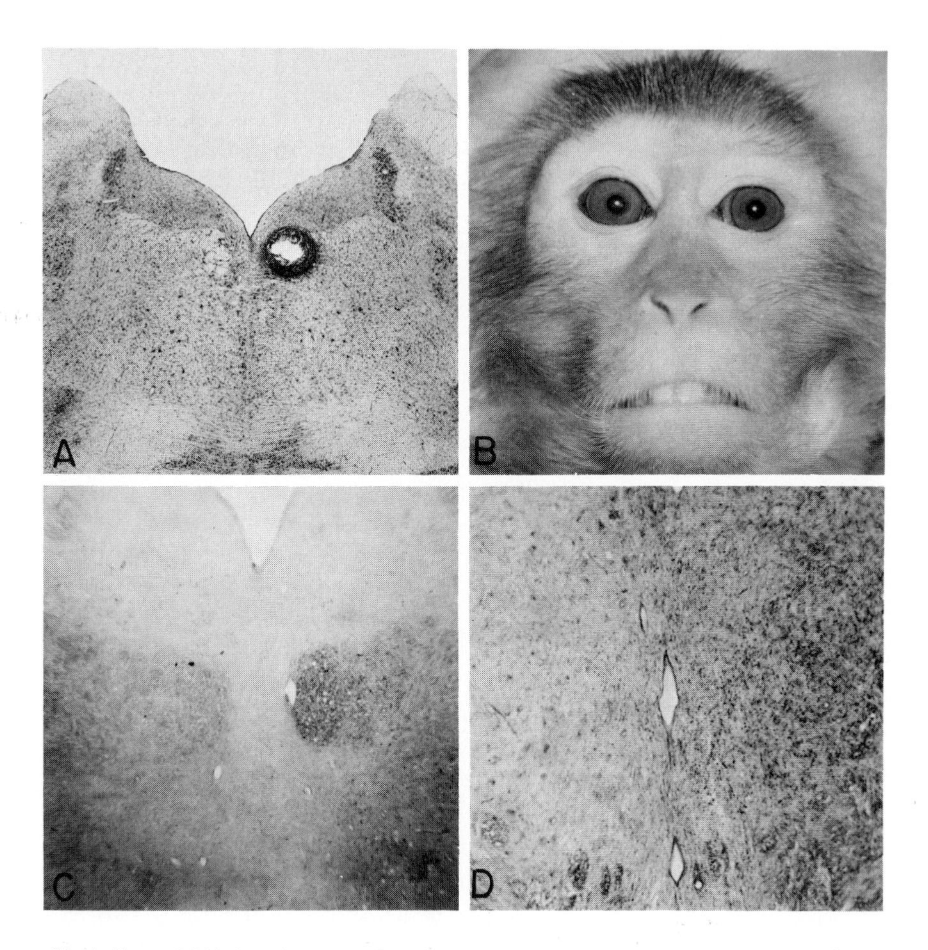

Fig. 9. Rhesus C-762. A, A discrete lesion in the right MLF rostral to the abducens nucleus. Cresyl violet stain, X7. B, Photograph of animal showing paresis of right ocular adduction on attempted left lateral gaze. C and D, Photomicrographs of degeneration confined to the right MLF (C) distributed differentially to the ventral nucleus of the oculomotor complex on the right (D). Nauta-Gygax stain, X30, X80.

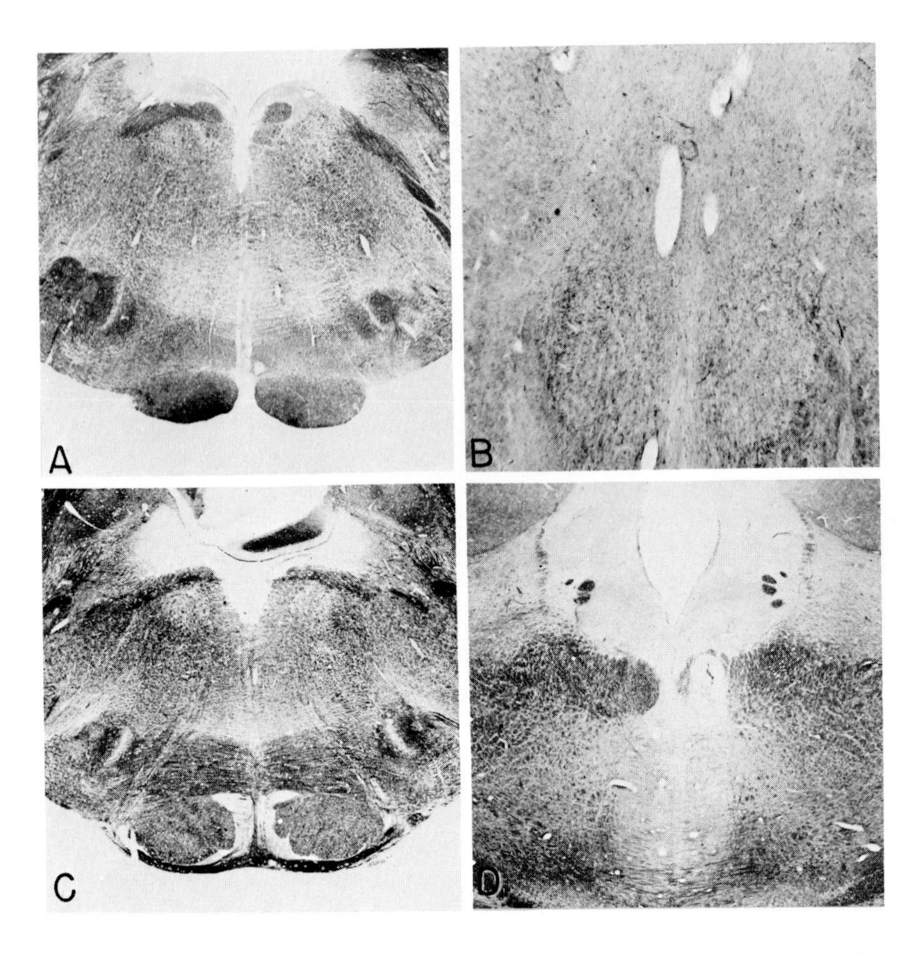

Fig. 10. A and B, Rhesus C-618. A discrete lesion involving only the most medial fibers of the MLF bilaterally at the level of the abducens nuclei (**A**), which produced bilateral paresis of ocular adduction on attempted lateral gaze to both the right and left, and degeneration terminating preferentially in the ventral nuclei of the oculomotor complex. Weil stain, X6; Nauta-Gygax stain, X30. C, Rhesus C-629. Bilateral destruction of the MLF at the level of the abducens nuclei which produced bilateral paresis of conjugate horizontal eye movements. D, Rhesus C-626. Unilateral lesion of the MLF caudal to the trochlear nucleus which did not impair conjugate horizontal eye movements. Weil stain, X6, X8.

which projects selectively upon cells of the ventral nucleus of the oculomotor complex on the same side as the paresis of ocular adduction (Fig. 9, c and d). With unilateral lesions in the MLF rostral to the abducens nucleus no degeneration is seen in the opposite MLF, or in any of the nuclei of the extraocular muscles contralaterally. The monocular horizontal nystagmus in the contralateral abducting eye was thought to be due to interruption of descending fibers in the MLF, possibly from the interstitial nucleus of Cajal, that project to the ipsilateral medial vestibular nucleus (Pompeiano and Walberg, 1957; Carpenter and Strominger, 1965). This hypothesis no longer seems tenable since discrete lesions in the interstitial nucleus do not produce contralateral monocular horizontal nystagmus, or nystagmus of any detectable kind.

One of the puzzling findings (Carpenter and McMasters, 1963) was that discrete lesions of the MLF near the trochlear nucleus did not produce detectable dissociation of horizontal eye movements or nystagmus (Fig. 10, d). Since no fibers of the MLF cross to the opposite side except in the immediate vicinity of the abducens nucleus, it is curious that MLF lesions near the trochlear nucleus do not produce the same syndrome as lesions in this bundle at more caudal levels. Anatomical findings associated with unilateral lesions of the MLF at the trochlear level reveal one important difference, namely that degeneration passing into the oculomotor complex projects to all somatic cell columns on the side of the lesion. Thus the degeneration in the oculomotor nuclear complex resulting from MLF lesions near the trochlear nucleus is not differentially or selectively distributed to the ventral cell column, as with lesions in the MLF at more caudal levels. It is important that degeneration resulting from unilateral MLF lesions at the trochlear level is strictly confined to somatic cell columns of the oculomotor complex on the side of the lesion and that no contralateral degeneration is seen.

One variant of the MLF syndrome produced in the monkey is of interest (Carpenter and McMasters, 1963). Relatively large bilateral lesions of the MLF at levels of the abducens nuclei produce virtually complete paresis of both ocular adduction and abduction (Fig. 10, c). These animals gaze straight ahead and show no lateral eye movements. They show what we have called a reptilian stare. Eye movements in a vertical plane are normal, and convergence is preserved. The paresis of ocular abduction does not seem to be as profound as the paresis of ocular adduction. No nystagmus was seen in these animals. This particular syndrome appears to be a combined anterior and posterior internuclear ophthalmoplegia, because no part of the abducens nuclei was involved by the lesion. Clinically posterior internuclear ophthalmoplegia is virtually impossible to distinguish from abducens nerve palsies. Experimental evidence suggests that posterior internuclear ophthalmoplegia is unlikely to occur as an isolated phenomenon. Degeneration resulting from lesions of the MLF between the abducens nuclei was confined to the MLF and the nuclei of the extraocular muscles. Degeneration was profuse bilaterally in the abducens nuclei, but no root fibers were degenerated. In the oculomotor complex degeneration was present bilaterally in the lateral somatic cell columns with the greatest concentration in the ventral nuclei.

Anatomical evidence (Carpenter, McMasters and Hanna, 1963) suggests an interrelationship between anterior internuclear ophthalmoplegia and lateral gaze paralysis. In the monkey localized lesions of the abducens nucleus produce paralysis of ipsilateral conjugate horizontal gaze in which both eyes are forcefully and persistently directed to the side opposite the lesion. Ocular convergence is not impaired and monocular horizontal nystagmus is sometimes seen. Ascending degeneration resulting from unilateral lesions in the abducens nucleus is primarily confined to the medial longitudinal fasciculi and is most profuse contralateral to the lesion. In the oculomotor complex terminal degeneration is most profuse in the contralateral ventral nucleus, the group which innervates the medial rectus muscle on that side. Thus, this syndrome seems to consist of two elements: (1) a lower motor neuron lesion of the abducens nucleus and (2) a lesion involving an internuclear fiber system. It is notable that the pareses of ocular adduction seen in this syndrome and in anterior internuclear ophthalmoplegia are both associated with ascending degeneration in the MLF which projects preferentially to the ventral nucleus of the oculomotor complex. This important feature of these syndromes differs only in that the paresis of ocular adduction occurs contralateral to lesions in the abducens nucleus and ipsilateral to lesions restricted to the MLF. This observation suggests that the same ascending system might be involved in both syndromes, but at different locations. In lateral gaze paralysis these fibers are interrupted prior to crossing to the opposite MLF; in the MLF syndrome the fibers are interrupted after they have decussated. These findings confirm other observations which indicate that virtually all ascending fibers of the MLF which decussate do so in the immediate vicinity of the abducens nucleus. Since most of the ascending fibers in the MLF rostral to the abducens nucleus are of vestibular origin, it initially was assumed that interruption of secondary vestibular fibers traversing the abducens nucleus and entering the opposite MLF accounted for the paresis of ocular adduction seen in these related syndromes. The fact that no lesion limited to a recognized subdivision of the vestibular nuclear complex produced paresis of contralateral ocular adduction (McMasters, Weiss and Carpenter, 1966) causes us to doubt this explanation. Further this doubt seemed to be supported by anatomical findings that no lesion in an individual vestibular nucleus produced ascending degeneration in the contralateral MLF which terminated profusely and selectively in the opposite ventral nucleus of the oculomotor complex. For these reasons it remains doubtful that the paresis of ocular adduction seen in anterior internuclear ophthalmoplegia and in paralysis of lateral gaze is a consequence of interruption of only ascending secondary vestibular fibers.

Accessory oculomotor nuclei

One of the so-called accessory oculomotor nuclei, the interstitial nucleus of Cajal, is considered to serve as a coordinating center for the control of rotatory movements of the head in a frontal plane and conjugate vertical and rotatory eye movements (Szentágothai, 1943, 1952; Hassler and Hess, 1954; Hyde and Eliasson, 1957; Hyde and Eason, 1959; Hyde and Toczek, 1962). Electrical stimulation in the region of the interstitial nucleus in unanesthetized (implanted electrodes or encéphale isolé preparations) and anesthetized animals evokes rotation of the head to the side stimulated and ocular torsion with contralateral and upward deviation of the eyes. Although eye movements are conjugate, the direction of ocular torsion is not constant; in many instances the ipsilateral eye turns in and the contralateral eye turns out, but the opposite also occurs (Szentágothai, 1943). According to Hyde and Eason (1959), ocular torsion in the cat averages about 20 degrees from the vertical.

Recently elegant physiological studies (Markham, Precht and Shimazu, 1966) have provided data concerning relationships of the interstitial nucleus to vestibular unit activity. These authors reported that stimulation of the interstitial nucleus produced: (1) ipsilateral inhibition of type I vestibular neurons, and (2) ipsilateral transynaptic activation of type II vestibular neurons. Type I vestibular neurons increase their resting discharge rate in response to angular acceleration in the direction of the recording side (i.e., ipsilateral rotation), while contralteral type I vestibular neurons decrease their discharge rate to this stimulus. Type II vestibular neurons behave in a reciprocal fashion to those of type I. Anatomical studies (Pompeiano and Walberg, 1957) have demonstrated that fibers from the interstitial nucleus project via the ipsilateral MLF to caudal portions of the medial vestibular nucleus. No other midbrain structures are known to project fibers to the vestibular complex. These investigations suggest that the interstitial nucleus preferentially inhibits ipsilateral type I vestibular neurons functionally related to the horizontal semicircular canal. Subsequent study of this question (Markham, 1968) confirmed the above observations and indicated that type I vestibular neurons related to the anterior semicircular canal show a less frequent and weaker inhibition in response to stimulation of the interstitial nucleus. These data have been interpreted as supporting the role of the interstitial nucleus in the performance of vertical and rotatory eye movements, in that descending impulses preferentially exert their strongest inhibitory drives upon vestibular neurons related to the horizontal semicircular canal. Thus, the suppression of horizontal eye movements would seem to facilitate vertical and rotatory eye movements.

The experiments of Szentágothai and Schab (1956) indicated that stimulation in the region of the central gray anterior to the aqueduct produced a marked exophthalmos and retractions of the nictitating membrane during the stimulation. The exophthalmos was reported to be more pronounced than that seen after stimulation of the cervical sympathetic trunk and could be elicited after transection of the sympathetic trunk. The protrusion of the eye during these experiments was thought to be due to inhibitory influences resulting from stimulation of the nucleus of Darkschewitsch. It was further demonstrated that stimulation in the region of the nucleus of Darkschewitsch completely inhibited normal labyrinthine reflexes. Because these authors found no degeneration in the oculomotor nucleus after lesions in the nucleus of Darkschewitsch, it was concluded that inhibitory influences from this nucleus must be conveyed to the oculomotor nucleus via intercalated neurons.

While the mechanism of this oculomotor inhibition remains unexplained, other authors (Scheibel, Markham and Koegler, 1961) have reported confirmatory evidence. These authors demonstrated that stimulation of the nucleus of Darkschewitsch produced: (1) slight protrusion of the eye, and (2) inhibition of physiologically produced nystagmus.

Nonvestibular afferent projections to the interstitial nucleus and the nucleus of Darkschewitsch are poorly understood, although fibers from a number of sources have been described. (See superior colliculus.) Cortical afferents to these nuclei have been described as originating from frontal (Szentágothai, 1943; Szentágothai and Rajkovits, 1958; Kuypers and Lawrence, 1967) and striate cortex (Mettler, 1935; Woodburne, Crosby and McCotter, 1946). According to Szentágothai and Rajkovits (1958), direct ipsilateral fibers from the motor cortex project to both the interstitial nucleus and the nucleus of Darkschewitsch in the cat. Studies in the monkey (Kuypers and Lawrence, 1967) indicated a significant projection from the precentral gyrus to the ipsilateral nucleus of Darkschewitsch. Frontal cortex rostral to the motor area projected a modest number of fibers to the ipsilateral interstitial nucleus, the nucleus of Darkschewitsch, and the nucleus of the posterior commissure. These authors found no corticofugal fibers projecting to these nuclei from temporal or occipital cortex. Pompeiano and Walberg (1957) found no projections to these nuclei from the cerebral cortex in the cat. In view of these observations based upon silver degeneration technics, it is difficult to explain projections to these nuclei from the striate cortex described by investigators who used the Marchi method.

Studies of cerebello-oculomotor fibers in the monkey (Carpenter and Strominger, 1964) suggest that a modest number of fibers from the dentate nucleus project to the contralateral accessory oculomotor nuclei.

It has been suggested (Muskens, 1914; Vogt and Vogt, 1919, 1920; Woodburne, Crosby and McCotter, 1946; Johnson and Clemente, 1959) that pallidofugal fibers may project to the interstitial nucleus. Recent more complete studies (Nauta and Mehler, 1966; Carpenter and Strominger, 1967) have failed to confirm this as a direct connection. These same investigations furnish no evidence that pallidofugal fibers terminate in the zona incerta. Physiological studies (Hassler and Hess, 1954; Hyde and Toczek, 1962) indicate that ocular torsion and head rotation, similar to that obtained from the interstitial nucleus, result from stimulation of the zona incerta. According to Hyde and Toczek (1962), ocular torsion resulting from stimulation of the interstitial nucleus is not abolished after lesions in the zona incerta, but lesions in the interstitial nucleus blocked ocular torsion obtained by stimulating the zona incerta. These data have been offered in support of the thesis that the zona incerta provides afferent fibers to the interstitial nucleus.

Recently attempts have been made to produce localized lesions in the interstitial nucleus, the nucleus of Darkschewitsch, and the posterior commissure in the monkey to determine the physiological effects of such lesions and to study the efferent projections of these nuclei. Electrodes were introduced into the cerebral hemispheres at an angle roughly perpendicular to the longitudinal axis of the brain stem. Because electrodes traverse medial regions of the thalamus, it was impossible to evaluate ascending degeneration, but this approach seemed to permit the best evaluation of degeneration in the midbrain and lower brain stem. The fact that the rostral part of the nucleus of Darkschewitsch curves downward in front of the interstitial nucleus (i.e., near the fasciculus retroflexus) made it extremely difficult to produce isolated lesions in the interstitial nucleus. Degeneration resulting from these lesions was studied by the Nauta and Gygax technic (1954).

Lesions in the interstitial nucleus of Cajal

Lesions in three monkeys destroyed significant portions of the interstitial nucleus rather selectively (Fig. 11). In one animal (C-1099) the lesion began in the oral pole of the nucleus of Darkschewitsch medial to the fasciculus retroflexus and passed ventrocaudally into the interstitial nucleus at the level of the posterior commissure. The lesion extended caudally in this nucleus to levels where the somatic cell columns of the oculomotor nucleus complex were first fully developed. Because the lesion involved primarily lateral portions of the interstitial nucleus, no part of the oculomotor nuclear complex was destroyed and direct injury to the MLF was minimal. Degeneration from this lesion was followed dorsally, around, and in, the lateral part of the central gray, into the ventral part of the posterior commissure (Fig. 12, a). Fibers crossing in the posterior commissure descended close to, but outside of, the central gray to enter the contralateral interstitial nucleus (Fig. 12, b). Moderate degeneration was seen in the ipsilateral nucleus of Darkschewitsch, but contralaterally this nucleus was free of degeneration except for a few fibers in extremely rostral portions. From the interstitial nucleus on both sides degenerated fibers entered the oculomotor complex and were distributed in a differential manner (Figs. 12, c and d). These fibers were distributed bilaterally and nearly symmetrically to parts of all of the lateral somatic cell columns, except for the ventral nuclei, cell groups which provide innervation for the medial recti muscles. In caudal portions of the oculomotor complex degeneration in the dorsal nuclei, cell groups which innervate the inferior recti muscles, greatly diminished and disappeared. Terminal degeneration present in the intermediate cell columns and in the medial nuclei extended the entire length of the oculomotor complex bilaterally. Degeneration passing to the visceral nuclei of the oculomotor complex was very sparse. The caudal central nucleus was virtually free of degenerated fibers.

At mesencephalic levels small amounts of degeneration were seen ipsilaterally in the nuclei of the posterior commissure, and the pretectal area. The rostral part of the superior colliculus was free of degeneration. Caudal portions of the ipsilateral superior colliculus contained degenerated fibers in the middle and deep gray and white strata which appeared to enter these

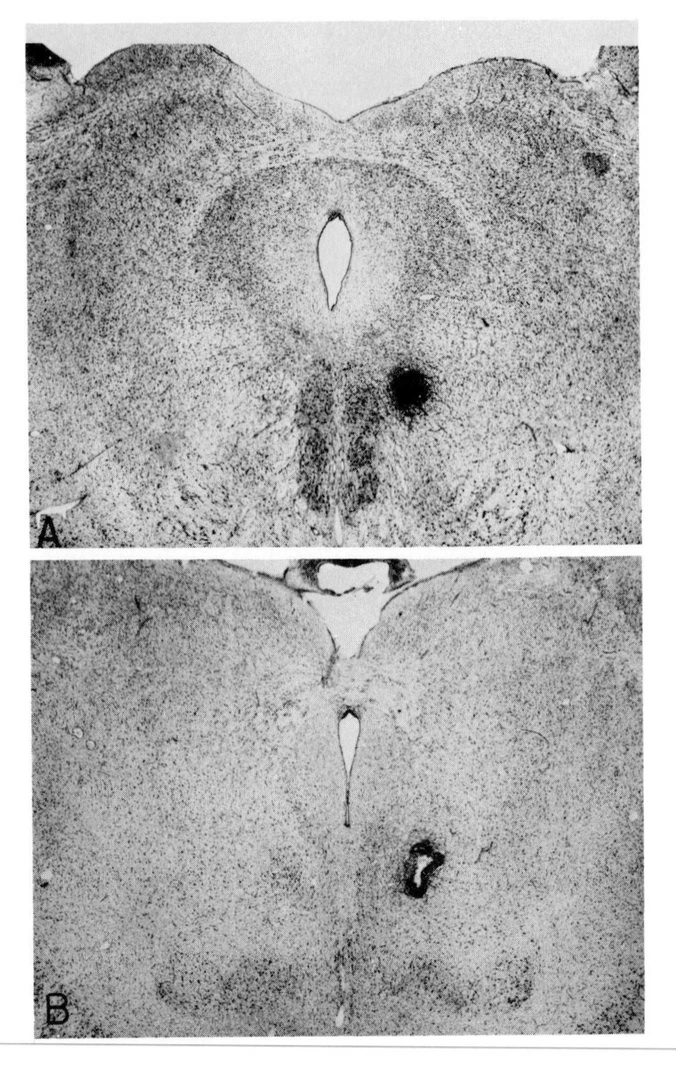

Fig. 11. Photomicrographs of lesions in the interstitial nucleus of Cajal. A, Rhesus C-1096, B, Rhesus C-1099. Cresyl violet stain, X8, X8.

layers from the lateral part of the central gray. No degeneration was seen in the stratum opticum, stratum cinereum or the stratum zonale. No degeneration was seen in the opposite superior colliculus or in the inferior colliculi.

Through caudal parts of the oculomotor complex degeneration was seen bilaterally in the MLF and in the ipsilateral central tegmental tract. Degeneration in the ipsilateral MLF was greatest in dorsal regions but

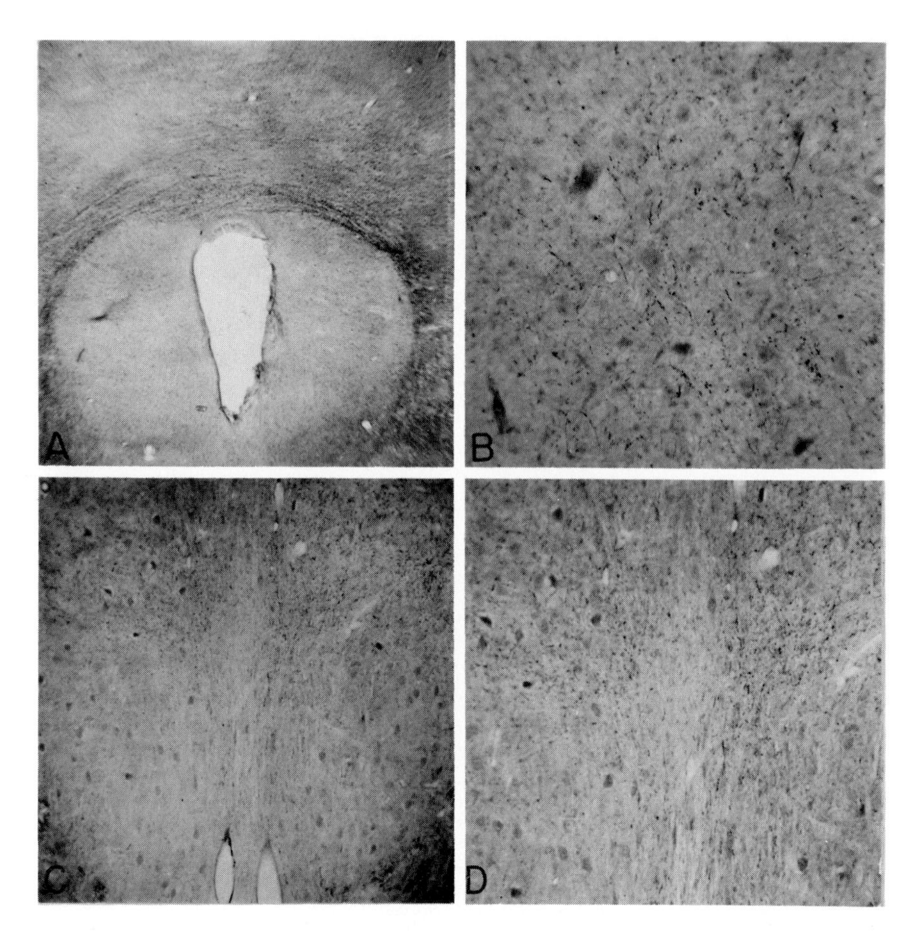

Fig. 12. **A, C,** and **D,** Rhesus C-1096. **A,** Degenerated fibers crossing in the ventral part of the posterior commissure. **C** and **D,** Degenerated fibers in portions of the medial nucleus and the intermediate cell column of the oculomotor complex bilaterally associated with virtually no degeneration in the ventral nuclei. **B,** Rhesus C-1099. Degenerated fibers traversing the contralateral interstitial nucleus. Nauta-Gygax stain, X22, X133, X52, X65.

extended along the entire medial border of this bundle; on the opposite side degenerated fibers occupied only a small dorsal area in the fasciculus. On both sides descending fibers projected into the trochlear nuclei and closely surrounded individual cells. Degeneration was most profuse on the side of the lesion.

Caudal to the trochlear nuclei degeneration was seen only in the dorsomedial part of the ipsilateral MLF and in the ipsilateral central tegmental tract. Degeneration in the ipsilateral MLF was most concentrated dorsally but was seen along the entire medial border of the bundle. At levels near the abducens nucleus degenerated fibers from the MLF migrated laterally towards the medial vestibular nucleus, and ventrally into the reticular formation. Degeneration within the ipsilateral medial vestibular nucleus was modest in amount and primarily localized to parts of the nucleus medial to the inferior vestibular nucleus. No terminal degeneration was found in the abducens nucleus. Terminal degeneration considered to arise from the interstitial nucleus was found ipsilaterally in: (1) the dorsal paramedian reticular nuclei, (2) the nucleus prepositus, and (3) the nucleus of Roller. Although descending degenerated fibers in the MLF projected to the medial accessory olivary nucleus, other evidence raised doubts concerning the origin of these fibers. Degenerated fibers of the interstitiospinal tract were traced in the anterior funiculus of the spinal cord to lumbar levels.

The descending degeneration in the central tegmental tract followed its classic course through the reticular formation. Some fibers of this tract coursed through, and perhaps terminated in, the pedunculopontine nucleus, but the largest group of fibers terminated in the ventral lamella of the principal olivary nucleus. A small number of fibers, appearing to descend with the central tegmental tract, entered the ipsilateral facial nucleus. These fibers were found in rostral parts of the facial nucleus where they were localized about cells of the dorsomedial and intermediate cell groups (Courville, 1966).

In two other animals (C-1091 and C-1096) with similar lesions findings were essentially the same, except for the presence of degeneration in the visceral nuclei and in rostral portions of the caudal central nucleus.

Observations and examination of these animals revealed differences which could be attributed to differences in the extent and location of the lesions. Two animals with lesions virtually restricted to the interstitial nucleus, displayed head tilt to the opposite side. In one of these animals (C-1099) head tilt was transient, lasting 5 days; head tilt in the other animal (C-1091) was more persistent but underwent attenuation. No disturbances of conjugate eye movements in any plane were seen in these animals. There was no nystagmus, disturbance of eyelid function, or impairment of convergence.

In rhesus C-1096 the lesion concomitantly involved a portion of the nucleus of Darkschewitsch. This animal exhibited marked head tilt to the opposite side for 6 days, but in addition showed mild bilateral lid retraction, impairment of upward gaze, and had a peculiar stare. The eyes were directed slightly downward most of the time. Eye movements in a horizontal plane were normal, as was convergence. No nystagmus was seen. Caloric responses to ice water produced normal horizontal nystagmus in all of these animals.

Lesions involving the nucleus of Darkschewitsch

Lesions in two monkeys (C-1095 and C-1102) selectively destroyed dorsal portions of the nucleus of Darkschewitsch without destroying any part of the interstitial nucleus, the MLF or the oculomotor complex (Fig. 13, a).

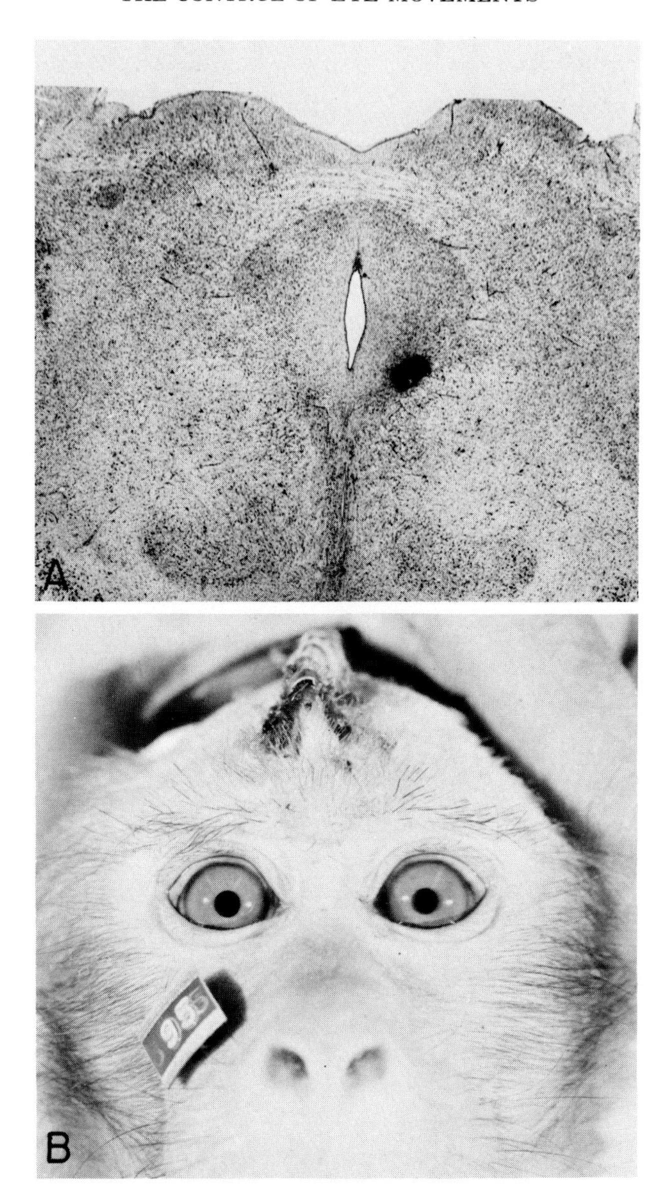

Fig. 13. Rhesus C-1095. A, Photomicrograph of lesion destroying the dorsal part of the nucleus of Darkschewitsch. Cresyl violet stain, X8. B, Photograph showing bilateral eyelid retraction and moderate downward deviation of the eyes. This animal also had limitations of vertical eye movements.

However, both of these lesions destroyed portions of the lateral central gray and fiber systems entering and leaving the posterior commissure.

Degeneration resulting from these lesions was similar. Dorsally projecting fibers crossed in the ventral part of the posterior commissure and passed to the contralateral interstitial nucleus. Only sparse degeneration was seen in the contralateral nucleus of Darkschewitsch. Degeneration in the ipsilateral interstitial nucleus was profuse. On both sides fibers entered the oculomotor complex via the interstitial nucleus. Degeneration in the oculomotor complex was not symmetrical and was less profuse than that associated with lesions of the interstitial nucleus. The ventral nucleus was free of degeneration bilaterally. The most consistent degeneration was seen in the intermediate cell column and in the medial nucleus. Although some parts of the dorsal nuclei contained degenerated fibers, the amount of degeneration in these nuclei in some sections was relatively modest. Degeneration in the visceral nuclei was moderate in one animal and scant in the other. Relatively scant degeneration was present in rostral parts of the caudal central nucleus. Bilateral degeneration was seen in the trochlear nuclei. Degeneration in the ipsilateral pretectum and caudal parts of the superior colliculus was similar to that described for lesions in the interstitial nucleus.

In sections of the brain stem caudal to the trochlear nuclei very scant degeneration was present in the dorsomedial part of the MLF. Most of these fibers appeared to project to portions of the medial accessory olive. No degeneration was seen in the abducens nucleus, the medial vestibular nuclei, the perihypoglossal nuclei, or the paramedian reticular nuclei, and no degenerated fibers projected to spinal levels.

Both of these animals exhibited lid retraction, impairment of upward eye movements, and one animal showed lid lag on downward gaze (Fig. 13, b). Horizontal eye movements were normal, as was ocular convergence. Neither animal had head tilt. Caloric stimulation produced normal horizontal nystagmus.

Lesions of the posterior commissure

Bilateral lesions interrupting ventrally crossing fibers in the posterior commissure in one animal (C-1112), produced a syndrome similar to that described in association with unilateral lesions involving the nucleus of Darkschewitsch (Fig. 14). The syndrome differed from that described above only in that convergence nystagmus was easily demonstrated and small amplitude vertical nystagmus (rapid phase down) also was seen. Optokinetic nystagmus could be elicited in vertical and horizontal planes. Degeneration resulting from these lesions was similar to that already described in that it was present bilaterally in the pretectum, the nuclei of the posterior commissure, and in the nuclei of Darkschewitsch and Cajal. In the oculomotor complex symmetrical degeneration was present throughout the lateral somatic cell columns, except for the ventral nuclei which contained no degeneration. Cells of the visceral nuclei were closely surrounded by terminal degenerated fibers throughout their extent. Rostral parts of the caudal central nucleus

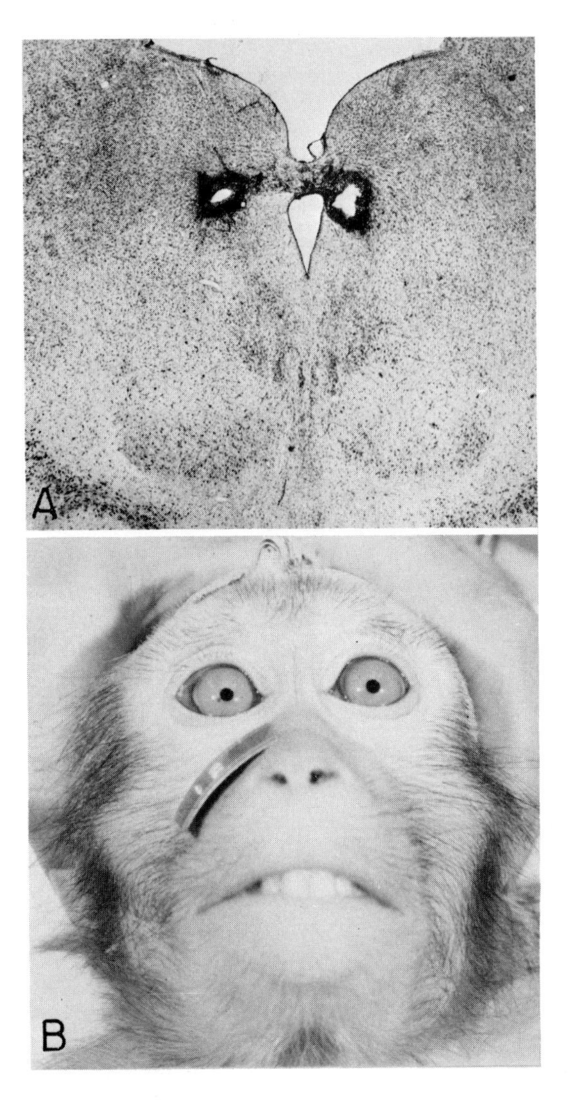

Fig. 14. Rhesus C-1112. **A,** Photomicrograph of bilateral lesions interrupting fibers crossing in the posterior commissure. Cresyl violet stain, X8. **B,** Photograph showing bilateral eyelid retraction and slight downward deviation of the eyes. This animal had restriction of vertical eye movements and convergence nystagmus.

contained moderate numbers of degenerated fibers, part of which seemed to be fibers of passage *en route* to the medial visceral cell columns. Degeneration was seen bilaterally and equally in the trochlear nuclei. Bilateral degeneration was seen in the middle and deep gray and white strata of the caudal parts of the superior colliculus. One additional finding not seen with other lesions was degeneration which projected bilaterally to the peripendicular nuclei. These fibers would appear to constitute, at least, a part of the so-called pretectal-tegmental tract (Bucher and Bürgi, 1952). None of these fibers could be traced into the substantia nigra, as reported by some authors (Tsai, 1925; Clark, 1932). Although a few fibers were degenerated bilaterally in the midbrain reticular formation, none of these appeared to descend to lower brain stem levels. No degeneration was seen in the MLF caudal to the trochlear nucleus. Sections of the pons, medulla and spinal cord revealed no degeneration.

These incomplete studies provide certain data concerning some of the efferent projections of the so-called accessory oculomotor nuclei. Discrete unilateral lesions of the interstitial nucleus produce bilateral, symmetrical and differential degeneration within the oculomotor complex, and bilateral degeneration in the trochlear nuclei, as reported by Szentágothai (1943). Fibers projecting to the oculomotor complex appear to be predominantly crossed. This suggestion is supported by the finding that a unilateral lesion in the interstitial nucleus, not involving the MLF, produces nearly symmetrical bilateral degeneration in specific parts of the oculomotor complex. A unilateral lesion in the interstitial nucleus destroys: (1) cells giving rise to fibers which cross to the opposite side via the posterior commissure, and (2) fibers from the contralateral interstitial nucleus in passage to subdivisions of the oculomotor complex on the side of the lesion. Because fibers arising in one interstitial nucleus cross in the ventral part of the posterior commissure and traverse the opposite interstitial nucleus, it is difficult to determine the proportion of uncrossed interstitio-oculomotor fibers, but their number would appear to be small. Thus, predominantly crossed interstitio-oculomotor fibers are distributed: (1) most profusely to the intermediate and medial cell columns, and (2) to rostral portions of the dorsal cell column. The projections to the caudal central and visceral nuclei are sparse and no fibers pass to the ventral cell column (Fig. 15). The interstitial nucleus does not project to the contralateral nucleus of Darkschewitsch.

Available evidence suggests that the interstitial nucleus projects fibers bilaterally to the trochlear nuclei. Following a unilateral lesion of the interstitial nucleus, degeneration is greatest in the ipsilateral trochlear nucleus, because this nucleus receives both crossed and uncrossed fibers. Ipsilateral fibers descend in the medial and dorsal parts of the MLF, while crossed fibers descend in the dorsolateral part of the MLF. Fibers descending in the contralateral MLF cross in the ventral part of the posterior commissure.

Fibers projecting caudally from the interstitial nucleus descend in the dorsomedial part of the MLF and project ipsilaterally to: (1) caudal portions of the medial vestibular nucleus, (2) the nucleus prepositus and the nucleus of Roller, and (3) the dorsal paramedian reticular nucleus of the medulla. Fibers of the interstitiospinal tract are uncrossed and descend at least to

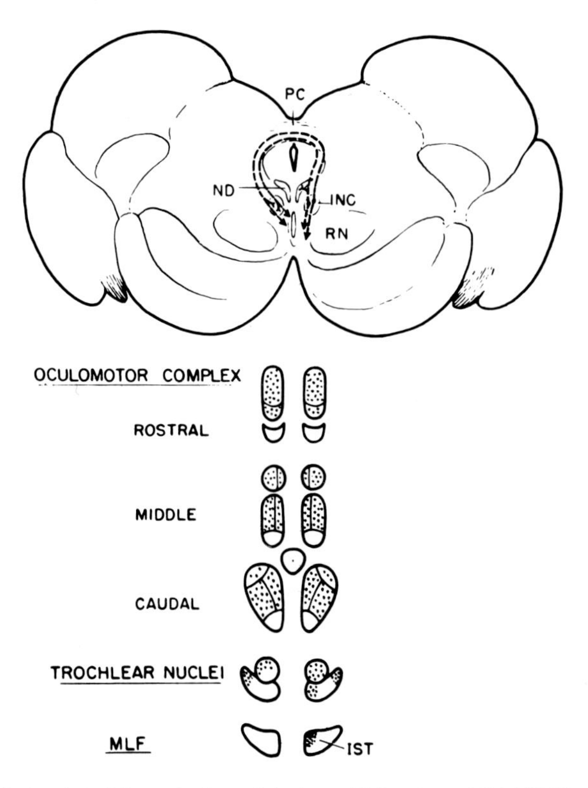

Fig. 15. Schematic drawing of the projections of the interstitial nucleus of Cajal (INC) to the oculomotor and trochlear nuclei. A lesion in the right interstitial nucleus produces degeneration which crosses in the ventral part of the posterior commissure (PC), passes ventrally outside of the central gray and traverses the contralateral INC *en route* to the oculomotor complex. In the oculomotor complex degeneration is bilateral in all somatic cell columns, except for the ventral nucleus. Degeneration is relatively less in caudal parts of the dorsal nucleus. Fibers descending in the lateral parts of the MLF project to the trochlear nuclei. Fibers of the interstitiospinal tract occupy a dorsomedial position in the ipsilateral MLF. No degeneration is seen in the contralateral nucleus of Darkschewitsch (ND).

lumbar spinal levels. It is uncertain as to whether fibers from the interstitial nucleus project to the ipsilateral medial accessory olivary nucleus, but lesions in the nucleus interrupt fibers terminating in that structure.

It has been reported by Szentágothai and Rajkovits (1958) that descending fibers from the interstitial nucleus terminate in the ipsilateral facial nucleus. Examination of our data suggests that these fibers descend with the central tegmental tract and terminate mainly in part of the dorsomedial and intermediate cell groups of the facial nucleus (Courville, 1966). Studies by Courville (1966a) tend to confirm this conclusion in that lesions in the perirubral reticular formation of the cat produced similar descending ipsilateral degeneration that terminated in the same subdivisions of the facial nucleus.

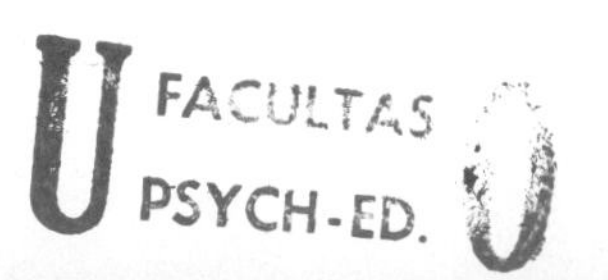

Conclusions concerning the efferent projections of the nucleus of Darkschewitsch are difficult to draw from these data since available lesions were not confined to this nucleus. However, the findings suggest that relatively few fibers project to the contralateral nucleus of Darkschewitsch and that no fibers project to the abducens, vestibular, perihypoglossal, or paramedian reticular nuclei, and none project to the spinal cord. The origin of fibers appearing to descend via the MLF to the medial accessory olivary nucleus could not be identified.

According to Szentágothai and Schab (1956) lesions in the nucleus of Darkschewitsch produce no degeneration in the oculomotor nuclei. Lesions in our animals involving this nucleus were not sufficiently discrete to provide data concerning this important point. It was our impression that all lesions destroying portions of the nucleus of Darkschewitsch concomitantly involved fibers of the interstitial nucleus which cross in the posterior commissure. The pattern of terminal degeneration in the oculomotor complex was similar to that observed with lesions in the interstitial nucleus but was less profuse and not symmetrical in distribution.

Observations from this study suggest that relatively discrete unilateral lesions in the interstitial nucleus produce primarily disturbance of head posture. Unilateral lesions involving the nucleus of Darkschewitsch, fibers from the interstitial nucleus which cross in the posterior commissure, and variable amounts of the lateral central gray substance appear to produce bilateral eyelid retraction and impairment of vertical eye movements, particularly those associated with upward gaze. Lesions involving fibers crossing in the ventral part of the posterior commissure produce a similar syndrome in the monkey, and appear to involve the same fiber systems.

REFERENCES

Allen, W. F. (1924). Distribution of the fibers originating from the different basal cerebellar nuclei. *J. Comp. Neurol.* **36**: 399-439.

Altman, J. (1962). Some fiber projections to the superior colliculus in the cat. *J. Comp. Neurol.* **119**: 77-95.

Altman, J., and Carpenter, M. B. (1961). Fiber projections of the superior colliculus in the cat. *J. Comp. Neurol.* **116**: 157-178.

Bennet, A. H. and Savill, T. (1889). A case of permanent conjugate deviation of the eyes and the head, the result of a lesion limited to the sixth nucleus. *Brain*. **12**: 102-116.

Benvenuti, E. (1901). Sulla patologia del ponte di varolio: Contributo clinico e anatomopatologico. *Ann. Nevrol.* (Naples). **19**: 97-130.

Blocq, P. and Guinon, G. (1891). Sur un cas de paralysie conjugée de la sixième paire. *Arch. Med. Exp. Anat. Path.* (Paris). **3**: 74-89.

Brodmann, K. (1905). Beiträge zur histologischen Lokalisation der Grosshirnrinde. III. Mitteilung: Die Rindenfelder der niederen Affen. *J. f. Psychol. u. Neurol.* **4**: 177-226.

Bucher, V. M. and Burgi, S. M. (1952). Some observations on the fiber connections of the di- and mesencephalon in the cat. II. Fiber connections of the pretectal region and the posterior commissure. *J. Comp. Neurol.* **96**: 139-177.

Brouwer, B. (1918). Klinisch-anatomische Untersuchungen uber den Oculomotoriuskern. *Z. ges Neurol. u. Psychiat.* **40**: 152-193.

Cajal, S. Ramon Y (1908). El ganglio intersticial del fasciculo longitudinal posterior en el hombre y diversos vertebrados. *Trav. Lab. Rech. Biol., Univ. Madrid.* **6**: 145-160.

Carpenter, M. B. and McMasters, R. E. (1963). Disturbances of conjugate horizontal eye movements in the monkey. II. Physiological effects and anatomical degeneration resulting from lesions in the medial longitudinal fasciculus. *Arch. Neurol.* **8**: 347-368.

Carpenter, M. B., McMasters, R. E. and Hanna, G. R. (1963). Disturbances of conjugate horizontal eye movements in the monkey. I. Physiological effects and anatomical degeneration resulting from lesions of the abducens nucleus and nerve. *Arch. Neurol.* **8**: 231-247.

Carpenter, M. B. and Strominger, N. L. (1964). Cerebello-oculomotor fibers in the rhesus monkey. *J. Comp. Neurol.* **123**: 211-230.

Carpenter, M. B. and Strominger, N. L. (1965). The medial longitudinal fasciculus and disturbances of conjugate horizontal eye movements in the monkey. *J. Comp. Neurol.* **125**: 41-66.

Carpenter, M. B. and Strominger, N. L. (1967). Efferent fibers of the subthalamic nucleus in the monkey. A comparison of the efferent projections of the subthalamic nucleus, substantia nigra and globus pallidus. *Am. J. Anat.* **121**: 41-72.

Clark, W. E. L. (1926). The mammalian oculomotor nucleus. *J. Anat.* **60**: 426-448.

Clark, W. E. L. (1932). An experimental study of the thalamic connections in the rat. *Phil. Trans. Roy. Soc.* Lond, B, **222**: 1-28.

Clark, W. E. L. (1936). The termination of ascending tracts in the thalamus of the macaque monkey. *J. Anat.* **71**: 7-40.

Cogan, D. G. (1956). *Neurology of the Ocular Muscles.* Charles C. Thomas, Springfield, Ill.

Cohen, B., Suzuki, J., and Bender, M. B. (1964). Eye movements from semicircular canal stimulation in the cat. *Ann. Oto., Rhinol. and Laryng.* **73**: 153-169.

Courville, J. (1966). The nucleus of the facial nerve: the relation between cellular groups and peripheral branches of the nerve. *Brain Research.* **1**: 338-354.

Courville, J. (1966a). Rubrobulbar fibers to the facial nucleus and the lateral reticular nucleus (nucleus of the lateral funiculus). An experimental study in the cat with silver impregnation methods. *Brain Research.* **1**: 317-337.

Crosby, E. C. (1950). The application of neuroanatomical data to the diagnosis of selected neurosurgical and neurological cases. *J. Neurosurg.* **7**: 566-583.

Crosby, E. C. (1953). Relations of brain centers to normal and abnormal eye movements in the horizontal plane. *J. Comp. Neurol.* **99**: 437-480.

Crosby, E. C., Humphrey, T., and Lauer, E. (1962). *Correlative Anatomy of the Nervous System.* pp. 731, Macmillan Co.

Darkschewitsch, L. (1889). Ueber den oberen Kern des N. oculomotorius. *Arch. f. Anat. u. Entwicklungsgesch.* (Anat. Abt.), pp. 107-116.

d'Espine, A. and Demole, V. (1917). Tubercules de la protuberance. *Arch. Med. Enf.* (Paris). **20**: 355-359.

Dow, R. W. and Moruzzi, G. (1958). *The Physiology and Pathology of the Cerebellum. Minneapolis: Univ. Minnesota Press.*

Fluur, E. (1959). Influences of semicircular ducts on extraocular muscles. *Acta Oto-Laryng.*, Suppl. **149**: 1-46.

Freeman, W. (1922). Paralysis of associated lateral movements of the eyes: A symptom of intrapontile lesion. *Arch. Neurol. and Psychiat.* **7**: 454-487.

Froment, J., Dechaume, J., and Colrat, A. (1930). Deux observations anatomo-cliniques de paralysie des mouvements associès de lateralité des yeux. *Rev. Otoneuroöphtal.* **8**: 713-727.

Garel, J. (1882). Nouveau fait de paralysie de la sixième paire avec déviation conjugée dans un cas d'hemiplegie alterne. *Rev. Med.* (Paris). **2**: 593-599.

Garey, L. J., Jones, E. G., and Powell, T. P. S. (1968). Interrelationships of striate and extrastriate cortex with the primary relay sites of the visual pathway. *J. Neurol. Neurosurg. Psychiat.* **31**: 135-157.

Gerebtzoff, M. A. (1936). Le pédoncule cérébelleux superieur et les terminations relles de la voie cérébello-thalamique. *Mem. Acad. Roy. Méd. Belg.* **25**: 1-58.

Gerebtzoff, M. A. (1941). Les bases anatomiques de la physiologie du cervelet. *La Cellule.* **49**: 73-166.

Hare, W. K., Magoun, H. W., and Ranson, S. W. (1937). Localization within the cerebellum of reactions to faradic cerebellar stimulation. *J. Comp. Neurol.* **67**: 145-182.

Hassler, R. and Hess, W. R. (1954). Experimentelle und anatomische Befunde über die Drehbewegungen und ihre nervösen Apparate. *Arch. f. Psychiat. u. Z. Neurol.* **192**: 488-526.

Holmes, G. (1921). Palsies of the conjugate ocular movements. *Brit. J. Ophthal.* **5**: 241-250.

Hoshino, T. (1921). Beitrage zur Funktion des Kleinhirnwurmes beim Kaninchen. *Acta Otolaryng.* Suppl. **2**: 1-72.
Hyde, J. E. and Eason, R. G. (1959). Characteristics of ocular movements evoked by stimulation of brain stem of cat. *J. Neurophysiol.* **22**: 666-678
Hyde, J. E. and Eliasson, S. G. (1957). Brain stem induced eye movements in cats. *J. Comp. Neurol.* **108**: 139-172.
Hyde, J. E. and Toczek, S. (1962). Functional relation of interstitial nucleus to rotatory movements evoked from zona incerta stimulation. *J. Neurophysiol.* **25**: 455-466.
Ingram, W. R. and Ranson, S. W. (1935). The nucleus of Darkschewitsch and nucleus interstitialis in the brain of man. *J. Nerv. and Ment. Dis.* **81**: 125-137.
Jefferson, G. (1958). Substrates for integrative patterns in the reticular core. In: *Reticular Formation of the Brain,* ed. Jasper, H. H., *et al.,* pp. 65-68. Boston: Little, Brown and Company.
Johnson, T. N. and Clemente, C. D. (1959). An experimental study of the fiber connections between the putamen, globus pallidus, ventral thalamus, and midbrain tegmentum in cat. *J. Comp. Neurol.* **113**: 83-101.
Klimoff, I. A. (1896). Concerning the connection of the cerebellum with the nucleus of the oculomotor nerve (in Russian). *Vrach. St. Petersburgh,* **17**: 1013-1014.
Klimoff, I. A. (1899). Ueber die Leitungsbahnen des Kleinhirns. *Arch. f. Anat. u. Entwicklungsgesch.* (Anat. Abt.), Leipzig, 11-27.
Knies, M. (1891). Ueber die centralen Störungen der willkurlichen Augenmuskeln. *Arch. f. Augenheilk.,* **23**: 19-51.
Kuypers, H. G. J. M. (1958). An anatomical analysis of cortico-bulbar connexions to the pons and lower brain stem in the cat. *J. Anat.* **92**: 198-218.
Kuypers, H. G. J. M. (1958a). Corticobulbar connexions to the pons and lower brain stem in man. An anatomical study. *Brain.* **81**: 364-388.
Kuypers, H. G. J. M. and Lawrence, D. G. (1967). Cortical projections to the red nucleus and the brain stem in the rhesus monkey. *Brain Research.* **4**: 151-188.
Lemmen, L. J., Davis, E. R., and Radnor, L. L. (1959). Observations on stimulation of the human frontal eye field. *J. Comp. Neurol.* **112**: 163-168.
Magoun, H. W., Hare, W. K., and Ranson, S. W. (1935). Electrical stimulation of the interior of the cerebellum in the monkey. *Am. J. Physiol.* **112**: 329-339.
Marburg, O. and Warner, F. J. (1947). The pathways of the tectum (anterior colliculus) of the midbrain in cats. *J. Nerv. and Ment. Dis.* **106**: 415-446.
Markham, C. H. (1968). Midbrain and contralateral labyrinth influences on brain stem vestibular neurons in the cat. *Brain Research.* **9**: 312-333.
Markham, C. H., Precht, W., and Shimazu, H. (1966). Effect of stimulation of interstitial nucleus of Cajal on vestibular unit activity in the cat. *J. Neurophysiol.* **29**: 493-507.
Mettler, F. A. (1935). Corticifugal fiber connections of the cortex of the Macaca mulatta. The occipital region. *J. Comp. Neurol.* **61**: 221-256.
Muskens, L. J. J. (1914). An anatomico-physiological study of the posterior longitudinal bundle in its relation to forced movements. *Brain.* **36**: 352-426.
Mussen, A. T. (1927). Experimental investigations on the cerebellum. *Brain.* **50**: 313-349.
Nauta, W. J. H. and Gygax, P. A. (1954). Silver impregnation of degenerating axons in the central nervous system. A modified technique. *Stain Tech.* **29**: 91-93.
Nauta, W. J. H. and Kuypers, H. G. J. M. (1958). Some ascending pathways in the brain stem reticular formation. In: *Reticular Formation of the Brain,* ed. Jasper, H. H. *et al.,* ch. 1, pp. 3-30. Boston: Little, Brown and Company.
Nauta, W. J. H. and Mehler, W. R. (1966). Projections of the lentiform nucleus in the monkey. *Brain Research.* **1**: 3-42.
Nyberg-Hansen, R. (1966). Sites of termination of interstitiospinal fibers in the cat. An experimental study with silver impregnation methods. *Arch. ital. Biol.* **104**: 98-111.
McMasters, R. E., Weiss, A. H., and Carpenter, M. B. (1966). Vestibular projections to the nuclei of the extraocular muscles. Degeneration resulting from discrete partial lesions of the vestibular nuclei in the monkey. *Am. J. Anat.* **118**: 163-194.
Papez, J. W. (1926). Reticulo-spinal tracts in the cat: Marchi method. *J. Comp. Neurol.* **41**: 365-399.
Papez, J. W. and Freeman, G. L. (1930). Superior colliculi and their fiber connections in the rat. *J. Comp. Neurol.* **51**: 409-439.
Pompeiano, O. and Walberg, F. (1957). Descending connections to the vestibular nuclei. An experimental study in the cat. *J. Comp. Neurol.* **108**: 465-502.

Peele, T. L. (1961). *The Neuroanatomical Basis for Clinical Neurology.* New York: McGraw-Hill Co.
Rasmussen, A. T. (1936). Tractus tecto-spinalis in the cat. *J. Comp. Neurol.* **63**: 501-525.
Riley, H. A. (1930). The central nervous system control of the ocular movements and the disturbances of this mechanism. *Arch. Ophth.* **4**: 640-661 and 885-910.
Sachs, E. and Fincher, E. F. (1927). Anatomical and physiological observations on lesions in the cerebellar nuclei in Macacus rhesus. *Brain.* **50**: 350-356.
Scheibel, A. B., Markham, C. H., and Koegler, R. (1961). Neural correlates of the vestibulo-ocular reflex. *Neurology.* **11**: 1055-1065.
Scheibel, M. E. and Scheibel, A. B. (1958). Structural substrates for integrative patterns in the brain stem reticular formation. **In**: *Reticular Formation of the Brain*, ed. Jasper, H. H. *et al.*, ch. 2, pp. 31-55. Boston: Little, Brown and Company.
Strong, O. S. and Elwyn, A. (1943). *Human Neuroanatomy.* Williams and Wilkins Co., Baltimore, Md. Ch. 14, p. 212.
Szentágothai, J. (1943). Die zentrale Innervation der Augenbewegungen. *Arch. Neurol. Psychiat.* **116**: 721-760.
Szentágothai, J. (1950). Recherches experimentales sur les voies oculogyres. *Semaine hôp.* (Paris), **26**: 2989-2995.
Szentágothai, J. (1950a). The elementary vestibulo-ocular reflex arc. *J. Neurophysiol.* **13**: 395-407.
Szentágothai, J. (1952). Die Rolle der einzelnen Labyrinthrezeptoren bei der Orientation von Augen und Kopf im Raume. Akademiai Kiado, Budapest. 129 pp.
Szentágothai, J. and Rajkovits, K. (1958). Der Hirnnervenanteil der Pyramidenbahn und der pramotorisch Apparat motorischer Hirnnervenkerne. *Arch. Psychiat. Nervenkr.* **197**: 335-354.
Szentágothai, J. and Schab, R. (1956). A midbrain inhibitory mechanism of oculomotor activity. *Acta physiol. Acad. Sci. hung.* **9**: 89-98.
Truex, R. C. and Carpenter, M. B. (1969). *Human Neuroanatomy.* 6th Ed. Williams and Wilkins Co., Baltimore, Md. 673 pp.
Tsai, C. (1925). The optic tracts and centers in the opossum, Didelphis virginiana. *J. Comp. Neurol.* **39**: 173-216.
Tsuchida, U. (1906). Ueber die Ursprungskerne der Augenbewegungsnerven. Arb. a. d. Hirnanat. Inst. Univ. Zurich, Bd. 2, p.1.
Van Gehuchten, A. (1898). Recherches sur l'origine réelle des nerfs craniens: I. Les nerfs moteur oculaires. *J. Belg. Neurol.* **3**: 114-129.
Van Gehuchten, A. (1904). Les connexions centrales du noyau de Deiters et les masses grises voisines (Faisceau vestibulospinal, faisceau longitudinal posterieur, stries medullairès). *Nevraxe* (*Louvain*), **6**: 19-73.
Vogt, C. and Vogt, O. (1919). Zur Kenntnis der pathologischen Veränderungen des Striatum und des Pallidum und zur Patho-Physiologie der dabei auftretenden Krankheitserscheinungen. S.-B. Heidelberger Akad. Wiss., Mth.-Nat. Kl. Abt. B., Biol. Wiss. Abh., **14**: 1-56.
Vogt, C. and Vogt, O. (1920). Zur Lehre der Erkrankungen des striären Systems. *J. Psychol. u. Neurol.* **25**: 627-846.
Walberg, F. (1957). Do the motor nuclei of the cranial nerves receive corticofugal fibers? An experimental study in the cat. *Brain.* **80**: 597-605.
Walker, A. E. and Weaver, T. A., Jr. (1940). Ocular movements from the occipital lobe in the monkey. *J. Neurophysiol.* **3**: 353-357.
Wallenberg, A. (1905). Sekundare Bahnen aus dem frontalen sensiblen Trigeminuskerne des Kaninchens. *Anat. Anz.* **26**: 145-155.
Warwick, R. (1953). Observations upon certain reputed accessory nuclei of the oculomotor complex. *J. Anat.* **87**: 46-52.
Wawick, R. (1953a). Representation of the extraocular muscles in the oculomotor nuclei of the monkey. *J. Comp. Neurol.* **98**: 449-504.
Warwick, R. (1954). The ocular parasympathetic nerve supply and its mesencephalic sources. *J. Anat.* **88**: 71-93.
Warwick, R. (1955). The so-called nucleus of convergence. *Brain.* **78**: 92-114.
Warwick, R. (1956). Oculomotor organization. *Ann. Roy. Coll. of Surg.* (*England*), **19**: 36-52.
Wernicke, C. (1877). Ein Fall von Ponserkrankung. *Arch Psychiat.* **7**: 513-538.
Winkler, C. (1927). *Manuel de Neurologie.* Tome 1^3. Erven F. Bohn. Haarlem.
Woodburne, R. T., Crosby, E. C., and McCotter, R. E. (1946). The mammalian midbrain and isthmus regions. Part II. The fiber connections. A. The relations of the tegmentum of the midbrain with the basal ganglia in Macaca mulatta. *J. Comp. Neurol.* **85**: 67-92.
Zimmerman, E. A., Chambers, W. W., and Liu, C. N. (1964). An experimental study of the anatomical organization of the cortico-bulbar system in the albino rat. *J. Comp. Neurol.* **123**: 301-324.

VESTIBULO-OCULAR RELATIONS

BERNARD COHEN

Eye movements induced by the vestibular apparatus and some aspects of vestibular nuclei organization will be briefly reviewed in this report. In addition, central pathways which connect the vestibular and oculomotor nuclei, particularly pathways through the pons responsible for horizontal eye movements induced by both visual and vestibular stimuli will be considered in detail. Patterns of eye movements induced by the semicircular canals have been described more comprehensively in a recent review (Cohen, 1970). Other facets of vestibulo-ocular relations have been reviewed elsewhere (Magnus, 1924; Camis and Creed, 1930; Dusser de Barenne, 1934; McNally and Stuart, 1942; Spiegel and Sommer, 1944; Wendt, 1951; Egmond *et al.*, 1952; Jansen and Brodal, 1954; Aschan *et al.*, 1956a; Neuro-otology, 1956; Brodal, 1958; Dow and Moruzzi, 1958; Gernandt, 1959; Rasmussen and Windle, 1960; Whitteridge, 1960; International Symposium on Problems in Otoneurology, 1961; Collegium Oto-Rhino-Laryngologicum, 1961; Japan Vestibular Society, 1963; Bender, 1964; Fields and Alford, 1964; International Vestibular Symposium, 1964; International Symposium on Vestibular and Oculomotor Problems, 1965; Role of the Vestibular Organs in the Exploration of Space, 1965; Kornhuber, 1966; Wolfson, 1966, de Reuck and Knight, 1967; Bender, 1969; Cawthorne *et al.*, 1969; Kornhuber, 1970).

I. EYE MOVEMENTS INDUCED BY THE VESTIBULAR APPARATUS

Sensory information which originates in the labyrinth is important for establishing the relationship of the head in space (Goltz, 1870; Breuer, 1874, 1875, 1889, 1891; Crum-Brown, 1874; Mach, 1875; Ewald, 1892; Camis and Creed, 1930). The sensory apparatus, the semicircular canals and the utricle and saccule, code head position and angular and linear head movements. Angular head movements are perceived primarily by the semicurcular canals (Lowenstein and Sand, 1940a, b; Egmond *et al.*, 1949, 1952; Groen *et al.*, 1952; Lowenstein, 1956; Ledoux, 1958; Money and Scott, 1962). The utricle and the saccule sense changes in linear velocity of the head or the static position of the head in space (Breuer, 1891; de Kleyn, 1920; Magnus, 1924; Benjamins and Huizinga, 1927; Versteegh, 1927; Tait and McNally, 1934; Hasegawa, 1935, 1937; McNally and Stuart, 1942; Lowenstein and Roberts, 1949; Jongkees, 1950). Eye movements induced by the vestibular apparatus may be viewed as a response of the nervous system to some aspect of this spatial relationship in an effort to promote vision (Dodge, 1923; Camis and Creed, 1930; Dusser de Barenne, 1934; McNally and Stuart, 1942; Gernandt, 1959; Jones and Milsum, 1965; Meiry, this volume).

For the most part eye movements induced by the vestibular apparatus are compensatory. That is, they oppose head movements or changes in head position and act to maintain the angle of the retina in space (Dodge, 1923; Bender *et al.*, 1965; Jones and Milsum, 1965; Bender and Feldman, 1967; Atkin and Bender, 1968). However, eye movements which are anticompensatory can also be induced by vestibular stimuli (Jones, 1964). It may be difficult to categorize vestibular reflexes for a number of reasons. Ocular and postural responses to vestibular stimuli either habituate or are considerably modified when stimuli are given repeatedly (Hood and Pfaltz, 1954; Fukuda *et al.*, 1958; McCabe, 1960; Crampton, 1962, 1964; Guedry, 1964, 1965; Collins and Updegraff, 1965; Brown and Crampton, 1966; Collins, 1966, 1969; Komatsuzaki *et al.*, 1969; Kornhuber, 1970). There is interaction of neck and vestibular reflexes (Barany, 1906; Magnus, 1924; Fukuda, 1961; Philipszoon, 1962; Jongkees and Philipszoon, 1964; Takemori and Suzuki, 1969; Biemond and de Jong, 1969). In addition, sensory information arising in other modalities, particularly vision, may suppress or block vestibular reflexes (McCabe, 1960; Collins, 1966). These topics are considered in greater detail elsewhere (Kornhuber, 1966, 1970).

Both the semicircular canals and the otolith organs exert a strong influence on the eyes and on eye muscles. Activity generated in semicircular canal nerves can reach eye muscles in about 1.5-3 msec (Dumont-Tyc and Dell, 1962; Cohen and Suzuki, 1963; Kumoi and Jampel, 1966; F. Ito *et al.*, 1969). When semicircular canal nerves are electrically stimulated, synchronous excitation of eye muscles can be produced at stimulation rates greater than 400/sec (Cohen and Suzuki, 1963). This is close to the fusion frequency of the fastest eye muscle fibers (Cooper and Eccles, 1930; Bach-y-Rita and Ito, 1966; Yamanaka and Bach-y-Rita, 1968). The excitatory drive of the otolith organs on the eye muscles can also be strong. When single utricular nerves were stimulated, the latency of contractions induced in eye muscles was about 5-7.5 msec (Suzuki *et al.*, 1969b). Allowing 2.5 msec as coupling time for activation of the contractile system (Cohen *et al.*, 1964), then about 2.5-5 msec is probably the minimum central latency of the reflex arc from otolith organs to eye muscles. Inhibition of eye muscles from semicircular canals or vestibular nerves is also carried over short latency pathways (Szentágothai, 1959, 1952; Cohen *et al.*, 1964; Richter and Precht, 1968; Baker *et al.*, 1969a, b).

Semicircular canals

Patterns of compensatory eye and head movements induced by the semicircular canals have been known in fish and birds for many years (Flourens,

1824; Lee, 1893, 1894; Ewald, 1892; Camis and Creed, 1930). Eye movements induced by the semicircular canals or by semicircular canal nerve stimulation have also been studied in mammals (Szentágothai, 1950, 1952; Fluur, 1959; Cohen and Suzuki, 1963; Suzuki *et al.*, 1964, 1969a; Suzuki and Cohen, 1964; Cohen *et al.*, 1966; Cohen, 1970). When an individual semicircular canal or its nerve are stimulated, eye movements are induced which lie in planes of space parallel to the plane of that canal. This is true regardless of the position of the eyes in the orbit or of the head on the neck (Cohen *et al.*, 1966).

The direction of eye movements induced by electrically stimulating individual ampullary nerves on the left side in an alert monkey is shown in Figure 1A-C. If two or more canals are simultaneously stimulated, the induced eye movements summate (Suzuki and Cohen, 1964; Suzuki *et al.*, 1964). Thus eye movements can be induced in every plane of space. If semicircular canal stimuli are of short duration, induced eye movements are brief and may be monophasic or biphasic (Cohen *et al.*, 1967a; Goto *et al.*, 1968). If the stimuli are of longer duration and animals are alert, nystagmus occurs. The slow phases of nystagmus induced by electrical stimulation of the left semicircular canals, i.e., by adding impulses to the ampullary nerves on the left side, are in the same direction as the eye movements shown in Figure 1 (Cohen *et al.*, 1965a). The quick phases of this nystagmus oppose the slow phases. If impulses in ampullary nerves are reduced instead of being increased (Ewald, 1892; Lowenstein and Sand, 1940a, b; Spiegel and Sommers, 1944), the slow phases of the induced nystagmus would be in opposite directions to the movements shown in Figure 1. Since the visual angle is the same in man as in monkey (Johnson, 1908; Imai, 1930), eye movements similar to those shown in Figure 1 would probably be induced by stimulation of individual semicircular canals in humans.

Semicircular canal function is most commonly studied in humans with caloric or rotatory stimuli. In normal individuals these stimuli do not excite individual canals. A caloric stimulus in one ear simultaneously activates all three semicircular canals on that side, although the response from the horizontal canal usually predominates. When both ears are simultaneously stimulated with hot or cold water, lateral canal responses are mutually inhibited, and vertical nystagmus is induced (Bárány, 1907; Shanzer and Bender, 1959). Angular rotation of the head, the natural or "adequate" stimulus for the semicircular canals, excites canals which lie in planes parallel to the plane of rotation. Therefore, at least two canals, one on each side, are simultaneously affected by a rotatory stimulus. A detailed description of the normal and pathological ocular and sensory responses to caloric and rotatory stimuli in man and in animals is beyond the scope of this review. A few of the many articles which deal with this subject include those by Bárány (1907), Dohlman (1925), Quix (1925), Dix and Hallpike (1952), Hallpike and Hood (1953), Carmichael *et al.*, (1956), Henriksson (1955a, b, 1956, 1967a, b), Aschan *et al.*, (1956a), Torok (1957, 1969) Stahle (1958), Shanzer and

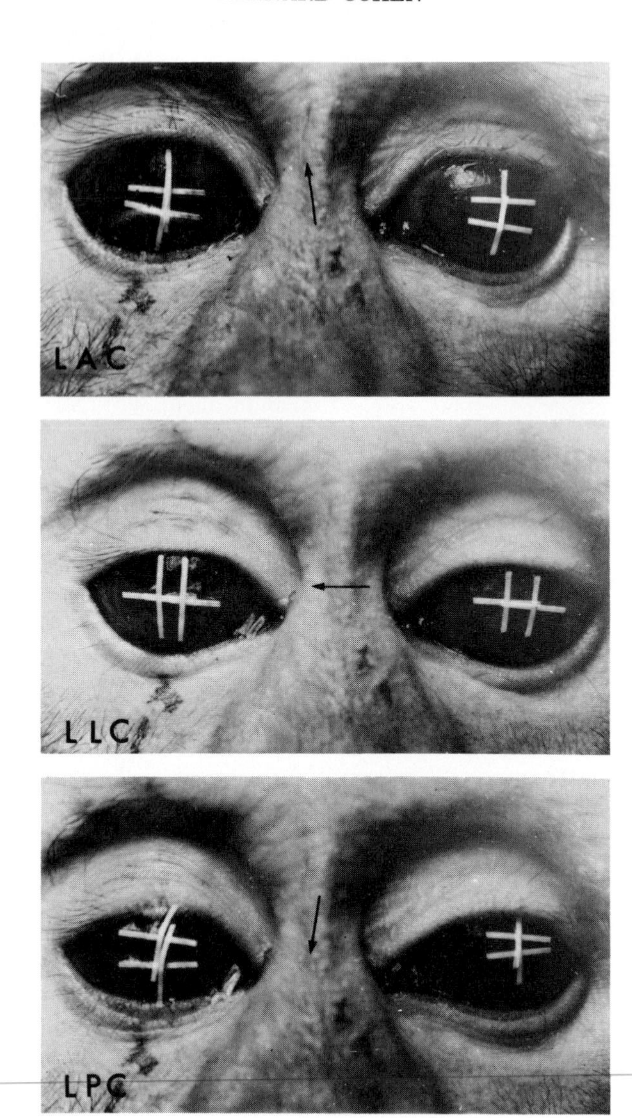

Fig. 1. Eye movements induced by electric stimulation of left anterior canal nerve (LAC), left lateral canal nerve (LLC) and left posterior canal nerve (LPC) in an alert monkey. A white cross on a blackened egg shell membrane covered the locally anesthetized cornea. The stimulus was a 50 msec train of 0.5 msec square waves at an intra-train frequency of 400/sec. Each photograph is a double exposure, one cross showing the position of the eyes at the beginning of stimulation, and the second the position of the eyes shortly after the end of stimulation. The arrows indicate the direction of movement. From the mid-position LAC induces upward counter-clockwise rotatory eye movements, LLC contralateral horizontal eye movements, and LPC downward counter-clockwise rotatory movements. From Suzuki, J. and Cohen, B. (1964). *Expl. Neurol.* **10**, 393-405. *Courtesy of Academic Press, Inc.*

Bender (1959), Jongkees *et al.* (1962), Japan Vestibular Society (1963), Jongkees and Philipszoon (1964), Jung and Kornhuber (1964), Kornhuber (1966), Jongkees (1967), Bender (1969), Cawthorne *et al.* (1969), Komatsuzaki *et al.* (1969).

Utricle and saccule

Eye movements induced by the otolith organs, the utricle and saccule, have been the subject of much controversy (Camis and Creed, 1930; McNally and Stuart, 1942; Bergstedt, 1961). The otolith organs compensate for static head tilt by inducing ocular counter-rolling (de Kleyn, 1920; Magnus, 1924; Benjamins and Huizinga, 1927; Lorente de No, 1928, 1931, Merton, 1956; Woellner and Graybiel, 1959, 1960; Miller, 1962; Azzena, 1966; Hannen *et al.*, 1966). The amount of compensatory counter-rolling against lateral head positions is relatively small. In recent studies in humans (Woellner and Graybiel, 1959; Miller, 1962; Hannen *et al.*, 1966) there was approximately 5-7° of static compensatory counter-rolling when subjects were tilted 45-90° to the right or left. Similar angles of compensatory counter-rolling were also found in the monkey (Cohen, Krejcova and Highstein, 1970). Examples of ocular counter-rolling against static head tilts of 45° to the left and right in a monkey are shown in Figure 2. Neck receptors do not induce significant amounts of counter-rolling against static head tilt (Cohen, Krejcova and Highstein, 1970).

Although compensatory counter-rolling against static tilt is relatively small, dynamic compensatory counter-rolling can be larger (Merton, 1958); Woellner and Graybiel, 1959; Jones, 1958; Hannen *et al.*,1966). For example,

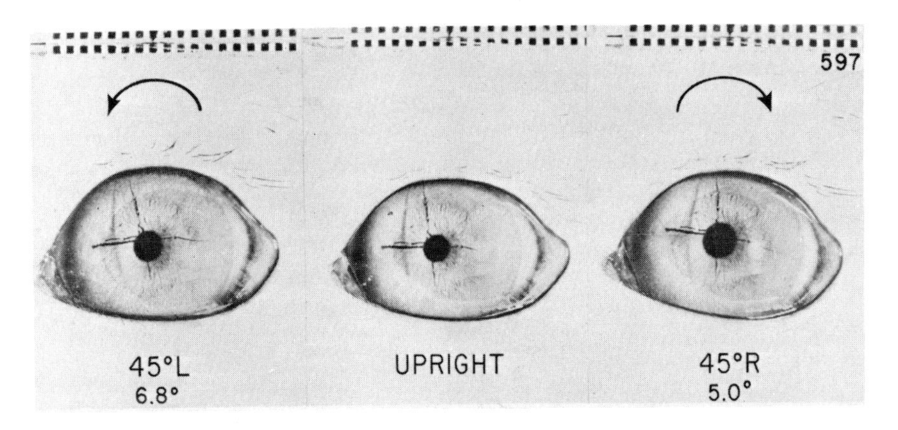

Fig. 2. Compensatory ocular counter-rolling in a monkey. The head and body were tilted together. A black cross tattooed on the cornea was used to indicate the position of the left eye. When the animal was 45° to the left (L), the eyes were rotated 6.8° in a counterclockwise direction. When the animal was 45° to the right (R) the eyes were torted 5° in a clockwise direction.

up to 20° of ocular torsion was induced during rotatory nystagmus when pilots rolled jet airplanes rapidly (Jones, 1958). Presumably the anterior and posterior semicircular canals and the otolith organs were simultaneously stimulated in these subjects. The otolith organs also respond to linear acceleration, and horizontal nystagmus has been induced in animals and in man by varying linear acceleration (Jongkees and Philipszoon, 1963, 1964; McCabe, 1964).

Although eye movements have been induced by natural stimuli which primarily excite the otolith organs, there have been relatively few studies of eye movements induced by mechanical or electrical stimulation of individual utricles or saccules in mammals. The four quadrants of the utricular macula were mechanically stimulated by Szentágothai (1964). He induced eye movements with oppositely-directed rotatory and vertical components from each of the four quadrants. He also electrically stimulated the utricular macula.

Patterns of eye movement induced by utricular nerve stimulation were recently studied in the alert cat by Suzuki *et al.*, (1969b). When the left utricular macula and its nerve were stimulated, the predominant component of eye movement was counter-clockwise rotation (Fig. 3). There was also some upward movement and adduction of the ipsilateral eye and depression and abduction of the contralateral eye. The vertical or horizontal components of movement varied somewhat depending on the parts of the macula or nerve which were stimulated. The direction of eye rotation reversed when the right utricular nerve was stimulated. Nystagmus in the coronal plane was also induced by repetitive stimulation of the utricular nerve. Quick phases of this nystagmus were oppositely-directed to the slow phases.

There is little detailed information about eye movements produced by the saccules. From anatomic considerations it seems likely that vertical and vertical-rotatory compensatory eye movements are produced by the saccules (Magnus, 1924; Benjamins and Huizinga, 1927; Hasegawa, 1937; McNally and Stuart, 1942; Miller, 1962). This is also suggested by findings of Jongkees and Philipszoon (1963) that nystagmus induced by varying linear acceleration was maximal when rabbits were in a lateral position which would most excite the saccules. This is a subject for further study.

Tests of otolith organ function usually depend on inducing vertigo or nystagmus by holding or moving the head into positions other than upright (Bárány, 1913; Nylén, 1924, 1950, 1953; Jongkees and Philipszoon, 1964; Bos *et al.*, 1964). Otolith organs responses can be demonstrated in normal individuals by administration of alcohol (Bárány, 1911; de Kleyn and Versteegh, 1930; Walter, 1954; Aschan *et al.*, 1956a, b; Bergstedt, 1961). Alcohol appears to reduce central inhibition, alllowing sensory information which originates in the otolith organs to be expressed as positional alcohol nystagmus (PAN). Compensatory counter-rolling against lateral head tilt is reduced after administration of alcohol (Miller and Graybiel, 1969).

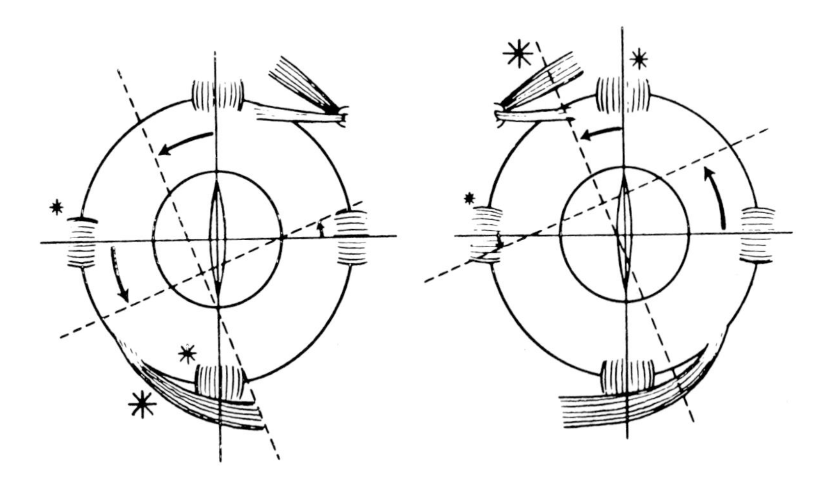

Fig. 3. Eye movements and eye muscle contractions induced by left utricular nerve stimulation in the cat. The solid cross shows the position of the eyes at the beginning of stimulation and the dashed cross the position of the eyes at the end of the induced movement. The arrows show the direction of movement. Counterclockwise tonic deviations and nystagmus with counterclockwise slow phases and clockwise quick phases were induced by left utricular nerve stimulation. The muscles most strongly activated during tonic deviations or slow phases of nystagmus are shown with large asterisks. They were the left superior oblique and right inferior oblique. The left superior rectus and right inferior rectus muscles also contracted (medium asterisks), and the left medial and right lateral rectus muscles were weakly activated (small asterisks). The other eye muscles were inhibited. Clockwise tonic deviations were not induced by left utricular nerve stimulation. From Suzuki, J., Tokumasu, K. & Goto, K. (1969b). *Acta oto-lar.* **68,** 350-362.

In man there are two phases of PAN (Aschan *et al.,* 1956a, b; Bergstedt, 1961). In the first phase (PAN I) the quick phases of nystagmus are geotropic, i.e., they are directed toward the ground. In the second phase (PAN II) the quick phases reverse direction and are apogeotropic. PAN II does not occur in most animals, but has been found in monkeys (Komatsuzaki *et al.,* 1969) and in some brown rabbits (Nohara *et al.,* 1966). PAN disappears after bilateral labyrinthectomy (de Kleyn and Versteegh, 1930; Aschan *et al.,* 1956b, 1964a; Suzuki *et al.,* 1968). Nito *et al.,* (1964, 1968) dispute that PAN originates in the utricle and saccule. They suggest instead that PAN is a response of the semicircular canals.

II. VESTIBULAR NUCLEI

The anatomy and central connections of the vestibular nuclei are summarized by Jansen and Brodal (1954), Brodal (1958), Dow and Moruzzi (1958), Brodal *et al.* (1962), Voogd (1964), Hauglie-Hanssen (1968),

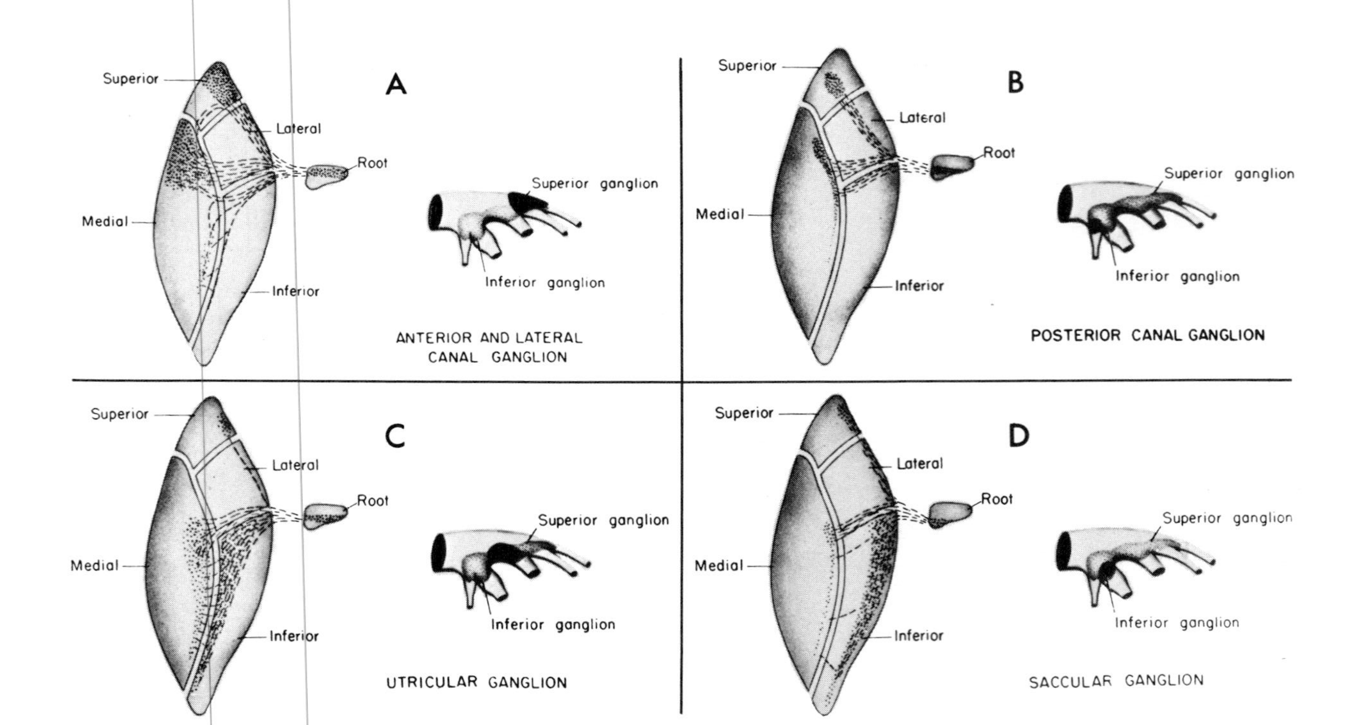

Fig. 4. Diagramatic representation of the central distribution of degeneration in the vestibular nuclei resulting from lesions of various parts of the vestibular ganglion. In A the lesion destroyed cells which innervate the anterior and lateral canals, in B the posterior canal, in C the utricle, and in D the saccule. Note that in A and B the most profuse central degeneration is present in the superior vestibular nucleus and in rostral parts of the medial vestibular nucleus, while in C and D the central degeneration is most profuse in the inferior vestibular nucleus and in caudal portions of the medial vestibular nucleus. From Stein, B. M. & Carpenter, M. B. (1967). *Am. J. Anat.* **120,** 281-318. *Courtesy of Wistar Institute Press.*

Sadjadpour and Brodal (1968) and the physiology of the vestibular nuclei by Brodal *et al.* (1962), Kornhuber (1966, 1970), and Precht (1970). Brodal, Pompeiano and Walberg (1962) have emphasized the discrete and particulate nature of the vestibular nuclei and of their afferent and efferent projections. From this they infer that the function of individual parts of the vestibular nuclei must be quite different.

Understanding of the function of the individual nuclei has been advanced by recent anatomical studies of Stein and Carpenter (1967) and Gacek (1968, 1969). They have shown that axons from the utricle and saccule end in different parts of the vestibular nuclei than do axons from the semicircular canals. Lorente de Nó (1933a) originally showed that there was a partially distinct and partially common central distribution of fibers from the cristae and maculae. Fig. 4A-D show a summary of some of the results of Stein and Carpenter. Neurons from the semicircular canals synapse primarily in the rostral medial and superior vestibular nuclei (Fig. 4A, B). Neurons from the utricle and saccule go mainly to the inferior and caudal medial vestibular nuclei (Fig. 4C, D).

These findings are of interest because they imply that activity arising in the semicircular canals and otolith organs is processed in areas of the vestibular nuclei which are largely separate from each other. In support of this idea, neurons in both the superior and medial vestibular nuclei respond during horizontal angular acceleration (Adrian, 1943; Duensing and Schaefer, 1958; Shimazu and Precht 1965) or semicircular canal nerve stimulation (Markham, 1968), while neurons in more caudal portions of the vestibular nuclei have been shown to respond to head tilt (Adrian, 1943; Duensing and Schaefer, 1959; Hiebert and Fernandez, 1965; Peterson, 1967; Fujita *et al.*, 1968).

Neural activity in vestibular nuclei during rotation

Changes in unit firing induced in the vestibular nuclei by natural and artificial stimulation of the vestibular apparatus and nerve have been reviewed in detail by Precht (1970). During horizontal angular acceleration, first order neurons in the ampullary nerve from the lateral canals increase their firing rate with ampullo-petal angular acceleration, and decrease it with ampullofugal acceleration (Lowenstein and Sand, 1940a, b). In the vestibular nucleus on the ipsilateral side, cells are both excited and inhibited by this stimulus (Gernandt, 1949; Ryu *et al.*, 1969). Of the cells which are excited on the ipsilateral side two types appear to be particularly important in processing incoming afferent information. These have been designated as tonic and kinetic cells (Shimazu and Precht, 1965; Precht and Schimazu, 1965). The tonic cells have continuous spontaneous activity which increases or decreases in response to rotation in the ipsilateral or contralateral directions, respectively. When the vestibular nerve is electrically stimulated, the latency of activation of tonic cells on the ipsilateral side indicates that they are excited over multisynaptic pathways (Precht and Shimazu, 1965).

Kinetic cells, on the other hand, are silent in the resting state and only increase their activity in response to strong rotation to the ipsilateral side. These cells are monosynaptically activated by stimulation of the ipsilateral vestibular nerve. Inhibitory postsynaptic potentials are induced in both tonic and kinetic cells by stimulation of the opposite vestibular nerve. This inhibition is mediated by commissural fibers which originate in the contralateral vestibular nuclei (Shimazu and Precht, 1966; Fredrickson *et al.*, 1966; Kasahara *et al.*, 1968; Mano *et al.*, 1968; Wilson *et al.*, 1968b). A smaller group of cells increase their firing rate by rotation in any direction (Gernandt, 1949). The role of tonic and kinetic units in inducing various types of compensatory eye movements is not clear at present (Precht, 1970).

Other aspects of vestibular physiology

There are still many unanswered questions about the physiology of the vestibular apparatus and nuclei. A few of these questions will be mentioned:

(1) There is a prominent efferent system which ends directly on sensory cells in the cristae and maculae (Wersäll, 1956, 1960; Engstrom, 1958, 1961; Ireland and Farkashidy, 1961; Gacek, 1960, 1966; Ades and Engstrom, 1965; Wersäll *et al.*, 1967; Hillman, 1969). The role of this efferent system in modulating vestibulo-ocular reflexes has not been clearly defined in mammals. The efferent fibers appear to mediate inhibition in the cat (Sala, 1965). In frogs efferent fibers which originate in the cerebellar cortex have also been shown to produce inhibition of afferent activity in the vestibular nerve (Llinás *et al.*, 1967; Llinás and Precht, 1969; Precht and Llinás, 1969b). Direct efferent fibers from the cerebellar cortex to the vestibular apparatus have not been found in mammals in electrophysiological studies (Precht and Llinás, 1969b).

(2) Several lines of evidence have shown that there is at least one integration of semicircular canal activity in the vestibulo-ocular reflex arc after the cupula (Cohen *et al.*, 1956a; Suzuki and Cohen, 1966; Precht, 1970; Robinson, this volume). Whether one of these integrations might take place in the vestibular nuclei and how it is accomplished is not known.

(3) There have been few studies of how or where neural activity responsible for vertical or rotatory eye movements induced by the vestibular apparatus is processed in the vestibular nuclei. Duensing (1968a, b) and Markham (1968) have shown that there are cells with reciprocal responses to rotation in the plane of the vertical canals in the vestibular nuclei. This suggests that cell types which process vertical canal information may be similar to those which have been described for lateral canals.

It is also not clear whether there is a separation of various parts of the vestibular nuclei which induce eye, head and body movements in various spatial planes. Recent experiments on eye movements induced by stimulation of the vestibular nuclei in the monkey have raised this possibility (Tokumasu *et al.*, 1969). In these studies mainly upward rotatory eye movements

(Fig. 5A) and nystagmus with upward rotatory slow phases were induced by stimulation of the superior vestibular nucleus. Horizontal movements were primarily induced by stimulation of the mid-portion of the vestibular complex, although there were also other types of movements which were induced from this region (Fig. 5B). Downward rotatory eye movements (Fig. 5C) and nystagmus with downward rotatory slow phases were mainly evoked by activation of the rostral portions of the medial and descending nuclei.

(4) The role of the individual vestibular nuclei in oculomotor function is still not well understood. Polysynaptic EPSP's and IPSP's have been recorded throughout the vestibular complex when the ipsilateral vestibular

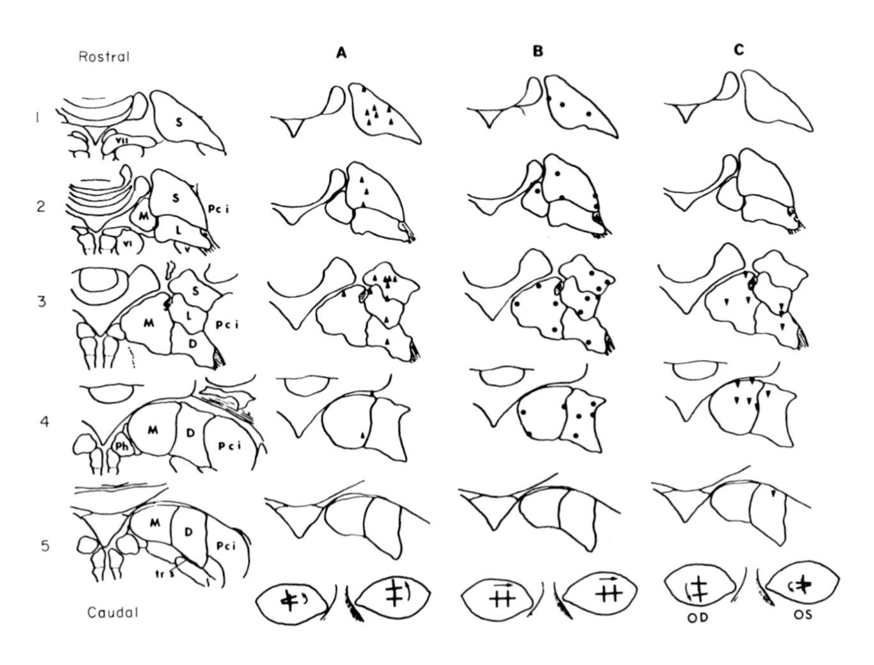

Fig. 5. Sites in the left vestibular nuclei from which eye movements were induced by stimulation with pulse trains. Trains were of 50 msec duration and were composed of 0.5 msec square waves at an intra-train frequency of 500/sec. Upward rotatory movements are shown in column A, horizontal eye movements in column B, and downward rotatory eye movements in column C. The rotatory component of movements induced by pulse trains stimulation of the left side were counterclockwise. A labeled drawing of these sections is on the left. Each section is 1 mm apart in the 45° stereotaxic plane. Abbreviations: S, superior vestibular nucleus; M, medial vestibular nucleus; L, lateral vestibular nucleus; D, descending vestibular nucleus; V, nucleus of spinal tract of trigeminal nerve; VI, abducens nucleus; VII, genu of the facial nerve; tr S, tractus solitarius, Ph, prepositus hypoglossal nucleus; Pci, inferior cerebellar peduncle. From Tokumasu, K., Goto, K. & Cohen, B. (1969). *Ann. Otol. Rhinol. Lar.* **78,** 1105-1119.

nerve is stimulated (Wilson *et al.*, 1966, 1968; M. Ito *et al.*, 1969; Kawai *et al.*, 1969). The superior and rostral medial vestibular nuclei receive afferent projections and code specific information from the semicircular canals (Brodal *et al.*, 1962; Precht and Shimazu, 1965; Shimazu and Precht, 1965; Stein and Carpenter, 1966; Markham, 1968; Gacek, 1969). The lateral vestibular nucleus appears to be most closely related to the otolith organs. Only the ventral portion of the lateral vestibular nucleus receives primary afferent vestibular projections (Walberg *et al.*, 1958; M. Ito *et al.*, 1964, 1969; Mugnaini *et al.*, 1967; Wilson *et al.*, 1967), although the dorsal part can be activated over polysynaptic pathways (Wilson *et al.*, 1967; M. Ito *et al.*, 1969). The dorsal portion seems most closely related to spinal cord function (Brodal *et al.*, 1962). The ventral portion has ascending and descending projections (Brodal *et al.*, 1962; Szentágothai, 1964; McMasters *et al.*, 1966; Wilson *et al.*, 1967), and horizontal nystagmus has been induced by stimulation in this region (Yules and Gault, 1966; Tokumasu *et al.*, 1969). However, primary afferents in this region may also have been activated in these studies. Cells in the lateral vestibular nucleus respond specifically to head tilt (Hiebert and Fernandez, 1965; Peterson, 1967; Fujita *et al.*, 1968). The majority of cells increase their firing rate when the ipsilateral side is down and decrease it when the contralateral side is down. Unit responses to semicircular canal stimulation on the other hand are nonspecific and the relationship between eye movements and semicircular canal-induced unit activity in the lateral vestibular nucleus is weak (Desole and Pallestrini, 1969). As noted, anatomical evidence suggests that the descending and caudal medial vestibular nuclei are also important in processing information from the otolith organs.

To evaluate the role of the individual vestibular nuclei in ocular reflexes, it would be of interest to know whether eye movements induced by individual semicircular canals or utricles and saccules would be differentially affected by lesion of different parts of the vestibular nuclei. Although ocular effects of lesions of the vestibular nuclei have been noted (Ferraro *et al.*, 1936, 1940; Ferraro and Barrera, 1936, 1938; Buchanan, 1940; Cranmer, 1951; Shanzer and Bender, 1959; Carpenter *et al.*, 1959), at present the symptoms and signs of localized lesions of the vestibular nuclei are not well defined (Jung and Kornhuber, 1964; Kornhuber, 1966; Bender, 1969; Cohen, 1970).

III. VESTIBULO-OCULAR PROJECTIONS

There are no neurons originating in the semicircular canals or in the otolith organs which project directly to eye muscle motor nuclei. Instead, a three neuron arc with an intermediate synapse in the vestibular nuclei or in the cerebellum is the most direct link between the vestibular apparatus and the eye muscles (Lorente de Nó, 1933b; Szentágothai, 1950). Most of the direct pathways from vestibular nuclei to eye muscle motor nuclei appear to lie in the region of the median longitudinal fasciculus (MLF). When the region of the MLF was destroyed in acute experiments, ocular responses induced by semicircular canal stimulation either disappeared or were markedly attenuated (Lorente de Nó, 1933b; Szentágothai, 1950, 1964).

Multisynaptic pathways also connect the vestibular nuclei to the eye muscles (Lorente de Nó, 1933b; Spiegel and Sommer, 1944; Szentágothai, 1950, 1964). Their importance is shown by the fact that after MLF destruction, slow tonic deviations and slow phases of nystagmus in vertical and horizontal planes are still produced by semicircular canal nerve and by caloric stimulation (Lorente de Nó, 1933b; Shanzer *et al.*, 1964; Shanzer, 1964; Cohen, Komatsuzaki and Alpert, unpublished data).

Monosynaptic and multisynaptic pathways between the vestibular and oculomotor nuclei end on different parts of oculomotor neurons in different types of synaptic terminals (Szentágothai, 1964). Heavily myelinated axons which connect vestibular and oculomotor nuclei via the MLF end in calyceal-like synapses which envelop the somata of oculomotor neurons (Szentágothai, 1964). It is probably possible to drive oculomotor motoneurons with considerable security at high rates through these synapses. Multisynaptic pathways from the reticular formation end in axodendritic synapses on these same motoneurons. In considering how vestibular information is processed in central structures, the site and function of both fast and slow pathways between vestibular and eye muscle motor nuclei have been considered.

Vestibulo-ocular pathway in brain stem and cerebellum

In support of the hypothesis that different regions of the vestibular nuclei are functionally discrete, their efferent connections are also largely separate. The medial and superior vestibular nuclei project ascending fibers into the MLF, to the abducens nuclei, and to the pontine reticular formation (Brodal and Pompeiano, 1957; Carpenter and McMasters, 1963; Szentágothai, 1964; Carpenter and Strominger, 1965; McMasters *et al.*, 1966; Wilson *et al.*, 1968a). Neurons from the reticular formation also end on oculomotor neurons (Lorente de Nó, 1933b; Scheibel and Scheibel, 1958; Szentágothai, 1964). Neither the superior nor the medial vestibular nuclei are important sources of afferent fibers to the cerebellum (Brodal *et al.*, 1962; Brodal, 1964a, b). Although vestibulo-cerebellar pathways may include fibers from the semicircular canals (Dow, 1936, 1938, 1939), semicircular canal-ocular pathways appear to lie primarily within the brain stem (Dow and Manni, 1958).

On the other hand the inferior vestibular nucleus has only meager direct projections through the brain stem to the oculomotor nuclei (Carpenter, 1960; Brodal *et al.*, 1962; McMasters *et al.*, 1966). Instead it projects mainly into the cerebellum (Fig. 6, Brodal and Torvik, 1957; Carpenter *et al.*, 1959; Carpenter, 1960). The coincidence of region of the inferior vestibular nuclei which receive projections from the utricle and saccule with those which project fibers into the cerebellum can be seen by comparing Figures 4C, D with

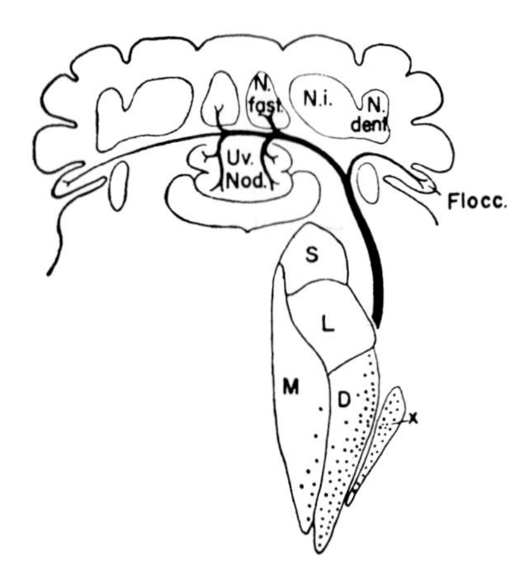

Fig. 6. Diagram summarizing site of origin of cells in the vestibular nuclei which project their axons into the cerebellum. From Brodal, A., Pompeiano, O. & Walberg, F. (1962). *The Vestibular Nuclei and Their Connections, Anatomy and Functional Correlations. Courtesy of Charles C. Thomas.*

Figure 6. From the cerebellum, direct cerebello-oculomotor fibers project to motoneurons of vertical eye muscles through the brachium conjunctivum (Carpenter and Strominger, 1964; Azzena and Giretti, 1967). In addition, the cerebellum projects into regions of the pontine reticular formation (Carpenter, 1959; Walberg *et al.*, 1962), and vestibular nuclei (Dow, 1936; 1938; Jansen and Brodal, 1954; Brodal *et al.*, 1962; Walberg *et al.*, 1962; Voogd, 1964; Angaut and Brodal, 1967) which in turn have monosynaptic or polysynaptic connections with the oculomotor nuclei.

Thus from the anatomic data there are two potential pathways over which activity induced in vestibular receptors might reach eye muscles. One carrying activity from the semicircular canals appears to lie primarily in the brain stem. It goes directly through the MLF and indirectly through the reticular formation to reach the oculomotor nuclei. The second carrying activity from the otolith organs can reach eye muscle motoneurons either through the medial or lateral vestibular nuclei, or might engage the cerebellum through the inferior vestibular nucleus, as an important link in this reflex arc.

There is little question that brain stem pathways are heavily utilized by activity arising in the vestibular system which reaches eye muscle motor nuclei. Prominent field potential changes are recorded in the brain stem at short latencies when vestibular nerves or individual semicircular canal nerves are stimulated (Gernandt, 1952, 1964; Gernandt *et al.*, 1959; Kumoi, 1965; Cook *et al.*, 1969). Pontine units respond to vestibular nerve stimulation (Potthoff *et al.*, 1967b; Gernandt, 1968), and are active during nystagmus induced by rotatory or caloric stimulation (Manni *et al.*, 1965; Gernandt, 1968) or after vestibular nuclei lesions (Duensing and Schaefer, 1957a, b).

On the other hand eye movements are readily induced by cerebellar stimulation in planes of space similar to those induced by semicircular canal nerve, vestibular nerve, or vestibular nuclei stimulation (Cohen *et al.*, 1965b). Cerebellar stimulation inhibits induced caloric nystagmus (Fernandez and Fredrickson, 1964). Field potential changes are evoked at short latency in the cerebellum by vestibular nerve stimulation (Dow, 1939), and Purkinje and granule cells are activated in the nodulus (Precht and Llinás, 1969a). Positional nystagmus, a sign of utriculo-ocular or sacculo-ocular reflex dysfunction, follows lesions of the cerebellum (Nylén, 1924, 1931, 1939; Spiegel and Scala, 1941; 1942; Fernandez, 1960; Fernandez and Fredrickson, 1964; Aschan *et al.*, 1964b; Grant *et al.*, 1964; Cohen *et al.*, 1969b). After cerebellar lesions caloric nystagmus may be relatively little affected while positional nystagmus may be prominent (Cohen *et al.*, 1969b). The major effect of cerebellar lesions on semicircular canal-induced nystagmus appears to be a loss of habituation on repeated stimulation (Singleton, 1967; Wolfe, 1968). Although these findings are consistent with the hypothesis that there may be a separation in pathways from otolith organs and semicircular canals, most of the evidence is indirect. Against this idea are findings by de Kleyn and Magnus (1920). They noted that all compensatory ocular reflexes were preserved in rabbits after cerebellar removal. This included counter-rolling produced by the otolith organs. Additional data are necessary before the role of the cerebellum in vestibular reflexes is better understood.

IV. PONTINE PATHWAYS FOR HORIZONTAL EYE MOVEMENTS

The vestibular organs respond to head movements in every spatial plane and compensatory eye and head movements are also induced in every spatial plane. Therefore, vestibulo-ocular pathways must carry activity which induces rotatory and vertical eye movements as well as horizontal eye movements. Pathways for downward or for rotatory eye movements probably terminate in the mesodiencephalon (Szentágothai, 1943; Hess *et al.*, 1946; Hassler and Hess, 1954; Hess, 1957; Hyde and Toczek, 1962; Pasik *et al.*, 1969). Lesions of the pretectum produce enduring paralysis of upward gaze, or of upward and downward gaze (Pasik *et al.*, 1966a, 1969a, b). The course of pathways which originate in the visual and vestibular systems and end in these regions is not entirely clear at present. Most of the direct projections for vertical eye movements induced by the vestibular system probably lie in the region of the MLF.

From the finding that lesions in the pretectum may affect vertical movements but leave horizontal movements intact (Pasik *et al.*, 1969a, b), or that lesions in the pons may affect horizontal eye movements and leave vertical movements intact (Bender and Shanzer, 1964; Pasik *et al.*, 1966a, 1969a, b; Cohen *et al.*, 1968), it would appear that there is a separation of neural activity which produces eye movements in various spatial planes at some point along oculomotor pathways. Pontine pathways from both the vestibular and

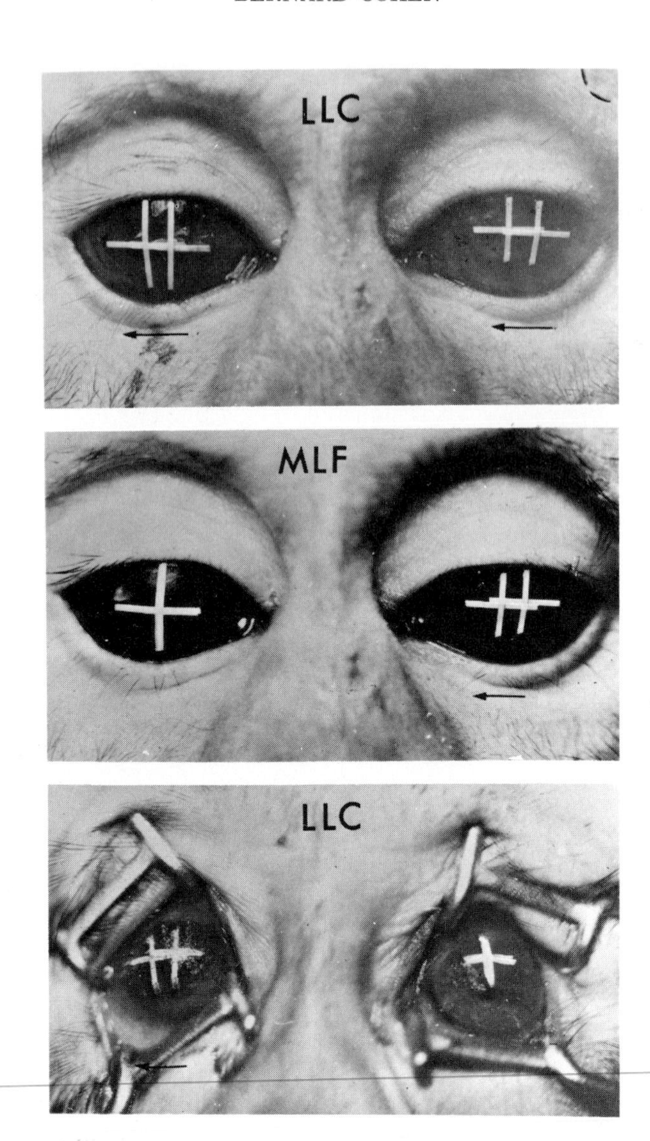

Fig. 7. Effects of a left MLF lesion on eye movements induced by left lateral canal nerve stimulation (LLC) in monkey. Top, conjugate horizontal eye movement to right induced by LLC stimulation before lesion. Middle, adduction of left eye induced by left MLF stimulation before lesion. Bottom, paralysis of adduction after MLF lesion. In response to LLC stimulation, the left eye now failed to move past the midline to the right. The right eye abducted normally, however. Double flash technique used in all three photographs. The underlying black arrows show the direction of movement.

visual systems which are important for producing horizontal eye movements will be discussed in the remainder of this report.

Direct pathways to the abducens nuclei

When impulses are added to one lateral semicircular canal nerve by electrical stimulation, ampullopetal angular acceleration, or caloric stimulation, the eyes initially move to the contralateral side (Fig. 7, top). Axons from cells in the vestibular nucleus on the side ipsilateral to the stimulus project across the brain stem to the contralateral abducens nucleus causing the opposite lateral rectus muscle to contract (Schaefer, 1965; Precht *et al.*, 1967, 1969; Baker *et al.*, 1969a, b). Electrical stimulation of the vestibular nerve also activates ipsilateral oculomotor nucleus motoneurons (Sasaki, 1963). Presumably some of the activated motoneurons in the 3rd nerve nucleus include cells in the ventral cell group which innervate the ipsilateral medial rectus muscle (Warwick, 1956, 1964). Ipsilateral lateral rectus motoneurons are concurrently inhibited by vestibular nerve stimulation or by appropriate angular acceleration (Schaefer, 1965; Richter and Precht, 1968; Precht *et al.*, 1969; Baker *et al.*, 1969b).

Two functional classes of units have been described in the abducens nucleus (Precht *et al.*, 1967, 1969; Horcholle and Dumont-Tyc, 1968, 1969). One group are the abducens motoneurons, themselves. Another group of cells does not project axons into the VI nerve. These cells are monosynaptically excited by ipsilateral vestibular nuclei stimulation and mediate inhibition onto abducens motoneurons. Motoneurons in the abducens nuclei have also been classified according to the types of muscle cells they innervate (Bach-y-Rita and Ito, 1966; Yamanaka and Bach-y-Rita, 1968; F. Ito *et al.*, 1969). This is considered by Bach-y-Rita and Peachey elsewhere in this volume.

The medial longitudinal fasciculus (MLF)

Axons connecting one vestibular nucleus to the contralateral abducens nucleus do not form a discrete bundle of fibers in crossing the midline, and there is no clear-cut clinical syndrome associated with interruption of these fibers. On the other hand direct projections from the vestibular nuclei to ipsilateral medial rectus motoneurons lie in the MLF, and eye findings which follow MLF lesions are characteristic. Because of its clinical importance, the role of the MLF in producing horizontal eye movements will be considered separately.

Afferent and efferent connections between the MLF and the vestibular nuclei have been described in this volume by Carpenter. Axons which ascend in the MLF from the vestibular system originate largely in the medial, lateral, and superior vestibular nuclei (Brodal and Pompeiano, 1957; Carpenter and McMasters, 1963; Szentágothai, 1964; McMasters *et al.*, 1966). The vestibular nuclei also receive descending projections through the MLF from the Interstitial Nuclei of Cajal (Pompeiano and Walberg, 1957). The descending fibers do not project to oculomotor neurons but instead excite inhibitory interneurons in the vestibular nuclei on the ipsilateral side. These primarily affect cells in the horizontal canal system (Markham *et al.*, 1966).

Portions of the vestibular nuclei which project through the MLF to the oculomotor, trochlear, and abducens nuclei in turn receive projections from the semicircular canals (McMasters *et al.*, 1966; Stein and Carpenter, 1967; Gacek, 1968, 1969). When individual semicircular canal nerves or vestibular nerves are stimulated, prominent potential changes are recorded at short latency in the region of the MLF on both sides of the brain stem (Cook *et al.*, 1969). These direct projections may be functionally related to rapid tonic deviations induced by the semicircular canals. The function of projections from the superior vestibular nucleus through the MLF is less certain (Szentágothai, 1964; McMasters *et al.*, 1966) and is considered by Carpenter in this volume.

The role which activity carried in the MLF plays in producing horizontal eye movements is still not entirely understood. It seems certain that the MLF is an important output pathway for activity causing adduction of the ipsilateral eye during horizontal eye movements. When one MLF is electrically stimulated, the ipsilateral eye adducts (Fig. 7, middle). Lesions of the MLF are followed by paralysis of adduction of the ipsilateral eye (Fig. 7, bottom; Spiller, 1924; Bender and Weinstein, 1944, 1950; Cogan, 1948; Cogan *et al.*, 1950; Smith and Cogan, 1959; Shanzer and Bender, 1959; Christoff *et al.*, 1960; Carpenter and McMasters, 1963; Bender and Shanzer, 1964; Carpenter and Strominger, 1965; Gonzalez and Reuben, 1967). There is also nystagmus in the contralateral eye when it abducts, and frequently spontaneous vertical nystagmus is present. Convergence is preserved, showing that the paralysis of adduction is supra-nuclear. This constellation of signs has been termed "anterior internuclear ophthalmoplegia." Except for paralysis of adduction of the ipsilateral eye, patterns of eye movements induced by semicircular canal nerve stimulation are generally maintained after lesions confined to the medial parts of the MLF (Shanzer, 1964; Shanzer *et al.*, 1964).

An electrolytic lesion which produced typical signs of the MLF syndrome in a monkey is shown in Fig. 8. The left MLF and left trochlear nucleus were destroyed (Fig. 8A), and fibers in the left MLF caudal to the lesion disappeared (Fig. 8B). Neurons in the ventral cell group of the left oculomotor nucleus lay close together and stained darkly, but there was no loss of these cells (Fig. 8C).

Initially in this animal the left eye did not cross the midline to the right in either slow or rapid eye movements. Later the adductive paresis was most manifest during rapid eye movements, i.e., during saccades and quick phases of nystagmus. Electrooculographic demonstration of the paresis of adduction in this monkey one year after lesion is shown in Figure 9. During both pendular rotation and OKN, the amplitude and maximum velocity of the quick phases to the left were approximately equal in both eyes. However, the amplitude and maximum velocity of the quick phases to the right in the left

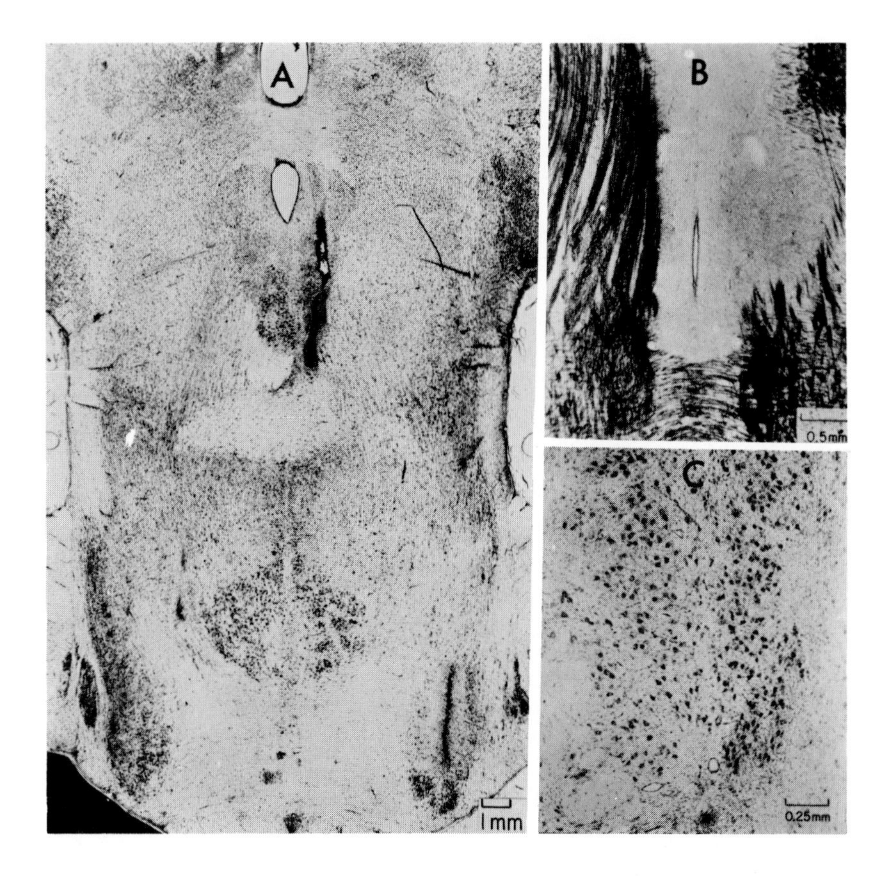

Fig. 8. Sections of brain stem of monkey 540 showing an electrolytic lesion of the left MLF and trochlear nucleus. Sections cut in vertical stereotaxic planes. Section A is through the center of the lesion. B. is caudal to it at the midpontine level, and C is rostral to it through the oculomotor nuclei. Cresyl violet and Weil stains.

eye were less than in the right eye (Fig. 9, OS & OS Vel, downward arrows). The duration of the quick phases in the left eye were also considerably prolonged. Carpenter and McMasters (1963) have also noted changes in eye movements after MLF lesions (See Carpenter this volume). Their findings that MLF lesions just rostral to the abducens nuclei did not produce permanent paralysis of adduction are similar to results in some of our animals. However they did not produce permanent paralysis of adduction by lesions in more rostral portions of the MLF. At present, there is no apparent explanation for this difference in findings.

It should be emphasized that the adductive paralysis after the MLF

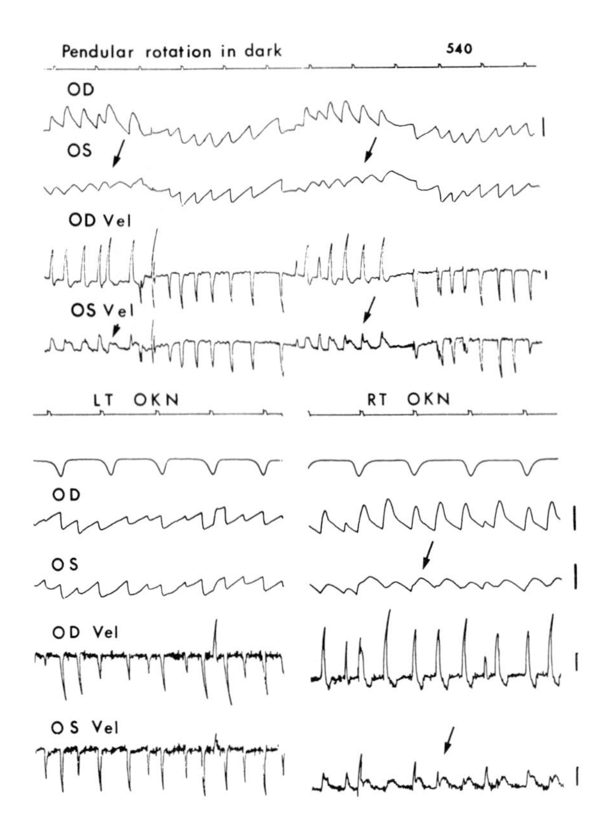

Fig. 9. Vestibular and optokinetic nystagmus (OKN) of monkey 540 one year after left MLF lesion shown in Figure 8. During pendular rotation the animal was rotated back and forth in darkness to induce vestibular nystagmus. Techniques for inducing OKN have been described in detail (Komatsuzaki *et al.*, 1969). The top trace in each recording is the time base (1 mark/sec). The second trace in OKN recordings registers the passage of drum stripes. The OKN drum was rotating at 90/sec. OD and OS refer to EOG recordings across right eye and left eye, respectively. The vertical bar on the right of the OD and OS traces is 10°. OD Vel and OS Vel are the differentiated recordings showing the velocity of the right and left eyes. The vertical bar on the right of the differentiated traces is 100°/sec. Note that the amplitude and velocity of quick phases of nystagmus to the left were of low amplitude and low maximum velocity (downward arrows)

lesion shown in Figure 9 was manifest during all types of rapid conjugate horizontal eye movements. This included spontaneous saccades and quick phases of nystagmus induced by visual and vestibular stimuli. This is also the case in humans after MLF lesions. Thus the MLF not only participates in eye movements induced by the vestibular apparatus, but is important for ipsilateral adduction during all types of rapid horizontal eye movements. This makes it unlikely that the paresis of adduction which was demonstrated in Figure 9 was due to destruction of the vestibular fibers which course through the MLF. Unless pathways from the visual system were to go through the vestibular nuclei, they could not gain access to neurons located in the vestibular nuclei which project through the MLF to medial rectus motoneurons during quick phases of OKN or during saccades. This seems unlikely for several reasons: (1) no such anatomic projections have been demonstrated; (2) changes in eye movements similar to those which follow MLF lesions are not caused by vestibular nuclei lesions (McMasters *et al.*, 1966). Therefore, there must be important extra-vestibular projections in the MLF or in the region of the MLF which end on oculomotor motoneurons. It is likely that destruction of these extra-vestibular projections is in large part responsible for the paralysis of adduction which has been described both clinically and experimentally.

Paramedian zone of the pontine reticular formation

If destruction of extra-vestibular axons in the MLF or in the region immediately adjacent to the MLF was responsible for the prolonged paresis of adduction during rapid eye movements, then the location of cells from which these axons arose is a matter of considerable interest. It is unlikely that these cells are located in the Interstitial Nucleus of Cajal, since destruction of the rostral brain stem does not produce adductive paralysis (Carpenter, this volume).

An alternative hypothesis is that they are situated in the paramedian zone of the pontine reticular formation (PPRF). The PPRF is not a discrete structure, but rather is a region of the pontine reticular formation which has been designated because of its apparent functional specificity (Bender and Shanzer, 1964). In the monkey the PPRF lies in the medial portions of Nucleus Reticularis Magnocellularis. It is bounded medially by the nuclei of the raphe and the MLF, dorsally by the brachium conjunctivum and gray matter of the floor of the fourth ventricle, and ventrally by the trapezoid body and roots of the abducens nerve. The lateral extent of this region is between 0.5 and 2 mm from the midline. Anteroposteriorly it extends from the trochlear to the abducens nuclei.

Anatomic evidence that cells in the PPRF project to medial rectus motoneurons through the MLF is generally lacking. The MLF's do not show striking degeneration after pontine lesions which produce conjugate gaze paralysis (Bender and Shanzer, 1964; Cohen *et al.*, 1968), but Nauta and Kuypers (1958) show two cases which had degeneration in the MLF after dorsal tegmental lesions (See their Figures 24-28, 34). Electrophysiological data provide some support for this idea. When the MLF was stimulated in the cat, field potential changes were induced on both sides of the pontine reticular formation at latencies less than 0.5 msec (Fig. 10A). In addition, cells on

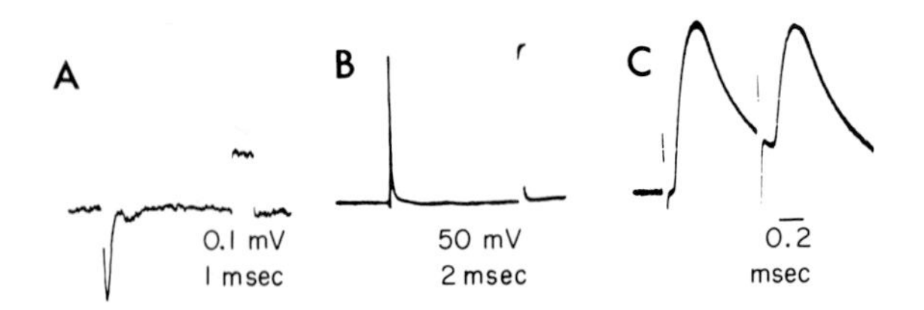

Fig. 10. A, Field potential changes induced in medial portions of the pontine reticular formation of cat by stimulation of the contralateral MLF at more rostral levels. B, C, Units in medial pontine reticular formation activated antidromically by MLF stimulation.

both sides of the PPFR were antidromically activated after MLF stimulation (Fig. 10B, C) (Nozue and Cohen, 1968). Thus there are cells located on both sides of the pontine reticular formation which project into the MLF or into the para-MLF region. Whether these cells end on medial rectus motoneurons and are active during rapid adductions has not been demonstrated.

Anatomic evidence that the PPRF contains neurons which project to oculomotor nuclei is stronger. Carpenter and McMasters (1963) noted retrograde changes in cells of Nucleus Reticularis Pontis Caudalis after a lesion in the region of the abducens nuclei which produced gaze paresis. Axons of neurons from the medial pontine reticular formation have been shown to project onto motoneurons in the oculomotor nucleus (Scheibel and Scheibel, 1958). Physiological data provide more support for the idea that portions of the pontine reticular formation are functionally linked to oculomotor and abducens nuclei. It will be reviewed in subsequent subsections.

Neuronal activity and potential changes in the PPRF before and during eye movements

Units on both sides of the pons are active during quick phases of nystagmus (Duensing and Schaefer, 1957a, b). In addition, gross potential changes in this region precede every rapid eye movement by 10-20 msec (Cohen and Feldman, 1968). Usually, but not invariably these potentials are of largest amplitude during saccades or quick phases of nystagmus to the ipsilateral side. Similar potentials which precede eye movements are not found elsewhere in the nervous system. It is postulated that these potential changes reflect activity in cells which generated these rapid eye movements (Cohen and Feldman, 1968).

In both the lateral geniculate body (LGB) and in the calcarine cortex of the monkey and the cat, there are potential changes which follow eye movements (Feldman and Cohen, 1967, 1968a, b; Brooks, 1968a, b). These are described elsewhere in this volume (Lehmann). When the pontine or mesencephalic reticular formation is stimulated, LGB potentials similar to those which accompany rapid eye movements are induced at short latency (Cohen and Feldman, 1968; Cohen *et al.*, 1969a). Presumably activity which produced the LGB potentials originated in the brain stem reticular formation.

Thus pontine potential changes which accompany rapid eye movements may also reflect activity in cells which produce potential changes in the lateral geniculate body which accompany rapid eye movements. Bizzi and Brooks (1963) have postulated a similar role for the PRF in generating PGO activity in cats during sleep.

Afferent input

There is both anatomic and physiologic evidence that the vestibular system projects into paramedian portions of the pontine reticular formation (Lorente de Nó, 1933b; Szentágothai, 1950, 1964; Gernandt and Thulin, 1952, Gernandt, 1964, 1968; Potthoff *et al.*, 1967a; Ladpli and Brodal, 1968). Information from a wide variety of other sensory modalities reaches units in the pontine reticular formation (Scheibel *et al.*, 1955; Potthoff *et al.*, 1967b). In addition, PPRF units are synaptically activated when parts of the brain which induce horizontal eye movements are stimulated (Cohen and Nozue, 1968). These include the vestibular system, the mesencephalic reticular formation, the fastigial nuclei, and the region of the MLF. Reticular formation units are also responsive to eye muscle stretch in both cat and goat (Cooper *et al.*, 1953; Fillenz, 1955; Whitteridge, 1960). It has recently been shown that unit activity in the pons generated by vestibular stimulation can be inhibited by eye muscle stretch (Gernandt, 1968). Thus there is interaction in the pontine reticular formation between afferent information from the vestibular system with that from ocular muscles themselves.

Stimulation

The direction of eye movements induced by electrical stimulation of the pons has been described in a number of reports (Monnier, 1945; Hyde and Eliasson, 1957; Bender and Shanzer, 1964). Horizontal eye movements are not induced by stimulation of lateral portions of the pontine reticular formation, but are induced when the medial pontine reticular formation, particularly the region of the PPRF, is electrically excited (Bender and Shanzer, 1964; Cohen *et al.*, 1967b). Examples of horizontal eye movements induced by PPRF stimulation are shown in Figure 11A, B. At the onset of stimulation the eyes moved conjugately to the right side. The latency of eye muscle activation after PPRF stimulation was short. In the animal whose records are shown in Figure 11C & D, the minimum latency of the onset of the potential change in the medial rectus muscle was 2.8 msec. If about 1 msec is allowed for synaptic delays at the oculomotor nucleus and medial rectus motor end plates, and about 0.5 msec for conduction along the third nerve, then only one or at most two neurons could be interposed between the PPRF stimulating electrode and eye muscle motor nuclei. This indicates that elements in the region of the PPRF lay close to eye muscle motoneurons in the projection pathway. In keeping with this, it was possible to drive eye muscle motor units synchronously at high frequencies by PPRF stimulation (Fig. 11D).

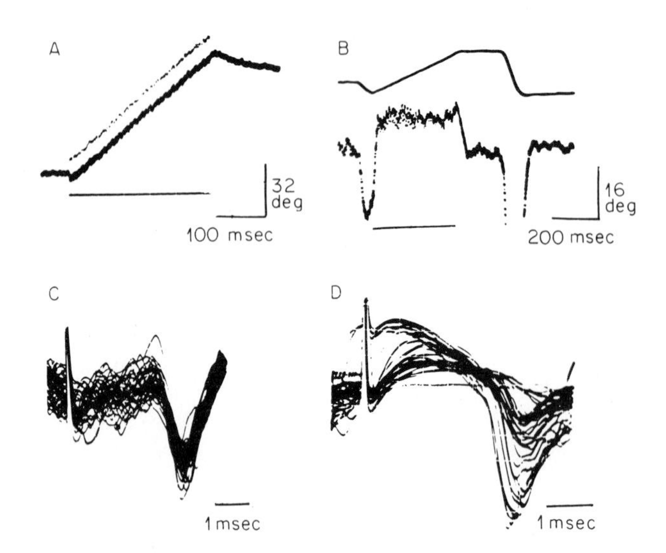

Fig. 11. A, B, Constant velocity eye movements induced by right PPRF stimulation. Single trace in A and upper trace in B is bitemporal EOG recorded with direct coupling. Lower trace in B is differentiated EOG. The duration of the stimulus is shown by the underlying horizontal bar. In A the stimulation frequency was 400/sec and in B 240/sec. C, D, Potential changes in left medial rectus muscle induced by right PPRF stimulation. 20 consecutive sweeps superimposed. PPRF stimulation was 1/sec in C and 100/sec in D.

Parenthetically, eye movements induced by PPRF stimulation are of interest because they are reproducibly of constant velocity over wide ranges of eye movement (Fig. 11A, B; Cohen *et al.*, 1967b). At various times during these constant velocity eye movements the extent of deviation must have been linearly related to the number of stimulating pulses which had been introduced up to that moment. This suggests that the stimulating pulses had been integrated by neural organizations in the pons which were activated by the stimulus. Stimulation of other parts of the nervous system with constant frequencies generally does not induce eye movements of constant velocity (Cooper and Eccles, 1930; Suzuki and Cohen, 1966; Robinson and Fuchs, 1969). Constant velocity movements frequently occur during pursuit movements and slow phases of caloric and optokinetic nystagmus. Whether PPRF stimulation activated input pathways to neural organizations which are also responsible for pursuit movements and slow phases is conjectural at present.

Effects of lesions

Changes in eye movements after PPRF lesions provide additional support for the hypothesis that the PPRF plays an important role in producing both slow and rapid horizontal eye movements. After unilateral lesions of

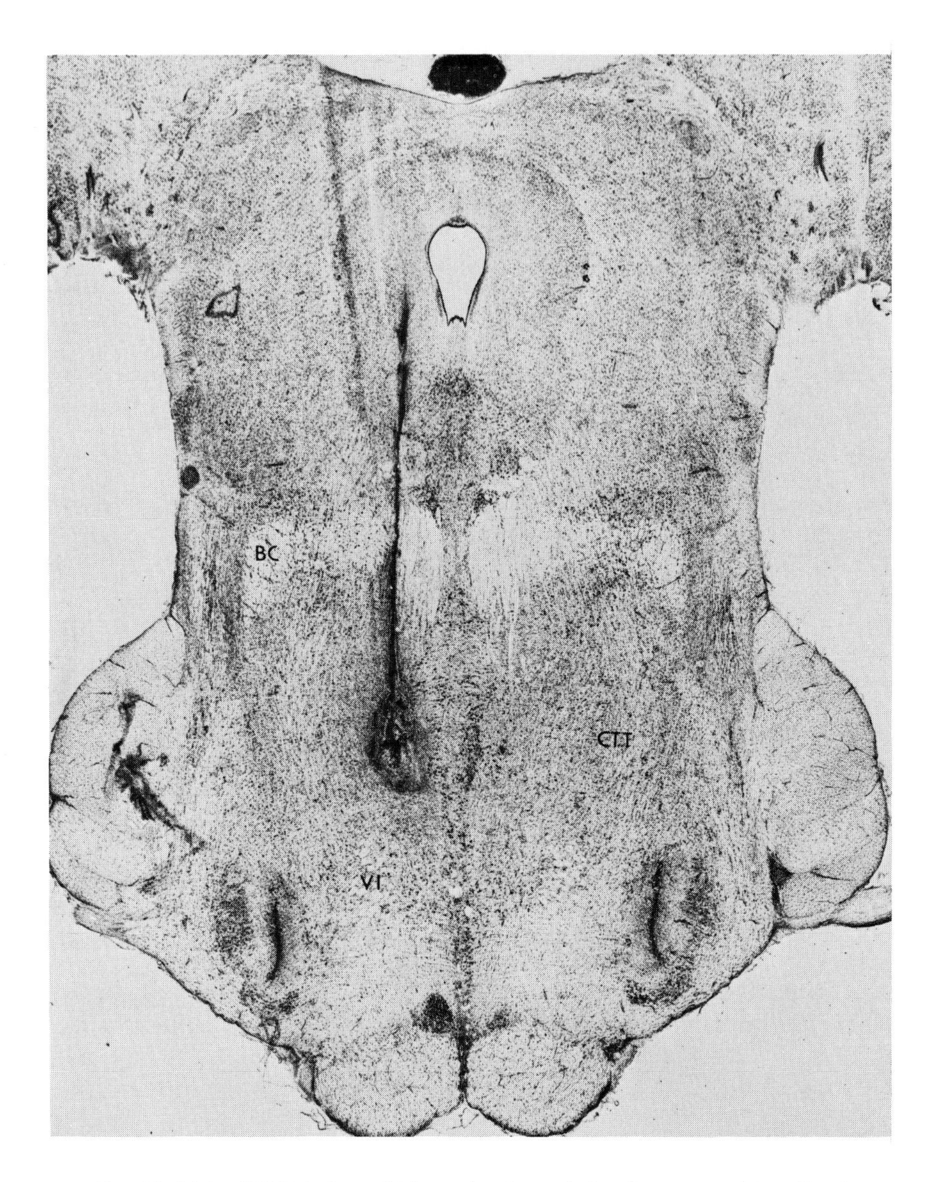

Fig. 12. Right PPRF lesion which produced paralysis of gaze to right. Cresyl violet stain. Section cut in vertical stereotaxic plane. Lesion is dorsal to VI nerve rootlets (VI) and trapezoid body, lateral to the nuclei of the median raphe, ventral to the brachium conjunctivum (BC), and medial to the central tegmental tract (CTT).

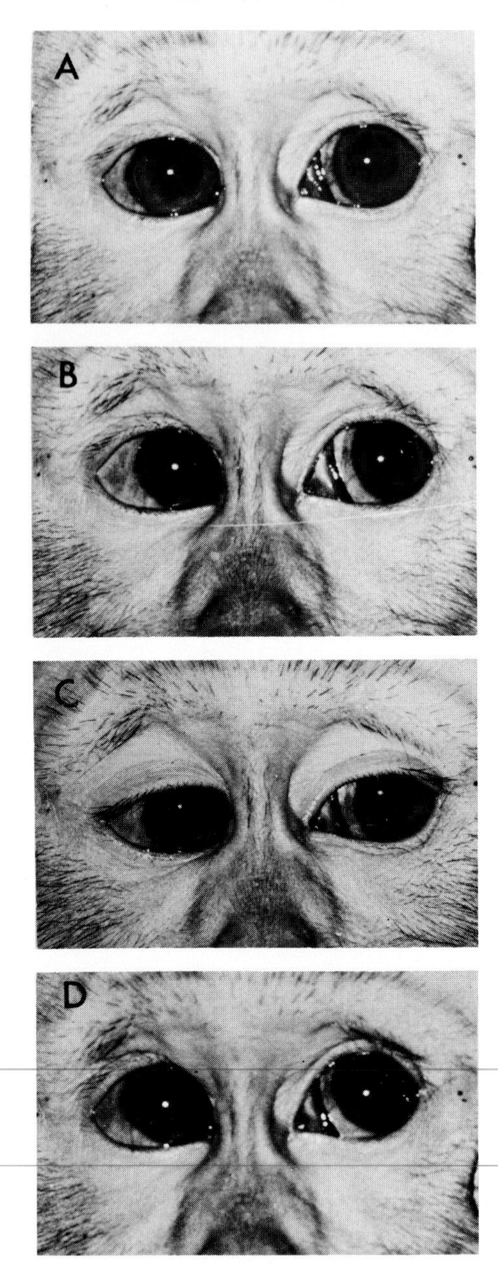

Fig. 13. Extent of horizontal excursion of eyes to right (A) and to left (B) after right PPRF lesion. Despite limited horizontal movement, downward (C) and upward (D) movement of the eyes were preserved.

the PPRF, there is paralysis of conjugate horizontal gaze to the ipsilateral side (Freeman, 1922; Shanzer *et al.*, 1958; Teng *et al.*, 1958; Shanzer and Bender, 1959; Bender and Shanzer, 1964; Cohen *et al.*, 1968). A lesion of the right paramedian zone of the pontine reticular formation which produced long lasting paralysis of conjugate gaze to the right in a monkey is shown in Figure 12. Before the lesion potential changes which preceded rapid eye movements were recorded through these electrodes, and constant velocity eye movements were induced by stimulation.

After the lesion the eyes were constantly to the left of the midline. The limits of excursion of the eyes to the left and right several days after a similar right PPRF lesion in another monkey are shown in Figure 13. Vertical movements were not impaired. The eyes did not cross to the right side of the midline for about six weeks. During this period, therefore, there were no eye movements or positions of fixation in the right hemifield of movement in either eye. In the left hemifield of movement quick phases of nystagmus and saccades to the right were initially absent and were defective for several months thereafter.

These defects are shown in Figure 14 which was recorded 32 days after a right PPRF lesion. The eyes moved mainly in the left hemifield of movement. In response to an optokinetic drum moving to the animal's right at 90°/sec, vigorous optokinetic nystagmus was induced to the left (Fig. 14A, Lt. OKN). The velocity of both the quick phases to the left (Vel) and of the slow phases to the right (SP Vel) were within normal limits. On the other hand during Rt OKN (Fig. 14B), the quick phases to the right were of small amplitude, high frequency, and low maximum velocity. Instead of nystagmus, there was a strong tonic deviation of the eyes to the left, i.e., in the direction of the slow phases. During pendular rotation in this animal, it was possible to induce tonic deviations to the left and to the right in the left hemifield of movement which were of the same velocity. Therefore, it seems likely that the primary defect in the left hemifield was in the quick phase rather than in the slow phase mechanism (Komatsuzaki and Cohen, unpublished data). Changes after PPRF lesions have been described in a previous report (Cohen *et al.*, 1968).

In some animals ipsilateral saccades and quick phases of nystagmus have been permanently abolished after lesions of the paramedian zone, although slow movements across the midline have recovered. In other animals with larger lesions all movements to the ipsilateral side were affected for long periods of time. Lorente de Nó (1933b) initially showed that all horizontal eye movements are lost after lesions in the pontine reticular formation on both sides. This was disputed by Spiegel and Price (1939), but has recently been corroborated by Bender and Shanzer (1964), McCabe (1965) and in our own studies (Komatsuzaki and Cohen, unpublished data). Vertical eye movements are usually normal after small lesions of the pons. Larger lesions which extend across the midline, however, can abolish eye movements in all directions (Freeman, 1922; Bender, 1960; Bender and Shanzer, 1964).

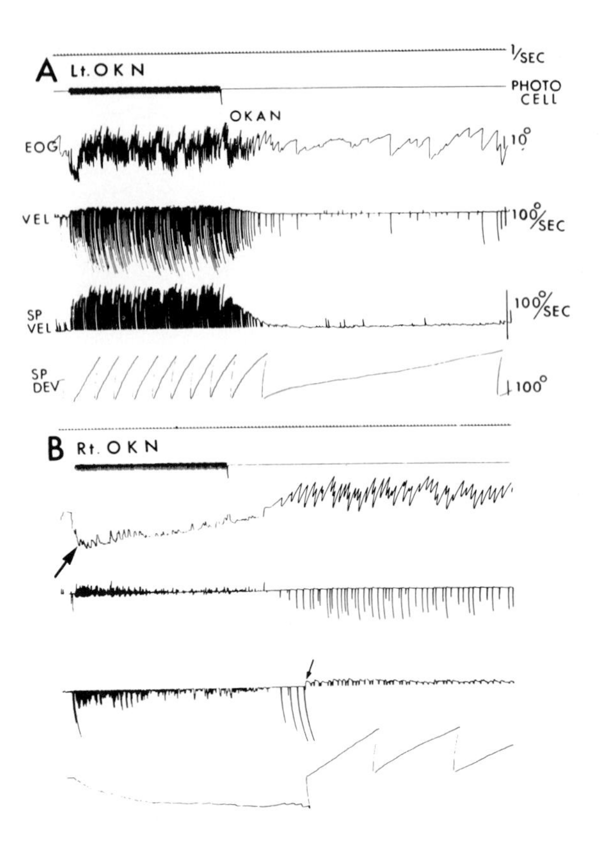

Fig. 14. Optokinetic nystagmus (OKN) recorded 32 days after a right PPRF lesion. From top to bottom in A & B the traces record the time base at 1 mark/sec, the passage of OKN drum stripes, the DC-EOG, the differentiated EOG (Vel), the differentiated EOG rectified and amplified to show slow phase eye velocity (SP Vel), and the integrated slow phase eye velocity showing total deviation of the eyes during slow phases (SD Dev). Calibration of each trace is given by the vertical bar on the right and is 10° for the EOG, 100°/sec for differentiated records, and 100° for integrated slow phase velocity. At the end of optokinetic stimulation the lights were extinguished and the animal was in complete darkness for the remainder of the recording. During this time optokinetic after-nystagmus (OKAN) was recorded. The upward arrow in B under the EOG shows the strong deviation of the eyes to the left induced by OKN drum movement to the left. At the downward arrow the direction of rectification was reversed so as to record the velocity of slow phases of the nystagmus to the left. From Cohen, B., Komatsuzaki, A. & Bender, M.B. (1968). *Archs Neurol., Chicago* **18,** 78-92. *Courtesy of American Medical Association Press.*

Carpenter *et al.*, (1963) have produced gaze paralysis after lesions in the region of the abducens nuclei. They note, however, that it is unlikely that this paralysis is produced by destruction of cells in the abducens nuclei. Rather they attribute it to interruption of axons of cells which lie outside the abducens nuclei but which pass through this region. There was no involvement of the right abducens nucleus in the monkey whose lesion is shown in Figure 12.

Lesions of similar size elsewhere in the nervous system do not cause conjugate gaze paralysis (Pasik *et al.*, 1959, 1960, 1966; Bender and Shanzer, 1964; Pasik and Pasik, 1964; Wagman, 1964; Harris *et al.*, 1967; Cohen *et al.*, 1968). Only after much larger lesions, such as after hemispherectomy (Pasik *et al.*, 1960; Pasik and Pasik, 1964), or in patients with large or expanding cerebral tumors can a similar type of gaze defect be produced, and it is usually temporary. Instead after cerebral lesions, gaze preference is more often found (Bender and Shanzer, 1964). During gaze preference due to cerebral lesions, the eyes are usually deviated to the same side, but can cross the midline in response to a vestibular or auditory stimulus (Pasik *et al.*, 1960; Jung and Kornhuber, 1964; Harris *et al.*, 1967). After lesions of the mesencephalic reticular formation the amplitude and velocity of quick phases can be equal in both directions and caloric nystagmus may be entirely normal. However, the slow phases of OKN with quick phases to the opposite side may be permanently defective (Harris *et al.*, 1967). After vestibular nuclei lesions either caloric nystagmus or positional nystagmus may be abnormal (Uemura and Cohen, unpublished data).

From the foregoing data it is possible to speculate on the role that neural organizations in each half of the pons play in producing horizontal eye movements. It seems likely that neural groups in each half of the PPRF contribute importantly to production of saccades and quick phases of nystagmus to the ipsilateral side in either hemifield of movement. In addition, each half of the pons appear to exert strong control over positions of fixation in the ipsilateral half field of movement, and to participate in inducing slow horizontal eye movements in both directions in that half field. Whether the changes in fixation and in slow eye movements are due to damage to neural groups or to interruption of afferent pathways to eye muscle motor nuclei is still not entirely clear. The former seems most likely. From these data it is apparent that neural groups which produce slow and rapid eye movements must be at least partially separate. It has been clear from the work of Westheimer (1954a, b) and Rashbass (1961) that this is likely to be the case.

The foregoing does not imply that all pathways or neural groups which produce horizontal eye movements lie in the PPRF. Direct pathways to abducens and oculomotor nuclei from the vestibular system which bypass the PPRF have been noted in this report. There may also be direct descending pathways from the visual system as well as ascending or descending multisynaptic pathways which reach oculomotor and abducens motoneurons by other routes. Neither does it imply that the PPRF is solely concerned with horizontal eye movements since potential changes are recorded in this area which precede vertical as well as horizontal eye movements. Furthermore, there are changes in vertical eye movements after large or bilateral PPRF lesions. However, the conclusion that the PPRF is the general locus of neural groups which play an important role in producing horizontal eye movements seems sound. Identification of the cells actually responsible for these movements and the characteristics of their neural activity is a matter for future study.

SUMMARY

(1) The vestibular system codes information about the relationship of the head to surrounding space and induces eye movements which promote vision. These eye movements lie in all spatial planes and are most commonly compensatory, i.e., they tend to oppose head deviations and maintain the angle of vision. Patterns and characteristics of eye movements induced by semicircular canals and otolith organs have been briefly described. When one canal or its nerves are activated, the eyes and head move in spatial planes parallel to the plane of the excited canal regardless of the position of the eyes in the orbit or of the head on the neck. Static head tilt activates the otolith organs which induce compensatory ocular counter-rolling. Eye movements induced by natural stimulation of individual utricles and saccules are not entirely clear. When utricular nerves are stimulated, conjugate rotatory eye movements are induced with intorsion of the ipsilateral eye and extorsion of the contralateral eye.

(2) The organization of the vestibular nuclei has been briefly considered. Data are still insufficient to permit an adequate description of the role of individual vestibular nuclei in oculomotor function. For the most part projections from the otolith organs and the semicircular canals end in different regions of the vestibular nuclei. This suggests that ocular reflexes induced by these receptors may be separately processed. In stimulation studies eye movements in different planes of space have been induced by stimulation of different parts of the vestibular nuclei. The effects of lesions of individual vestibular nuclei on vestibulo-ocular reflexes are not well understood.

(3) There are two potential pathways by which activity in vestibular nuclei can reach eye muscle motor nuclei. One lies in the brain stem, the other in the cerebellum. It seems likely that much of the activity from the semicircular canals which reaches eye muscle motor nuclei travels through the brain stem. Anatomical evidence and findings after cerebellar lesions suggest that pathways through the cerebellum might participate in utriculo-ocular and sacculo-ocular reflexes.

(4) Pathways from vestibular nuclei to eye muscle motor nuclei through the brain stem which mediate activity for horizontal eye movements have been considered in detail. Activity from vestibular nuclei can reach appropriate oculomotor nuclei via direct commissural fibers, the median longitudi-

nal fasciculus (MLF), or through the pontine reticular formation. Direct pathways from the vestibular system which mediate activity for vertical gaze appear to lie in the region of the MLF, but the location of multisynaptic pathway which carry this activity is still obscure.

The role of the MLF in producing horizontal eye movements is of interest because of the characteristic oculomotor findings which occur after it is destroyed. After MLF lesions, one of the salient changes in eye movements is paralysis or paresis of ipsilateral adduction during rapid eye movements, i.e., during saccades and quick phases of nystagmus. All rapid adductive eye movements are similarly affected whether induced by vestibular or by visual stimuli. It seems unlikely that destruction of the prominent vestibular projections through the MLF to the medial rectus motoneurons is primarily responsible for the adductive paresis during rapid eye movements. Instead it is postulated that there is a separate extra-vestibular projection in the MLF or in the region of the MLF which carried activity responsible for these deviations.

Evidence that neural organizations and pathways important for producing horizontal eye movements are located in the paramedian zone of the pontine reticular formation (PPRF) has been reviewed. There is anatomical evidence that neurons in this region project to oculomotor neurons. Unit activity and gross potential changes in the PPRF lead rapid horizontal eye movements. Cells in the PPRF are synaptically activated by stimulation of parts of the brain which induce horizontal eye movement. Eye movements are induced at short latency by stimulation of the PPRF. After PPRF lesions there is paralysis of conjugate gaze to the ipsilateral side. From the data which has been presented, it seems likely that neural organizations which generate rapid horizontal eye movements lie in the PPRF. In addition, pathways or neural groups important for producing slow eye movements also appear to be located in the PPRF.

ACKNOWLEDGEMENT

I should like to acknowledge the collaboration of Drs. Jack Alpert, Atsushi Komatsuzaki, Hana Krejcova and Michihiko Nozue in experiments on the MLF, pontine reticular formation and counter-rolling, and the assistance of Mr. David Borras, Mr. Edward Murray and Mrs. Diana Cabrera.

REFERENCES

ADES, H.W. & ENGSTROM, H. (1965). Form and innervation of the vestibular epithelia. **In** *The Role of the Vestibular Organs in the Exploration of Space,* NASA SP-77, Washington, D.C.

ADRIAN, E.D. (1943). Discharges from vestibular receptors in the cat. *J. Physiol.* **101,** 389-407.

ANGAUT, P. & BRODAL, A. (1967). The projection of the "vestibulo-cerebellum" onto the vestibular nuclei in the cat. *Archs ital. Biol.* **105,** 441-479.

ASCHAN, G., BERGSTEDT, M. & STAHLE, J. (1956a). Nystagmography. *Acta oto-lar.* Suppl. **129,** 1-103.

ASCHAN, G. BERGSTEDT, L., GOLDBERG, L. & LAURELL, L. (1956b). Positional nystagmus in man during and after alcohol intoxication. *Quart. J. Alcohol. Dis.* **17,** 381-405.

ASCHAN, G., BERGSTEDT, M. & GOLDBERG, L. (1964a). Positional alcohol nystagmus in patients with unilateral and bilateral labyrinthine destructions. *Confin. Neurol.* **24,** 80-102.

ASCHAN, G., EKVALL, L. & GRANT. G. (1964b). Nystagmus following stimulation in the central vestibular pathways using permanently implanted electrodes. *Acta oto-lar.* Suppl. **192,** 63-77.

ATKIN, A. & BENDER, M.B. (1968). Ocular stabilization during oscillatory head movements; Vestibular system dysfunction and the relation between head and eye velocities. *Archs. Neurol.,* Chicago, **18,** 559-566.

AZZENA, G.B. (1966). Otolithic influences on the unitary discharge of the oculomotor nucleus. *Brain Res.* **2,** 218-232.

AZZENA, G.B. & GIRETTI, M.L. (1967). Responses of the oculomotor units to deep cerebellar stimulation. *Brain Res.* **6,** 523-534.

BÁRÁNY, R. (1906). Augenbewegungen durch Thoraxbewegungen ausgelost. *Zentbl. Phyiologie,* **20,** 298-302.

BÁRÁNY, R. (1907). *Physiologie und Pathologie des Bogengangapparates beim Menschen.* Leipzig u. Vienna: Franz Deuticke.

BÁRÁNY, R. (1911). Experimentelle alcohol intoxication. *Monatschr. f. Ohrenh.* **45,** 959-962.

BÁRÁNY, R. (1913). Dauernde Veranderugen des spontanen Nystagmus bei Veranderungen der Kopflage. *Monatschr. f. Ohrenh.* **47,** 481.

BENDER, M.B. & WEINSTEIN, E.A. (1944). Effects of stimulation and lesion of the medial longitudinal fasciculus in the monkey. *Archs. Neurol. Psychiat.,* Chicago **52,** 106-113.

BENDER, M.B. & WEINSTEIN, E.A. (1950). The syndrome of the median longitudinal fasciculus. *Proc. Assoc. R.es. Nerv. Ment. Dis.* **28,** 414-420.

BENDER, M.B. (1960). Comments on the physiology and pathology of eye movements in the vertical plane. *J. Nerv. & Ment. Diseases,* **130,** 454-466.

BENDER, M.B. (Ed.). (1964). *The Oculomotor System.* New York: Harper & Row (Hoeber).

BENDER, M.B. & SHANZER, S. (1964). Oculomotor pathways defined by electric stimulation and lesion in the brain stem of monkey. **In** Bender, M.B., *The Oculomotor System.* New York: Harper & Row (Hoeber).

BENDER, M.B., FELDMAN, M. & ATKIN, A. (1965). Optic illusions in lesions of the vestibular system. **In** *Proceedings of the International Symposium on Vestibular and Oculomotor Problems.* Tokyo: Nippon Hoechst.

BENDER, M.B. & FELDMAN, M. (1967). Visual illusions during head movement in lesions of the brain stem. *Archs Neurol.* Chicago **17,** 354-364.

BACH-Y-RITA, P. & ITO, F. (1966). In vivo studies on fast and slow muscle fibers in cat extraocular muscles. *J. Gen. Physiol.* **49,** 1177-1198.

BAKER, R.G., MANO, N. & SHIMAZU, H. (1969a). Intracellular recording of antidromic responses from abducens motoneurons in the cat. *Brain Res.* **15,** 573-576.

BAKER, R.G., MANO, N. & SHIMAZU, H. (1969b). Postsynaptic potentials in abducens motoneurons induced by vestibular stimulation. *Brain Res.* **15,** 577-580.

BENDER, M.B. (1969). Disorders of eye movements. **In** *Handbook of Clinical Neurology*. Amsterdam: North Holland Publishing Co.

BENJAMINS, C.E. & HUIZINGA, E. (1927). Untersuchungen uber die Funktion des Vestibular apparates bei der Taube. *Pflugers Arch. ges. Physiol.* **217,** 105-123.

BERGSTEDT, M. (1961). Studies of positional nystagmus in the human centrifuge. *Acta oto-lar.* Suppl. **165,** 1-144.

BIEMOND, A. & DE JONG, J.M.B.V. (1969). On cervical nystagmus and related disorders. *Brain* **92,** 437-458.

BIZZI, E. & BROOKS, D.C. (1963). Functional connections between pontine reticular formation and lateral geniculate nucleus during deep sleep. *Archs ital. Biol.* **101,** 666-680.

BOS, J.H., JONGKEES, L.B.W. & PHILIPSZOON, A.J. (1964). On the direction of spontaneous and positional nystagmus. *Confin. Neurol.* **24,** 103-116.

BREUER, J. (1874). Uber die Funktion der Bogangange des Ohrlabyrinthes. *Med. Jahrb.* **4,** 72-124.

BREUER, J. (1875). Beitrage fur Lehre von statischen Sinne (Gleichgewichtsorgan, Vestibularapparat des Ohrlabyrinths. *Med. Jahrb.* **5,** 86-156.

BREUER, J. (1889). Neue Versuche an den Ohrbogengagen. *Pfluger Arch. ges. Physiol.* **44,** 135-152.

BREUER, J. (1891). Uber die Funktion der Otolithen-Apparate. *Pflugers Arch. ges. Physiol.* **48,** 195-306.

BRODAL, A. & POMPEIANO, O. (1957). The origin of ascending fibres of the medial longitudinal fasciculus from the vestibular nuclei. An experimental study in the cat. *Acta Morph. Neerl. Scand.* **1,** 306-328.

BRODAL, A. & TORVIK, A. (1957). Uber den Ursprung der sekundaren vestibulocerebellaren Fasern bei der Katz. Eine experimentell-anatomische Studie. *Arch. Psychiat. Nervenkr.* **195,** 550-567.

BRODAL, A. (1958). *The Reticular Formation of the Brain Stem, Anatomical Aspects and Functional Correlations.* Springfield, Ill. Charles C. Thomas.

BRODAL, A., POMPEIANO, O. & WALBERG, F. (1962). *The Vestibular Nuclei and Their Connections, Anatomy and Functional Correlations.* Springfield, Ill., Charles C. Thomas.

BRODAL, A. (1964a). Anatomical organization and fiber connections of the vestibular nuclei **In** *Neurological Aspects of Auditory and Vestibular Disorders.* Springfield, Ill., Charles C. Thomas.

BRODAL, A. (1964b). Anatomical observations on the vestibular nuclei with special reference to their relations to the spinal cord and cerebellum. *Acta oto-lar.* Suppl. **192,** 24-51.

BROOKS, D.C. (1968a). Waves associated with eye movement in the awake and sleeping cat. *Electroen. Neurophysiol.* **24,** 532-541.

BROOKS, D.C. (1968b). Localization and characteristics of the cortical waves associated with eye movement in the cat. *Expl. Neurol.* **22,** 603-613.

BROWN, J.H. & CRAMPTON, G.H. (1966). Concomitant visual stimulation does not alter habituation of nystagmic, oculogyral or psychophysical responses to angular acceleration. *Acta oto-lar.* **61,** 80-91.

BUCHANAN, A.R. (1940). Nystagmus and eye deviations in guinea pigs with lesions in the brain stem. *Laryngoscope* **50,** 1002-1011.

CAMIS, M. & CREED, R.S. (1930). *The Physiology of the Vestibular Apparatus.* London: Oxford Univ. Press (Clarendon).

CARPENTER, M. B. (1959). Lesions of the fastigial nuclei in the rhesus monkey. *Am. J. Anat.* **104,** 1-34.

CARPENTER, M. B., BARD, D. S. & ALLING, F. A. (1959). Anatomical connections between the fastigial nuclei, the labyrinth and the vestibular nuclei in the cat. *J. comp. Neurol.* **111**, 1-26

CARPENTER, M.B. (1960). Fiber projections from the descending and lateral vestibular nuclei in the cat. *Am. J. Anat.* **107,** 1-22.

CARPENTER, M.B., ALLING, F.A. & BARD, D.S. (1960). Lesions of the descending vestibular nucleus in the cat. *J. comp. Neurol.* **114,** 39-50.

CARPENTER, M.B., MCMASTERS, R.E. & HANNA, G.R. (1963). Disturbances of conjugate horizontal eye movements in the monkey. I. Physiological effects and anatomical degeneration resulting from lesions of the abducens nucleus and nerve. *Archs Neurol.,* Chicago **8,** 231-247.

CARPENTER, M.B. & MCMASTERS, R.E. (1963). Disturbances of conjugate horizontal eye movements in the monkey. II. Physiological effects and anatomical degeneration resulting from lesions of the medial longitudinal fasciculus. *Archs Neurol.,* Chicago **8,** 347-368.

CARPENTER, M.B. & STROMINGER, N.L. (1964). Cerebello-oculomotor fibers in the rhesus monkey. *J. comp. Neurol.* **123,** 211-230.

CARPENTER, M.B. & STROMINGER, N.L. (1965). The medial longitudinal fasciculus and disturbances of conjugate horizontal eye movements in the monkey. *J. comp. Neurol.* **125,** 41-66.

CAWTHORNE, T., DIX, M.R. HALLPIKE, C.S. & HOOD, J.D. (1956). The investigation of vestibular function. *Br. med. Bull.* **12,** 131-142.

CAWTHORNE, T., DIX, M.R., HOOD, J.D. & HARRISON, M.S. (1969). Vestibular syndromes and vertigo. In *Handbook of Clinical Neurology,* vol. 2, ed. Vinken, P.J. & Bruyn, G.W. Amsterdam: North Holland Publishing Co.

CHRISTOFF, N., ANDERSON, P., NATHANSON, M. & BENDER, M.B. (1960). Problems in anatomic analysis of lesions of the median longitudinal fasciculus. *Archs Neurol.* Chicago **2,** 293-304.

COGAN, D.G. (1948). *Neurology of the Ocular Muscles.* Springfield, Ill., Charles C. Thomas.

COGAN, D.G., KUBIK, C.S. & SMITH, W.L. (1950). Unilateral internuclear ophthalmoplegia. Report of eight clinical cases with one post-mortem study. *Archs Ophthal.,* Chicago 44, 783-796.

COHEN, B. & SUZUKI, J. (1963). Eye movements induced by ampullary nerve stimulation. *Am. J. Physiol.* **204,** 347-351.

COHEN, B., SUZUKI, J. & BENDER, M.B. (1964). Eye movements from semicircular canal nerve stimulation in the cat. *Ann. Otol. Rhinol. Lar.* **73,** 153-169.

COHEN, B., SUZUKI, J. & BENDER, M.B. (1965a). Nystagmus induced by electric stimulation of ampullary nerves. *Acta oto-lar.* **60,** 422-436.

COHEN, B., GOTO, K., SHANZER, S. and WEISS, A.H. (1965b). Eye movements induced by electric stimulation of the cerebellum in the alert cat. *Expl. Neurol.* **13,** 145-162.

COHEN, B., TOKUMASU, K. & GOTO, K. (1966). Semicircular canal nerve, eye and head movements: The effect of changes in initial eye and head position on the plane of the induced movement. *Archs Ophthal.,* Chicago **76,** 523-531.

COHEN, B., GOTO, K. & TOKUMASU, K. (1967a). Return eye movements, An ocular compensatory reflex in the alert cat and monkey. *Expl. Neurol.* **17,** 172-185.

COHEN, B., KOMATSUZAKI, A. & HARRIS, H.E. (1967b). Characteristics of pontine pathways for conjugate gaze. *Trans. Amer. Neurol. Assoc.* **92,** 219-220.

COHEN, B., KOMATSUZAKI, A. & BENDER, M.B. (1968). Electrooculographic syndrome in monkeys after pontine reticular formation lesions. *Archs Neurol.,* Chicago **18,** 78-92.

COHEN, B. & FELDMAN, M. (1968). Relationship of electrical activity in pontine reticular formation and lateral geniculate body to rapid eye movements. *J. Neurophysiol.* **31,** 806-817.

COHEN, B. & NOZUE, M. (1968). The pontine reticular formation and horizontal eye movements. *Proc. of Int. Union of Physiol. Sci.* **7,** 89.

COHEN, B., FELDMAN, M. & DIAMOND, S.P. (1969a). Effects of eye movement, brain stem stimulation, and alertness on transmission through the lateral geniculate body of monkey. *J. Neurophysiol.* **32,** 583-594.

COHEN, B., KOMATSUZAKI, A. & ALPERT, J. (1969b). Positional nystagmus after lesions of the cerebellum. *Proc. IX Int. Congr. Neurol.* **193,** 198-199.

COHEN, B., KREJCOVA, H. & HIGHSTEIN, S. (1970). Ocular counter-rolling induced by static head tilt in the monkey. *Fed. Proc.* **29, 454.**

COHEN, B. (1970). Vestibulo-ocular reflex arcs. Chapt. 4.4 **In** *The Vestibular System,* vol. VI, *Handbook of Sensory Physiology,* ed., Kornhuber, H.H. Springer (In press).

Collegium Oto-Rhino-Laryngologicum. (1961). *Acta oto-lar.* Suppl. **163.**

COLLINS, W.E. & UPDEGRAFF, B.P. (1966). A comparison of nystagmus habituation in the cat and the dog. *Acta oto-lar.* **62,** 19-26.

COLLINS, W.E. (1966). Vestibular responses from figure skaters. *Aerospace Med.* **37:** 1098-1104.

COLLINS, W.E. (1969). Modification of vestibular nystagmus and "vertigo" by means of visual stimulation. *Trans. Amer. Acad. Ophthal. Otolaryng.* **72,** 962-979.

COOK, W.A. Jr., CANGIANO, A. & POMPEIANO, O. (1969). An electrical investigation of the efferent pathway from the vestibular nuclei. *Archs ital. Biol.* **107:** 235-274.

COOPER, S. & ECCLES, J.C. (1930). The isometric response of mammalian muscle. *J. Physiol.* **69:** 377-385.

COOPER, S., DANIEL, P.M. & WHITTERIDGE, D. (1953). Nerve impulses in the brain stem of the goat. II. Responses with long latencies obtained by stretching the extrinsic eye muscles. *J. Physiol.* **120:** 491-513.

CRAMPTON, G.H. (1962). Directional imbalance of vestibular nystagmus in cat following repeated unidirectional angular acceleration. *Acta oto-lar* **55:** 41-48.

CRAMPTON, G.H. (1964). Habituation of ocular nystagmus of vestibular origin. **In** Bender, M.B., *The Oculomotor System.* New York: Harper & Row (Hoeber).

CRANMER, R. (1951). Nystagmus related to lesions of the central vestibular apparatus and the cerebellum. *Ann. Otol. Rhinol. Lar.* **60:** 186-196.

CRUM-BROWN, A. (1874). On the sense of rotation and the anatomy and physiology of the semi-circular canals of the inner ear. *J. Anat. Physiol.* 8:327-331.

DEKLEYN, A. (1920). Tonischer Labyrinthreflex auf die Augenmuskeln. *Pflugers Arch. ges Physiol.* **178:** 179-192.

DEKLEYN, A. & MAGNUS, R. (1920). Uber die Unabhangigkeit der Labyrinthreflexe vom Kleinhirn und uber die Lage der Zentren fur die Labyrinthreflexe im Hirnstamm. *Pflugers Arch. ges. Physiol.* **178:** 124-178.

DEKLEYN, A. & VERSTEEGH, C. (1930). Experimentelle Untersuchungen uber den sogenannten Lagennnystagmus wahrend akuter Alkoholvergiftung beim Kaninchen. *Acta oto-lar.* **14:** 356-377.

DEREUCK, A.V.S. & KNIGHT, J. (Eds.) (1967). *Myotatic, Kinesthetic, and Vestibular Mechanisms.* Boston: Little Brown & Co.

DESOLE, C. & PALLESTRINI, E.A. (1969). Responses of vestibular units to stimulation of individual semicircular canals. *Expl. Neurol.* **24:** 310-324.

DEVITO, R.V., BRUSA, A. & ARDUINI, A. (1956). Cerebellar and vestibular influences on Deitersian units. *J. Neurophysiol.* **19:** 241-253.

DIX, M.R. & HALLPIKE, C.S. (1952). The pathology, symptomatology and diagnosis of certain common disorders of the vestibular system. *Proc. R. Soc. Med.* **45:** 341-354.

DODGE, R. (1923). Adequacy of reflex compensatory eye-movements including the effects of neural rivalry and competition. *J. exp. Psychol.* **6:** 169-181.

DOHLMAN, G. (1925). Physikalische und physiologische Studien zur Theorie des Kalorischen Nystagmus. *Acta oto-lar.* Suppl. **5:.**

DOW, R.S. (1936). The fiber connections of the posterior parts of the cerebellum in the rat and cat. *J. Comp. Neurol.* **63:** 527-548.

DOW, R.S. (1938). Effect of lesions in the vestibular part of the cerebellum in primates. *Archs Neurol. Psychiat.,* Chicago **40:** 500-520.

DOW, R.S. (1939). Cerebellar action potentials in response to stimulation of various afferent connections. *J. Neurophysiol.* **2:** 543-555.

DOW, R.S. & MORUZZI, G. (1958). *The Physiology and Pathology of the Cerebellum.* Minneapolis: Univ. of Minn. Press.

DOW, R.S. & MANNI, E. (1964). The relationship of the cerebellum to extraocular movements. **In:** Bender, M.B., *The Oculomotor System.* New York: Harper & Row (Hoeber).

DUENSING, F. & SCHAEFER, K.P. (1957a). Die Neuronenaktivitat in der Formatio reticularis des Rhombencephalons beim vestibularen Nystagmus. *Arch. Psychiat.* **196:** 265-290.

DUENSING, F. & SCHAEFER, K.P. (1957b). Die "locker gekoppelten" Neurone der Formatio reticularis des Rhombencephalons beim vestibularen Nystagmus. *Arch. Psychiat.* **196:** 402-420.

DUENSING, F. & SCHAEFER, K.P. (1958). Die Aktivitat einzelner Neurone im Bereich der Vestibulariskerne bei Horizontalbeschleunigungen unter besonderer Berucksichtigung des vestibularen Nystagmus. *Arch. Psychiat. Nervenkr.* **198:** 225-252.

DUENSING, F. & SCHAEFER, K.P. (1959). Uber die Konvergerz verscheidener labyrintharer Afferenzen auf einzelne Neurone des Vestibulariskerngebietes. *Arch. Psychiat. Nervenkr.* **199:** 345-371.

DUMONT-TYC, S. & DELL, P. (1962). Facilitating and inhibiting constituents of the vestibulo-ocular reflex. *J. Physiol., Paris* **54:** 331-332.

DUSSER DE BARENNE, J.G. (1934). The labyrinthine and postural mechanism. **In** *Handbook of General Experimental Psychology.* Massachusetts: Clark Univ. Press.

EGMOND, A.A.J.V., GROEN, J.J. & JONGKEES, L.B.W. (1949). The mechanism of the semicircular canal. *J. Physiol.* **110:** 1-17.

EGMOND, A.A.J.V., GROEN, J.J. & JONGKEES, L.B.W. (1952). *The Function of the Vestibular Organ.* Basel: S. Karger.

ENGSTROM, H. (1958). On the double innervation of the sensory epithelia of the inner ear. *Acta oto-lar.* **49:** 109-118.

ENGSTROM, H. (1961). The innervation of the vestibular sensory cells. *Acta oto-lar.* Suppl. **163:** 30-40.

EWALD, J.R. (1892). *Physiologische Untersuchungen uber das Endorgan des Nervus octavus.* Wiesbaden: Bergmann.

FELDMAN, M. & Cohen, B. (1967). Eye movement responses in the calcarine cortex after retinal ablation. *Physiologist* **10:** 168.

FELDMAN, M. & COHEN, B. (1968a). Eye movement responses in the visual system of the monkey before and after retinal ablation. *Proc. Int. Union of Physiol. Sci.* **7:** 132.

FELDMAN, M. & COHEN, B. (1968b). Electrical activity in the lateral geniculate body of the alert monkey associated with eye movements. *J. Neurophysiol.* **31:** 455-466.

FERNANDEZ, C. (1960). Interrelations between flocculonodular lobe and vestibular system. **In** *Neural Mechanism of the Auditory and Vestibular Systems.* Springfield, Ill.: Charles C. Thomas.

FERNANDEZ, C. & FREDRICKSON, J.M. (1964). Experimental cerebellar lesions and their effect on vestibular function. *Acta oto-lar.* Suppl. **192:** 52-62.

FERRARO, A. & BARRERA, S.E. (1936). Effects of lesions of the juxta-restiform body (I.A.K. bundle) in Macacus rhesus monkeys. *Archs Neurol. Psychiat., Chicago* **25:** 13-29.

FERRARO, A. BARRERA, S.E. & BLAKESLEE, G.A. (1936). Vestibular phenomena of central origin. *Brain* **59:** 466-482.

FERRARO, A. & BARRERA, S.E. (1938). Differential features of "cerebellar" and vestibular phenomena in Macacus rhesus: Preliminary report based on experiments on 300 monkeys. *Archs Neurol., Chicago* **39:** 902-918.

FERRARO, A., PACELLA, B.L. & BARRERA, S.E. (1940). Effects of lesions of the medial vestibular nucleus. An anatomical and physiological study in Macacus rhesus monkeys. *J. comp. Neurol.* **73:** 7-36.

FIELDS, W.S. & ALFORD, B.R. (eds.) (1964). *Neurological Aspects of Auditory and Vestibular Disorders.* Springfield, Ill.: Charles C. Thomas.

FILLENZ, M. (1955). Responses in the brain stem of the cat to stretch of extrinsic ocular muscles. *J. Physiol.* **128:** 182-199.

FLOURENS, M. (1824). *Recherches Experimentales sur les Proprietes et les Fonctions du Systeme Nerveux dans les Animaux Vertebres.* Paris: Crevot.

FLUUR, E. (1959). Influences of semicircular ducts on extraocular muscles. *Acta oto-lar.* Suppl. **149.**

FREDRICKSON, J.M., SCHWARZ, D. & KORNHUBER, H.H. (1966). Convergence and interaction of vestibular and deep somatic afferents upon neurons in the vestibular nuclei of the cat. *Acta oto-lar.* **61:** 168-188.

FREEMAN, W. (1922). Paralysis of associated lateral movements of the eyes: A symptom of intrapontile lesion. *Archs Neurol. Psychiat., Chicago* **7:** 454-487.

FUJITA, Y., ROSENBERG, J. & SEGUNDO, J.P. (1968). Activity cells in the lateral vestibular nucleus as a function of head position. *J. Physiol.* **196:** 1-18.

FUKUDA, T., HINOKI, M. & TOKITA, T. (1958). Static and kinetic labyrinthine reflex. *Acta oto-lar.* **49:** 467-477.

FUKUDA, T. (1961). Studies on human dynamic posture from the viewpoint of postural reflexes. *Acta oto-lar.* Suppl. **161.**

GACEK, R.R. (1960). Efferent component of the vestibular nerve. **In** *Neural Mechanisms of the Auditory and Vestibular Systems,* ed. Rasmussen, G.L. & Windle, W.F., pp. 276-284, Springfield, Ill.: Charles C. Thomas.

GACEK, R.R. (1966). The vestibular efferent pathway. **In** *The Vestibular System and its Diseases,* ed. Wolfson, R.J., pp. 99-115. Philadelphia: Univ. of Pennsylvania Press.

GACEK, R.R. (1968). Neuroanatomical pathways of the vestibular system. *Ann. oto-rhino-lar.* **77:** 676-685.

GACEK, R.R. (1969). The course and central termination of first order neurons supplying vestibular end organs in the cat. *Acta oto-lar.* Suppl. **254:** 1-66.

GERNANDT, B.E. (1949). Response of mammalian vestibular neurons to horizontal rotation and caloric stimulation. *J. Neurophysiol.* **12:** 173-184.

GERNANDT, B.E. & THULIN, C.A. (1952). Vestibular connections of the brain stem. *Am. J. Physiol.* **171:** 121-127.

GERNANDT, B.E., IRANYI, M. & LIVINGSTON, R.B. (1959). Vestibular influences on spinal mechanisms. *Expl. Neurol.* **1:** 248-273.

GERNANDT, B.E. (1959). Vestibular mechanisms. **In** *Handbook of Physiology,* vol. 1. Washington, D.C.: American Physiological Society.

GERNANDT, B.E. (1964). Vestibular connections in the brain stem. **In** Bender, M.B., *The Oculomotor System.* New York: Harper & Row (Hoeber).

GERNANDT, B.E. (1968). Interactions between extraocular myotatic and ascending vestibular activities. *Expl. Neurol.* **20:** 120-134.

GOLTZ, F. (1870). Uber die physiologische Bedeutung der Bogengange des Ohrlabyrinths. *Pfluger Arch. ges. Physiol.* **3:** 172-192.

GONZALEZ, C. & REUBEN, R.N. (1967). Ocular electromyography in the syndrome of the medial longitudinal fasciculus: Patterns of inhibition and excitation. *Am. J. Ophthal.* **64:** 916-926.

GOTO, K., TOKUMASU, K. & COHEN, B. (1968). Return eye movements, saccadic movements, and the quick phase of nystagmus. *Acta oto-lar.* **65:** 426-440.

GRANT, G., ASCHAN, G. & EKVALL, L. (1964). Nystagmus produced by cerebellar lesions. *Acta oto-lar.* Suppl. **192:** 78-84.

GROEN, J.J., LOWENSTEIN, O. & VENDRIK, A.J.H. (1952). The mechanical analysis of the responses from the end-organs of the horizontal semicircular canal in the isolated elasmobranch labyrinth. *J. Physiol.* **117:** 329-346.

GUEDRY, F.E. Jr. (1964). Visual control of habituation to complex vestibular stimulation in man. *Acta oto-lar.* **58:** 377-389.

GUEDRY, F.E. Jr. (1965). Psychophysiological studies on vestibular function. **In** *Contributions to Sensory Physiology,* vol. 1, ed. Neff, D.W. New York: Academic Press.

HALLPIKE, C.S. & HOOD, J.D. (1953). The speed of the slow component of ocular nystagmus induced by angular acceleration of the head: its experimental determination and application to the physical theory of the cupular mechanism. *Proc. R. Soc. B.* **141:** 216-230.

HANNEN, R.A., KABRISKY, M., REPLOGLE, C.R., HARTZLER, V.L. & ROCCAFORTE, P.A. (1966). Experimental determination of a portion of the human vestibular system response through measurement of eyeball counterrol. *IEEE Trans. Biomed. Engin.* **13:** 65-70.

HARRIS, H.E., KOMATSUZAKI, A. & COHEN, B. (1967). Oculomotor deficits after lesions of the mesencephalic reticular formation in monkeys. *Physiologist* **10:** 195.

HASEGAWA, T. (1935). Labyrinthreflexe nach Abschleuderung der Otolithenmembranen. *Pfluger Arch. ges. Physiol.* **236:** 589-593.

HASEGAWA, T. (1937). Die statokinetische Funktion des Sacculus. *Zeitschrift fur Hals-Nasen- und Ohrenheilkunde* **43:** 129-132.

HASSLER, R. & HESS, W.R. (1954). Experimentelle und anatomische Befunde uber die Drehbewengungen und ihre nervosen Apparate. *Arch. Psychiat. Nervenkr.* **192:** 488-526.

HAUGLIE-HANSSEN, E. (1968). Intrinsic neuronal organization of the vestibular nuclear complex in cat. *Ergbn. Anat. EntwGesch.* **40:** 1-105.

HENRIKSSON, N.G. (1955a). An electrical method for registration and analysis of the movements of the eyes in nystagmus. *Acta oto-lar.* **45:** 25-41.

HENRIKSSON, N.G. (1955b). The correlation between the speed of eye in the slow phase of nystagmus and vestibular stimulus. *Acta oto-lar.* **45:** 120-136.

HENRIKSSON, N.G. (1956). Speed of slow component and duration in caloric nystagmus. *Acta oto-lar.* Suppl. **125.**

HENRIKSSON, N.G., LUNDGREN, A., LUNDGREN, K. & NILSSON, A. (1967a). New techniques of otoneurological diagnosis. I. Analysis of eye movements. **In** *Myotatic, Kinesthetic and Vestibular Nystagmus,* ed. de Reuck, A.V.S. & Knight, J., pp. 219-230. Boston: Little Brown & Co.

HENRIKSSON, N.G., JOHANSSON, G. & OSTLUND, H. (1967b). New techniques of otoneurological diagnosis. II. Vestibulo-spinal and postural patterns. **In** *Myotatic, Kinesthetic and Vestibular Mechanisms,* ed. de Reuck, A.V.S. & Knight, J., pp. 231-237. Boston: Little Brown & Co.

HESS, W.R., BURGI, S. & BUCHER, V. (1946). Motorische Funktion des Tektal und Tegmentalgebietes. *Mschr. Psychiat. Neurol.* **112:** 1-52.

HESS, W.R. (1957). *The Functional Organization of the Diencephalon.* New York: Grune & Stratton.

HIEBERT, T.G. & FERNANDEZ, C. (1965). Dietersian responses to tilt. *Acta oto-lar.* **60:** 180-190.

HILLMAN, D.E. (1969). Light and electron microscopical study of the relationships between the cerebellum and the vestibular organ of the frog. *Expl. Brain Res.* **9:** 1-15.

HOOD, J.D. & PFALTZ, C.R. (1954). Observations upon the effects of repeated stimulation upon rotation and caloric nystagmus. *J. Physiol.* **124:** 130-144.

HORCHOLLE, G. & DUMONT-TYC, S. (1968). Unites oculomotrices au cours du nystagmus. *Expl. Brain Res.* **5:** 16-31.

HORCHOLLE, G.B. & DUMONT-TYC, S. (1969). Phenomenes synaptiques du nystagmus. *Expl. Brain Res.* **8:** 201-218.

HYDE, J.E. & ELIASSON, S.G. (1957). Brainstem induced eye movements in cat. *J. comp. Neurol.* **108:** 139-172.

HYDE, J.E. and TOCZEK, S. (1962). Functional relation of interstitial nucleus to rotatory movements evoked from zona incerta stimulation. *J. Neurophysiol.* **25:** 455-465.

IMAI, R. (1930). Studies on the angle gamma of the eye. *Acta Soc. Ophthal. Jap.* **34:** 117-210.

International Symposium on Problems in Otoneurology. (1961). *Acta oto-lar* Suppl. **159.**

International Symposium on Vestibular and Oculomotor Problems. (1965). Tokyo: Nippon Hoechst Ltd.

International Vestibular Symposium. (1964). *Acta oto-lar.* Suppl. **192:**

IRELAND, P.E. & FARKASHIDY, J. (1961). Studies on the efferent innervation of the vestibular endorgans. *Trans. Amer. Otol. Soc.* **49:** 20-30.

ITO, F., BACH-Y-RITA, P. & YAMANAKA, Y. (1969). Extraocular muscle intracellular and motor nerve responses to semicircular canal stimulation. *Expl. Neurol.* **24:** 438-449.

ITO, M., HONGO, T., YOSHIDA, M., OKADA, Y. & OBATA, K. (1964). Intracellularly recorded antidromic responses of Deiter's neurones. *Experientia (Basel)* **20:** 295-296.

ITO, M., HONGO, T. & OKADA, Y. (1969). Vestibular-evoked postsynaptic potentials in Deiter's neurones. *Expl. Brain Res.* **7:** 214-230.

JANSEN, J. & BRODAL, A. (1954). *Aspects of Cerebellar Anatomy.* Oslo: Johan Grundt Tanum Forlag.

Japan Society of Vestibular Research. (1963). Contribution to the vestibular physiology and vestibular test. *Acta oto-lar.* Suppl. **179:**

JOHNSON, G.L. (1900). Contributions to the comparative anatomy of the mammalian eye, chiefly based on ophthalmoscopic examination. *Phil. Trans. R. Soc.* **194:** 1-82.

JONES, G.M. (1958). Vestibular interference with vision in flight. *Proc. R. Soc. Med.* **52:** 185-186.

JONES, G.M. (1964). Predominance of anti-compensatory oculomotor response during rapid head rotation. *Aerospace Med.* **35:** 965-968.

JONES, G.M. & MILSUM, J.G. (1965). Spatial and dynamic aspects of visual fixation. *IEEE Trans. Biomed. Engin.* **BME-12:** 54-62.

JONGKEES, L.B.W. (1950). On the function of the saccule. *Acta oto-lar.* **38:** 18-26.

JONGKEES, L.B.W. (1961). On positional nystagmus. *Acta oto-lar.* Suppl. **159:** 78-83.

JONGKEES, L.B.W., MAAS, J.P.M. & PHILIPSZOON, A.J. (1962). Clinical nystagmography. A detailed study of electro-nystagmography in 341 patients with vertigo. *Pract. Otorhino-laryng. (Basel)* **24:** 65-93.

JONGKEES, L.B.W. & PHILIPSZOON, A.J. (1963). The influence of position upon the eye-movements provoked by linear accelerations. *Acta oto-lar.* **56:** 414-419.

JONGKEES, L.B.W. & PHILIPSZOON, A.J. (1964). Electro-nystagmography. *Acta oto-lar.* Suppl. **189:** 1-111.

JONGKEES, L.B.W. (1967). The examination of the vestibular organ. *Progress in Brain Research* vol. 23, *Sensory Mechanisms,* ed. Zotterman, Y., pp. 155-168. Amsterdam: Elsevier Publishing Co.

JUNG, R. & KORNHUBER, H.H. (1964). Results of electro-nystagmography in man: The value of optokinetic, vestibular, and spontaneous nystagmus for neurologic diagnosis and research. **In** Bender, M.B., *The Oculomotor System.* New York: Harper & Row (Hoeber).

KASAHARA, M., MANO, N., OSHIMA, T., OZAWA, S. & SHIMAZU, H. (1968). Contralateral short latency inhibition of central vestibular neurons in the horizontal canal system. *Brain Res.* **8:** 376-378.

KAWAI, N., ITO, M., AND NOZUE, M. (1969). Postsynaptic influences on the vestibular non-Deiters' nuclei from primary vestibular nerve. *Expl. Brain Res. 8,* 190-200.

KOMATSUZAKI, A., HARRIS, H.E., ALPERT, J. & COHEN, B. (1969). Horizontal nystagmus of rhesus monkeys. *Acta oto-lar* **67:** 535-551.

KORNHUBER, H.H. (1966). Physiologie und Klinik des zentralvestibularen Systems (Blick- und Stutzmotorik). *Hals Nasen-Ohren-Heilkunde Band III,* Teil **3:** 2150-2351.

KORNHUBER, H.H. (Ed.) (1970). *The Vestibular System,* vol. VI. *Handbook of Sensory Physiology.* Springer (In press).

KUMOI, T., HOSOMI, H., MATSUMURA, H., AMATSU, M. & ASAI, R. (1965). An analysis of the vestibular evoked potentials in response to stimulation of the vestibular nerve branches. **In** *International Symposium on Vestibular and Oculomotor Problems,* pp. 45-50. Tokyo: Nippon Hoechst.

KUMOI, T. & JAMPEL, R.S. (1966). Influence of lateral rectus muscle contractions on the abducens nerve discharge evoked by vestibular nerve stimulation. *Expl. Neurol.* **15:** 180-191.

LADPLI, R. & BRODAL, A. (1968). Experimental studies of commissural and reticular formation projection from the vestibular nuclei in the cat. *Brain Res.* **8:** 65-96.

LEDOUX, A. (1958). Les canaux semicirculaires. *Acta oto-rhino-lar. belg.* **12:** 109-348.

LEE, F.S. (1893). A study of the sense of equilibrium in fishes. I. *J. Physiol.* **15:** 311-348.

LEE, F.S. (1894). A study of the sense of equilibrium in fishes. II. *J. Physiol.* **17:** 192-210.

LLINÁS, R., PRECHT, W. & KITAI, S. (1967). Cerebellar purkinje cell projection to the peripheral vestibular organ in the frog. *Science* **158:** 1328-1330.

LLINÁS, R. & PRECHT, W. (1969). The inhibitory vestibular efferent system and its relation to the cerebellum in the frog. *Expl. Brain Res.* **8:** 16-29.

LORENTE DE NÓ, R. (1928). *Labyrinthreflexe auf die Augenmuskeln.* Vienna. Urban.

LORENTE DE NÓ, R. (1931). Ausgewahlte Kapitel aus der vergleichenden Physiologie des Labyrinthes. Die Augenmuskelreflexe beim den Kaninchen und ihre Grundlagen. *Ergebn. Physiol.* **32:** 73-242.

LORENTE DE NÓ, R. (1933a). Anatomy of the eighth nerve. The central projection of the nerve endings of the internal ear. *Laryngoscope* **43:** 1-38.

LORENTE DE NÓ, R. (1933b). Vestibulo-ocular reflex arc. *Archs Neurol. Psychiat., Chicago* **30:** 245-291.

LOWENSTEIN, O. & SAND, A. (1940a). The mechanism of the semicircular canal. *Proc. R. Soc. B.* **129:** 256-275.

LOWENSTEIN, O. & SAND, A. (1940b). The individual and integrated activity of the semicircular canals of the elasmobranch labyrinth. *J. Physiol.* **99:** 89-101.

LOWENSTEIN, O. & ROBERTS, T.D.M. (1949). The equilibrium function of the otolith organs of the thornback ray (Raja clavata). *J. Physiol.* **110:** 392-415.

LOWENSTEIN, O, (1956). Peripheral mechanism of equilibrium. *Br. med. Bull.* **12:** 114-118.

MACH, E. (1875). *Grundlinien der Lehre von den Bewegungsempfindungen.* Leipzig: Engelmann.

MAGNUS, R. (1924). *Korperstellung.* Berlin: Springer.

MANNI, E. AZZENA, G.B., CASEY, H. & DOW, R.S. (1965). Influence of the labryinth on unitary discharge of the oculomotor nucleus and some adjacent formations. *Expl. Neurol.* **12:** 9-24.

MANNI, E. & DESOLE, C. (1966). Responses of oculomotor units to stimulation of single semicircular canal units. *Expl. Neurol.* **15:** 206-219.

MANO, N., OSHIMA, T. & SHIMAZU, H. (1968). Inhibitory commissural fibers interconnecting the bilateral vestibular nuclei. *Brain Res.* **8:** 378-382.

MARKHAM, C.H., PRECHT, W. & SHIMAZU, H. (1966). Effect of stimulation of interstitial Nucleus of Cajal on vestibular unit activity in the cat. *J. Neurophysiol.* **29:** 493-507.

MARKHAM, C.H. (1968). Midbrain and contralateral labyrinth influences on brain stem vestibular neurons in the cat. *Brain Res. 9,* 312-333.

McCabe, B.F. (1960). Vestibular suppression in figure skaters. *Am. Acad. Ophthal. Otolaryng.* **64:** 264-268

McCABE, B.F. (1964). Nystagmus response of the otolith organs. *Laryngoscope* **74:** 372-381.

McCABE, B.F. (1965). The quick component of nystagmus. *Laryngoscope* **75:** 1619-1646.

McMASTERS, R.E., WEISS, A.H. & CARPENTER, M.B. (1966). Vestibular projections to the nuclei of the extraocular muscles: Degeneration resulting from discrete partial lesions of the vestibular nuclei in the monkey. *Am. J. Anat.* **118:** 163-194.

McNALLY, W.J. & STUART, E.A. (1942). Physiology of the labyrinth reviewed in relation to sea sickness and other forms of motion sickness. *War Medicine* **2:** 683-771.

MERTON, P.A. (1956). Compensatory rolling movements of the eye. *J. Physiol.* **132:** 25P-27P.

MERTON, P.A. (1958). Compensatory rolling movements of the eyes. *Proc. R. Soc. Med.* **52:** 184-185.

MILLER, E.F. (1962). Counter-rolling of the human eyes produced by head tilt with respect to gravity. *Acta oto-lar* **54:** 479-501.

MILLER, E.A. & GRAYBIEL, A. (1969). Effects of drugs on ocular counter-rolling. *Clin. Pharmacol. & Therap.* **10:** 92-99.

MONEY, K.E. & SCOTT, J.W. (1962). Functions of separate sensory receptors of non-auditory labyrinth of the cat. *Am. J. Physiol.* **202:** 1211-1220.

MONNIER, M. (1946). Le formations reticulees tegmentales; equilibration des postures du regard de la tete et du tronc. *Rev. Neurol.* **78:** 422-452.

MUGNAINI, E., WALBERG, F. & BRODAL, A. (1967). Mode of termination of primary vestibular fibres in the lateral vestibular nucleus. An experimental electron microscopical study in the cat. *Expl. Brain Res. 4,* 187-211.

NAUTA, W.J.H. & KUYPERS, H.G.J.M. (1958). Some ascending pathways in the brain stem reticular formation. **In** *Reticular Formation of the Brain,* ed. Jasper, H.H. *et al.,* pp. 3-30. Boston: Little, Brown & Co.

Neuro-otology. (1956). *Br. med. Bull.* **12:** 91-160.

NITO, Y., JOHNSON, W.H., MONEY, K.E. & IRELAND, P.E. (1964). The non-auditory labyrinth and positional alcohol nystagmus. *Acta oto-lar.* **58:** 65-67.

NITO, Y., JOHNSON, W.H. & IRELAND, P.E. (1968). Positional alcohol nystagmus in the cat. *Ann. Otol. Rhinol. Lar.* **77:** 111-125.

NOHARA, K. (1966). Influence of alcohol administration upon labyrinthine function in rabbits. *J. Tokyo Woman's Med. College* **36:** 240-256.

NOZUE, M. & COHEN, B. (1968). The median longitudinal fasciculus (MLF) and horizontal eye movements. *Fed. Proc.* **27:** 451.

NYLÉN, C.O. (1924). Some cases of ocular nystagmus due to certain position of the head. *Acta oto-lar* **6:** 106-137.

NYLÉN, C.O. (1931). A clinical study on positional nystagmus in cases of brain tumor. *Acta oto-lar.* Suppl. **15.**

NYLÉN, C.O. (1939). Oto-neurologic diagnosis of tumors of the brain. *Acta oto-lar.* Suppl. **13.**

NYLÉN, C.O. (1950). Positional nystagmus: A review and future prospects. *J. Lar. Otol.* **64:** 295-310.

NYLÉN, C.O. (1953). The posutre test. *Acta oto-lar.* Suppl. **109:** 125-130.

PASIK, P., PASIK, T. & KRIEGER, H.P. (1959). Effects of cerebral lesions upon optokinetic nystagmus in monkeys. *J. Neurophysiol.* **22:** 297-304.

PASIK, P., PASIK, T. & BENDER, M.B. (1960). Oculomotor function following cerebral hemidecortication in the monkey. *Archs Neurol. Chicago* **3:** 298-305.

PASIK, P. & PASIK, T. (1964). Oculomotor functions in monkeys with lesions of the cerebrum and the superior colliculi. **In** Bender, M.B., *The Oculomotor System.* New York: Harper & Row (Hoeber).

PASIK, P., PASIK, T. & BENDER, M.B. (1966a). The pretectal syndrome in monkeys. *Trans. Am. Neurol. Assoc.* **91:** 316-318.

PASIK, T., PASIK, P. & BENDER, M.B. (1966b). The superior colliculi and eye movements. *Archs Neurol. Chicago* **15:** 420-436.

PASIK, P., PASIK, T. & BENDER, M.B. (1969a). The pretectal syndrome in monkeys: I. Disturbances of gaze and body posture. *Brain* **92:** 521-534.

PASIK, T. PASIK, P. & BENDER, M.B. (1969b). The pretectal syndrome in monkeys. II Spontaneous and induced nystagmus, and 'lightning" eye movements. *Brain 92,* 871-884.

PETERSON, B.W. (1967). Effect of tilting on neurons in the vestibular nuclei of the cat. *Brain Res.* **6:** 606-609.

PHILIPSZOON, A.J. (1962). Compensatory eye movements and nystagmus provoked by stimulation of the vestibular organ and the cervical nerve roots. *Pract. Otorhinolaryng.* **24:** 193-201.

POMPEIANO, O. & WALBERG, F. (1957). Descending connections to the vestibular nuclei. An experimental study in cat. *J. comp. Neurol.* **108:** 465-503.

POTTHOFF, P.C., BURANDT, H.R. & Richter, H.P. (1967a). Neuronale Reaktionen in Pons und Mesencephalon der Katze nach galvanischer Labyrinthpolarissation. *Arch. Ohr. Nas. Kehlkopfheilk.* **189:** 262-280.

POTTHOFF, P.C., RICHTER, H.P. & BURANDT, H.R. (1967b). Multisensorische Konvergenzen an Hirnstammneuronen der Katze. *Arch. Psychiat. Nervenkr.* **210:** 36-60.

PRECHT, W. & SHIMAZU, H. (1965). Functional connection of tonic and kinetic vestibular neurons with primary vestibular afferents. *J. Neurophysiol.* **28:** 1014-1028.

PRECHT, W., GRIPPO, J. & RICHTER, A. (1967). Effect of horizontal angular acceleration on neurons in the abducens nucleus. *Brain Res.* **5:** 527-531.

PRECHT W., RICHTER, A. & GRIPPO, J. (1969). Responses of neurones in cat's abducens nuclei to horizontal angular acceleration. *Pfluger Arch. ges. Physiol.* **309:** 285-309.

PRECHT W. & LLINÁS, R. (1969a). Functional organization of the vestibular afferents to the cerebellar cortex of frog and cat. *Expl. Brain Res.* **9:** 30-52.

PRECHT, W. & LLINÁS, R. (1969b) Comparative aspects of the vestibular input to the cerebellum. In *Neurobiology of Cerebellar Evolution and Development,* ed. Llinas, R., pp. 677-699. Chicago: American Medical Assoc. Press.

PRECHT, W. (1970). The physiology of the vestibular nuclei. Chapter 4.2 **In** *The Vestibular System,* vol. VI, *Handbook of Sensory Physioloby,* ed., Kornhuber, H.H. Springer (In press).

QUIX, F.H. (1925). The function of the vestibular organ and the clinical examination of the otolithic apparatus. *J. Lar. Otol.* **40:** 425-443.

RASHBASS, C. (1961). The relationship between saccadic and smooth tracking eye movements. *J. Physiol.* **159:** 326-338.

RASMUSSEN, G.L. & WINDLE, W.F. (Eds.), (1960). *Neural Mechanisms of the Auditory and Vestibular Systems.* Springfield, Ill.: Charles C. Thomas.

RICHTER, A. & PRECHT, W. (1968). Inhibition of abducens motoneurones by vestibular nerve stimulation. *Brain Res.* **11:** 701-705.

ROBINSON, D.A. & FUCHS, A.F. (1969). Eye movements evoked by stimulation of frontal eye fields. *J. Neurophysiol.* **32:** 637-648.

Role of the Vestibular Organs in the Exploration of Space. (1965). *NASA SP-77.* Washington, D.C.

RUPERT, A., MOUSHEGIAN, G. & GALAMBOS, R. (1962). Microelectrode studies of primary vestibular neurons in cat. *Expl. Neurol.* **5:** 100-109.

RYU, J.H., MCCABE, B.F. & FUNSAKA, S. (1969). Types of neuronal activity in the medial vestibular nucleus. *Acta oto-lar.* **68:** 137-141.

SADJADPOUR, K. & BRODAL, A. (1968). The vestibular nuclei in man. *Journal fur Hirnforschung* **10:** 299-323.

SALA, O. (1965). The efferent vestibular systems. *Acta oto-lar.* Suppl. **197:**

SASAKI, K. (1963). Electrophysiological studies on oculomotor neurons of the cat. *Jap. J. Physiol.* **13:** 287-302.

SCHAEFER, K.P. (1965). Die Erregungsmuster einzelner Neurone des Abducens-Kernes beim Kaninchen. *Pfluger Arch. ges. Physiol.* **284:** 31-52.

SCHEIBEL, M.E., SCHEIBEL, A.B., MOLLICA, A. & MORUZZI, G. (1955). Convergence interaction of afferent impulses on single units of reticular formation. *J. Neurophysiol.* **18:** 309-331.

SCHEIBEL, M.E. & SCHEIBEL, A.B. (1958). Structural substrates for integrative patterns in the brain stem reticular core. **In** *Reticular Formation of the Brain,* ed. Jasper, H.H. *et al.,* pp. 31-55. Boston: Little, Brown & Co.

SHANZER, S., TENG, P., KREIGER, H.P. & BENDER, M.B. (1958). Defects in optokinetic after-nystagmus in lesions of the brain stem. *Am. J. Physiol.* **194:** 419-422.

SHANZER, S. & BENDER, M.B. (1959). Oculomotor responses on vestibular stimulation of monkeys with lesions of the brain stem. *Brain* **82:** 669-682.

SHANZER, S. (1964). Effects of semicircular canal stimulation in monkeys with lesions of the medial longitudinal fasciculus (MLF). *Fed. Proc.* **23:** 414.

SHANZER, S., GOTO, K., COHEN, B. & BENDER, M.B. (1964). Median longitudinal fasciculus and vertical eye movements. *Trans. Am. Neurol. Assoc.* **89:** 225-226.

SHIMAZU, H. & PRECHT, W. (1965). Tonic and kinetic responses of cat's vestibular neurons to horizontal angular acceleration. *J. Neurophysiol.* **28:** 991-1013.

SHIMAZU, H. & PRECHT, W. (1966). Inhibition of central vestibular neurons from the contralateral labyrinth and its mediating pathway. *J. Neurophysiol.* **29:** 467-492.

SINGLETON, G.T. (1967). Relationships of the cerebellar nodulus to vestibular function: a study of the effects of nodulectomy on habituation. *Laryngoscope* **77:** 1579-1620.

SMITH, J.L. & COGAN, D.G. (1959). Internuclear ophthalmoplegia: A review of fifty-eight cases. *Archs Ophthal.* **61:** 687-794.

SPIEGEL, E.A. & PRICE, J.B. (1939). Origin of the quick component of labyrinthine nystagmus. *Archs Otolar.* **20:** 576-588.

SPIEGEL, E.A. & SCALA, N.P. (1941). Vertical nystagmus in cerebellar lesions. *Archs Ophthal.* **26:** 661-669.

SPIEGEL, E.A. & SCALA, N.P. (1942). Positional nystagmus in cerebellar lesions. *J. Neurophysiol.* **5:** 247-260.

SPIEGEL, E.A. & SOMMER, I. (1944). *Neurology of Ear, Ear, Nose and Throat.* New York: Grune & Stratton.

SPILLER, W.G. (1924). Ophthalmoplegia internuclearis anterior: A case with necropsy. *Brain* **47:** 345-357.

STAHLE, J. (1958). Electro-nystagmography in the caloric and rotatory tests. *Acta oto-lar.* Suppl. **137.**

STEIN, B.M. & CARPENTER, M.B. (1967). Central projections of portions of the vestibular ganglia innervating specific parts of the labyrinth in the rhesus monkey. *Am. J. Anat.* **120:** 281-318.

SUZUKI, J., COHEN, B. & BENDER, M.B. (1964). Compensatory eye movements induced by vertical semicircular canal stimulation. *Expl. Neurol.* **9:** 137-160.

SUZUKI, J. & COHEN, B. (1964). Head, eye, body and limb movements from semicircular canal nerves. *Expl. Neurol.* **10:** 395-405.

SUZUKI, J. & COHEN, B. (1966). Integration of semicircular canal activity. *J. Neurophysiol.* **29:** 981-995.

SUZUKI, J., GOTO, K., KOMATSUZAKI, A. & NOZUE, M. (1968). Otolithic influences on tonus changes of the extraocular muscles. *Ann. Otol.* **77:** 959-970.

SUZUKI, J., GOTO, K., TOKUMASU, K. & COHEN, B. (1969a). Implantation of electrodes near individual vestibular nerve branches in mammals. *Ann. Otol.* **78:** 815-826.

SUZUKI, J., TOKUMASU, K. & GOTO, K. (1969b). Eye movements from single utricular nerve stimulation in the cat. *Acta oto-lar.* **68:** 350-362.

SZENTÁGOTHAI, J. (1943). Die zentrale innervation der Augenbewegungen. *Arch. Psychiat. Nervenkr.* **116:** 721-760.

SZENTÁGOTHAI, J. (1950). The elementary vestibulo-ocular reflex arc. *J. Neurophysiol.* **13:** 395-407.

SZENTÁGOTHAI, J. (1952). *Die Rolle der einzelnen Labyrinthrezeptoren bei der Orientation von Augen und Kopf im Raume.* Budapest: Akademiai Kiado.

SZENTÁGOTHAI, J. (1964). Pathways and synaptic articulation patterns connecting vestibular receptors and oculomotor nuclei. **In** Bender, M.B., *The Oculomotor System.* New York: Harper & Row (Hoeber).

TAIT, J. & MCNALLY, W.J. (1934). Some features of the action of the utricular maculae (and of the associated action of the semicircular canals) of the frog. *Phil. Trans. R. Soc.* **224:** 241-286.

TAKEMORI, S. & SUZUKI, J. (1969). Influences of neck torsion on otolithogenic eye deviations in the rabbit. *Ann. Otol.* **78:** 640-647.

TENG, P., SHANZER, S. & BENDER, M.B. (1958). Effects of brain stem lesions on optokinetic nystagmus in monkeys. *Neurology* **8:** 22-26.

TOKUMASU, K., GOTO, K. & COHEN, B. (1969). Eye movements from vestibular nuclei stimulation in monkeys. *Ann. Otol. Rhinol. Lar.* **78:** 1105-1119.

TOROK, N. (1957). The culmination phenomenon and frequency pattern of thermic nystagmus. *Acta oto-lar.* **48:** 530.

TOROK, N. (1969). Nystagmus frequency versus slow phase velocity in rotatory and caliric nystagmus. *Ann. Otol.* **78:** 625-639.

VERSTEEGH, C. (1927). Ergebnisse partieller Labyrinthextirpation bei Kaninchen. *Acta oto-lar.* **11:** 393-408.

VOOGD, J. (1964). *The Cerebellum of the Cat. Structure and Fibre Connections.* Philadelphia: F.A. Davis Co.

WAGMAN, I.H. (1964). Eye movements induced by electric stimulation of cerebrum in monkeys and their relationship to bodily movements. In Bender, M.B., *The Oculomotor System.* New York: Harper & Row (Hoeber).

WALBERG, F., BOWSHER, D. & BRODAL, A. (1958). The termination of primary vestibular fibers in the vestibular nuclei in the cat. An experimental study with silver methods. *J. comp. Neurol.* **110:** 391-419.

WALBERG, F., POMPEIANO, O., WESTRUM, L.E. & HAUGLEI-HANSSEN, E. (1962). Fastigio-reticular fibers in the cat. *J. comp. Neurol.* **119:** 187-199.

WALTER, H.W. (1954). Alkoholmissbrauch und Alkohollagenystagmus. *Deutsch Z. Ges. Gerichtl. Med.* **43:** 232-241.

WARWICK, R. (1956). Oculomotor organization. *Ann. R. Coll. Surg.* **19:** 36-52.

WARWICK, R. (1964). Oculomotor organization. In Bender, M.B. *The Oculomotor System.* New York: Harper & Row (Hoeber).

WENDT, G.R. (1951). "Vestibular Functions". In *Handbook of Experimental Psychology.* New York: John Wiley & Sons.

WERSÄLL, J. (1956). Studies on the structure and innervation of the sensory epithelium of the cristae ampullares in the guinea pig. *Acta oto-lar.* Suppl. **126.**

WERSÄLL, J. (1960). Electron micrographic studies of vestibular hair cell innervation. In *Mechanisms of the Auditory and Vestibular Systems,* chapt. 18, ed. Rasmussen, G.L. & Windle, W.F., pp. 247-257. Springfield, Ill.: Charles C. Thomas.

WERSÄLL, J., GLEISNER, L. & LUNDQUIST, P.G. (1967). Ultrastructure of the vestibular end organs. In *Myotatic, Kinetic, and Vestibular Mechanisms,* ed. de Reuck, A.V.S. & Knight, J., pp. 105-116. Boston: Little, Brown & Co.

WESTHEIMER, G. (1954a). Mechanism of saccadic eye movements. *Archs Ophthal.* **52:** 710-724.

WESTHEIMER, G. (1954b). Eye movement responses to a horizontally moving visual stimulus. *Archs Ophthal.* **52:** 932-941.

WHITTERIDGE, D. (1960). Central control of eye movements. In *Handbook of Physiology,* vol. 2. Washington, D.C.: American Physiological Society.

WILSON, V.J., KATO, M., THOMAS, R.C. & PETERSON, B.W. (1966). Excitation of lateral vestibular neurons by peripheral afferent fibers. *J. Neurophysiol. 29,* 508-529

WILSON, V.J., KATO, M., PETERSON, B.W. & WYLIE, R.M. (1967). A single-unit analysis of organization of Deiter's Nucleus. *J. Neurophysiol.* **30:** 603-619.

WILSON, V.J., WYLIE, R.M. & MARCO, L.A. (1968a). Organization of the medial vestibular nucleus. *J. Neurophysiol.* **31:** 166-185.

WILSON, V.J., WYLIE, R.M. & MARCO, L.A. (1968b). Synaptic inputs to cells in the medial vestibular nucleus. *J. Neurophysiol.* **31:** 176-185.

WOELLNER, R.C. & GRAYBIEL, C.A. (1959). Counter-rolling of the eyes and its dependence on the magnitude of gravitational or inertial force acting laterally on the body. *J. appl. Physiol.* **14:** 632-634.

WOELLNER, R.C. & GRAYBIEL, C.A. (1960). The loss of counter-rolling of the eyes in three persons presumably without functional otolith organs. *Ann. Otol. Rhinol. Lar.* **69:** 1006-1012.

WOLFE, J. (1968). Evidence for control of nystagmic habituation by folium-tuber vermis and fastigial nuclei. *Acta oto-lar.* Suppl. **231.**

WOLFSON, R.J. (Ed.) (1966). *The Vestibular System and its Diseases.* Philadelphia: Univ. of Pennsylvania Press.

YAMANAKA, Y. & BACH-Y-RITA, P. (1968). Conduction velocities in the abducens nerve correlated with vestibular nystagmus in cat. *Expl. Neurol.* **20:** 143-155.

YULES, R.B. & GAULT, F.P. (1966). The relationship of nystagmus to lateral vestibular nuclei stimulation. *Expl. Neurol.* **15:** 475-483.

EEG, EVOKED POTENTIALS, AND EYE AND IMAGE MOVEMENTS

DIETRICH LEHMANN

Eye movements are the results of commands emanating from the brain. In many instances, the voluntary or involuntary decision to send an eye movement command is based on afferent information which represents either changes in the outside world, or specific activity of other centers in the central nervous system. Such eye movements may be explained teleologically. In other cases, eye movements may be initiated by spontaneous activity of some control centers, or they may be triggered as an accidental side effect of other complex processes in the central nervous system, and thus, teleological explanations may not be adequate.

I will attempt to outline the present knowledge about cerebral EEG phenomena which precede, accompany, or follow eye and image movements. The emphasis of this report will be on observations in humans.

The topic described in the title touches upon several areas of investigation. Many publications have appeared in some of these areas, e.g. in sleep research. Other areas, e.g. the pre-eye-motion potentials, are just beginning to yield data. This survey will not be a complete review; rather it attempts to illustrate the present state of research by selective discussions.

A. Preference for Certain Eye Movements in Wakefulness and Different EEG Sleep Stages

Wakefulness and the different stages of sleep in the normal adult human are accompanied by certain wave patterns of the spontaneous electroencephalogram (EEG); the wave patterns are felt to reflect the general functional

Supported by USPHS, NIH grant NB 06038.

states of the brain or different levels of vigilance. The different patterns are reasonably well described by the frequency distribution of their waves. It is of interest to note that specific types of eye movements are preferentially associated with wakefulness and the different sleep stages (see Dement 1964). Pursuit movements, saccades, drift and tremor are the classes of eye movements observed in wakefulness, and slow and rapid eye movements have been described during specific sleep stages.

Polygraphic recordings which monitor EEG, eye movements, head muscle, and neck muscle activity in humans during sleep (Dement and Kleitman, 1957; Jouvet, 1967) suggest the differentiation of three combinations of sleep characteristics: 1) drowsiness (initial stage 1 sleep), 2) slow wave sleep (stages 2,3 and 4), and 3) paradoxical sleep (stage 1 with rapid eye movements =REM). In mammals and man, initial stage 1 is seen at the onset of sleep, whereas slow wave sleep stages 2,3 and 4, and paradoxical sleep (stage 1 REM) alternate periodically during the night. The change from one stage to the other often is a gradual, stepwise process, and not all phenomena change simultaneously. One manifestation of a certain stage of sleep may precede another manifestation of the same stage by many seconds.

Scalp EEG recordings during drowsiness (initial stage 1) and paradoxical sleep (stage 1 REM) show a low voltage, irregular pattern with a predominance of 5 - 7 cps rhythms. Clusters of sharp waves were observed from depth electrode recordings in the pons, lateral geniculate, and visual cortex of cats during paradoxical sleep (see Jouvet 1967); these pontine-geniculate-occipital waves will be discussed in section D. The slow wave sleep stages are dominated by higher amplitudes of slow (1 - 3 cps) scalp EEG rhythms.

The tonic activity of head and neck muscles is continuous in drowsiness, decreases somewhat in slow wave sleep, and disappears completely with the onset of paradoxical sleep; typically, occasional jerks of skeletal muscles ("twitches") appear in the latter stage.

The eye movements during the initial sleep stage 1 are slow (about 0.2 - 0.6 cps) horizontal oscillations (Kuhlo and Lehmann, 1964; Dement, 1964), which are usually conjugate, smooth, and often continuous ("pendular deviations", Fig. 1). These slow eye movements are unlike eye movements observed during wakefulness without the presence of a target in adequate motion. On the other hand, the pendular deviations are similar to eye movements under drugs which induce general anaesthesia (Burford, 1941; Rashbass; 1961), and similar to eye movements in cases of cerebral lesions (Kornhuber, 1966). It was suggested that pendular deviations may be caused by free-running mechanisms of pursuit movements. We note here that very vivid visual hallucinations are commonly experienced during the initial sleep stage 1; however, later recall of these "hypnagogic hallucinations" is poor (Oswald 1962; Kuhlo and Lehmann, 1964).

Typically, there are very few eye movements during the slow wave sleep stages 2,3 and 4. An occasional brief awakening with some EEF alpha waves

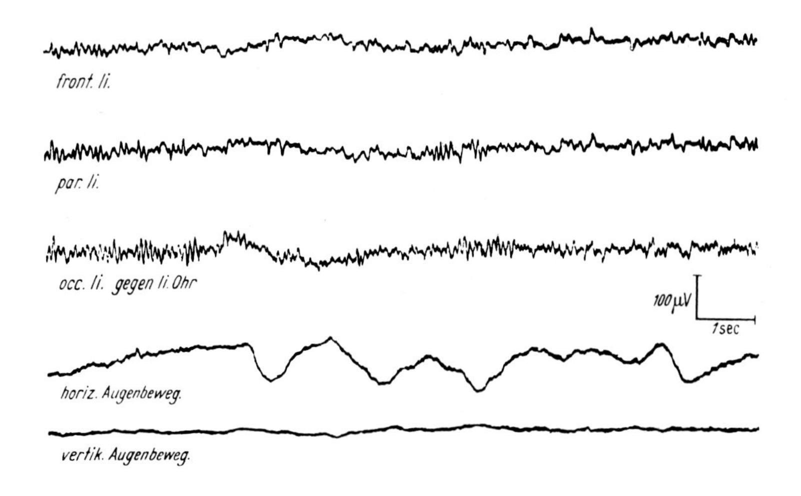

Fig. 1. EEG and eye movements during drowsiness (initial sleep stage 1.) Upper three traces: Frontal, parietal and occipital EEG vs. left ear. Fourth and fifth trace: Horizontal and vertical eye movement recordings, respectively. EEG alpha disappears, and low voltage irregular EEG appears, accompanied by slow horizontal eye movements. (From W. Kuhlo and D. Lehmann, *Arch. Psychiat. Nervenkr.* **205:** 687-716, 1964; by permission of Springer Verlag, Berlin).

may be followed by a short epoch of slow eye oscillations, especially in stage 2.

In paradoxical sleep, rapid eye movements (REM) dominate the recordings. These eye movements resemble to some extent fixation saccades; they are conjugate, and occur without directional preference about 60 to 70 times per minute; typically, they occur in bursts of five or more movements (Jouvet, 1967). Very few slow eye movements are seen during paradoxical sleep. The bursts of rapid eye movements are very often preceded - particularly at the beginning of a stage 1 REM period - by a short run of fairly regular, approximately 3 cps waves which are best seen over frontal areas (saw-toothed waves, Schwartz and Fischgold, 1960; Berger *et al.,* 1962). The functional significance of the saw-toothed waves is not known. Differences of the characteristics of rapid eye movements in sleep and wakefulness were reported in cats (Jeannerod and Mouret, 1963) and in monkeys (Fuchs and Ron, 1968). The latter authors found, for example, that the histograms of angular velocities of eye movements were rather constant during REM sleep, but quite different from histograms obtained during wakefulness. During REM sleep, there were intermediate angular velocities of eye movements between the range of the saccades and slow pursuit movements of wakefulness. Visual inspection of the eye movement recording exhibited "round shouldered saccades" during REM sleep which are not seen during wakefulness. Further, the rapid eye movements during paradoxical sleep showed a peculiar tendency to complete loops, the eye position returning after 3 to 11 eye movements (within an average time of 2.5 sec) to the point of origin; an average of seven such loops occurred per minute during paradoxical sleep. No loops of eye movements were observed during wakefulness.

A relatively high incidence of dream reports after awakening of a subject from paradoxical sleep had led to the hypothesis that paradoxical sleep is specifically associated with dreaming (Dement and Kleitman, 1957). It was speculated that the bursts of rapid eye movements result from the sleeper's attempt to follow dream images which move in the visual field (Dement, 1964). This theory was not universally accepted (Dement, 1967) for various reasons, e.g. because it had been observed that rapid eye movements persisted during paradoxical sleep in decorticate humans who are not likely to be able to detect visual shapes (Jouvet *et al.,* 1961). It has also been pointed out (e.g. by Oswald, 1962) that images tend to be experienced as parts, not wholes, and that they are oriented in the visual field, not in real space, so that eye movements do not change the "fixation" point. Besides, if dream images solicit REM, why do the impressive hypnagogic images of initial stage 1 sleep fail to invite rapid eye movements? Several other hypotheses about the nature and function of the rapid eye movements in paradoxical sleep were published. Provision of afferent stimulation for structural differentiation and maturation of the central nervous system was suggested as a function of REM sleep by Roffwarg *et al.* (1966). Berger (1969) proposed the hypothesis that the periodic innervation of the oculomotor system during REM sleep maintains a state of facilitation for binocularly coordinated eye movements. Let us consider at this point that "twitching" of face, hand or foot muscle groups is a typical feature in paradoxical sleep. These twitches do not copy purposeful movements, and REMs may very well be analogous events, since the oculomotor nuclei are anatomically analogous to other cranial motor nerve nuclei which mediate the typical motor manifestations of REM sleep (loss of tone and twitching) to head and neck muscles.

B. Eye Position and the Generation of Alpha EEG Patterns

The most prominent and common wave pattern in electroencephalograms recorded from the scalp of normal adult humans during relaxed wakefulness with closed eyes, is the so-called alpha EEG (8 to 12 cps waves over occipital regions of the head). The first descriptions of the human EEG reported the very impressive phenomenon of quick disappearance ("blocking") of alpha EEG after eye opening in a lighted room, after tactile or auditory stimuli, after other attention-attracting events, and during intention to act (Berger, 1930). Alpha, and the blocking reaction of alpha, is observed in a wide range of animals, although alpha is not as prominent in some animals as it is in man. Numerous workers have investigated the blocking ("desynchronization") of cortical EEG alpha, and its relation to attention. It was shown that activation of the reticular formation of the brainstem results in desynchronization of the cortical EEG and behavioral arousal (see Jasper *et al.,* 1958). For thirty years the presence of EEG alpha had been considered more or less as a direct sign of relaxed wakefulness, and desynchronization as the manifestation of attentional states, reflecting general brain conditions.

Since 1965 several reports have appeared which linked the occurrence of alpha EEG activity to oculomotor functions. Mulholland and Evans (1965) reported that there was a marked increase in the occurrence of alpha when the eyes were rolled upwards instead of looking ahead; this effect persisted when a closed loop experimental design was used, where the subject's alpha turned on a brilliant light of a radio program, and EEG desynchronization extinguished the stimulus (Fig. 2); these are experimental conditions which classically counteract the EEG patterns which triggered them. The authors argued that keeping the eyes elevated obviously requires continuous attention; thus, lack of attention was less likely to be the crucial factor for occurrence of alpha than eye orientation. Extreme eye deviations are required to produce the alpha enhancement, and upwards and downwards orientation of the eyes is effective (Fenwick and Walker, 1968). Later observations indicated that release of accommodation and convergence also enhanced alpha (Mulholland and Evans, 1966; Dewan, 1967). Mulholland (1968) hypothesizes that the state of the systems which control the tracking eye movements, and the "triad of accommodation" (pupil diameter, vergence, and lens accommodation) is crucial for the occurrence of EEG alpha or EEG desynchronization. He proposes an afferent-efferent sensory-oculomotor theory of desynchronization of the occipital EEG: maximum afferent visual information and maximum eye position control occur with open eyes in a patterned environment, resulting in desynchronization (activation of the maximal number of single units), whereas the lack of visual input and the lack of eye position control with closed eyes does not produce desynchronization, and consequently, alpha EEG occurs. The close physical relationship of oculomotor pathways and the activating reticular formation (Bender and Shanzer, 1964; Carpenter, 1969) is felt to be of importance in this context.

However, alpha enhancement by eye positioning is not reliably reproducible in the same subject (Mulholland and Evans, 1965); the mechanism apparently includes factors which are not yet understood. Further, power spectrum analysis of the human EEG during alpha blocking showed different results for alpha blocking caused by eye opening, and for alpha blocking caused by mental arithmetic (Glass and Kwiatkowski, 1968), suggesting that mental activity is an important factor in alpha suppression.

C. EEG Potentials Which Precede Eye Movements

The cortex contains well known areas which play a dominant role in the control of limb muscle activity. The scalp EEG recorded from such areas in humans has been shown to exhibit potential changes which precede voluntary activity of the skeletal muscles by a constant time interval.

Classically, it was assumed that the frontal eye fields (area 8) are relay

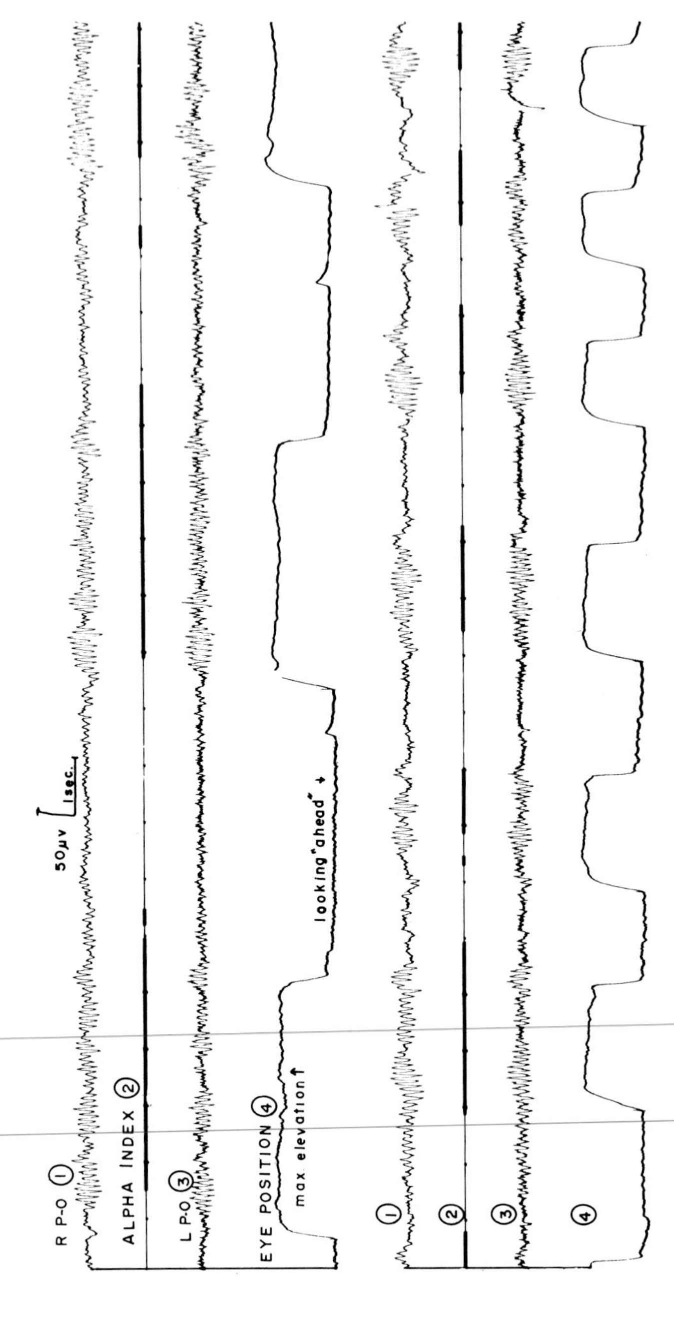

Fig. 2. Human alpha EEG and eye position in darkness. (1) right parietal-occipital and (3) left parietal-occipital EEG; (2) auditory feedback to subject during occurrence of alpha; (4) vertical eye position. (After T. Mulholland, p. 101 in: Evans, C.R. and Mulholland, T.B., *Attention in Neurophysiology*, Butterworths, London 1969; by permission of the publisher).

stations in the motor control of eye movements: electrical stimulation of this area in anesthetized patients causes slow eye movements; however, Robinson and Fuchs (1969) have demonstrated that in unanesthetized animals such stimulation causes contralateral single saccades in 96% of all stimulations, and never smooth, vergence or centering movements or nystagmus. On the other hand, single cell recordings from area 8 in unanesthetized monkeys failed to show cells which discharged prior to an eye movement; the units fired after the onset of an eye movement, or showed steady activity when the eyes were immobile and oriented in a specific direction (Bizzi, 1967).

In spite of the negative results in the search for the cortical single unit representation of eye movement control, scalp EEG phenomena in humans have been observed phase-locked with, and prior to the onset of, saccadic eye movements. Gaarder *et al.* (1966) describe that an alpha-like component of the spontaneous EEG is phase-locked to involuntary saccades before and after the saccade. They hypothesize that the saccades may be paced by the alpha cycle which thereby paces information input and processing.

Scott and Bickford (1967) mentioned the recording of slow scalp EEG potential changes prior to eye movements. Barlow and Cigánek (1969) reported a slow occipital scalp negativity (recorded O_z P_z without further attempts for localization) which precedes the onset of all voluntary saccades by approximately 200 msec in different visual stimulus conditions and in darkness. It is very interesting that no potential was found prior to involuntary (compensatory) eye movements during passive movements of the head (28°) while fixating a stationary bright spot (Fig. 3). The authors observe that the interval between active eye movements was approximately 3 seconds in their study and that therefore expectancy (Walter *et al,* 1964) may play a role in the generation of the prepotential. Hillyard and Galambos (in press) investigated the contingent negative variation (CNV, Walter *et al,* 1964) preceding voluntary eye movements. They showed that the CNV was not related to the size of the subsequent eye movement, but reflected the speed of the movement.

Becker *et al.* (1968) describe changes of averaged scalp EEG potentials which precede eye movements in humans (Fig. 4). The authors distinguish (1) the "readiness potential" which builds up slowly (the illustration shows the potential onset at about 700 msec before the start of the eye movement), is surface negative, and shows a bilateral distribution, largest over precentral areas; (2) the "premotion positivity," starting approximately 150 msec before eye movements, again with bilateral distribution, and considerable individual differences (seen in about 50% of the subjects). These results indicate that the general cortical EEG signs which are associated with execution of limb movements are present also before eye movements, whereas a localized motor potential prior to eye movements is not detectable on the scalp. The lack of such localized scalp EEG changes is in agreement with Bizzi's findings which were mentioned above. However, further developments in the EEG studies can be expected.

We examined the scalp EEG in experiments with human subjects who were asked to perform horizontal saccades voluntarily, without command, in

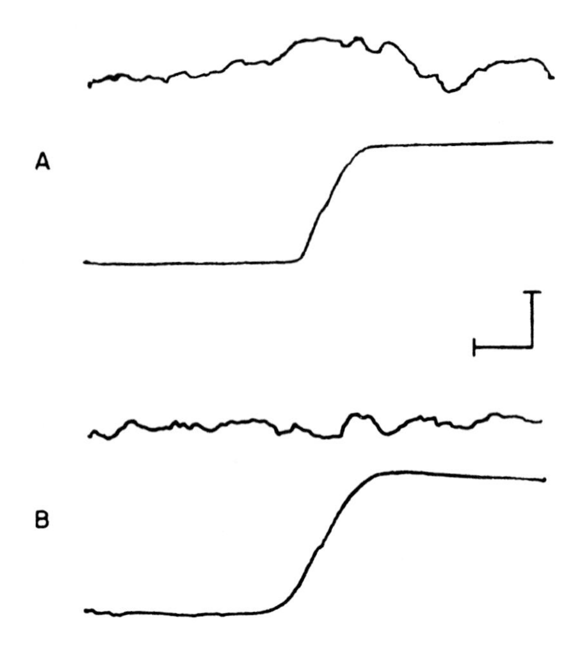

Fig. 3. (A) Averaged EEG potentials preceding and following voluntary eye movements; fixation spot on oscilloscope screen moved congruously with eye. (B) Averaged EEG potentials preceding and following involuntary (compensatory) eye movements (stationary fixation spot and passive head movements). Upper traces: Parietal-occipital EEG, upward deflection indicates parietal positivity; lower traces: Oculogram. Calibration: 100 msec, 4 μV. (From T.S. Barlow and L. Cigánek, *Electroenceph. clin. Neurophysiol.* **26:** 183-192, 1969; by permission of Elsevier Publishing Co., Amsterdam).

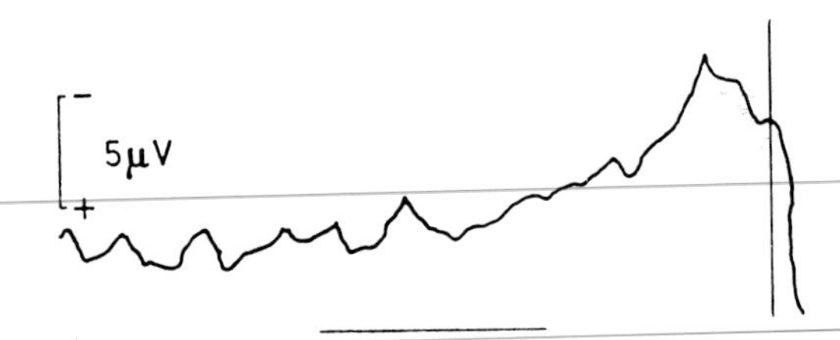

Fig. 4. Averaged brain potential (with premotion positivity) preceding eye movements to the right. Recording vertex vs. left ear. Up = vertex negative. Average of 50 recordings. The vertical line indicates onset of eye movement. Time calibration: 500 msec. (After W. Becker *et al., Naturwissenschaften* **55:** 550, 1968; by permission of Springer Verlag, Berlin).

total darkness, at a rate of one saccade per approximately 10 seconds. A decrease in amplitude of the occipital alpha EEG($O_1 - P_1$) was seen before, and an increase after the saccade. The EEGs were processed so that the alpha waves were represented by an envelope curve connecting all peaks of the waves (see inset in Fig. 5); then the wave envelopes during 2 sec before until 2 sec after saccades were averaged. A typical result shown in Fig. 5 demonstrates the decrease of alpha EEG prior to the saccade, and a surge of alpha peaking at about 500 msec after the eye movement. It is of interest that this alpha envelope curve is similar in its time course to Barlow and Cigánek's EEG averages. This is in good agreement with the findings of Caspers and Schulze (1959) that EEG synchronization (in our case, alpha) is associated with a positive shift of the DC potential, and desynchronization (in our case, absence of alpha) with a negative DC shift.

Depth EEG potentials which precede the onset of saccadic eye movements by 10-20 msec were recorded from the paramedian zone of the pontine reticular formation in the alert monkey (Cohen and Feldman, 1968). An example is shown in Fig. 6. The potentials are multiphasic, and their configuration depends on the direction of the rapid eye movement.

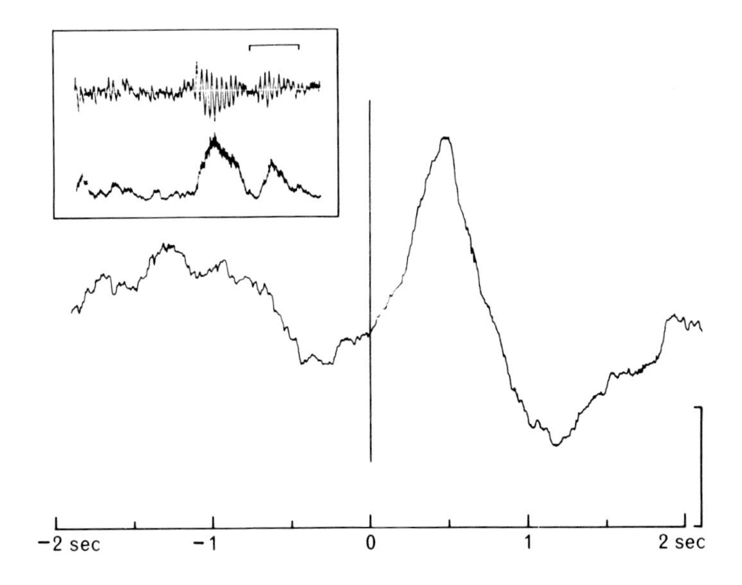

Fig. 5. Averaged alpha EEG envelope from 2 sec before to 2 sec after 30 horizontal, voluntary saccades in darkness. Vertical line at time 0=onset of eye movements. Parietal-occipital EEG recording. Increase of average indicates increased occurrence of alpha. Amplitude calibration: 20 μV, the time axis indicates zero voltage level. Inset (upper left) illustrates the translation of alpha EEG (upper trace) into envelope curve (lower trace). Time calibration: 1 sec.

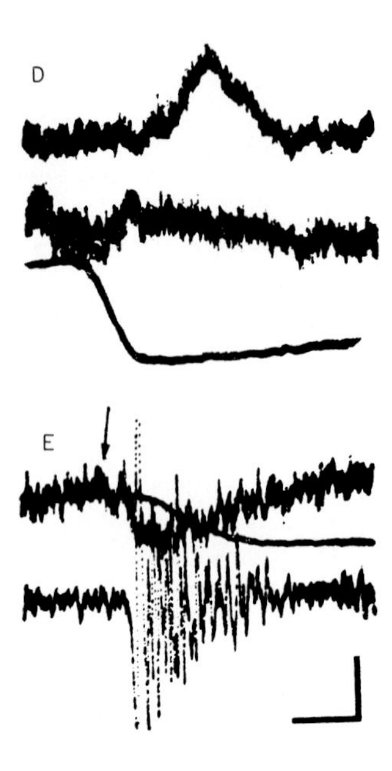

Fig. 6. Rapid eye movements in alert monkeys, and recordings from lateral geniculate body and pons. D: lateral geniculate body (upper trace); paramedian pontine reticular formation (middle trace); eye movement recording of quick phase of nystagmus on darkness (lower trace). E: paramedian pontine reticular formation (upper trace); eye movement recording (middle trace), electromyogram from right medial rectus muscle (lower trace). Arrow indicates initial pontine potential. Time calibration: 40 msec for D, 20 msec for E. Amplitude calibration: 100 μV. (From B. Cohen and M. Feldman, *J. Neurophysiol.* **31:** 806-817, 1968; by permission of Charles C. Thomas, Springfield, Ill.).

D. Pontine-Geniculate-Occipital Waves: The Question of Efference Copy

During paradoxical sleep (EEG stage 1 sleep with rapid eye movements) monophasic EEG waves can be recorded from the pons (Jouvet *et al.,* 1959), from oculomotor nuclei (Brooks and Bizzi, 1963), from the lateral geniculate body (Mikiten *et al.,* 1961; Brooks and Bizzi, 1963), and from the occipital cortex (Mouret *et al.,* 1963). The waves are often called pontine-geniculate-occipital (PGO) waves (Delorme *et al.,* 1965). They occur at a fairly constant daily rate of 14,000 ± 3,000 waves/day, and the onset of PGO waves precedes other signs of paradoxical sleep by some 30 to 40 sec (in cats, see Jouvet, 1969). PGO waves which are recorded from the different anatomical structures grossly coincide in time (Fig. 7). Bizzi and Brooks (1963) reported a time lag of maximally 5 msec between wave occurrence in the pons and lateral geniculate - but either structure may lead the other; on the other hand, stimulation of the pontine reticular

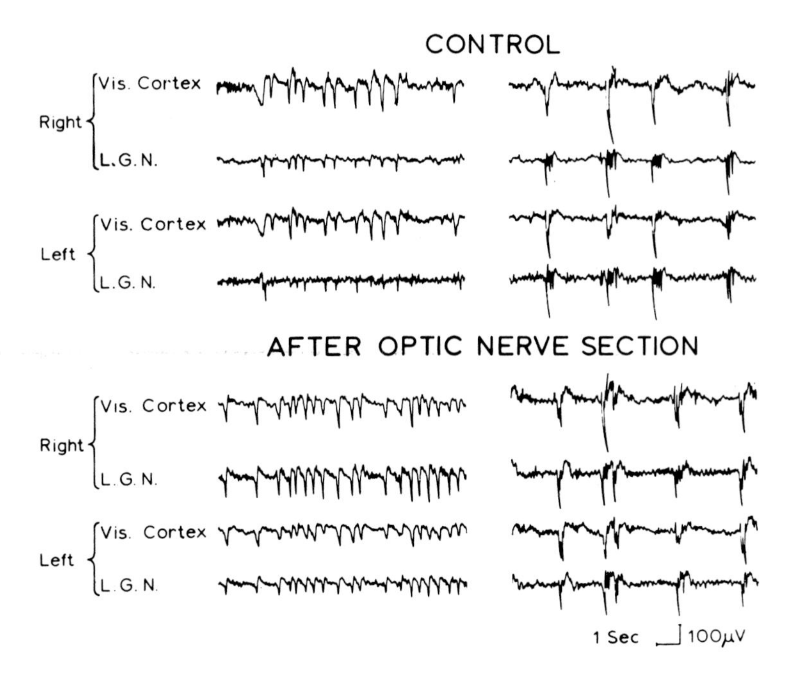

Fig. 7. PGO waves during arousal before, and one day after bilateral section of the optic nerve in cat. Records on the left: alert with eye movements. Records on the right: in paradoxical sleep. (From D.C. Brooks, *Electroenceph. clin. Neurophysiol.* **23:** 134-141, 1967; by permission of Elsevier Publishing Co., Amsterdam).

formation caused geniculate waves during REM sleep, but stimulation of the lateral geniculate body did not cause waves in the pons in cats (Bizzi and Brooks, 1963).

Spontaneous, individual PGO waves coincide with individual rapid eye movements during paradoxical sleep and wakefulness (Brooks, 1968a, 1968b; Cohen and Feldman, 1968; Feldman and Cohen, 1968), although there is no constant relation between characteristics of the saccade, and shape or amplitude of the PGO waves (Brooks, 1968b; Feldman and Cohen, 1968). PGO waves do not depend on visual or motor afferences generated by eye movements or eye muscle contractions, and rather reflect the efferent motor command, because the waves persist after enucleation (Michel *et al.,* 1964), transection of the optic nerves (Fig. 7, Brooks[1], 1967), and flaxedil paralysis of the animal

[1]Brooks (1970, pers. common.) feels that the cortical waves are abolished by the transection.

(Brooks, 1968a; Feldman and Cohen, 1968); similarly, PGO waves are not seen when the eyeball is moved passively in darkness (Feldman and Cohen 1968). These conditions are contrary to the conditions which allow so-called Lambda waves (visually evoked EEG potentials) to occur in the visual cortex of animals and man: Lambda waves follow active or passive eye movements when structured visual input is present, and they are not recorded in darkness (see Scott and Bickford, 1967, and the review in Section F). Therefore, "lambda waves" and "PGO waves" refer to different phenomena. PGO waves may contain lambda wave components when recorded in conditions which allow visual input. This latter problem arises in the interpretation of occipital waves related to eye movements during wakefulness in illuminated surrounds (Calvet *et al.*, 1965; Brooks, 1968b).

PGO waves occur after the onset of rapid eye movements. Feldman and Cohen (1968) found a latency of 40 msec between the onset of eye muscle activity and the onset of the geniculate wave in the alert monkey, in darkness (Fig. 8). The authors noted a small wave preceding the geniculate wave when the monkey was allowed to see. Brooks (1968b) used a photographic technique with 48 frames/sec to record eye movements, and estimated a latency of about 30 msec between onset of eye movement and onset of the occipital wave in the

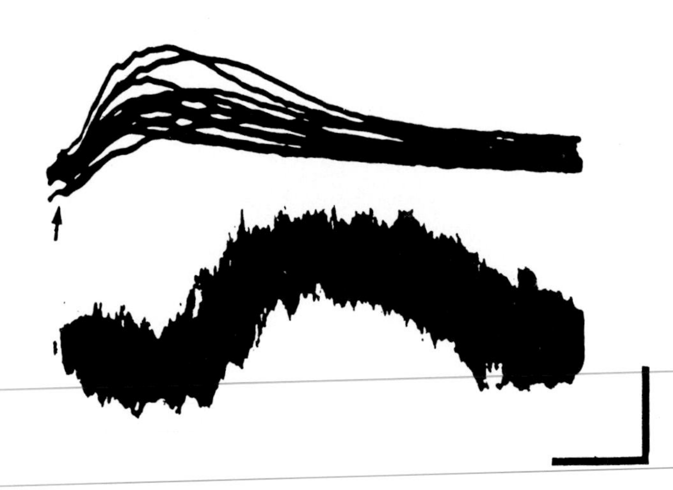

Fig. 8. Eye movements (upper trace) and geniculate waves (lower trace) during 10 consecutive quick phases of caloric nystagmus (monkey) in the dark. EMG of right lateral rectus muscle was used as trigger. Calibrations: time 40 msec; amplitudes, 30° deviation (upper trace), 100 μV (lower trace). (From M. Feldman and B. Cohen, *J. Neurophysiol.* **31:** 455-566, 1968; by permission of Charles C. Thomas, Springfield, Ill.).

alert cat (apparently, these recordings were obtained in an illuminated room, and visual input may have influenced the result). However, acoustic and tactile stimuli applied in darkness give rise to PGO waves as well, even without concomitant eye movements (e.g. Feldman and Cohen, 1968), although a very rapid habituation of these waves was observed during repetitive stimulation.

There are differences in opinion about the nature of PGO waves. Potentials related to eye movements in the absence of visual input have been differentiated into potentials observed during sleep (PGO waves), and potentials observed during wakefulness (eye movement potentials, Jeannerod and Sakai, 1970), emphasizing different characteristics of the potentials in the two recording conditions; e.g. Jeannerod and Sakai (1970) describe PGO waves during sleep which precede individual eye movements by a short latency.

The possible relation between PGO waves and the postulated suppression of visual perception during saccades was discussed in several papers (e.g. Brooks, 1968b; Feldman and Cohen, 1968). It appears that the latencies of PGO waves are quite sufficient to influence the final percept, although they may be too long to interfere with the transfer of information at the level of the lateral geniculate body. Thus, PGO waves may carry a correction signal in the sense of the proposed efference copy (Holst and Mittelstaedt, 1950), interfering at a higher level. On the other hand, Bizzi (1966) demonstrated presynaptic inhibition at the geniculate level during rapid eye movements in sleep, and Kawamura and Marchiafava (1968) showed that presynaptic LGB inhibition started before, and ended after the execution of tracking eye movements in acute cat experiments.

E. EEG Potentials Evoked by Image Movements on the Retina

When a light spot or a pattern moves on the retina, the light or dark areas of the stimulus will fall on receptive fields which, before the movement, had not received the same input. Consequently, retinal, geniculate, and cortical cells are activated or inhibited (See Grüsser and Grüsser-Cornehls, 1969). Indeed, the majority of cortical single cells in the cat will be most easily activated by moving visual stimuli (Hubel and Wiesel, 1965). Theoretically, one may expect that such moving stimuli are not effective in recordings which reflect the simultaneous activity of many neurons (as it is presumably the case in EEG recordings), since the movement of the stimulus across the retina will activate consecutive retinal areas which, in turn, continuously will activate new cortical single units: a momentary response time-locked to an event which is continuous in time is *per se* not possible. However, it has been shown that images which move on the retina while the eye is fixed, and fixed targets which are scanned actively by the moving eye, evoke EEG potentials time-locked to the onset of the eye movement or image movement. These responses essentially are reported as similar to a flash-evoked response, with the usual occipital negativity between 60 to 90 msec latency, followed by a positivity around 110-150 msec, and a tendency for a late negativity around 250 msec.

The finding of cortical EEG responses evoked by stimuli which move passively or actively on the retina can be explained by the assumption that the moving retinal stimulus corresponds to a potential maximum of occipital EEG evoked activity migrating on the cortex; if an EEG electrode allows recording of activity from a small area of cortex, and the movement of the EEG potential maximum on the scalp covers a much larger area, then one may see a potential maximum at a certain latency. This condition is, however, unlikely. It is more likely that only the activity generated by the passage of the stimulus across the fovea is picked up by scalp EEG electrodes, since generally the foveal representation on the cortex is larger and closer to the scalp than much of the representation of the retinal periphery.

Barlow and Cigánek (1968) compared EEG responses evoked by light spots of 40 msec exposure time with responses evoked by moving light spots. They found comparable EEG wave forms as responses to foveal light flashes, and to light spots moving from the retinal periphery to the fovea; however, the movement responses were delayed by about 40 msec - the time for the stimulus movement from retinal periphery to fovea, suggesting that the result was a

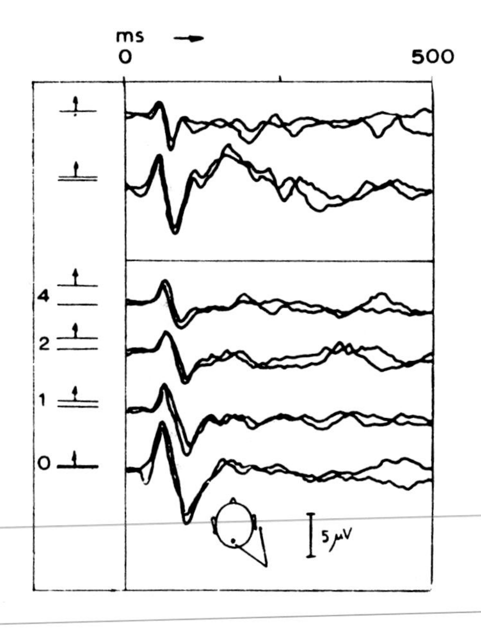

Fig. 9. Averaged EEG response evoked by moving line. The left column indicates the stimulus condition, the right column shows the responses, recorded as demonstrated. The second trace illustrates enhancement by the presence of a reference line; the enhancement of the response is inversely related to the initial separation of the two lines (lower four traces). (From D. M. MacKay and W.J. Rietveld, *Nature (Lond.)* **217:** 677-678, 1968; by permission of Macmillan & Co., Ltd., London).

foveal on-response. Dawson *et al.* (1968) showed that moving spot stimuli evoke an averaged EEG response of the same or greater magnitude than those evoked by stationary light flash stimuli of much greater intensity (however, the light flashes were of much shorter duration than the moving stimuli). MacKay and Rietveld (1968) used a line, moving vertically, as stimulus. The evoked EEG response was larger when a stationary reference line was added to the stimulus display; decrease of the distance between moving line and stationary reference line increased the amplitude of the response (Fig. 9). When both stimulus lines moved in opposite directions, an EEG response was obtained which was similar to the response to movement of one line at twice the velocity. Increase in spatial frequency of the stimulus pattern increased the size of the response, but the direction of the stimulus movement on the retina had no effect on the wave-shape of the EEG response, contrary to Barlow and Ciganek's observations.

F. EEG Potentials Evoked by Eye Movements Across Patterned Visual Fields (Lambda Waves)

Some human subjects show positive sharp waves in their occipital scalp EEG during alpha blocking when observing a patterned target (Gastaut, 1951; Evans, 1952). These so-called lambda waves follow eye movements, and are not found when the subject has his eyes closed, when he is in darkness, or when he observes a uniform field (see Scott *et al.*, 1967). Lambda waves were also recorded from animals (Scott *et al.*, 1968). Most of the lambda wave reports apparently described EEG responses evoked by an eye movement which causes an image displacement on the retina during the observation of a patterned target. (No EEG response is seen when the target moves with the eye, i.e., when the target image remains stationary on the retina [Barlow and Ciganek, 1968]). However, reports on lambda waves may very well include cortical potentials which are independent from visual input and which follow eye movements. These potentials (pontine-geniculate-occipital waves) were discussed in section D.

Gaarder *et al.* (1964) averaged the EEG which follows involuntary saccades in humans observing a patterned fixation target (20 min arc, or 5 degree arc); evoked potentials were obtained which show the usual main features of visually evoked potentials in humans to flash stimuli (Fig. 10).

Scott and Bickford (1967) used a larger, complex picture target and asked the subject to scan it. Again, typical evoked responses were seen after eye movements; similar potentials were recorded when the eyeball was moved passively, by tapping; the potentials were absent when the same procedure was used in darkness (Fig. 11). The authors emphasize that the potentials are similar when obtained without perceptual blurring during involuntary saccades, and with perceptual blurring when tapping the eyeball. Scott and Bickford conclude therefore that an anti-blur mechanism is not likely to be reflected by the potentials.

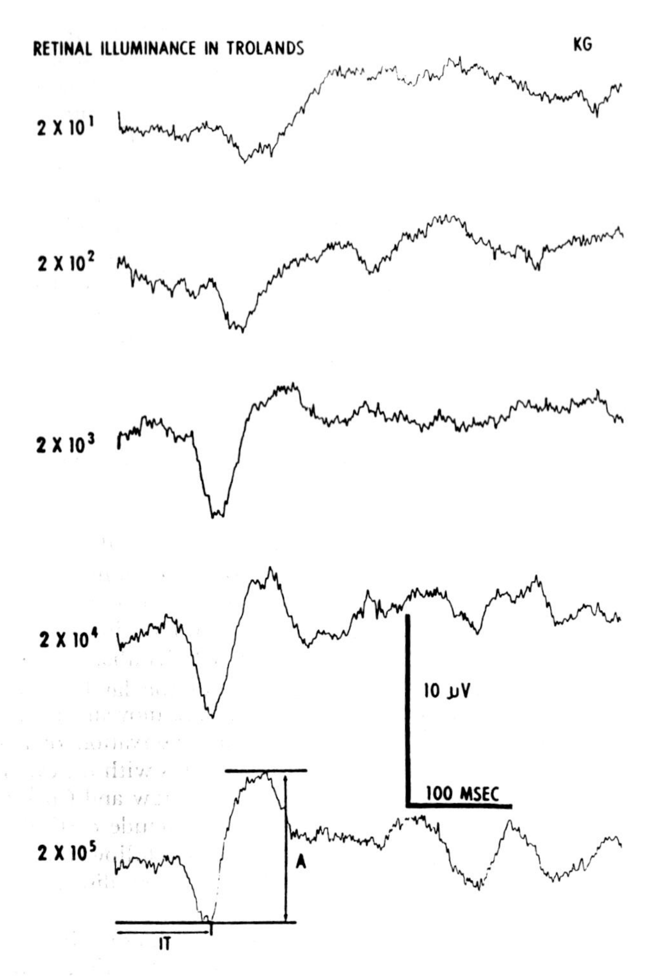

Fig. 10. Averaged EEG potentials following 50 spontaneous saccades during fixation of a five degree target at different levels of illuminance. Recording: inion vs 5 cm anterior to inion, anterior electrode positive = up. (From K. Gaarder *et al., Science,* **146:**1481-1483, 1964; by permission of Amer. Assoc. for the Advancement of Science, Washington, D.C.).

Rémond *et al.* (1965) studied characteristics of averaged lambda responses in humans, using voluntary and spontaneous saccades. Lambda waves are localized over occipital areas (Fig. 12). The localization of the stimulus pattern within one half of the visual field resulted in lambda waves which were larger over the hemisphere contralateral to the stimulus. The latency of the different components of the response depended on the intensity of the

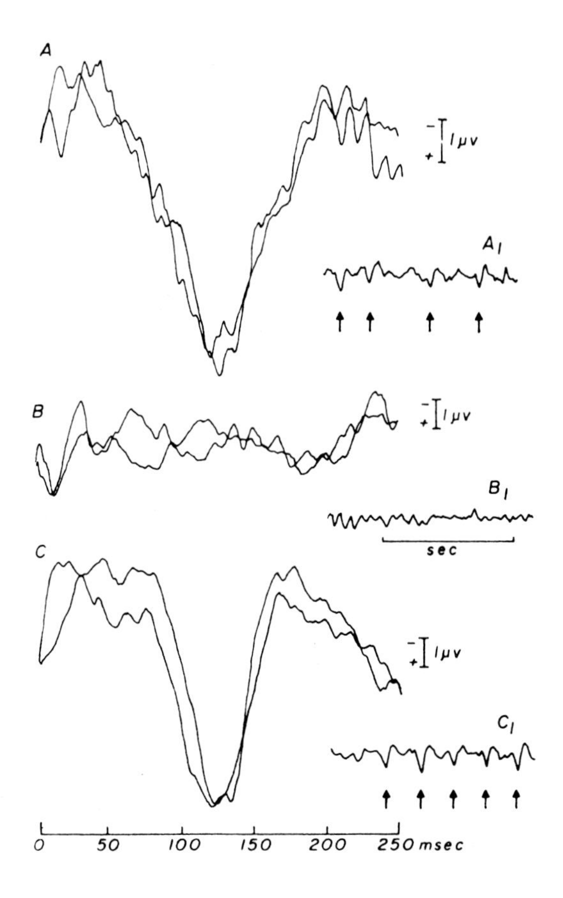

Fig. 11. Averaged parieto-occipital EEG potentials (two sets, of 20, superimposed). A. Tapping outer canthus of eye during fixation of stimulus card. B: Similar tapping in darkness. C: Scanning of complex stimulus card. Insets A, B, and C show raw EEG with lambda waves (arrows). (From D.F. Scott and R.G. Bickford, *Science* **155:** 101-102, 1967; by permission of Amer. Assoc. for the Advancement of Science, Washington, D. C.).

illumination of the target. However, the direction of the eye movements had no effect on the resulting waveshape.

The report of Gaarder *et al.* (1964) also described systematic changes of the response as a function of the illuminance of the target. The authors proposed that data handling in the visual system is discontinuous, and that each saccade produces a package of information represented by the evoked response. This theory was supported by further experiments where voluntary saccades were used for the retinal image displacement and as trigger signal for the averaging

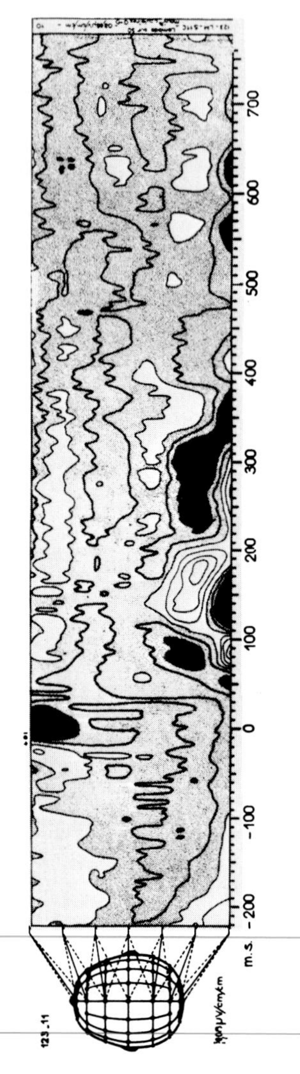

Fig. 12. EEG data ("lambda waves") averaged during the execution of 50 eye movements of 10 degree amplitude across a complex target field. The maximum of the eye movement artifact is seen at time 0 msec. The distribution of the electrical charge was computed from measurements obtained from a chain of nine electrodes along the midline of the head, as indicated at left. The change of the field distribution along the recording line is illustrated as a function of time up to 770 msec after the eye movements. White: current sources. Black: current sinks. (A conventionally recorded lambda wave would represent a horizontal slice of the graph shown here). (From A. Remond *et al., Rev. Neurol.* **113:** 193-226, 1965; by permission of Masson et Cie, Paris).

process (Gaarder, 1968). Differences in size and shape of the responses were found in different experimental conditions, e.g., larger EEG responses were seen with larger size of the saccade.

An illuminated dot was used as target by Barlow and Ciganek (1969) who averaged EEG responses in a condition where the eye moved while the target was stationary, and compared them with responses which were averaged when the target moved and the eye was fixed. The latter condition produced evoked responses with latencies 50 - 100 msec shorter than the "eye moving" condition. The authors felt that this difference could not be accounted for by slight differences in the displacement of the image on the retina, and they suggest that the finding might be related to the time course of the amplitude decrease of potentials evoked during eye movement (see Section G).

Extreme sensitivity of the brain to the observation of geometrical patterns has been reviewed by Bickford and Klass (1964); seizure discharges in the EEG, and clinical epileptic seizures can be triggered in some patients by such simple stimuli.

G. EEG Potentials Evoked During Saccades, and the Saccadic Suppression of Perception

A passive movement of the eyeball (tapping) lets us see a moving world; why do we not see the world move when a voluntary or involuntary saccade occurs? The theory of the efference copy (Helmholtz, 1962; Holst and Mittelstaedt, 1950) postulates a cancellation of the visual percept received during the time of saccadic eye movement. The postulated perceptual suppression was investigated in psychophysical experiments where light flashes are presented during saccadic eye movements. The results are still partially contradictory, and range from reports of no perceptual change (during involuntary saccades, Krauskopf *et al.*, 1966) to some elevation of threshold (0.5 log units during involuntary saccades with light flashes in stabilized vision, Beeler, 1967) to reports of considerable suppression (with voluntary and involuntary saccades in normal vision, Zuber and Stark, 1966). The thresholds during smooth pursuit movements, incidentally, approximate the thresholds during times without eye movements (Starr *et al.*, 1969).

Several workers have investigated EEG responses evoked during voluntary saccades. Changes of the responses during the saccades were described by all groups. Michael and Stark (1967) did not see a reduction of amplitude, but reported definite modifications of the shape of the response 60 msec before, and at the beginning of the saccade (The EGG waveshape accompanying eye movements without flash presentations was subtracted from the response to light flashes before the evaluation).

Foveal presentation of light flashes was used by Duffy and Lombroso (1968) who found that the average power of the response waveform decreased to a minimum of 20% of the norm response 40 msec before onset of the saccade, then slowly increased up to 200 msec after the start of the eye movement. Gross *et al.* (1967) attempted to avoid retinal blur by the presentation of an

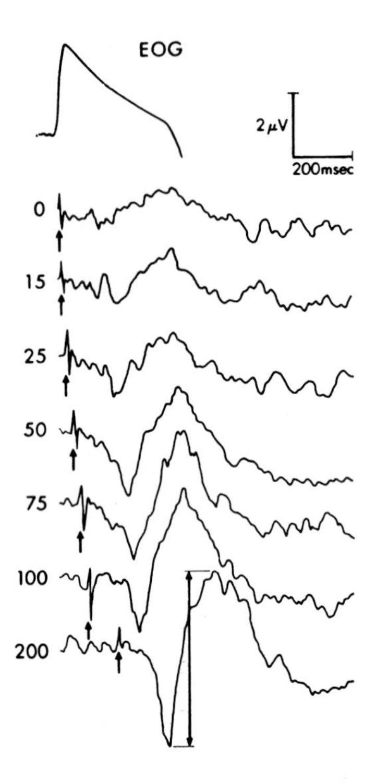

Fig. 13. Averaged EEG responses evoked by test light flashes at different times after initiation of eye movement. Vertical arrows indicate the presentation of the light flashes; the numbers in the margin give the delay in msec between initiation of eye movement and presentation of flash. Occipital versus linked ear electrodes. Occipital positivity = up. (From E.G. Gross *et al, Electroenceph. clin. Neurophysiol.* **22:** 204-209, 1967; by permission of Elsevier Publishing Co., Amsterdam).

alternating pattern of horizontal stripes. The EEG responses were almost absent when the target was presented at the beginning of a saccade; the responses increased with increasing latency of the target presentation after the onset of the eye movement, and were largest at 200 msec latency (Fig. 13). Potentials accompanying eye movements alone were subtracted out, as in the study discussed above. The authors concluded that blocking of the response cannot be cortical, since not even the first component of the response was observed during suppression. They also report very little suppression of responses to diffuse light flashes, and argue that the suppression effect is pattern specific. This conclusion was not supported by Chase and Kalil (1968) in a study which investigated the effect of diffuse flashes of different intensities, and of horizontal stripe patterns of different spatial frequencies. With dim flashes or high spatial frequency of the stripes, no evoked response could be detected at the onset of eye movements. Increase of flash intensity, or wider black and white stripes, however, caused discrete EEG responses.

Obviously, the evoked EEG responses show graded attenuation as a function of the time of stimulus presentation relative to the occurrence of the saccade, but the responses are also powerfully influenced by other experimental conditions as e.g. intensity of the stimulus. We notice that a basically common shape of the EEG responses - a major positivity at about 130-150 msec latency - is observed by most investigators in spite of widely different experimental conditions and electrode placements.

At this stage it is difficult to assess the functional significance of the observed attenuations of the evoked activity. It has been argued that the attenuation reflects the effect of centrally controlled presynaptic inhibition described at the geniculate level during tracking eye movements (Kawamura and Marchiafava, 1968). Evidence for the existence of the efference copy may be the single unit discharges associated with eye movements in the frontal eye field (Bizzi, 1967, 1968), and the observation of pontine-geniculate-occipital EEG sharp waves during rapid eye movements. Effects of such activity are seen in the modification of evoked EEG responses, and of occipital single unit activity (Wurtz, 1968) during eye movements. However, since stimuli during saccades still elicit cortical responses and percepts in many stimulus conditions, we must conclude that the perceptual constancy of our surround is ensured by processes at higher analysis levels, above the detection problem.

H. The Effect of Stabilization of Retinal Images

Motions of the retinal image which are caused by eye movements (pursuit movements, drift, and tremor) can be eliminated by several techniques which result in spatial stabilization of the image on the retina. Pattern changes in the on-going scalp EEG are associated with the fluctuations of perception of stabilized retinal images. The changes of the scalp EEG precede the perceptual fading or reappearing of the stabilized image, and therefore, the perceptual fluctuations were concluded to be caused by central processes (Lehmann *et al.*, 1965; Kessey and Nichols, 1967). Induced changes of the EEG were accompanied by changes of visibility of the stabilized image (Keesey and Nichols, 1969).

EEG responses evoked by intermittant presentation of an image stabilized on the retina may be expected to be different from the EEG responses evoked by the same image in normal vision, since the information reaching the central areas and the processing task for the brain must be different in the two conditions; further, since the stabilized image tends to fade perceptually, this may be reflected by the evoked potentials.

Riggs and Whittle (1967) examined monocularly evoked parieto-occipital potentials in two subjects during stabilized and normal presentation of alternating stripe patterns. Each stripe changed from black to white and back at a relatively high frequency (about 24 cps) so that the stabilized condition allowed perceptual fading. Conventional flash stimulation of the target at 7 - 21 cps was also used. In spite of sometimes virtually complete disappearance of the stimulus, and under different frequency, intensity, and wave length conditions, no difference was observed in the EEG potentials which were averaged in the stabilized and normal viewing condition.

A dichoptic experimental design was used in evoked potential experiments with humans by Lehmann *et al.* (1967), in order to assess effects of retinal stabilization versus normal viewing conditions. Light flashes of constant parameters (3.2/sec) were shown to one eye of the subject, while the other eye observed a continuously illuminated cross target or a uniform dark field in normal or in stabilized vision. The continuously illuminated target by itself does not give rise to evoked potentials; if, however, the afference generated by the monocular target influences the state of the central processor which receives input from both eyes, then this influence should be demonstrable by the central responsiveness to test flashes presented to the other eye. Evoked EEG potentials were averaged from parieto-occipital electrodes. The mean amplitude of the monocularly evoked potentials during contraocular observation of the cross target in normal vision was about 70% of the amplitude which was obtained during contraocular darkness. On the other hand, the mean evoked potential amplitude during observation of the stabilized cross image was 90% of the mean amplitude during contraocular darkness. In other words, the monocularly evoked potentials obtained with the contraocular target in normal vision exhibited only 75% of the amplitude of potentials which were recorded with the target seen in stabilized vision.

The experimental design used the response-evoking light flashes as indicators of available central capacity, reasoning that increase in amplitude of the response indicates time-locked participation of more neural elements. The results suggest that the cortical capacity, which is required in normal vision to incorporate information concerning head and eye movements into a meaningful percept of a retinal image, may not be used when the image is stationary on the retina; thus, extra capacity becomes available to participate in the generation of EEG potentials evoked by monocular light flashes when the other eye sees a target as a stabilized image instead of the normal viewing condition.

ACKNOWLEDGEMENT

The author is obliged to the Brain Information Service, UCLA, for assistance in the literature search.

REFERENCES

BARLOW, J.S. & CIGÁNEK, L. (1969). Lambda responses in relation to visual evoked responses in man. *Electroenceph. clin. Neurophysiol.* **26,** 183-192.

BECKER, W., DEECKE, L., HOEHNE, O., IWASE, K., KORNHUBER, H.H. & SCHEID, P. (1968). Bereitschaftspotential, Motorpotential und praemotorische Positivierung der menschlichen Hirnrinde vor Willkürbewegungen. *Naturwissenschaften* **55,** 550.

BEELER, G.W., Jr., (1967). Visual threshold changes resulting from spontaneous saccadic eye movements. *Vision Res.* **7,** 769-776.

BENDER, M.B. & SHANZER, S. (1964). Oculomotor pathways defined by electrical stimulation and lesions in the brain stem. **In:** M.B. Bender (Ed). *The Oculomotor System,* New York, Harper & Row, pp. 81-140.

BERGER, H. (1930). Über das Elektrenkephalogramm des Menschen. *J. Psychol. Neurol.* **40,** 160-179 [English translation in: *Electroenceph. clin. Neurophysiol.* Suppl. **28,** 1969. p. 75-93]

BERGER, R.J. (1969). Oculomotor control: A possible function of REM sleep. *Psychol. Rev.* **76,** 144-164.

BERGER, R.G., OLLEY, P. & OSWALD, I. (1962). The EEG, eye movements and dreams of the blind. *Quart. J. exp. Psychol.* **14,** 183-186.

BICKFORD, R.G. & KLASS, D.W. (1964). Eye movement and the electroencephalogram. **In:** M.B. Bender (Ed). *The Oculomotor System,* New York, Harper & Row, pp. 293-302.

BIZZI, E. (1966). Changes in the orthodromic and antidromic response of optic tract during the eye movements of sleep. *J. Neurophysiol.* **29,** 861-870.

BIZZI, E. (1967). Discharge of frontal eye field neurons during eye movements in unanesthetized monkeys. *Science* **157,** 1588-1590.

BIZZI, E. (1968). Discharge of frontal eye field neurons during saccadic and following eye movements in unanesthetized monkeys. *Exp. Brain Research* **6,** 69-80.

BIZZI, E. & BROOKS, D.C. (1963). Functional connections between pontine reticular formation and lateral geniculate nucleus during deep sleep. *Arch. ital. Biol.* **101,** 666-680.

BROOKS, D.C. (1967). Effect of bilateral optic nerve section on visual system monophasic wave activity in the cat. *Electroenceph. clin. Neurophysiol.* **23,** 134-141.

BROOKS, D.C. (1968a). Waves associated with eye movement in the awake and sleeping cat. *Electroenceph. clin. Neurophysiol.* **24,** 532-541.

BROOKS, D.C. (1968b). Localization and characteristics of the cortical waves associated with eye movement in the cat. *Exp. Neurol.* **22,** 603-613.

BROOKS, D.C. & BIZZI, E. (1963). Brain stem electrical activity during sleep. *Arch. ital. Biol.* **101,** 648-665.

BURFORD, G. (1941). Involuntary eyeball motion during anesthesia and sleep: Relationship to cortical rhythmic potentials. *Anesth. Analg.* **20,** 191-199.

CALVET, J., CALVET, M.C., & LANGLOIS, J.M. (1965). Diffuse cortical activation waves during so-called desynchronized EEG patterns. *J. Neurophysiol.* **28,** 893-907.

CARPENTER, M.B. (1969). Central oculomotor pathways [This Symposium].

CASPERS, H. & SCHULZE, H. (1959). Die Veraenderungen der corticalen Gleishcpannung waehrend der natuerlichen Schlaf-Wach-Perioden beim freibeweglichen Tier. *Pflügers Arch. ges. Physiol.* **270,** 103-120.

CHASE R. & KALIL, R. (1968). Visual evoked responses to flashes and pattern shifts during voluntary eye movements. Paper presented at EPA, Washington, D.C.

COHEN, B. & FELDMAN, M. (1968). Relationship of electrical activity in pontine reticular formation and lateral geniculate body to rapid eye movements. *J. Neurophysiol.* **31,** 806-817.

DAWSON, W.W., PERRY, N.W., Jr. & CHILDERS, D.G. (1968). Flash and scan stimulation of retinal fields and evoked response production. *Electroenceph. clin. Neurophysiol.* **24,** 467-473.

DELORME, F., JEANNEROD, M. & JOUVET, M. (1965). Effects remarquables de la réserpine sur l'activité EEG ponto-géniculo-occipitale. *Compt. Rend. Soc. Biol.* (Paris). **159,** 900-903.

DEMENT, W.C. (1964). Eye movements during sleep. **In:** M.B. Bender (Ed) *The Oculomotor Ssytem,* New York, Harper & Row, pp. 336-416.

DEMENT, W.C. (1967). Possible physiological determinants of a possible dream-intensity cycle. *Exp. Neurol. Suppl.* **4,** 38-55.

DEMENT, W.C. & KLEITMAN, N. (1957). Cyclic variations in EEG during sleep and their relation to eye movements, body motility, and dreaming. *Electroenceph. clin. Neurophysiol.* **3,** 673-690.

DEWAN, E.M. (1967). Occipital alpha rhythm, eye position and lens accommodation. *Nature* (Lond.) **214,** 975-977.

DUFFY, F.H. & LOMBROSO, C.T. (1968). Electrophysiological evidence for visual suppression prior to the onset of a voluntary saccadic eye movement. *Nature* (Lond.) **218,** 1074-1075.

EVANS, C.C. (1952). Some further observations on occipital sharp waves (lambda waves). *Electroenceph. clin. Neurophysiol.* **4,** 371.

FELDMAN, M. & COHEN, B. (1968). Electrical activity in the lateral geniculate body of the alert monkey associated with eye movements. *J. Neurophysiol.* **31,** 455-466.

FENWICK, P.B.C. & WALKER, S. (1968). The effects of eye position on the alpha rhythm. *Electroenceph. clin. Neurophysiol.* **25,** 508.

FUCHS, A.F. & RON, S. (1968). An analysis of rapid eye movements of sleep in the monkey. *Electroenceph. clin. Neurophysiol.* **25,** 244-251.

GAARDER, K. (1968). Interpretive study of evoked responses elicited by gross saccadic eye movements. *Percept. Motor Skills* **27,** 683-703.

GAARDER, K., KORESKO, R. & KROPFL, W. (1966). The phasic relation of a component of alpha rhythm to fixation saccadic eye movements. *Electroenceph. clin. Neurophysiol.* **21,** 544-551.

GAARDER, K., KRAUSKOPF, J., GRAF, V., KROPFL, W. & ARMINGTON, J.C. (1964). Averaged brain activity following saccadic eye movement. *Science* **146,** 1481-1483.

GASTAUT, Y. (1951). Un signe électroencéphalographique peu connu: les points occipitales survenant pendant l'ouverture des yeux. *Rev. neurol.* **84,** 640-643.

GLASS, A. & KWIATKOWSKI, A.W. (1968). Normal power spectral density changes in the EEG during mental arithmetic and eye opening. *Electroenceph. clin. Neurophysiol.* **25,** 507.

GROSS, E.G., VAUGHAN, H.G. & VALENSTEIN, E. (1967). Inhibition of visual evoked responses to patterned stimuli during voluntary eye movements. *Electroenceph. clin. Neurophysiol.* **22,** 204-209.

GRÜSSER, O.J. & GRÜSSER-CORNEHLS, U. (1969). Neurophysiologie des Bewegungssehens: Bewegungsempfindliche und richtungsspezifische Neurone im visuellen System. *Ergebn. Physiol.* **61,** 178-265.

HELMHOLTZ, H. VON. (1962). *Treatise on physiological optics.* vol. 3. New York, Dover.

HILLYARD, S.A. & GALAMBOS, R. Eye movement artifact in the CNV. *Electroenceph. clin. Neurophysiol.* (In Press).

HOLST, E. VON & MITTELSTAEDT, H. (1950). Das Reafferenzprinzip. *Naturwissenschaften* **37,** 464-476.

HUBEL, D.H. & WIESEL, T.N. (1965). Receptive fields and functional architecture in two nonstriate visual areas (18 and 19) of the cat. *J. Neurophysiol.* **28,** 229-289.

JASPER, H.H., PROCTOR, L.D., KNIGHTON, R.S., NOSHAY, W.C. & COSTELLO, R.T. (Eds.). (1958). *Reticular formation of the brain.* Henry Ford Hospital Intern. Symposium, no. 7. Boston, Little, Brown.

JEANNEROD, M. & MOURET, J. (1963). Étude comparative des movements ocularies observés chez le chat au cours de la veille et du sommeil. *J. Physiol.* (Paris). **55,** 268.

JEANNEROD, M. & SAKAI, K. (1970). Occipital and geniculate potentials related to eye movements in the unanesthetized cat. *Brain Res.* (In press).

JOUVET, M. (1967). Neurophysiology of the states of sleep. *Physiol. Rev.* **47,** 117-177.

JOUVET, M. (1969). Biogenic amines and the states of sleep. *Science.* **163,** 32-41.

JOUVET, M., MICHEL, F. & COURJON, J. (1959). Sur un stade d'activité électrique cérébrale rapide au cours du sommeil physiologique. *Compt. Rend. Soc. Biol.* (Paris). **153,** 1024-1028.

JOUVET, M., PELLIN, B. & MOUNIER, D. (1961). Étude polygraphique des differentes phases du sommeil au cours des troubles de conscience chroniques. *Rev. Neurol.* **105,** 181-186.

KAWAMURA, H. & MARCHIAFAVA, P.L. (1968). Excitability changes along visual pathways during eye tracking movements. *Arch. ital. Biol.* **106,** 141-156.

Keesey, U.T. & Nichols, D.J. (1967). Fluctuations in target visibility as related to the occurrence of the alpha component of the electroencephalogram. *Vision Res.* **7,** 859-879.

Keesey, U.T. & Nichols, D.J. (1969). Changes induced in stabilized image visibility by experimental alteration of the ongoing EEG. *Electroenceph. Clin. Neurophysiol.* **27,** 248-257.

Kornhuber, H.H. (1966). Physiologie and Klinik des zentralvestibulaeren Systems. **In:** Berendes, Link, and Zöllner (Eds.) *Hals-Nasen-Ohrenheilkunde.* vol. III/3, pp. 2150-2351. Stuttgart, Thieme.

Krauskopf, J., Graf, V. & Gaarder, K. (1966). Lack of inhibition during involuntary saccades. *Amer. J. Psychol.* **79,** 73-81.

Kuhlo, W. & Lehmann, D. (1964). Das Einschlaferleben und seine neurophysiologischen Korrelate. *Arch. Psychiat. Nervenkr.* **205,** 687-716.

Lehmann, D., Beeler, G.W. Jr., & Fender, D.H. (1965). Changes in patterns of the human electroencephalogram during fluctuations of perception of stabilized retinal images. *Electroenceph. clin. Neurophysiol.* **19,** 336-343.

Lehmann, D., Beeler, G.W., Jr. & Fender, D.H. (1967). EEG responses to light flashes during the observation of stabilized and normal retinal images. *Electroenceph. clin. Neurophysiol.* **22,** 136-142.

Mackay, D.M. & Rietveld, W.J. (1968). Electroencephalogram potentials evoked by accelerated visual motion. *Nature* (Lond.) **217,** 677-678.

Michael, J.A. & Stark, L. (1967). Electrophysiological correlates of saccadic suppression. *Exp. Neurol.* **17,** 233-246.

Michel, F., Jeannerod, M., Mouret, J., Rechtschaffen, A. & Jouvet, M. (1964). Sur les méchanismes de l'activité de pointes au niveau du système visual au cours de la phase paradoxale du sommeil. *Compt. Rend. Soc. Biol.* (Paris). **158,** 103-106.

Mikiten, T.H., Niebyl, P.H. & Hendley, C.D. (1961). EEG desynchronization during behavorial sleep associated with spike discharges from the thalamus of cat. *Fed. Proc.* **20,** 327.

Mouret, J., Jeannerod, M. & Jouvet, M. (1963). L'activité électrique du système visuel au cours de la phase paradoxale du sommeil chez le chat. *J. Physiol.* (Paris). **55,** 305-306.

Mulholland, T. (1968). Feedback electroencephalography. *Activ. nerv. sup. (Praha)* **10,** 410-438.

Mulholland, T. & Evans, C.R. (1965). An unexpected artifact in the human electroencephalogram concerning the alpha rhythm and the orientation of the eyes. *Nature* (Lond.) **207,** 36-37.

Mulholland, T. & Evans, C.R. (1966). Oculomotor function and the alpha activation cycle. *Nature* (Lond.) **211,** 1278-1279.

Oswald, I. (1962). *Sleeping and Wakefulness.* Amsterdam, Elsevier.

Rashbass, C. (1961). The relationship between saccadic and smooth tracking eye movements. *J. Physiol.* (Lond.) **159,**326-338.

Rémond, A., Lesèvre, N. & Torres, F. (1965). Étude chronotopographique de l'activité occipitale moyenne recueillie sur le scalp chez l'homme en relation avec les déplacements du regard (complex lambda). *Rev. Neurol.* **113,** 193-226.

Riggs, L.A. & Whittle, P. (1967). Human occipital and retinal potentials evoked by subjectively faded visual stimuli. *Vision Res.* **7,** 441-451.

Robinson, D.A. & Fuchs, A.F. (1969). Eye movements and frontal eye fields. *J. Neurophysiol.* **32,** 637-648.

Roffwarg, H.P., Muzio, J.N. & Dement, W.C. (1966). Ontogenetic development of the human sleep-dream cycle. *Science.* **152,** 604-619.

Schwartz, B.A. & Fischgold, H. (1960). Introduction à l'étude polygraphique du sommeil de nuit. *Vie méd.* **41,** 39-40.

Scott, D.F. & Bickford, R.G. (1967). Electrophysiologic studies during scanning and passive eye movements in humans. *Science.* **155,** 101-102.

SCOTT, D.F., GROETHUYSEN, U.G. & BICKFORD, R.G. (1967). Lambda responses in the human electroencephalogram. *Neurology* (Minneap.). **17,** 770-778.

SCOTT, D.F., LICHTENHELD, F.R. & BICKFORD, R.G. (1968). Lambda wave studies on the EEG of animals. *Arch. Neurol.* **18,** 574-582.

STARR, A., ANGEL, R. & YEATES, H. (1969). Visual suppression during smooth following and saccadic eye movement. *Vision Res.* **9,** 195-197.

WALTER, W.G., COOPER, R., ALDRIDGE, V. J., MCMALLUM, W.C. & WINTER, A.L. (1964). Contingent negative variation; an electric sign of sensory-motor association and expectancy in the human brain. *Nature* (Lond.). **203,** 380-384.

WURTZ, R.H. (1968). Visual cortex neurons: Response to stimuli during rapid eye movements. *Science.* **162,** 1148-1150.

ZUBER, B.L. & STARK, L. (1966). Saccadic suppression: Elevation of visual threshold associated with saccadic eye movements. *Exp. Neurol.* **16,** 65-79.

SUPRANUCLEAR DISORDERS OF OCULAR CONTROL SYSTEMS IN MAN
Clinical, Anatomical, and Physiological Correlations—1969

WILLIAM F. HOYT and ROBERT B. DAROFF

The significant developments in the physiology and bio-mechanics of eye movements recorded in other chapters of this book originate from scientists working in widely differing disciplines, sometimes without knowledge of one another's endeavors. Their new definitions and still evolving conceptions of the systems controlling eye movement call for revisions of much traditional neurologic doctrine as formulated from clinical and neuropathologic observations. Our major aims in the preparation of this chapter were two-fold; firstly, to provide the clinician with a re-appraisal of the supranuclear ocular motor syndromes and signs in terms of current physiological concepts; and secondly, to share with our colleagues in physiology and bioengineering the tempting opportunities for useful collaborative investigations of various defective eye movement control systems exemplified in patients with clinical involvement of the cerebrum, cerebellum, or brain stem.

We purposely included the year "1969" in the title of this review. Much of what will follow is speculative, although based on what seems supported by current physiological, anatomical and clinico-pathological correlation. Future advances in these areas will undoubtedly contradict some of our conceptions and, hopefully, validate others. We will welcome either equally.

The various types of ocular motor disorders are discussed in terms of horizontal, vertical and vergence movements, with a final section on para- and internuclear disorders. A separate section is not included for the most commonly encountered abnormality of ocular movement—nystagmus. Limitation of space precluded its consideration as a specific entity, although several varieties of nystagmus are discussed. Contemporary clinical and physiological reviews of this subject are available elsewhere (Kornhuber, 1966; Walsh and Hoyt, 1969).

THE ANATOMICAL SUBSTRATE FOR CONJUGATE SACCADIC AND PURSUIT CONTROL SYSTEMS

The anatomy of the ocular motor system is presented in detail by Carpenter elsewhere in this volume. Despite the possible redundancy, a brief review will be provided as a necessary prelude to our clinical discussions.

Horizontal saccades are probably represented cortically in the contralateral frontal lobe although each hemisphere is capable of initiating ipsilateral saccades as well (Robinson and Fuchs, 1969). Pursuit movements originate cortically in occipital-parietal (peristriate) visual association areas. Both types of eye movements, in the horizontal plane, ultimately are regulated in the pontine paramedian reticular formation just ventral to the medial longitudinal fasciculi (Bender and Shanzer, 1964; Cohen *et al.*, 1968).

Uncertainty and controversy characterize the exact course of the corticopontine pathways. For saccades, experimental studies (Brucher, 1966; Bender and Shanzer, 1964) and clinical evidence suggest that descending corticofugal fibers from the frontal eye field are initially grouped in the anterior limb of the internal capsule and adjacent globus pallidus. Thereafter, the fibers separate into two bundles. The major pathway courses caudo-medially passing along the ventrolateral surface of the thalamus amidst the zona incerta and Forel's fields. In the rostral midbrain these fibers are situated primarily in the ipsilateral reticular formation. They decussate, according to Baucher (1966), in the upper pons (close to the level of the trochlear nucleus that Bender established from his physiological data), and terminate in the contralateral pontine tegmentum, near the vestibular and abducens nuclei.

A second bundle of fibers descends through the internal capsule and cerebral peduncle to the basis pontis before it turns dorsally to enter the pontine tegmentum. This pathway constitutes *Dejerine's aberrant pyramidal system* (Dejerine, 1926). The significance of this system as the major corticofugal pathway for horizontal gaze, although dismissed by Brucher (1966), retains uncritical acceptance by some (Kemper *et al.*, 1967; Halsey, *et al.*, 1967). However, the ventral brain stem lesions alleged to have produced paresis of horizontal gaze have always involved the tegmentum as well, and no discernable effect on eye movements follows isolated ventral brain stem lesions in monkey (Bender and Shanzer, 1964) and man (Bucy, *et al.*, 1964).

Experimental lesions in the occipital cortex consistently produce degenerative changes in the ipsilateral superior colliculus (Garey, *et al.*, 1968). Although it is not absolutely certain that the occipito-collicular pathway subserves horizontal pursuit movements, available clinical evidence suggests that it does. The occipito-collicular projections (internal sagittal stratum) lie medial to the optic radiation and apparently pass into the retro-lenticular portion of the internal capsule, through the pulvinar, and then to the brachium of the ipsilateral superior colliculus (Holmes, 1936). These fibers probably leave the colliculus within the medial tectospinal tract, coursing ventrally around the periaqueductal gray and the medial longitudinal fasciculus, and crossing to the opposite side of the midbrain tegmentum in the dorsal fountain decussation or the decussation of Meynert (Crosby, *et al.*, 1962). Then they join the fiber projections from the frontal area mediating saccades and together decussate at the ponto-mesencephalic junction. We propose, therefore, that the occipito-pontine tract must undergo a second decussation. This inference is compatible with clinical evidence (to be discussed later) that horizontal pursuit movements are regulated by the ipsilateral occipital cortex.

Cortical representation and descending pathways for vertical saccades and pursuit probably course with the horizontal gaze systems. Bender's (1960) contention that vertical gaze systems are bilaterally represented seems valid for levels above the rostral mesencephalon. The anatomical substrate for vertical movements will be discussed in more detail in the section on clinical disorders of vertical gaze.

Similarly, remarks on the anatomy of ocular vergence are included in the section describing clinical disorders of this system.

CLINICAL DISORDERS OF SUPRANUCLEAR CONTROL SYSTEMS FOR HORIZONTAL EYE MOVEMENTS

Fronto-Mesencephalic disorders

Tonic deviation of the eyes, a frequent manifestation of cerebral lesions, is traditionally separated by clinicians into "irritative" and "paralytic" types. "Irritative" deviations are usually a sign of seizure activity that drives the eye to the opposite side. "Paralytic" deviations are ipsilateral to the lesion and are associated with gross impairment of conjugate ocular movements to the opposite side. Such deviations are assumed to result from disinhibition of antagonists of the non-functioning yoke muscles (Bielschowsky, 1935). Tonic deviation has been described with destructive lesions in several areas of the hemisphere (Cotte-Rittaud and Courjon, 1962; Bender, 1962; David and Hacaen, 1947; and Gastaut, 1960), but is usually associated with contralateral hemiplegia and indicates involvement of the ipsilateral fronto-mesencephalic pathway (Holmes, 1921). The responsible lesion usually lies in the hemispheric white matter rather than the cortex (Bender, 1962). If the pathologic process is limited to a frontal lobe, sparing the posterior portions of the hemisphere and brain stem, the abnormality of conjugate gaze involves only the saccadic system.

A. Unilateral lesions

The following description of clinical signs in a patient with an acute right-sided frontal lesion illustrates unilateral fronto-mesencephalic defects of conjugate eye movements. The patient, in addition to left-sided weakness or paralysis of his limbs, will have no random saccades toward the left of the mid-position, not even during REM sleep (Appenzeller and Fischer, 1968). Similarly, he will be unable to initiate a saccade to the left in response to a command or to visual or auditory stimuli. The eyes usually deviate tonically to his right, particularly if he is obtunded (Cogan, 1964). When so deviated and commanded to look to the left, his eyes will jerk quickly to the mid-position. This saccadic movement from the eccentric to the mid-position probably is initiated from his intact hemisphere.

The integrity of the "final common pathway" for lateral gaze can be determined by evoking a deviation in the paretic direction in response to appropriate vestibular (cold water irrigated into the left ear canal, or warm water into the right canal) and oculocephalic stimulation. The latter is performed by rapidly turning the patient's head to the right, causing his eyes to deviate in the opposite direction. It was once thought that influences from proprioceptive receptors in the neck muscles upon the ocular motor system were minimal in man, and that evoked eye movements from this "doll's head" maneuver were primarily vestibular in origin (Ford and Walsh, 1940), but demonstration of normal oculocephalic reflexes in patients who have no response to caloric testing negates this conclusion (DeKleyn and Stenvers, 1941; Jampel and Quaglio, 1964; and Plum and Posner, 1966).

The caloric-induced tonic ocular deviation is absent in normal awake subjects, but occurs bilaterally in patients with depressed levels of consciousness of whatever cause (Nathanson *et al.*, 1957). Since it occurs in the direction of impaired saccades in patients with suprapontine lesions, the pontine reticular formation would appear to be disinhibited by lesions of the fronto-mesencephalic system.

When sufficiently alert, the patient can execute normal pursuit of objects moving horizontally in either direction. Optokinetic testing with targets moving to his left evokes normal nystagmus. Targets moving to his right cause smooth tonic deviation of his eyes into full right gaze without evidence of rapid movements toward the left. This involuntary deviation is due to uninterrupted ocular pursuit reflexes. Absence of the fast phases of optokinetic nystagmus (OKN) suggests that these reflex saccades depend upon the same anatomic substrate as voluntary saccades. This clinical inference is supported by laboratory studies in subhuman primates by Pasik and Pasik (1964a) and by Brucher (1966). The patient with interruption of his right fronto-mesencephalic pathway may also retain normal OKN left-directed saccades to, but not beyond, his midposition of gaze (Silberpfennig, 1941).

The situation with regard to the fast phase of vestibular nystagmus, the other major reflex saccade, is variable. Authoritative observers have stressed the combined loss of vestibular fast phase and voluntary saccades in the direction away from the lesion (Meyers, 1925; Merwarth and Feiring, 1939; Silberpfennig, 1939; Gastaldi, 1953; Cogan, 1956). For example, irrigation of cold water in the right auditory canal of a patient with a right-sided lesion would induce tonic ocular deviation to the right with absence of fast phases in the direction of his gaze paresis. However, we have observed patients who retained the fast phase of caloric-induced nystagmus despite loss of other saccades (optokinetic and voluntary) in the same direction. We have termed this phenomenon *dissociated saccadic palsy.* The dissociated loss of saccadic function implies that vestibular saccades (quick phases) can be generated, probably in the rostral tegmentum of the midbrain, without the participation of a fronto-mesencephalic system.

The ocular signs of a lesion in the fronto-mesencephalic system are usually referred to as a voluntary or frontal *"gaze"* palsy, but, in our opinion, *"saccadic palsy"* would be more descriptive. The clinical characteristics of these conjugate defects provide valuable information about the cerebral control of saccades. Unilateral *saccadic palsy* is usually caused by an acute lesion (Bender, 1962) and only rarely by a slowly progressive process such as a neoplasm, even when confined to the frontal lobe (Huber, 1961). Despite persistence of other neurologic deficits, the *saccadic palsy* is transient. After a period varying from days to weeks, normal voluntary saccades return. During recovery, the patient is able to make progressively larger saccades into his paretic field of gaze but, unable to maintain this deviation, his eyes drift back again towards center. This slow retrograde drift is interrupted by a phasic jerking in the intended direction of regard (Cogan, 1956), a nystagmus termed *"gaze-paretic"* and possessing a unique character due to its slow (1-2 per second) frequency (Jung and Kornhuber, 1964). As recovery continues, the excursion of the initial eye movement gradually increases, retrograde drift and nystagmus decrease, and finally full saccadic function returns. These rehabilitated saccades probably are initiated by motor systems in the intact (ipsilateral) hemisphere. Previous damage in this hemisphere may preclude the "take-over" of saccadic control; in this case *saccadic palsy* would persist (Cogan, 1965). If, alternatively, a fronto-mesencephalic lesion occurs later in the "compensating" hemisphere, bilateral and enduring *saccadic palsy* ensues (Cogan, 1964, 1956; Holmes, 1938). The capacity of a single hemisphere to assume control of horizontal saccadic movements in both directions is well exemplified clinically in patients who have undergone complete hemispherectomy (Volk and Bruell, 1956; Gassel and Williams, 1963).

Incomplete unilateral fronto-mesencephalic involvements cause *saccadic paresis* evidenced clinically by gaze-paretic nystagmus. This jerking movement of the eyes is phenomenologically identical to the paretic nystagmus already described during recovery of a *saccadic palsy.* Both of us have observed another sign of *saccadic paresis* that has received but scant mention elsewhere (Holmes, 1930); in deviating away from the damaged frontal lobe, the eyes execute a series of small jumps or jerks before reaching their goal. These *"hypometric saccades"* also occur in extrapyramidal and cerebellar system disorders.

B. Bilateral lesions

Bilateral disruption of the fronto-mesencephalic systems results in the often-described clinical syndrome of bilateral loss of saccadic eye movements with preservation of pursuit, vestibular and oculocephalic movements (Holmes, 1921, 1930, 1936, 1938; Ford and Walsh, 1940; Cogan, 1956; Kestenbaum, 1961). Credit for the first description of the syndrome belongs to Gowers (1879). Bilateral lesions of the fronto-mesencephalic systems usually cause complete bilateral *saccadic palsy*—voluntary, optokinetic and vestibular. Cold caloric irrigation of either ear induces tonic ipsiversive conjugate deviation. In most cases vertical saccades are also defective. They may be totally lost, paretic during voluntary or reflex activity, paretic in one vertical direction or, occasionally, entirely normal. Bilateral *saccadic palsy* "releases" the ordinarily latent occipital fixation reflexes and produces a clinical sign aptly termed *"spasm of fixation"* by Holmes (1930). The patient's eyes seem to "lock-on" to an object and remain there until fixation is interrupted again by one or several blinks. With the lids closed, a head deviation toward the new object of regard carries the eyes to the new fixation.

Starr (1967) studied a patient with Huntington's chorea by employing techniques of electro-oculography, cinematography and electromyography (EMG). There was total *saccadic palsy* bilaterally with preservation of slow vestibular and pursuit movements. EMG of the extraocular muscles during attempted saccades disclosed slowness of recruitment in the agonist and concomitant lag of inhibition in the antagonist. When the patient moved his eyes between two fixation points, the duration of the movement was greatly slowed, being more than 10 times normal. Starr (1969) reflected, "The patient willed a saccade but only smooth following occurred."

Previous reports of unilateral as well as bilateral lesions causing *saccadic palsy* described the ability of some of the patients to move their eye from one position to another along a series of interposed and closely placed points, particularly if these points are joined by lines (Ford and Walsh, 1940; Holmes, 1938). Ford and Walsh's report inferred that the willed movements represented small-amplitude visually evoked saccades. However, Holmes (1938) described a patient's reading habits in such a way as to suggest that the smooth pursuit system was involved. Further, Starr's recording of his patient's eyes during reading showed *slow drifts* across the lines of print, not saccadic jumps.

Starr (1967) suggested that the loss of saccades resulted from lesions in the caudate nucleus. The pathology in Huntington's chorea is not limited to the caudate nucleus however, but involves deep hemispheric white matter diffusely as well as the frontal cortex (Denny-Brown, 1962; Blackwood *et al.*, 1963). Although caudate degeneration is prominant in all afflicted patients, very few develop the gross *saccadic palsy* manifested in Starr's patients.

Much of the confusion surrounding the entity described above, and related ocular motor defects, could be avoided if non-descriptive eponyms such as "Gowers' ophthalmoplegia" were replaced with a more meaningful and concise terminology. For the syndrome of acquired, and total, bilateral loss of saccades with preserved ocular pursuit, we propose the term *"global saccadic paralysis."*

C. Ocular motor apraxia

Attempts to classify several closely related ocular motor disorders, the so-called "apraxias of gaze," are seriously hampered by a lack of data from appropriate eye movement recordings. We must depend, therefore, on simple descriptions of the syndromes. Our inferences are uncertain at best. Specifically, the problem here centers on the exact nature of "random eye movements." Patients have been described who could not execute voluntary or reflex saccades, but retained "random eye movements." Since clinical accounts of preserved "random eye movements" seldom mention their speed, proper conceptualization and classification of the ocular motor apraxias must await adequate eye movement recording and analysis.

An *apraxia* in neurologic parlance usually indicates an absent or impaired purposeful movement despite the demonstrable integrity of the neural structures directly subserving that movement. The disorder is classically regarded as one of a "higher" level of function than the primary motor modality (Waltz, 1961). Recently Geschwind (1965) applied the concept of "disconnection" to the apraxias. Pathologically, a disconnection syndrome results from lesions which disrupt cortico-cortical relationships. The site of the lesion may be in the white matter association pathways or in cortical association areas which constitute obligatory way stations between primary sensory and motor cortices.

Holmes (1930, 1936, 1938) described patients with random eye movements who had bilateral fronto-mesencephalic lesions and the typical features of *global saccadic paralysis.* If the random eye movements were saccades, the term *"acquired apraxia of saccades"* would be descriptively appropriate. Since the fast phases of caloric and optokinetic nystagmus were absent in these patients, the presence of random saccades would imply spontaneous discharges from the brainstem paramedian reticular formation or direct impulses impinging upon it from undetermined sources. However we doubt that the random eye movements in Holmes' patients were saccadic.

Another variety of *ocular motor apraxia* includes the loss of ocular pursuit and voluntary saccades. The random eye movements in patients with this disorder probably are saccades, since the vestibulo-ocular reflexes are normal. OKN is absent because ocular pursuit is defective. The disturbance is usually bilateral, but unilateral cases also occur (Cogan and Adams, 1953). Since this syndrome involves all voluntary ocular movements, it should be designated *"acquired apraxia of gaze."* Waltz (1961) reported a bilateral example of this disorder in a patient with a left-sided frontal lobe lesion. This case lends support to Geschwind's (1965) notion that the "memories" of movement in both directions are contained in the dominant hemisphere.

Congenital ocular motor apraxia, as described by Cogan (1952), is typically characterized by loss of pursuit and all saccadic movements. However, cases with normal pursuit movements have been reported (Cogan, 1952; Altrocchi and Menkes, 1960; Cogan, 1966). Vertical movements are often affected in acquired apraxias, but rarely in the congenital variety. Another distinguishing feature is the dramatic "fixation spasms." Afflicted children employ characteristic head thrusts, usually with a blink, to change fixation. Initially, the head overshoots the target markedly, then returns slowly. As the child grows up, he accomplishes fixation shifts with improved facility and his head movements become less obvious (Cogan, 1952; Reed and Israels, 1956; Robles, 1966). We are unaware of any postmortem study of this disorder but teratoma of the lateral ventricle, absence of the corpus collosum and megalocephally have been shown radiologically.

Other rare types of ocular motor apraxia are forms of *saccadic dissociations* such as the case reported by Stenvers (1925). The patient had a right frontal tumor and could not look to the left on command but was able to initiate a saccade to fixate upon an object in his left visual field. This suggests a disconnection of the appropriate frontal region from all other cortical areas except the ipsilateral peristriate area. A similar *saccadic dissociation* involved prompt saccadic response toward an unexpected sound in Holmes' (1930, 1936) patient with bilateral saccadic palsy. Here the disconnection spared the pathway between the auditory and fronto-mesencephalic system.

Occipito-Mesencephalic disorders

Various tonic deviations, disorders of ocular pursuit and optokinetic nystagmus, impaired fixation, and certain complex "apraxias" comprise the disorders of the occipito-collicular systems that subserve functions of fixation and pursuit. The ocular pursuit system is sensitive, vulnerable and, clinically, the most frequently disturbed. The prototype of abnormalities of this system is the degradation of smooth tracking into a series of small step-like saccades traditionally termed "cogwheel eye movements," or more precisely, *"saccadic pursuit."* The sign occurs bilaterally during states of fatigue, inattention, or impaired consciousness as well as in diffuse cerebral, cerebellar, or brain stem disease. It is the first ocular motor effect produced by sedative or anticonvulsive drugs (Walsh and Hoyt, 1969; Rodin, 1964; Hermann *et al.*, 1962). The same *saccadic pursuit* phenomenon occurs when a normal subject attempts to track an object moving at speeds exceeding 45° per second (Von Noorden and Mackensen, 1962). These and other types of saccades are affected in diseases of fronto-mesencephalic systems. For example, a patient with *global saccadic paralysis* does not develop *saccadic pursuit* when following rapidly moving objects or when narcotized with one of the barbiturate drugs (Starr, 1967).

A. Deviations

Irritative lesions in the occipital lobe may produce adversive (contralateral) ocular deviations, a manifestation of seizure (Bender *et al.*, 1957; Cotte-Rittaud and Courgon, 1962). Ipsilateral deviation with paralysis of all contralateral movements is rare but may occur briefly after an acute occipital lobe lesion. Although in most instances it only represents a deficiency of visual exploration in the hemianopic field of vision, its occurrence in a congenitally blind patient is noteworthy (Holmes, 1921). A shock-like state, termed "diaschisis" by von Monakow (1914), is the sudden inhibition that occurs in remote portions of a neural system as a response to acute deafferentation. This phenomenon explains transcallosal visual inhibition following unilateral occipital injury and it must also explain many other enigmatic and transient neurologic effects of acute cerebral lesions.

B. Pursuit and optokinetic nystagmus

Eye movement disorders usually do not occur with lesions limited to the calcarine cortex (unless the disease is bilateral and impairs central vision and optic fixation reflexes). The abnormalities to be discussed here result from involvement of peristriate cortex and its descending corticofugal projections through the deep white matter and posterior thalamus. Lesions involving this projection usually are associated with contralateral homonymous hemianopia. Consequently, studies of ocular motor defects in patients with occipital-parietal hemianopias are particularly relevant (Kestenbaum, 1961; Gassel and Williams, 1963; Cords, 1929; Jung and Kornhuber, 1964); saccades are normal but pursuit movements are predictably defective. Total inability to pursue an object in one or both directions (*"pursuit palsy"*) is exceedingly rare as an isolated abnormality (Raff, 1967), but saccadic pursuit is an expected finding. This sign is present in conjugate gaze *toward the side of the lesion.* A patient with a deep posterior hemispheric lesion on the right side exhibits normal smooth pursuit movements to his left and the jerky saccadic pursuit to his right. The patients generally have unilateral impairment of evoked optokinetic nystagmus and the defective response appears when the targets move *towards the side of the lesion.* The mechanism of the optokinetic abnormality is admittedly complex, controversial, and partly unresolved (Brucher, 1966; Davidoff, *et al.*, 1966; Hood, 1967; Pasik and Pasik, 1964b), but we tentatively agree with Gassel and Williams (1963) that impaired pursuit function is the underlying cause of OKN failure from posterior hemispheric lesions.

Mowrer (1936) concluded from clinical and experimental observations that "each hemisphere *normally* mediates movement of ocular pursuit towards the homolateral side (as well as saccadic movements in the opposite direction)." Our observations confirm this conclusion. In contrast Kestenbaum (1961) postulated contralateral cerebral control of pursuit movements, suggesting that a normal pursuit required "adequate regulating counter impulses" to the opposite side; absence of "counter impulses" was his explanation for cogwheel pursuit.

"Spasticity of conjugate gaze" (Cogan, 1964), an oblique or horizontal ocular deviation evoked during forceable lid closure (Barany, 1913), signifies a mid-cerebral (temperoparietal) lesion opposite the deviation (Smith, Gay and Cogan, 1959). Cogan regards the phenomenon as a sign of innervational "hypertonus" causing the eye to veer away from the lesion; he suggests this hypertonus may account for the observed ipsilateral impairment of pursuit and OKN (Cogan, 1964). Gassel and Williams (1963) termed the phenomenon "tonic ocular motor imbalance," and attempted to correlate it with the frequently associated defects of pursuit and OKN responses. They found the relationship less than conclusive but could offer no alternative to Cogan's theory.

C. Disturbances of fixation

Holmes (1936, 1938) described an uncommon occipito-collicular sign that usually appears in only one field of gaze. If the patient is asked to look at an object on that side, "he moves his eyes promptly towards it, but he fails to keep them directed steadily on it." This failure of fixation occurs in patients whose vision is normal. The lesions that impair fixation, according to Holmes, involve the region of the pulvinar or brachium of the superior colliculus.

D. Occipito-parietal apraxias of gaze (pursuit palsy)

Large biparietal lesions cause disconnection of occipito-frontal integration and also destroy the control systems for pursuit, fixation, and visually-evoked saccades (Holmes, 1918a; Holmes and Horrax, 1919). The eyes move about erratically and only seem to reach the new point of fixation by chance. Largely because of the latter sign, this disorder of ocular movement has been regarded as an ocular motor apraxia. Loss of the near reflex and the blink response to visual threat are additional signs of the syndrome.

A final form of ocular motor apraxia is that described by Balint in 1909 and more recently expounded by Hecaen and deAjuriaguerra (1954) and Waltz (1961). This type occurs in association with major bilateral posterior hemispheric involvement. The findings in each reported case of Balint's syndrome vary. Also, the associated visual field and mental defects cause such severe perceptual disturbances that eye movement analysis becomes confusing. Therefore, we consider that it is probably an oversimplification to regard Balint's "syndrome" as an uncomplicated "apraxia" of gaze (Cogan and Adams, 1955; Stieglmayr, 1967).

Diffuse hemispheric and upper brain stem disease

A. Roth-Bielschowsky syndrome and midbrain lesions of the paramedian reticular formation (MPRF)*

In diffuse hemispheric disease, particularly when the upper brain stem is affected, both the fronto-mesencephalic and the occipito-mesencephalic systems are characteristically disrupted. Selective impairments are infrequent where the frontal and occipital pathways converge toward the subthalamic and upper midbrain levels. In those instances in which both systems are involved the Roth-Bielschowsky syndrome is produced (Cogan, 1956; Kestenbaum, 1961). The patient cannot initiate a saccade or pursuit in either direction. The defect of the pursuit system explains the lack of any optokinetic responses. Oculocephalic reflexes are markedly hyperactive as are the caloric-induced responses (fast phases are absent). Vertical gaze may also be paralyzed. Localization of the most minute and focal lesions accountable for a

*Because of its common usage, we utilize the eponymic designation "Roth-Bielschowsky Syndrome" rather than *global paralysis of gaze.*

patient's signs is a favorite clinical exercise in neurology. The contralateral midbrain paramedian reticular formation (MPRF) ventrolateral to the medial longitudinal fasciculus (MLF) is the precise area for loss of both saccades and pursuit in the same direction. A unilateral lesion there will paralyze horizontal gaze in the opposite direction. The intact pons accounts for the caloric and oculocephalic deviation to the side of impaired gaze.

The almost obligatory associated disruption of adjacent structures, however, namely the overlying MLF and laterally placed oculomotor nerve fascicles, account for the rarity of pure defects. Therefore, a left MPRF lesion usually co-exists with a left internuclear ophthalmoplegia (MLF involvement) and/or a left oculomotor nerve palsy. Either of these associated conditions paralyzes adduction of the ipsilateral eye and hence partially masks supranuclear aspects of the gaze palsy. Failure of the contralateral eye in abduction will be the sole supranuclear manifestation of the MPRF defect.

An interesting finding with large midbrain tegmental lesions involving the oculomotor nuclei and MPRF bilaterally is the absence of ocular divergence (due to unopposed abducens tonus), usually associated with isolated bilateral third nerve palsies. Apparently the abducens motoneurons, deprived of suprasegmental influence, have diminished tonic activity.

Lesions of the MPRF in monkeys have yielded contradictory results. Whereas Bender and Shanzer's (1964) and Shanzer and Bender's (1959) experiments are compatible with our clinical impression, later work from the same institution demonstrated no contralateral gaze defect with unilateral MPRF lesions (Harris *et al.*, 1967).

B. Progressive supranuclear palsy

Steele *et al.*,(1964) described a unique degenerative disease of the nervous system which they called "Progressive Supranuclear Palsy" (PSP). The process usually becomes evident in the presenium and is invariably progressive, leading to death within several years. The clinical manifestations include supranuclear ophthalmoplegia, pseudobulbar palsy, dysarthria, masked facial expression, dystonic rigidity of the neck and upper trunk and dementia. Ophthalmoplegia, pyramidal tract signs, and dementia distinguish this entity from Parkinsonism, which it resembles superficially. The ophthalmoplegia initially affects vertical gaze, specifically saccades and pursuit in the downward direction. PSP is perhaps the only progressive disorder with primary initial involvement of downward movements. Subsequent to the vertical impairment, a gradual loss of willed horizontal saccades and then of pursuit ensues (David *et al.*, 1968). Intact horizontal pursuit movements permit tonic slow phase OKN deviation in early stages of the illness. Eventually, when all gaze is paralyzed, there are no optokinetic responses. Oculocephalic maneuvers induce full horizontal deviation but the severe neck rigidity frequently precludes vertical manipulation. Tonic deviation with loss of the fast phase of nystagmus invariably results from caloric stimulation. Ultimately therefore, the ophthalmoplegia of PSP progresses to a complete Roth-Bielschowsky syndrome involving both vertical and horizontal movements.

Pathological studies point to involvement of various parts of the basal ganglia and brain stem. Of prime import are the regions of the zona incerta, subthalamus, midbrain paramedian reticular formation and periaqueductal gray. Behrman *et al.*, (1969) also found cerebellar lesions, limited to the dentate nuclei. Saccadic impairment may be attributed to the zona incerta lesions; the periaqueductal pathology disrupts the pursuit system by interrupting the tectotegmental pathway. The midbrain tegmental and possibly dentate nuclei lesions affect both eye movement systems. The location of the lesions appropriately explains the ophthalmoplegia; yet it has been suggested that the eye movement difficulty represents simply a Parkinsonion-like rigidity. David *et al.*, (1968) contend that there is direct involvement of eye movement control systems in PSP. Their conviction is substantiated by experience with L-Dopa (Wagshul and Daroff, 1969), which may significantly lessen the rigidity and bradykinesia of PSP but which fails to affect the ophthalmoplegia.

C. Perservation and tonic reflex devaition

"Tonic reflex deviation of the eyes" or *"Gaze perseveration"* is a rare and curious phenomenon described by Denny-Brown (1962, 1969). The abnormality is seen usually in mute, unresponsive patients with diffuse cerebral disease, often with asymmetrical posterior hemispheric signs. The eyes are deviated tonically to the side of the posterior lesion but may be attracted to a moving object in the contralateral field of vision. Once so moved, the eyes remain "locked" to the contralateral side for up to ten minutes, despite subsequent removal of the fixation object. Denny-Brown regards *gaze perseveration* as pathophysiologically similar to oculogyric crises.

Parkinsonism

The anatomical connections of the extrapyramidal system, and specifically the basal ganglia (caudate, putamen, globus pallidum and subthalamic nuclei) and substantia nigra, have been described succinctly by Carpenter (1966a) and Nauta (1966), to which reference is made for details.

Clinical findings in patients with extrapyramidal disease attributed to the basal ganglia suggest, but do not prove, participation of the latter in the systems controlling conjugate gaze. Saccadic (cogwheel) pursuit movements, oculogyric spasms, and the loss of voluntary saccadic movements are examples of conjugate gaze abnormalities associated clinically with diffuse disease of the basal nuclei and their connections. It is not clear whether disease of these subcortical systems 1) interrupts centrifugal gaze pathways passing near or through the basal ganglia or 2) affects gaze modifying systems from the basal ganglia.

Parkinson's disease, the most common and familiar of the extrapyramidal disorders of motor control, occurs in middle or late life and is a syndrome of tremor, rigidity, and akinesia. The fundamental pathological process, of unknown etiology, produces nerve-cell degeneration principally in the substantia nigra and variably in the globus pallidus (Earle, 1966).

Ocular motor disorders in Parkinsonism are well known, and include infrequency of blinking, a "staring" expression, jerkiness of following movements of the eyes, and occasional attacks of oculogyric spasms. Recently these extrapyramidal defects of ocular motor control have been investigated by clinical electrophysiological techniques.

Loeffler *et al.,* (1966) made a detailed EMG study of defects in function of the lid muscles in patients with Parkinsonism. The electrical activity of the levator palpebrae superior and the orbicularis oculi was recorded during tremors, forced lid closure and blinks, revealing a variety of abnormal innervation patterns. The abnormal slowness of blinks and "apraxia" of lid opening were further described by Goldstein and Cogan (1965) as well as Strang (1969), who prefers the term "lid-drop" to "apraxia" in his analysis of levator motor problems as a complication of pallidal or thalamic surgery for Parkinsonism.

Akinesia and bradykinesia of ocular movement in Parkinsonism are manifest as inertia in initiating normal quick shifts of gaze and slowness of willed eye movements (voluntary saccades) respectively. When the patient attempts to make a rapid saccade to either side, his eyes respond with a series of halting, stepwise jerks (hypometric saccades) that finally bring them in line with the new position of fixation.

EMG analyses of agonist and antagonist rectus muscles during horizontal voluntary saccades have delineated the electrical activity of such hypometric saccades (Slatt, Loeffler and Hoyt, 1966). More recently Highstein, Cohen and Mones (1969) have investigated the defects of saccadic eye movements in Parkinson's disease by electrooculography, and present evidence on the abnormally slow velocities of such movements, including the small hypometric saccades.

Pursuit movements of the eyes are also defective in Parkinsonism. If the target moves slowly, the eyes may follow smoothly, but if the target moves more rapidly, smooth pursuit converts into irregular and frequent saccades. The reflex retinal input employed in the pursuit system seems to overcome the akinesia and inertia of starting a gaze movement, but when one of the eyes loses fixation on the target or must change direction, the akinesia and bradykinesia of the saccadic system prevents or impedes the normally accurate and rapid execution of the corrective movement. These defects in ocular pursuit were studied electromyographically by Slatt, Loeffler, and Hoyt (1966). The recruitment of muscle units in pursuit movements was more synchronous than that occurring during voluntary saccades.

Even during fixation of a stationary object, the ocular motor control system of the patient with Parkinson's disease is faulty. During fixation in the primary position (straight ahead) the eyes tend to drift and then to flick back again at amplitudes that sometimes can be observed with magnification. EMG recordings of this phenomenon of *ocular motor impersistance* (Slatt, Loeffler, and Hoyt, 1966) reveal a spindle-like pattern of innervation instead of an abrupt burst of activity representing a saccade. In Parkinsonism, it may be that the sensory input from the retinas cannot maintain, or assist the ocular motor system in maintaining, an exact and synchronized motor response.

Pontine lesions of the paramedian reticular formation (PPRF)

Descending fiber systems for horizontal gaze aggregate in the midbrain paramedian reticular formation, decussate in the lower midbrain and upper pontine tegmentum (Bender and Shanzer, 1964; Brucher, 1966), and terminate in the pontine paramedian reticular formation (PPRF) through which all ipsilateral horizontal conjugate eye movements are mediated. The indispensability of the PPRF for all horizontal eye movement is overwhelmingly supported by clinical (Freeman, 1922; Holmes, 1931; Reese and Yaskin, 1941; Freeman and Ammerman, 1943; Madonick, 1951; Jung and Kornhuber, 1964; Appenzeller and Fischer, 1968) and experimental evidence (Bender and Shanzer, 1964; Teng, *et al.*, 1958; Shanzer and Bender, 1959; Nozue and Cohen, 1968; Cohen and Feldman, 1968; and Cohen *et al.*, 1968). In contrast to the transient nature of the gaze palsy with unilateral cerebral disease, conjugate gaze palsies from PPRF lesions usually persist (Bielschowsky, 1935; Cogan, 1956).

Bilateral PPRF lesions at *the level of the abducens nuclei* cause paralysis of all horizontal versions: saccadic or pursuit, reflex or voluntary. The lack of reflex ocular deviation with caloric stimulation is of particular importance. It indicates that the vestibulo-ocular relfex arc traverses, or is at least strongly dependant upon, the PPRF. Chronic bilateral PPRF lesions cause gaze-evoked nystagmus upon looking upward but do not impair the range of movement in this direction. Acute bilateral lesions, however, may result in transient vertical gaze paralysis. "Spastic convergence" secondary to divergence inertia is another sign occasionally associated with bilateral PPRF lesions.

An EMG study of bilateral pontine paralysis of horizontal ocular movement was performed by Esslen and Papst (1961) in a man with a brainstem tumor. The recordings showed minimal facilitation of agonist muscles with absence of inhibition in antagonist muscles. The authors stressed the lack of reciprocal inhibition and excitation between medial and lateral rectus muscles, and the continuous high voltage "spastic" hyperactivity of motor units – particularly in medial rectus muscles.

Unilateral PPRF lesions at the level of the abducens nucleus abolish ipsilateral saccades and pursuit movements. With a left sided lesion, cold caloric stimulation of the left external auditory canal evokes no response; stimulation on the right causes ipsilateral tonic deviation without producing vestibular saccades toward the left. Similarly, optokinetic stimulation with targets moving toward the patient's right induces a tonic ocular pursuit without left-beating saccades; OKN stimulation in the other direction evokes fast and slow responses. However, as Cohen *et al.*, (1968) demonstrated, the slow phase occurs only in the functioning field of gaze, (e.g. never crosses midline). Apparently the intact PPRF on the right performs this function. Simon and Gay (1964) reported impaired OKN responses as targets move away from the side of the pontine lesion in cases without frank impairment of lateral gaze.

More rostral pontine lesions cause identical defects in horizontal movements of the eyes except that caloric and oculocephalic responses are preserved. Thus a left PPRF lesion *rostral to the abducens nucleus* leads to the findings outlined above for the more caudal lesion, except that cold caloric stimulation in the left ear will produce deviation of the eyes toward the syringed ear canal (left) with a superimposed fast phase to the right.

Gaze paretic nystagmus is seen with incomplete PPRF lesions.

Cerebellar and cerebellar system disorders

Anatomical and physiological concepts of cerebellar function have recently been reviewed by Evarts and Thach (1969). The specific role of the cerebellum in the control of ocular movement has a voluminous bibliography, much of which is included in the reviews of Dow and Moruzzi (1958) and Dow and Manni (1964). Many aspects of ocular motor pathophysiology of cerebellar lesions in man remain obscure, partly due to the remarkable functional compensation, particularly in youth, that follows major cerebellar resections (Wania and Walsh, 1959). Indeed one of us (R.B.D.) followed a patient with almost complete replacement of the cerebellar vermis by metastatic carcinoma who had no obvious eye movement disorder. Further, "pure" cerebellar disease is a clinical rarity. Cerebellar tumors usually compress the brainstem and their clinical manifestations frequently are combinations of cerebellar and brainstem dysfunction. The most common conditions affecting the cerebellum are multiple sclerosis and occlusive vascular disease; both usually involve the brainstem concurrently. Since it is often impossible clinically to distinguish the ataxias of cerebellar and brainstem origin, neurologists have resorted to the less specific term, *cerebellar system disease.* Cerebellar system disease can impair any or all of the subsystems for eye motor control, including controls of conjugate position, fixation, pursuit and saccades.

A. Conjugate deviation and paresis

Acute lesions of the cerebellar hemisphere cause gaze palsy, or paresis, and conjugate ocular deviation, (Spiller, 1910). From clinical observations, ipsilateral gaze impairment has been variously contended to be of purely cerebellar origin (Holmes, 1917; Meyers, 1931), due to brain stem compression (Bucy and Weaver, 1941), or primarily cerebellar and secondarily brain stem (Fisher *et al.*, 1965).

The ocular motor effects of discrete cerebellar lesions have been assessed following stereotactic ablations (for surgical treatment of limb motor disorders). Krayenbühl and Siegfried (1969) found no clinical ocular motor deficit after coagulation of the dentate nucleus provided the nucleus interpositus was spared. Nashold and collaborators (1969; Nashold and Slaughter, 1969) reported a case in which transient ipsilateral ocular motor paresis followed a lesion involving the left nucleus interpositus and medial portion of the dentate; normal gaze was present after several months.

There is no serious doubt that acute lesions of the deep medial portion of a cerebellar hemisphere can produce profound, but temporary, ipsilateral gaze palsy without affecting reflex tonic deviation. As the lesion progresses and compresses the pontine tegmentum, the reflex movements of the eyes will be unobtainable.

The pattern of ocular disturbances is similar in static unilateral cerebellar and cerebral lesions. Both lesions spare reflex movements in the acute phase and both pass through a period of jerking unsteady gaze, *gaze paretic nystagmus,* as recovery proceeds (Cogan, 1956). This similarity suggests that the cerebellar gaze impairment may result from disruption of cerebello-frontal connections. The nucleus interpositus and dentate project in the brachium conjunctivum (the superior cerebellar peduncle), through the contralateral red nucleus, to the thalamus and finally the frontal cortex (Crosby *et al.,* 1962; Evarts and Thach, 1969).

Initiation of movement is currently considered to be one of the major functions of the cerebellum. Evarts and Thach (1969) hypothesize that cerebellar cortical computations of patterns of muscle activity would normally be relayed from the nuclear output to the cerebral cortex via the thalamus. Alternatively, the experiments of Mehler *et al.,* (1958) suggest the possibility of inhibition of the descending fronto-mesencephalic system at the level of the zona incerta in acute cerebellar nuclear dysfunction. Both possibilities involve loss of cerebellar influence on the descending frontal system for voluntary saccades. The concomitant loss of ipsilateral pursuit function would appear related to the vulnerability of the smooth pursuit system with lesions in various areas of the central nervous system, including the cerebellum.

A third mechanism for the production of the gaze palsy of acute cerebellar hemispheric lesions involves the connection of the cerebellar nuclei with the ipsilateral pontine paramedian reticular formation (PPRF) via the uncrossed cerebello-tegmental fascicles within the brachium conjunctivum (Crosby *et al.,* 1962; Carpenter and Strominger, 1964). This provides a more direct explanation for involvement of both saccadic and pursuit movements (*diaschisis* of the ipsilateral PPRF).

B. Nystagmus with cerebellar lesions

The existence of any "purely" cerebellar form of nystagmus has been denied by Schaller (1921) and minimized by others (Riley, 1930). These authors all claimed that co-existing brain stem involvement always explained nystagmus in patients with cerebellar syndromes.

Slow nystagmus evoked by ipsilateral gaze occurs transiently with incomplete or resolving acute cerebellar hemispheric lesions (Holmes, 1917; Cogan, 1956). This gaze-paretic nystagmus directed toward the lesion is the only type of cerebellar nystagmus that occurs unequivocally with a focal cerebellar lesion in man. Holmes mentioned concomitant rapid contralateral jerk nystagmus in his patients, but brain stem compression was probably implicated in that an identical pattern of nystagmus characterizes large cerebello-pontine angle tumors (Kornhuber, 1969).

Nystagmus evoked by particular head positions—*positional nystagmus* (PN) has been considered to result from midline cerebellar lesions among other diverse etiologies. However, Bergstedt (1961) found the sign in 34.6% of normals. We share the opinion expressed by Salmon (1969) that positional nystagmus has no localizing significance.

C. Hypometric saccades and cogwheel pursuit movements

Kornhuber (1968) distinguishes two eye signs that seem to indicate different areas of involvement within the cerebellum. In diffuse lesions and intoxications, the pursuit movements become cogwheeled but the saccadic system is unaffected. Cerebellar cortical atrophy causes the opposite effect; pursuit is normal but saccadic refixations are performed in several steps instead of the usual single movement. These "hypometric" saccades are frequently of reduced velocity (Kornhuber, 1969; Fuchs and Kornhuber, 1969; Kornhuber, 1968), and the eyes approach the new fixation point with a heavily over-damped trajectory (Fig. 1). Similar abnormal saccadic movements have been noted in Parkinsonism (Highstein *et al.*, 1969), incomplete fronto-mesencephalic lesions (Holmes, 1930), leukodystrophy (von Noorden and Preziossi, 1966), and secondary to diazepan (Valium) intoxication (Aschoff, 1968). Hypometric saccades consisting of small individual jerks of normal (fast) velocity are frequently seen in healthy subjects (Weber and Daroff, in preparation).

Fuchs and Kornhuber (1969) found short latency evoked responses in several areas of cerebellar cortex after ocular muscle stretch in cats. The projection sites of these eye muscle afferents coincide in part with known projection areas from the frontal lobe saccadic system and the striate cortex. The cerebellar regions also produce eye movements when electrically stimulated. A proprioceptive feed-back loop for the control of eye movements, mediated by the cerebellum, was proposed. Disturbances of this loop by a cerebellar cortical lesion result in slow hypometric saccades.

D. Opsoclonus ("Saccadomania")

This bizarre phenomenon is a distinct ocular motor disorder consisting of involuntary, repetitive, chaotic, irregular, unpredictable, multi-directional

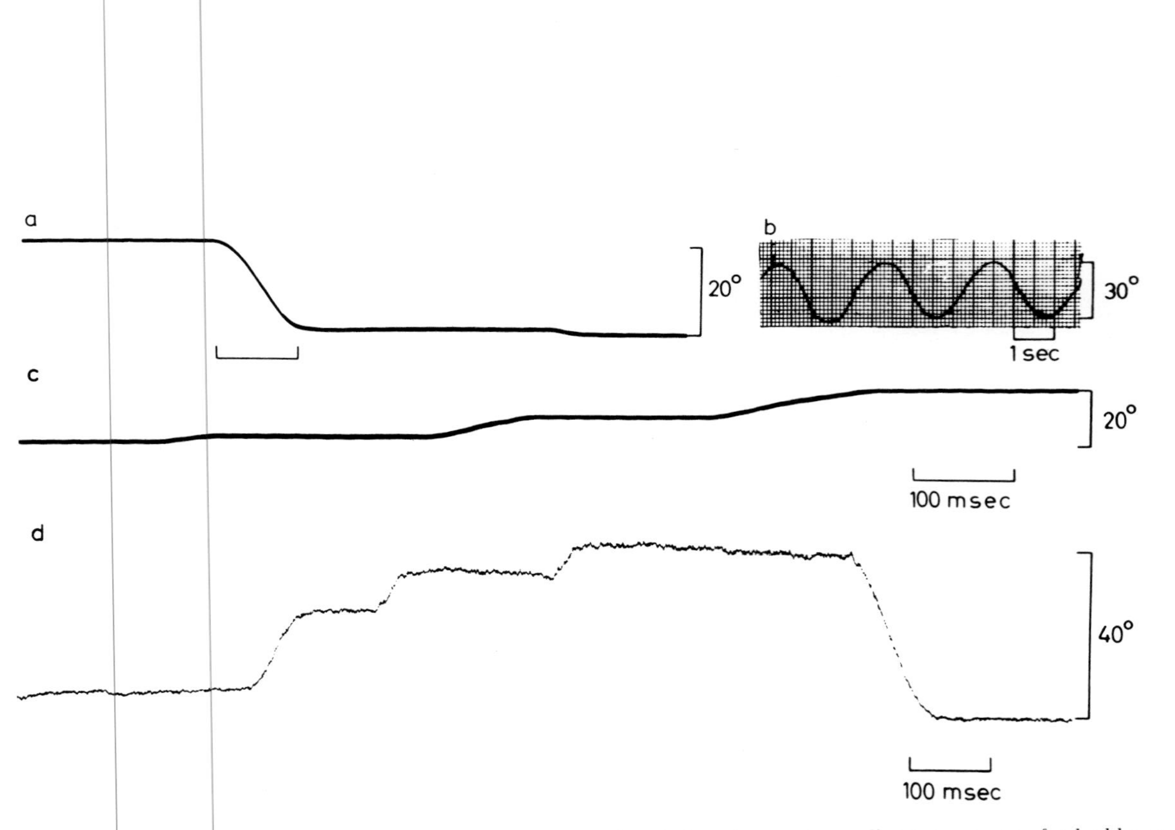

Fig. 1. Hypometric Saccades. This composite of electro-oculograms is from Kornhuber. a) normal saccadic eye movement of a healthy person, b) normal smooth pursuit eye movement in a patient with cerebellar cortical atrophy, c) slow hypometric saccade in the same patient shown in b. Note that three separate movements are required to attain the 20° and each individual movement is extremely slow. d) hypometric saccade in a patient with unilateral cerebellar astrocytoma. The three individual saccades in this movement are of normal velocity and we think this particular form of hypometric saccades may be a normal variant. (From Kornhuber, H., 1969).

saccades. It has been variously termed "dancing eyes," "acute ocular oscillations," "ataxic conjugate movements of the eyes," "chaotic agitation," and "myoclonie oculare encephalitique," but we prefer either "opsoclonus" or *"saccadomania."* The abnormality is usually continuous, persisting even during sleep (Smith and Walsh, 1960). In cases where it is intermittent, it is precipitated by attempts at visual fixation (Winkler *et al.*, 1966; Baringer *et al.*, 1968). The movements are seemingly conjugate, but careful analysis of an electro-oculogram by one of us (R.B.D.) revealed small but definite disconjugate features.

Opsoclonus is commonly associated with limb muscle tremulousness, myoclonus, and mild ataxia as part of a post-infectious encephalopathy (Smith and Walsh, 1960; Winkler *et al.*, 1966; Baringer *et al.*, 1968; Cogan, 1968a). This syndrome belongs to a spectrum of disorders designated "vasculomyelinopathies" by Poser (1969). Total recovery from the opsoclonus is usual after several weeks. Occasionally the brainstem involvement is severe, leading to coma and death (Cogan, 1954).

In infancy, opsoclonus and generalized limb myoclonus may follow a protracted course for several years with frequent remissions and exacerbations (Dyken *et al.*, 1968). Abnormalities in immunoglobulins and the therapeutic efficacy of adrenal steroids suggest an underlying auto-immune process.

Since 1968, several cases of opsoclonus and acute cerebellar ataxia have been reported in children who harbored an occult neuroblastoma (Solomon and Chutorian, 1968; Davidson *et al.*, 1968; Bray *et al.*, 1969). When the neoplasm was removed, the opsoclonus usually disappeared. The relationship between the neuroblastoma and opsoclonus is unclear. Bray *et al.*, (1969) proposed several possibilities, the most likely being a metabolite liberated by the tumor which is toxic to the cerebellum.

Opsoclonus and cerebellar ataxia may occur in adults as a nonmetastatic complication of a distant carcinoma. Three such cases have been examined histopathologically. Alessi (1940) reported a case with a known carcinoma of the uterus. Necropsy revealed demyelination around the dentate nuclei and mild loss of Purkinje cells as well as diffuse white matter gliosis. Ross and Zeman's (1967) patient as well as that of Ellenberger *et al.*, (1968) also had cerebellar damage.

In summary, although opsoclonus occurs in several different disease states, cerebellar ataxia usually co-exists and, where pathological studies have been performed, they have almost always shown involvement of the cerebellum, especially the dentate nucleus.

E. Ocular dysmetria

Ocular dysmetria is a frequent eye sign of cerebellar system disorders. It is provoked by refixation saccades, and consists of an initial conjugate "overshoot" followed either by a single corrective return to the new target or, more commonly, a brief small amplitude rapid oscillation before the eyes come to rest.

A detailed study of the eye movement disorder in one patient disclosed that the pattern was analogous to the performance of a regulator having a delay in the use of its error signal (Higgins and Daroff, 1966). The cerebellum receives afferents from ocular muscle stretch receptors (Fuchs and Kornhuber, 1969) and abolition or slowing of the integration of such signals could account for the over-shoot and minimally damped oscillation (dysmetria) in cerebellar system disorders.

F. Pendular macro-oscillations: cerebellar "kippdeviationen"

An occasional symptom of an acute unilateral cerebellar lesion is an exaggerated overshoot followed by pendular oscillations of the eyes, not unlike the performance of a critically underdamped control system. The oscillations are evoked by any saccade, large or small. In the three cases that we have observed, the phenomenon persisted for two to three weeks following the onset of cerebellar dysfunction. As recovery took place, the wide-angle oscillations diminished in number and frequency and the eye movements resembled ordinary ocular dysmetria. Each of our patients had marked cerebellar ataxia with unilateral intention "tremor" (of arm and leg) on the side of the lesion. There was no paresis of conjugate ocular movements in horizontal or vertical directions and no evidence of brainstem ocular motor disorder other than minimal gaze-evoked vertical nystagmus in one patient. All patients were alert and spoke without dysarthria. The neurologic examination in each suggested the presence of a large lesion involving a cerebellar hemisphere.

When these patients made a horizontal saccade of any type (large or small, to the right or left, reflex or voluntary) both eyes moved immediately and maximally to the intended direction and then swung back to the opposite side, oscillating back and forth until the patient, in desperation, closed his eyes. The oscillations covered a wide range (approximately 50°) and the velocity was relatively slow. The rate was about 1.0 cycles per second. Slow pursuit movements were executed normally in all directions. OKN responses were abnormal in that all horizontal or vertical saccadic movements evoked the uncontrolled horizontal pendular oscillations.

A more common type of horizontal conjugate oscillation occurs in less pronounced forms in normal subjects or in patients with chronic cerebellar system disease. This type of pendular deviation is suppressed by visual fixation reflexes and is "released" by darkness or lid closure (Fig. 2). Its amplitude is somewhat less (10° to 30°) and its frequency is greater (2.5/sec) than the previously described macro-oscillation. Kornhuber (1966) described this form of horizontal to-and-fro eye movement as "*Kippdeviationen*" and attributed its occurrence to normal or pathologic disinhibition of the rostral mesencephalic reticular formation, which becomes manifest when visual inhibitory controls are suspended.

If Kornhuber's (1966) explanation is correct, perhaps the pendular macro-oscillations in our patients with acute cerebellar lesions represented an

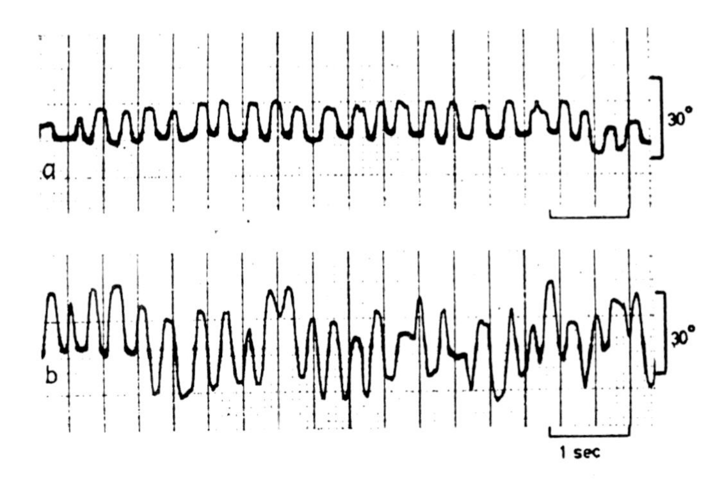

Fig. 2. "Kippdeviationen" with acute cerebellar encephalitis (a) with eye open in the dark; (b) with closed eyes. The oscillations in these tracings are, according to Dr. Kornhuber, disinhibited (exaggerated), spontaneous microsaccades that are apparently underdamped, occur continuously during waking hours, and at a frequency of 2.5 cycles per second (From Kornhuber, H. 1966).

exaggerated form of "*Kippdeviationen*" in which oscillating phasic activity in the rostral mesencephalic tegmentum was the consequence of acute and asymmetric release from inhibitory cerebellar control.

G. Ocular flutter

This is a descriptive term covering several different types of ocular instability with a similar clinical appearance. It occurs apparently spontaneously during fixation and consists of several rapid, small amplitude, horizontal pendular oscillations (Cogan, 1954). Rarely, the abnormality may be monocular (Goldberg and Jampel, 1963). Flutter commonly coexists with ocular dysmetria in cerebellar system lesions and may represent a dysmetric oscillation provoked by subtle vergence movements (Higgins and Daroff, 1966). In patients who also have tremor, the eye and limb movements have similar frequencies (approximately 11 cycles/sec) but are not in phase (Brumlik and Means, 1969).

H. Skew deviation

This refers to a vertical divergence of the optic axes seen frequently in patients with acute asymmetrical cerebellar system disease. It is an imbalance of static eye position or of the vertical vergence mechanism rather than a movement disorder and has been reviewed clinically by Smith *et al.*, (1964) and Walsh and Hoyt (1969).

CLINICAL DISORDERS OF THE SUPRANUCLEAR SYSTEMS FOR VERTICAL OCULAR MOVEMENT

Electrical stimulations of the brain and vertical eye movements

Stimulation of the frontal lobe in unanesthetized patients often evokes contralateral deviation of the eyes, occasionally with an upward or downward component (Penfield and Boldrey, 1937). However, pure vertical deviations (upward or downward) are rarely found upon unilateral stimulation of the frontal cortex. On the other hand, vertical (upward) deviations can be evoked by simultaneous bilateral stimulation of frontal eye fields in monkeys (Pasik and Pasik,1964a; Bender, 1960).

The development of techniques for stereotactic implantation of stimulating electrodes in subcortical areas of human patients has resulted in several reports of electrically induced vertical eye movements. Wycis and Spiegel (1958) obtained vertical nystagmus from pretectal stimulation ventral to the posterior commissure. Spiegel *et al.*, (1964) produced vertical deviations from stimulation in the fields of Forel. Nashold and Gills (1967) elicited convergence and downward deviation from the posterior sensory nucleus of the thalamus in one patient, but found no correlation between stimulation and lesion in the same area.

Periodic "spasms" of vertical gaze

A. Oculogyric crises

Conjugate spasmodic deviations of the eyes, usually in the vertical plane, have been termed oculogyric crises, oculogyric spasms, oculogyric seizures, visual fits, and tonic eye fits. This disorder of ocular movement occurred frequently among victims of the 1918 influenza epidemic, usually associated with the multiple stigmata of postencephalitic Parkinsonism. Similar eye signs may occur in petit mal epilepsy and in a variety of other conditions (Stern, 1928; Walsh and Hoyt, 1969). The oculogyric crisis commences with upward rolling of the eyes, sometimes obliquely toward the right or the left. The ocular deviation is usually tonic but can be clonic as well. Deviation to the side is rare as is deviation downward (Stern, 1927) or convergence deviation (van Bogaert, 1927). Sometimes by great effort the patient can return his eyes to the mid-position, but only for a moment or two. The eyelids usually remain open, sometimes with rhythmical jerking in the levator muscles, sometimes with repetitive twitching in the orbicularis oculi. Kyrieleis (1931) recorded the occurrence of mydriasis, anisocoria, or blurring of vision during attacks. There are also associated head and facial movements.

Each oculogyric spasm lasts several moments; the eyes then descend to the horizontal and, a few moments later, roll upward again. This sequence continues during the length of the "crisis," usually one to two hours. The patient almost always remains conscious throughout and is able to perform commands and answer questions. A few patients have described visual or auditory hallucinations, anxiety, mental confusion, or even stupor during the period of the attack (Jelliffe, 1929; Wilson, 1954).

The varied theories that have been offered to explain oculogyric crises are as yet unsupported by clinical neurophysiological studies. Jelliffe's theory of the obsessive compulsive nature of oculogyric crises was favored during the 1920's. However, Hall, in 1931, studied the positions of the eyes of 206 normal subjects during sleep and found that they varied in about the proportions of the directions of deviation reported in patients with oculogyric crises. From this he proposed that the crises came about by a mechanism similar to or perhaps identical to the tonic phase of sleep.

More recently, Onuaguluchi (1961), from his detailed study of 67 patients, proposed that several factors were concerned in the production of the attacks: (a) a cerebral cortical lesion producing impaired cortical inhibition; (b) a brainstem lesion causing weakness of the extraocular muscles; and (c) excessive sources of vestibular stimulation such as the presence of hard wax in the external auditory canal. He concluded that these three factors caused facilitation of the reticular activating system of the brainstem and diencephalon, resulting in the abnormal vestibulo-ocular reflex responsible for tonic upward-gaze spasms.

Denny-Brown (1962) related oculogyric crises to other pathophysiological phenomena with tonic deviations of head and eyes.

On the basis of electrical stimulation and ablation studies, Klemme (1941) implicated the motor and pre-motor cortex in the generation of oculogyric crises. Wycis and Spiegel (1958) produced temporary remission with partial ablation of the periaqueductal grey and mesencephalic tegmentum. Some response of oculogyric crises to coagulating lesions of the pallidum (Hassler *et al.*, 1960), and of the thalamus and especially the posterior limb of the internal capsule (Gillingham, 1962; Gillingham and Kalyanaraman, 1965) has been reported. Matiar (1955) proposed hypothalmic imbalance and impairment of the autonomic nervous system as underlying factors. L-Dopa therapy is said to abolish (Calne *et al.*, 1969) or significantly reduce the oculogyric attack (Yahr *et al.*, 1969).

B. Vertical deviation of the eyes during seizures; eye "fits"

The oculogyric "seizures" observed in children with petit mal epileptic episodes differ significantly from the oculogyric crises associated with postencephalitic Parkinsonism: (a) they usually occur in children having no overt signs of neurological disease; (b) they last only for seconds; (c) they tend to consist of clonic instead of tonic upward movements; (d) they are often associated with a lapse in consciousness but without a loss of postural control; and (e) they may occur as minor spells in intervals between major motor seizures. The two forms of involuntary upward deviation do share some common characteristics. Both can be accompanied by autonomic and limbic symptomatology involving the pupils, heart rate, breathing, orofacial movements, or behavioral disturbances. Both may have associated blinking or fluttering movement of the eyelids.

Some cases of oculogyric seizures are induced by specific sensory stimuli. Whitty (1960) described a 7½ year old girl who had petit mal attacks when she ran from shadow into bright sunlight. There would be a momentary arrest of movement with staring and then clonic upward movement of the eyes. The child would deliberately induce her attacks by running into the sunlight or by blinking rapidly. We observed a child with similar photogenic oculogyric seizures which she induced by waving a finger before her eyes while she stared at the sun.

Shanzer and co-workers (1965) investigated a curious form of reflex epilepsy wherein voluntary sustained (3 seconds) deviation of the eyes to the right induced eyelid fluttering, ocular deviation upward with shimmering movements, twisting of the face to the left, and jerking of the fingers and toes on the right.

One of us (W.F.H.) observed a 10 year old girl with a calcified lesion of the right thalamus and mild stigmata of congenital hemiplegia who suffered from attacks of sudden and total blindness. During each episode, her vision faded for 2-4 minutes, her pupils dilated widely, her eyes turned up, and clonic spasms of the left arm and face appeared; she never lost consciousness or the ability to speak coherently. This association of transient visual loss and oculogyric seizures is rare but has also been described in patients with postencephalitic oculogyric attacks.

With simultaneous motion pictures of eye movements and EEG recordings Bickford and Klass (1964) were able to establish that turning movements of the eyes occur 10-30 milliseconds before the spike-and-wave discharge appears in the EEG. This may be evidence that the spike-and-wave discharge is a secondary event in the sequence, or at least that its reception from scalp electrodes is delayed in comparison with the beginning of each eye movement. Often the 3 per second spike-and-wave discharges correspond exactly with the rate of myoclonic jerking of circumorbital and lid muscles (Bickford and Klass, 1964).

C. Tonic vertical deviation of the eyes in healthy neonates

In 1955, Lebensohn described tonic downward deviation of the eyes in an infant. The deviation was present at all times when the baby was awake but the eyes returned to a level position during sleep and rolled upward freely when the head and neck were flexed forward. By two years of age, the tonic ocular deviation was no longer present and the patient had perfectly normal ocular movements. Walsh and Hoyt (1969) described two neonates with similar tonic downward deviation of the eyes for the first few weeks after birth.

Lebensohn believed that his patient had birth trauma; there was no evidence of injury in the infants observed by Walsh and Hoyt. One of us (W.F.H.) examined an eight month old infant with tonic-clonic oculogyric episodes that had been noted daily for six months. Each episode lasted for about one hour during which the eyes turned upward in gross clonic jerking movements accompanied by blinking. Occasionally, for short periods, the eyes would remain in tonic upward deviation. When the child was suddenly alerted she would immediately return her eyes to the straight ahead position, search about briefly, and then let her eyes drift upward once again. There was no crying or abnormal head movement associated with the oculogyric jerking of the eyes or with the alerting response. Horizontal ocular pursuit was abnormally jerky in both directions. Fast and slow phases of vestibular nystagmus were normal horizontally and vertically (as tested by rotation). Ocular motor function was normal by age 18 months; oculogyric spells no longer occurred.

In contrast to the vertical oculogyric seizures of petit mal and to post-encephalitic oculogyric crises, the tonic vertical deviation of neonates was unassociated with poor health, was temporary, and could be stopped by an alerting stimulus. The etiology of this abnormality of vertical ocular control is unknown.

D. Familial periodic vertical nystagmus

In 1962, Sogg and Hoyt recorded the cases of a father and son who suffered from attacks of vertical upward jerking nystagmus since infancy. The father's attacks were usually precipitated by fatigue or emotional upset, but could also be triggered by sustained upward gaze; this, together with a defect of downward saccadic movements during OKN tests, suggested a supranuclear derangement. Since the original report (Sogg and Hoyt, 1962), two more sons born to this family have manifested the same affliction of periodic disturbance of vertical ocular control. This familial periodic vertical nystagmus consists of a variable clonic upward jerking movement with blinking of the lids and hyperextension of the neck.

White (1969) has recently described a family of 62 members (five generations) in which 23 had periodic nystagmus, vertigo and ataxia; the nystagmus was downward in one member.

The neurophysiological or perhaps neurochemical explanation of these distinctive and inherited disorders of vertical ocular control and associated bulbar activities is completely obscure.

E. Spastic downward deviation of eyes in the comatose patient

A patient with acute thalamic hemorrhage may have extreme downward deviation of the eyes. Associated findings include small unreactive pupils, impaired vertical eye movements when tested by oculocephalic maneuvers, and hemiparesis (Fisher, 1967). We have observed a 3 month old infant, with intermittent hydrocephalus from a midline tumor involving the septum pellucidum and thalamus, who developed tonic downward deviation with convergence each time the intraventricular pressure became elevated. Another young patient displayed these signs during post-traumatic coma from midbrain contusion; at times her eyes made spontaneous clonic convergence movements. Similar forced down-gaze spasms occur during coma in some of the metabolic encephalopathies; reflex ocular movements are greatly slowed but not abolished.

With an implanted electrode, Nashold and Gills (1967) obtained tonic downward ocular deviation during stimulation of a patient's thalamus (13 mm. lateral to the midsagittal plane). It would seem likely that most lesions producing forced downward deviation in convergence represent acute involvement of the pretectum and rostral midbrain, since in each instance there was an associated paresis of vertical gaze.

Spastic downward deviation is to be differentiated from "*ocular bobbing*," a phasic disorder consisting of abrupt downward jerks of the eyes followed by a slow upward return to the mid-position. Ocular bobbing usually occurs in gravely ill, stuporous or comatose patients with extensive disease of the pons, causing total paralysis of spontaneous and reflex horizontal eye movements. The downward jerks tend to be arhythmic and unpredictable, but in rare cases are regular (Fisher, 1964; Daroff and Waldman, 1965). Several features distinguish "bobbing" from *vertical ocular myoclonus*, namely: irregularity of rate, two components of unequal velocity, lack of synchronous associated movements of midline structures (palate, pharynx, trachea, etc.), and occasional lack of conjugacy and persistance of deviated position downward. The two disorders, ocular bobbing and myoclonus, are distinct clinically; interchangeable usage of these terms (Yap *et al.*, 1968) is misleading.

Vertical gaze disorders from lesions in the periaqueductal, pretectal, posterior commissural, and subthalamic areas

Lesions in the rostrodorsal midbrain and posterior third ventricle produce an array of distinctive neuro-ophthalmological signs, implicating supranuclear control systems for vertical deviation of the eyes, eyelid posture and blinking, pupillary and ciliary muscle activity, and ocular vergence. The vertical ocular motor disturbances caused by periaqueductal lesions are of particular clinical importance. (It is now firmly established that the superior colliculi have no function in mediating vertical eye movements (Pasik *et al.*, 1966 and 1969; Balthasar, 1968)).

A. Paralysis of the vertical saccadic system (with preservation of pursuit)

Fronto-mesencephalic systems controlling voluntary and reflex saccadic movements in the vertical plane can be damaged selectively. The patient can lose his ability to glance upward, downward, or both, while retaining the capacity to pursue objects moving vertically. Optokinetic responses are distinctive in this variety of supranuclear saccadic palsy: the eyes deviate smoothly until they reach the limit of gaze, and here they remain as if locked in position by the vertically moving visual stimuli. This tonic deviation in the direction of the target movement (slow phase) has been described previously with horizontal saccadic palsy and reflects, in both situations, absence of corrective fast phases (saccades). Occasionally the palsy involves vertical saccadic movements in one direction only. For example, upward-moving optokinetic stimuli may evoke only conjugate upward deviation of the eyes, while optokinetic testing in the opposite direction produces normal responses—the patient having lost only downward saccades. Appropriate vestibular stimulation will evoke tonic upward deviation without a fast phase downward. Vertical oculocephalic responses are often difficult to elicit in such cases, due to an associated dystonia of the neck.

Absence of vertical saccadic movements, often in one direction only, occurs in young children as a congenital anomaly. When the palsy is acquired during adult life and particularly when there is loss of *downward* saccades, the patient's visual handicap is profound. He is simply unable to "look" where he is stepping and walking.

The anatomical site of the lesion or lesions causing isolated paralysis of downward gaze is not yet clear. André Thomas *et al.*, (1933) presented a case in which neuropathological findings implicated the ventrolateral mesencephalic (periaqueductal) reticular formation in a down-gaze palsy. Recent evidence that such palsies result from lesions in the prerubral zone is derived from studies of stereotactic lesions (Nashold and Gills, 1967) and electrical stimulation (Spiegel *et al.*, 1964).

B. Monocular supranuclear elevator palsy with rostral midbrain lesions

Vertical diplopia occurs frequently as an early sign of pretectal or periaqueductal disease, and also during the stages of resolution of a conjugate vertical gaze palsy. It is evidence for asymmetrical elevator paresis of the two eyes, and is important to the question of the existence of monocular (supranuclear) paresis of elevation. Many so-called congenital double-elevator palsies, occurring frequently with congenital ptosis, represent supranuclear anomalies of ocular motor excitation and inhibition (Esslen and Pabst, 1961).

Acquired monocular elevator palsy with retention of Bell's phenomenon was described by Bielchowsky in 1935, and later by Man (1967). A recent clinical investigation of seven cases by Jampel and Fells (1968) characterizes this syndrome in detail. The authors stressed that these palsies should not be termed "skew deviation," for the eyes are straight in the horizontal plane of fixation and only move disjunctively as the patient looks upward. They proposed that a discrete vascular lesion in the pretectal region of the midbrain caused the signs in their patients. Evidence for this was the occurrence of pupillary anomalies (in 3 cases) and convergence paresis in one case.

The superior rectus muscle appears to be the predominant elevator throughout the range of horizontal gaze with the inferior oblique playing only a minor role (Jampel, 1962; Boeder, 1961). Accepting Warwick's (1953) concept of the oculomotor nucleus, Jampel and Fells (1968) contend that monocular elevation paresis can be caused by a lesion affecting mainly the central neural connections of the superior rectus muscle. Complete paralysis of elevation probably also includes involvement of the inferior oblique connections. Such lesions could be confined to or include the contralateral superior rectus subnucleus, but it is more likely that they are in the pretectal area close to the oculomotor nucleus. Here both the crossed and uncrossed supranuclear fibers to the superior rectus and the inferior oblique subnuclei are in close proximity.

C. Impaired vertical gaze, convergence–retraction nystagmus, and associated signs of the sylvian aqueduct syndrome

1. Clinical Observations. Although paresis of upward gaze was recognized by Parinaud (1883) as a sign of rostral brainstem involvement, Koerber (1903) was the first to describe and name a unique clinical feature of certain supranuclear vertical palsies, namely *nystagmus retractorius.* Koerber described two patients with impaired vertical gaze associated with rhythmical retraction of the globes into the orbits. A few years later Salus (1910) and then Elschnig (1913) encountered similar findings, each in a patient with involvement of the region of the sylvian aqueduct and the fourth ventricle.

Primary components of the sylvian aqueduct (Koerber–Salus–Elschnig) syndrome include impairment of vertical gaze (saccadic or saccadic and pursuit), retraction–convergence nystagmus evoked by upward saccades, dissociated or total pupillary areflexia, and associated signs reflecting the extent of the rostral mesencephalic disease (pseudobulbar reflexes, emotional lability, etc.).

The syndrome usually develops in an orderly manner when it results from a dorsally-placed tumor (commonly a pinealoma). Initially the patient complains of blurred distant vision, "eye strain," and occasionally transient episodes of vertical diplopia. Gradually the pupillary size increases and the reaction to light becomes slowed; pupillary constriction during accommodative effort is usually normal, or almost so. Paresis of vertical ocular movement begins as a subtle restriction, followed by progressive diminution, of amplitude. Gaze-evoked vertical nystagmus rarely precedes the limitation of voluntary movement. Voluntary vertical saccades may attain less range than pursuit movements in the early stage.

Before the restriction of upward gaze is gross, subtle deficiencies in vertical control cause subjective difficulties that disturb the patient. Each time he initiates a saccade in an upward direction, his eyes first converge and then diverge to regain fusion. As the disturbance increases, every saccadic eye movement, horizontal or vertical, is accompanied by a convergence of the optic axes with a delayed return of the eyes to the parallel position. Most patients with the sylvian aqueduct syndrome complain about their inability to read rapidly; this is at least partially explained by the addition of convergence to every saccadic movement. The abnormality consequent to a single saccade is visible grossly when the patient executes a large upward "flick" of his eyes to center (the primary position). As the eyes complete the movement they seem to wobble or "swim" back and forth rapidly for just an instant in the horizontal direction, and even retract clonically into the orbit once or twice. In our experience this ocular motor sign is a hallmark of the sylvian aqueduct syndrome and of periaqueductal involvement.

An effective way to elicit retraction nystagmus has been stressed by Smith *et al.*, (1959), among others. With downgoing optokinetic targets, retraction jerks will be evoked by each fast phase (upward saccade) of the nystagmus. This method will evoke the sign in virtually all patients with vertical gaze paralysis from a lesion of the rostro-dorsal midbrain.

Reflex vestibular stimulation also causes easily detectable retraction or convergence jerking of the eyes. When upward postrotatory nystagmus is evoked, intense retraction–convergence jerks of 3–4 per second, of regular amplitude and form, result; downward postrotatory nystagmus usually is normal.

Rapid *lateral* gaze movements, like the vertical saccades, may induce spurious convergence. This combination produces differing manifestations in each eye: 1) The adducting eye exhibits *adduction clonus and drift,* a rapid movement of the adductor (due to summation of the saccadic contraction and the "convergence" jerk) with overshoot of the target, followed by a brief series of clonic twitches and then a slow drift back to the fixation target. 2) The abducting eye presents *pseudoabducens paresis.* There is a slow or damped movement of the abductor; if the target is at full lateral gaze the eye will stop short, as in the case of a paretic lateral rectus. These two signs are clearly demonstrated when the patient attempts to observe OKN stimuli moving away from the eccentric position of gaze; the abducted eye moves very little while the adducted eye displays a definite rhythmic nystagmus. The above phenomena may mimic a *Lutz posterior internuclear ophthalmoplegia* (a sign to be discussed in the last section of this chapter).

Bell's phenomenon (elevation of the eyes during forced lid closure) has been employed to distinguish supranuclear and peripheral restrictions of upward gaze, supposedly being affected only in the latter. However, we have not found Bell's maneuver effective in most patients with the sylvian aqueduct syndrome, in conformity with observations of Nashold and Gills (1967), Jampel and Fells (1968) and, in monkeys, Pasik *et al.*,(1969).

2. Lesions causing the sylvian aqueduct syndrome. Pathoanatomical and Stereotactic Evidence. The importance of the lateral pretectal zone of the midbrain at the rostral-lateral portion of the tegmentum for the integration of vertical conjugate gaze in humans is beyond question (Balthasar, 1966). Experimental studies extending back to the work of Hensen and Voelkers (1878) and including the more refined investigations of Szentágothai (1943, 1950a) stressed the significance of the periaqueductal nuclei, particularly the nucleus of Cajal, in the mediation of vertical ocular functions. Detailed clinical–pathological studies of focal infarcts in the rostrolateral midbrain provided supporting evidence for the role of Cajal's nucleus in man (Balthasar and Hopf, 1966). While some of these periaqueductal lesions were discrete and unilateral (Schuster, 1921; van Gehuchten, 1949; Freund, 1913), most involved larger areas of the brain and were often distributed bilaterally (Bárány, 1913; Elschnig, 1913).

From results of stereotactic lesions in 15 monkeys, Pasik *et al.*, (1969) concluded that the posterior commissure and its nuclei are concerned with the mediation of upward movements, while the nucleus of Cajal (as well as the superior colliculus and other structures) is not essential for vertical eye movements. Correlation of ocular motor defects one week post-lesion with histological determination of the lesions revealed that ten animals with palsy of upward gaze had either destruction or secondary degeneration of the posterior commissure and its nuclei. In contrast, these structures were essentially intact in the five monkeys with normal ocular motor function.

The effect of a unilateral lesion in *man* was studied by Nashold and Gills (1967) following focal stereotactic lesions in the rostral lateral tegmentum of the midbrain. These lesions were employed in the treatment of intractable pain; they were *strictly unilateral* and were located at the rostrocaudal level of the posterior commissure, extending rostrally 5 mm. to the level of the pineal recess, and laterally from the border of the periaqueductal gray matter to include the spinothalamic and quintothalamic tracts (4–6 mm). The complex of ocular signs produced resembled the sylvian aqueduct syndrome in most details. The signs in eight patients included: 1) paralysis of upward gaze–eight patients, 2) retraction–convergence nystagmus–seven patients, 3) transient vertical nystagmus–three patients, 4) pathological lid retraction–three patients, and 5) pupillary abnormalities–four patients.

Most of the ocular findings associated with stereotactic lesions of the mesencephalic tegmentum were transient but the paralysis of upward gaze and nystagmus retractorius persisted as fixed abnormalities. The results of this study indicate that defects in vertical gaze can be produced by *unilateral* rostral midbrain lesions in man.

3. Clinical electrophysiological studies. Although it is evident that the lesions causing the Koerber-Salus-Elschnig syndrome are in the region of the sylvian aqueduct, relatively little is known of the pathophysiological mechanism responsible for these peculiarly characteristic eye movements. In 1961, Segarra and Ojeman reviewed the various hypotheses and supporting evidence for each. These were: 1) that retraction movements resulted from some type of "diffuse spread" of voluntary impulses to all ocular motor nuclei (Elschnig, 1913); 2) that only the medial and lateral recti contracted simultaneously and no vertical activity was necessary (Bielchowsky, 1935); and 3) that retraction nystagmus was a result of an exaggerated stretch reflex (Wilke, 1941).

Esslen and Papst (1961) provided important EMG evidence regarding the innervational disturbance responsible for the paralysis of vertical gaze. They found dense, high-voltage motor-unit activity in both the superior rectus and inferior rectus while the eye at "rest" was in the primary position of gaze. This excessive tonic activity resembles continuous spastic innervation, a result of disinhibition of oculomotor neurons. Such disinhibition presumably results from interruption of supranuclear inhibitory pathways or other systems that control the excitability of oculomotor neurons. From recordings during attempted upward and downward movements, Esslen and Papst (1961) showed clearly that supranuclear paralysis of gaze stems from the desynchronization or blocking of excitatory and inhibitory impulses destined for the appropriate cell groups in the oculomotor nucleus. In a study of retraction nystagmus and vertical gaze palsy (a 65 year old patient with a bronchiogenic carcinoma metastatic to the periaqueductal area), they demonstrated faulty recruitment of motor units in the superior rectus during attempted upward gaze; a pathological co–innervation of the remaining three rectus muscles (the medial, inferior and lateral rectus) accounted for the jerking retraction of the eye. The most pronounced co-innervation occured in the medial rectus and explained the distinct tendency of the eyes to converge during the retraction movements. Gay, Brodkey and Miller (1963) also performed a detailed EMG evaluation of three patients with typical retraction nystagmus. Their findings confirmed those of Esslen and Papst (1961) and added several details. Co-contraction of all ocular muscles, including the obliques, is demonstrated in their recordings.

The EMG findings of Gay *et al.*, (1963) provided evidence refuting earlier hypotheses as to the mechanism underlying retraction nystagmus. There was no evidence for a "spread" of innervation (Elschnig, 1913) or an exaggerated stretch reflex (Wilke, 1941); the vertical eye muscles were included in the activity (cf. Bielschowsky, 1935). The co-firing patterns during retraction nystagmus were completely synchronous and had a form that was more typical of saccadic discharges (voluntary or evoked) than of true convergence. Gay and co-workers theorized that a lesion in the substrate mediating voluntary upward gaze (a bilateral frontal–lobe function) might cause bilateral innervation of horizontal rotators of the eye during an intense voluntary effort to look up. However, this theory fails to explain why the cofiring of retraction occurs with appropriate vestibular stimulation and even during rapid horizontal ocular movements. It would appear instead that the physiological defect in the sylvian aqueduct syndrome involves a general arrest in the cortico-mesencephalic inhibitory systems that normally modulate the excitability of various groups of neurons in the ocular motor pool.

It is tempting to relate the abnormal phasic co-firing of convergence-retraction nystagmus to characteristics of normal human saccadic eye movements recorded electromyographically in a study by Tamler *et al.*, (1959). EMG recordings of all extraocular muscles during a saccade in any direction revealed a burst of activity in the agonist, complete inhibition of the antagonist, and coactivity of the auxillary muscles. Brief co–contraction, according to these investigators, is a normal characteristic of saccades; perhaps it represents the substrate upon which the abnormal phasic coactivity observed in the sylvian aqueduct syndrome is superimposed.

We have analyzed the ocular movements in this syndrome with electro-oculography (Figs. 3 and 4) and our findings are in general agreement with those of Atkin and Bender (1964). The eyes show no evidence of horizontal

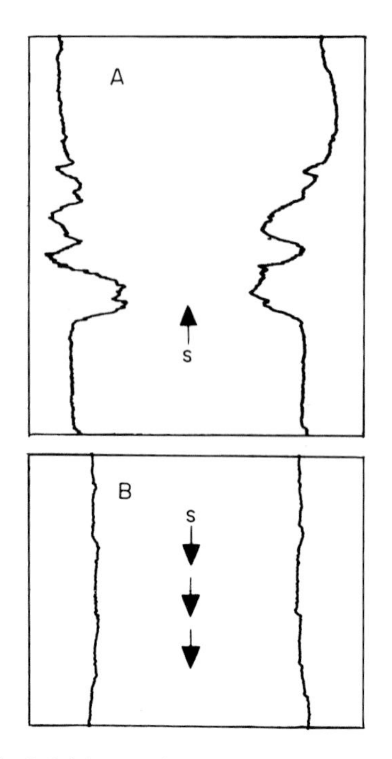

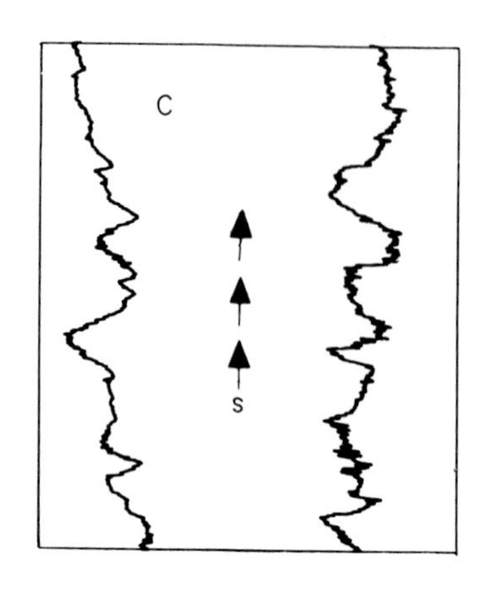

Fig. 3. Sylvian aqueduct syndrome. Electro-oculograms (DC) of horizontal eye movements (so-called convergence nystagmus) evoked by vertical saccades. **A.** One voluntary saccade (S↑)– directed upward from down gaze position to center – evokes, for about 1 second, a series of irregular wandering disjunctive asymmetric convergence–divergence movements in the horizontal plane. **B.** A series of optokinetic evoked saccades (S↓↓) downward does not alter the horizontal parallelism of the eyes. **C.** Upward OKN saccades (S↑↑) cause horizontal irregular asynchronous oscillatory eye movements and a convergence of the optical axes. The so-called convergent–retraction nystagmus is completely disconjugate with irregular amplitude, rate and direction.

vergence movements during stimulation with upward moving OKN stimuli (Fig. 3b). The jerking vergence movements of the eyes evoked by down-moving stripes have the following characteristics (Fig. 3c): 1) The average position of the eye varies from mild to moderate convergence with only occasional divergent movements to the baseline; 2) The recordings of the movement of the two eyes show a preponderance of a "mirror image" convergence–divergence movement with occasional rapid conjugate movements; 3) Convergence–divergence movements are highly irregular in amplitude and rate. They are rarely rapid, and are accompanied by simultaneous elevations of the lids.

Horizontal OKN stimuli evoke normal-appearing fast and slow movements in the eye that adducts in the fast phase (Fig. 4c). The movements of the fellow eye are damped (slowed) in every fast phase and tend to drift over a greater distance during each slow phase; as a result, the eye progressively

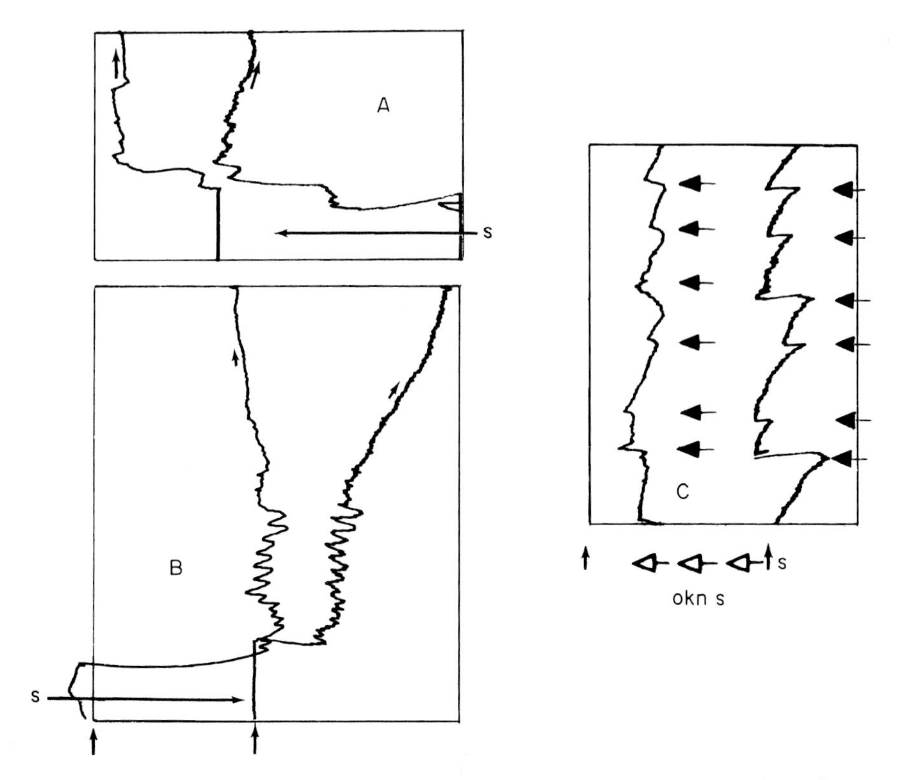

Fig. 4. Sylvian aqueduct syndrome. Electro-oculograms (DC recordings) of horizontal 30° to 40° centering saccades, A and B, and OKN saccades from right to center, C. (All recordings show right eye on right, left eye on left, with time scale running from below upward). A. Horizontal saccade to center starting in right gaze, (←—S). The adducting eye starts first, hesitates midway, completes saccade, oscillates rapidly for 0.75 seconds, and then diverges slightly. The left eye begins abduction 0.1 seconds late, hesitates, then abducts moving conjugately with the right eye, overshoots slightly and oscillates slightly. It fails to move as far as the right eye and does so more slowly. One and one-half seconds later the visual axes are still converged (top of record). B. Centering (horizontal) saccade from left gaze to midline (S—→): again the abducting eye (right eye) starts later and moves about 1/3 as far as the adducting eye (left eye). As the saccade ends, both eyes oscillate about 1 second, and finally the right eye diverges (for about 1½ seconds) until the two eyes are parallel (top of record). C. OKN saccades (to left, ←←← S) (marked with black arrows) with eyes initially deviated 15° to the right. The adducting right eye (right tracing) makes rapid saccades to left but their amplitudes are variable; some are small and others large. The abducting left eye (left tracing) is late in beginning and markedly damped in the performance of OKN saccades. During continuation of the OKN stimuli (not demonstrated in the tracing) the adducting eye converges while the abducting eye remains relatively immobile.

converges toward its fellow. Large horizontal saccades toward the center are disjunctive and unequal in amplitude; the adducting eye (the laterally deviated eye) starts first and travels farther than the abducting eye. The two eyes, now in a converged attitude, go through a rapid series of low amplitude convergence oscillations for about one second; about 12 oscillations occur before the esotropic eye drifts laterally to the straight ahead position during the next 1.0–1.5 seconds (Fig. 4a and b).

These electronystagmographic findings clearly show the effects of co-innervation of antagonists on the performance of saccadic horizontal eye movements and demonstrate the overwhelming damping effect by the medial rectus on any voluntary saccade performed by its antagonist. Certainly this damping by a co-contracting medial rectus plus a relative acceleration of the fellow (adducting) eye and the slow return of the eye to a parallel position constitutes a major handicap for the patient. It explains his subjective sensation of slow "focusing" after large amplitude refixation movements. The perceptual delay can last almost 3 seconds. The failure of normal inhibition of the medial rectus during maximal abduction of the eye can restrict full lateral movement and create the clinical appearance of a weak lateral rectus. As mentioned previously, this finding has been observed repeatedly with rostral midbrain lesions and has been termed a pseudo sixth–nerve palsy.

Vertical gaze disorders with lesions in the pontine tegmentum

Vertical gaze–evoked nystagmus is a common sign in patients with bilateral (diffuse or focal) involvement of the pontine tegmentum. It is also regularly associated with bilateral internuclear ophthalmoplegia (see final section of this chapter). Paralysis of vertical gaze does not occur with unilateral involvements of the pontine tegmentum. On the other hand, unilateral lesions in the region of the middle cerebellar peduncle can produce pronounced skew deviation.

Bender and Shanzer (1960, 1964) studied the effect of bilateral lesions in the paramedian reticular formation of the pontine tegmentum of monkeys. The lesions not only resulted in bilateral paresis of horizontal ocular movements, but also caused as severe a paralysis of all vertical movements as do pretectal lesions.

The present authors doubted that bilateral lesions of the pontine paramedian reticular formation of man would produce such a paralysis of vertical gaze. Recently, however, one of us (W.F.H.) observed a 60–year old man with a right horizontal gaze palsy and ipsilateral facial paresis of gradual onset; vertical gaze was normal. Neuroradiological studies revealed a discrete mass elevating the floor of the fourth ventricle near the facial eminence. At operation a cystic tumor was found to the right of the midline immediately in front of the stria medullaris. It was partially removed with minimal trauma; its inferior capsule was stripped from the floor of the ventricle. Postoperatively, the patient awakened promptly and could speak. At that time, he had a nearly total ophthalmoplegia with preserved pupillary reactions and lid function. Tonic deviation of his eyes occurred when his left ear canal was irrigated with cold water (the right side was non-reactive). Within 24 hours he had regained 50% of vertical gaze and had gaze–evoked vertical nystagmus. Thirty–six hours later his eye movements had returned to their preoperative state. Edema of the pontine tegmentum adjacent to the site of resection must have occurred to produce effects on the uninvolved side. His ophthalmoplegia, sparing the lids but involving all remaining gaze functions, represented an example of what Bender and Shanzer had found in their experimental studies.

Several more cases of acute postoperative vertical gaze paresis were found which had persisted 24 to 48 hours, often with skew deviation. In no instance had the dorsal midbrain or the caudal aqueduct been manipulated by the surgeon.

It is possible that some of the acute postinfectious external ophthalmoplegias (with associated signs of ataxia, areflexia, and previous history of a "flu-like" illness 10–14 days before) represent a similar bilateral involvement of the paramedian pontine reticular formation (Fisher, 1956; Smith and Walsh, 1957; Goodwin and Poser, 1963; and Van Allen and MacQueen, 1964). These patients have no spontaneous eye movements at the acute stage of their illness but as the palsy clears they begin to regain first horizontal, and then vertical movements accompanied by paretic gaze-evoked nystagmus. Several toxic ophthalmoplegias cause similar signs and recover in the same sequence.

Vertical gaze disorders with lesions in the medulla oblongata

Only brief mention is made here of the relatively minor role of cervico-medullary disease in disordered control of vertical gaze. Involvement of the medial longitudinal fasciculi and the paramedian reticular system may cause instability of vertical gaze, expressed frequently as *down-beating nystagmus* (Cogan, 1968b). One of us (R.B.D.) has noted this sign to be particularly specific for cervico-medullary junction pathology (Arnold-Chiari malformation; basilar invagination) if the down-beating nystagmus is of greater amplitude during extremes of lateral than straight downward gaze.

Occasionally a constant vertical nystagmus in the primary position of gaze, and rarely a skew deviation with vertical diplopia, result from disorders of the cervical-vestibular postural systems (Moberg *et al.,* 1962; Grant, 1966; Bjerver and Silfverskiold, 1968).

CLINICAL DISORDERS OF SYSTEMS CONTROLLING OCULAR VERGENCE

Only man and primates possess the capacity to move both eyes freely and all the while fixate binocularly, maintain a clear image, appreciate stereopsis, and vary the point of focus in any frontal plane from a near point to infinity. Performance of these tasks requires a precise physiological linkage of accommodation, convergence and pupillary constriction—a triad that has been termed *the near-response, the near reflex, and the near synkinesis.* These integrated controls impart to man the tools with which he acquires his three-dimensional concept of space. Understanding of the anatomy and physiology of vergence–accommodation control is a requisite for interpretation of normal and abnormal ocular motor functions. It is precisely because of its complexity, the subjective nature of the end–points used to test it, and the technical problems involved in recording each of its parts that clinical information about its supranuclear disorders is disappointingly scant and poorly quantitated.

In normal binocular vision, accommodation and convergence operate in unison. The basic stimuli for the binocular adjustment for near vision are: 1) change in the vergence of the light reaching the two foveas, and 2) temporal disparity of the two images relative to the two foveas. The relationship of convergence and accommodation is not absolutely fixed, but under normal conditions a unit change in one is accompanied by a unit change in the other.

However, the elements of the near reflex are not exclusively dependent on each other; any one of the three functions can be abolished without interference with the others. Convergence or accommodation may be eliminated selectively by the use of prisms or lenses, and pupillary constriction alone can be blocked by small doses of weak atropine–like drugs without noticeable cycloplegia. Accommodation, convergence, and pupillary constriction are associated movements and are not linked to one another in the manner usually referred to by the term "reflex." They are controlled, synchronized, and associated by supranuclear connections that can be independent.

Vergence movements and brain stimulation

Convergence of the eyes of monkeys was early produced by bilateral stimulation of corresponding areas in frontal lobes or occipital eye fields (Mott and Schafer, 1890). More recently, Jampel (1959) elicited asymmetrical convergence movements (variably associated with miosis, accommodation, or both) upon unilateral stimulation of points in the primate preoccipital cortex. The convergence was usually manifested by adduction of the ipsilateral eye, although unequal adduction of both eyes frequently occurred. Jampel concluded that symmetrical convergence movements are synthesized bilaterally at the highest level of nervous activity, the cerebral cortex. Thence they are projected independently to both sides of the pretectum and rostral mesencephalic reticular formation where they are further integrated with other elements of the ocular motor system. Unilateral cortical stimulation in the human also occasionally produces convergence (Rasmussen and Penfield, 1948). That convergence can be obtained by stimulating the cortex is evidence against a separate "center" for convergence (the so–called nucleus of Perlia) within the oculomotor nucleus.

Jampel (1959) recorded accommodative changes in the primate eye induced by faradic stimulation of overlapping areas of the preoccipital (peristriate) cortex. Accommodation was usually obtained in both eyes by unilateral cortical stimulation; it was always accompanied by convergence and often by pupillary constriction.

Accommodation, inward movement of the eye (unilateral adduction), and pupillary constriction have resulted from stimulation of areas deep within the brain of monkeys and humans. Bender and Weinstein (1953) applied minute currents to the monkey brain and obtained adduction of the ipsilateral eye from an area of the tegmentum lying ventro–laterally at the rostral end of the midbrain. As they moved their electrode toward the midline and more ventrally, head and eye movements became more complex. By increasing the stimulating current at points near the midline, they obtained bilateral adduction responses.

In man, adduction of the ipsilateral eye has been obtained most commonly from stimulation of the prerubral fields of Forel and the oral pole of the red nucleus (Spiegel *et al.,* 1964; Nashold and Gills, 1967). Convergence and downward deviation of the eyes occurred with stimulation of the posterior sensory thalamus 13 mm lateral to the midline; convergence and ipsilateral tilting of the head resulted from stimulations in the midbrain at the level of the inferior colliculus (ventral and lateral to the aqueduct); and convergence and slight downward deviation of the eyes resulted from stimulation of an area at the mesencephalic–pontine junction 4–5 mm laterally and ventrally from the aqueduct (Nashold and Gills, 1967).

Supranuclear lesions and vergence "spasm"

Clinically, the terms "spastic," "spasm." "spasticity" and the like are used freely to cover a wide variety of conditions of dissimilar origin, many of which are not presently understood. Spasm of convergence, usually associated with spasm of accommodation, is often encountered in hysterical individuals, but it also occurs in patients who seem entirely stable. It often disappears when a cycloplegic agent is used. Convergence "spasm" has been described in patients with basilar inflammation, following head trauma, and as a consequence of hyperopia with abnormality of the A/C ratio (Walsh and Hoyt, 1969). Cogan (personal communication) observed spasm of the near reflex lasting 5–10 seconds following brief hyperextension of the neck in a 17 year old girl who had an Arnold–Chiari malformation and basilar impression. Consistently after each hyperextension of her neck, both eyes would converge sharply and the pupils would constrict. The mechanism of this "spasm" was never clarified.

Convergence spasms, clonic convergence jerks, and convergence–retraction nystagmus occur in combination with vertical gaze palsies. That these abnormalities of ocular movement are indeed "spastic" phenomena is evidenced by EMG data. However, convergence phenomena in the sylvian aqueduct syndrome should be regarded as "pseudo–convergence," for the innervational disorder in these cases is quite different from the pattern of innervation in normal convergence. The same applies to paradoxical convergence occurring in some congenital ocular motor syndromes with anomalous patterns of innervation, and to the peculiar tonic convergence and downward deviation of the eyes described by Fisher (1967) in comatose patients with thalamic hemorrhage.

Spasticity of medial rectus muscles in acute bilateral internuclear ophthalmoplegia (i.e., bilateral MLF lesions (see final section)) causes diplopia and inertia of divergence following fixation on a nearby object (the near response). Similar convergence "spasm" causes inertia of divergence in patients with bilateral pontine gaze palsy.

Supranuclear paralysis of divergence

In 1940, Bender and Savitsky described divergence paralysis in a patient with a single minute hemangioma in the periaqueductal gray matter at the level between the superior and inferior colliculus (revealed at autopsy). Chamlin and Davidoff (1950) described paralysis of divergence in patients with increased intracranial pressure from cerebral tumor, pseudotumor cerebri, or subdural hematoma; surgical intervention promptly relieved the symptom. These patients did not exhibit the secondary deviation phenomenon that characterizes a nuclear or peripheral abducens palsy. A variety of other neurological disorders have been accompanied by divergence palsy (Lyle, 1954; Walsh and Hoyt, 1969).

Divergence paralysis occurs suddenly and gives rise to homonymous diplopia and convergent strabismus. There is no apparent weakness of the lateral rectus muscles. The diplopia is characterized by a constant displacement of the images in all fields at points equidistant from the eyes, usually in the far field of vision. The clinical phenomenon of acute esotropia for distance with normal binocular vision at near is incontestable. Burian and Miller (1958) provide an interesting discussion of the differential diagnosis and provide a useful list of references.

Cyclic disorders of vergence; circadian strabismus

A fascinating phenomenon that may be related to divergence paresis, and is as poorly understood, is the so–called "*cyclic esotropia*" or "*alternate-day–esotropia*." In this disorder of vergence the patient, usually a young child, manifests esotropia and often experiences diplopia for 24–hour periods; these alternate with 24–hour periods during which ocular motor functions are perfectly normal (Costenbader and Mousel, 1964). Richter (1968) termed the condition "clock–mechanism" esotropia and likened it to other congenital and acquired 24 to 48 hours cyclic phenomena in man. None of the children had associated neurological disease and peculiarly, all were cured by operation on the medial rectus muscles.

Windsor and Berg (1960) described non-comitant *vertical cyclic deviation* in a boy in whom several transitions from one phase of the cycle to the other were observed and recorded. In this child, symptomatic phases caused diplopia and resembled superior oblique palsy; cycles could be modified by administration of barbiturates.

Supranuclear paralysis of convergence

Paralysis of convergence is defined as an inability to converge the visual axes but with no weakness of the medial rectus muscles during the performance of lateral gaze. Such paralysis may arise as a result of organic disease such as encephalitis, multiple sclerosis, vascular occlusion and other involvements of the rostral midbrain. It occurs commonly as a result of cerebral concussion, and rarely with bilateral parieto-occipital lesions (Holmes, 1918b). Intermittent horizontal diplopia and convergence paralysis occur in some patients afflicted with narcolepsy.

The condition is manifest by diplopia (crossed horizontal images) during gaze at nearby objects. Since convergence can be controlled voluntarily, "functional" paresis manifest by hysterical patients and malingerers poses a difficult problem in differential diagnosis. Bielschowsky (1935) defined the criteria for true convergence paresis as 1) definite evidence of intracranial disease; 2) sudden onset; 3) signs and symptoms tested at various times must be consistent; 4) there must be accommodation and constriction of the pupils even though the attempted convergence does not result in eye movement; and 5) a base-out prism will not cause an eye movement in a true paresis, whereas it will in functional illness.

Several cases of bilateral occipital injury and convergence palsy were reported by Holmes in 1918. Feigenbaum and Kornbleuth (1946) described a patient with paralysis of convergence and bilateral homonymous "ring" scotomas caused by bilateral occipital lobe injuries. They concluded that the peristriate cortex had been damaged bilaterally resulting in the failure of convergence. Jampel (1959) offered experimental evidence from monkeys supporting the clinical concept that bilateral occipital lesions result in "paresis" of convergence.

In an EMG evaluation of total convergence paresis in a patient with diffuse brain-stem and cerebellar disease, Esslen and Papst (1961) recorded the absence of medial rectus excitation and lateral rectus inhibition during accommodative effort. The EMG of the medial rectus showed abnormally high-voltage tonic activity; a normal interference pattern appeared in the medial rectus during lateral gaze.

PARA- AND INTERNUCLEAR DISORDERS OF OCULAR MOTOR INTEGRATION

Paranuclear disorders of excitation and reciprocal inhibition

Disorders of the paranuclear elements of the reticular formation, the interneurons, distort normal excitatory and inhibitory coordination of ocular muscles, resulting in bizarre and paradoxical eye movements, usually in young children. The signs of these innervational defects are more subtle when acquired as sequelae of acute or chronic brain stem disease. The anomaly of innervation usually affects the muscles of one eye, sometimes in combination with muscles of the lid, face or jaw. While the neuronal or synaptic defects in interneurons have not been established, ocular EMG findings reported during the past decade confirm gross alterations in patterns of reciprocal innervation of affected muscles. These EMG studies of anomalous ocular innervation also provide interesting data regarding inhibitional processes in ocular motor activity.

A. Paradoxical innervation of agonist and antagonist

The retraction syndromes and related ocular motor defects. Clinically, the anomaly called Duane's retraction syndrome (Duane, 1905) usually consists of congenital "paresis" of the lateral rectus muscle and retraction of the eye during attempted adduction. Limitation of abduction on the affected side is usually severe, but when it is incomplete there is greater mobility of the eye in the upper and lower fields of lateral gaze. The retraction movement of the globe occurring during adduction may be obvious or subtle. The movement is accompanied by narrowing of the palpebral fissure and often by oblique upward (rarely downward) deviation of the eye. Adduction is usually complete but in rare cases is severely limited (Huber *et al.*, 1964). The patient often prefers to hold his head in a position that allows gaze toward the side of the unaffected eye.

The retraction syndrome has been reported in association with a wide variety of congenital defects of the brain and body (Walsh and Hoyt, 1969). The syndrome occurs most often in girls and, peculiarly, most often on the left side. Bilateral involvement is not uncommon; familial occurrence is frequent.

Other hereditary brain stem innervational anomalies and "palsies" of bulbar muscles have many pathophysiological features in common with Duane's retraction syndrome and may even be associated with it in the same or other family members. Hereditary laryngeal abductor paralysis (Plott, 1964) and hereditary mirror movements (Regli *et al.*, 1967) are developmental motor abnormalities with similar pathological co-innervation of antagonistic muscle pairs.

In early descriptions of the congenital syndromes of defective ocular abduction and retraction (Sinclair, 1895; Friedenwald, 1896; Turk, 1899, and Duane, 1905), the underlying mechanism was considered to be a peripheral anomaly involving orbital and connective tissue. However, recent EMG studies have provided evidence that the retraction phenomenon is a result of paradoxical supranuclear (brain stem) innervation of both horizontal rectus muscles and various combinations of vertically-acting ocular muscles (Breinin, 1957; Papst and Esslen, 1960; Sato, 1960; Burger, 1963; Blodi *et al.*, 1964; Huber *et al.*, 1964; and Zauberman *et al.*, 1967). Further, not only is the affected muscle present, but it usually has a functioning nerve supply; however it may contract as the eye moves *away* from its normal field of action. EMG observations indicate that several different anomalies of neuromuscular innervation produce clinical signs of retraction syndrome (Zauberman *et al.*, 1967).

Esslen and Papst (1961) defined several variants of Duane's syndrome: 1) Paradoxical innervation between the lateral and inferior rectus muscles. In this type, abduction is restricted and there is convergence during upward gaze and divergence during downward gaze. 2) Paradoxical innervation between the lateral and superior rectus. Here convergence occurs during downward gaze, and divergence during upward gaze. The lateral and superior recti fire simultaneously and abduction is impaired in the horizontal plane. Retraction is absent in these first two varieties. 3) Paradoxical innervation between the lateral rectus and several eye muscles. Here, the clinical signs are similar to those in the typical retraction syndrome. The lateral rectus fires maximally during ocular movement in several directions, e.g., during contraction of the medial rectus, inferior rectus or superior rectus. Lateral rectus innervation is less effective during horizontal abduction and the range of movement is limited.

We have examined a patient with ocular findings corresponding to Esslen and Papst's third category of congenital abductor palsy and, in addition, retraction of the affected eye during downward and lateral gaze. Examination showed: 1) straight eyes in the primary position, 2) absence of abduction of the left eye during attempted gaze to the left, 3) normal right conjugate gaze, 4) no retraction of the left eye or narrowing of the palpebral fissure during adduction, 5) oblique upward and lateral movement of the left eye during upward gaze with the right eye fixing, 6) oblique downward and lateral movement of the left eye during downward gaze with the right eye fixing, and 7) *full abduction of the left eye* during voluntary lateral gaze with the eyes depressed and, associated with this movement, retraction of the globe resembling the down-gaze retraction described recently by Khodadoust and van Noorden (1967).

Esslen and Papst's EMG study of this type of anomaly showed absence of recruitment of motor units in the left lateral rectus during voluntary gaze toward the right or left, and anomalous co-innervation of the left lateral rectus and superior rectus during upward gaze with co-innervation of lateral and inferior rectus in downward gaze.

Ocular EMG recordings by Blodi *et al.*,(1964) revealed a variety of inappropriate muscle discharges in several cases of congenital abduction "paresis." These included anomalous co-firing of the medial rectus during attempted abduction, and, in another patient, co-inhibition of the medial and lateral recti during attempted adduction, so that the eye moved upward. The electro-oculographic data recorded by Cenacchi and Bertoni (1967) from a patient with a bilateral retraction syndrome revealed further complexities of this anomaly, including anomalous nystagmoid movements in response to vestibular stimulation.

If the innervational deficit underlying this variety of the retraction syndrome is indeed supranuclear, its complexity is truly baffling. Within a single patient it would require defects in connections of various sub-nuclei of both the left and right third nuclei plus the left sixth nucleus. While some cases of

Duane's syndrome may be the result of paranuclear or interneuronal defects, we feel that the more complex cases may rather be due to a peripheral anomaly of distribution of one third nerve (e.g., to the superior, lateral and inferior recti), coupled with dysplasia of the abducens nerve and nucleus. Hoyt and Nachtigäller (1965) summarized anatomical evidence in favor of peripheral anomalies of nerves supplying the paradoxically innervated rectus muscles typified by Duane's syndrome. Further, an extra branch of the third nerve can substitute for an aplastic abducens nerve (Tillack and Winer, 1962; and Bremer, 1921). Zauberman and co-workers (1967) obtained EMG records in one case consistent with a peripherally determined innervational anomaly.

Rarely, the ocular EMG record shows sparse low-voltage potentials or absent potentials, suggesting that the muscle is denervated or dysplastic (Orlowski and Wojtowicz, 1962).

In addition to the congenital anomaly of abduction with retraction, there have been occasional reports of other congenital ocular motor defects with retraction. A *vertical retraction* syndrome, reported in two siblings by Khodadoust and von Noorden (1967), included variable limitation of vertical gaze and ocular retraction in downward gaze.

Zweifach *et al.*, (1969) described a congenital syndrome of bilateral horizontal gaze paresis that may include *monocular vergence retraction.* Two of their five patients showed this sign during attempts to look to the side. This effect evoked a vergence movement with pupillary constriction (the near reaction) and retraction of the eye on the side of the intended gaze. The monocular retraction phenomenon indicated anomalous co-innervation of horizontal rectus muscles.

B. Inverse reciprocal innervation in lateral gaze; "perverted" ocular movements

Bárány (1930) and Burian and Cahill (1952) reported patients with a bizarre congenital ocular motor syndrome manifesting paradoxical divergence during lateral gaze, clinically referred to as congenital supranuclear adduction palsy. All of their patients had unilateral limitation of adduction and other evidence of ipsilateral congenital ophthalmoplegia, without lid or pupillary involvement. Lateral gaze toward the involved side produced striking divergence of the non-fixing eye. Gaze toward the uninvolved side first produced adduction in the non-fixing eye and then normal abduction as the fixing eye crossed the midline. Vertical gaze was usually normal. Tests with the rotating chair or optokinetic drum provoked striking ocular divergence jerks alternating with symmetrical ocular convergence during the slow phases. The reverse stimuli (vestibular or OKN) produced normal conjugate jerk-type nystagmus. In one patient, the involved eye would not adduct beyond the midline, elevate, or abduct fully. EMG study of the activity in the lateral rectus muscle of this patient showed subnormal firing with paradoxical excitation during contralateral gaze and no increase in tonus during ipsilateral gaze.

Although Burian and Cahill's (1952) electro-oculographic recording of the anomalous vergence movements (divergence and return) showed approximately symmetrical rapid divergence jerks and equally slow convergence return movements, the common denominator in these cases was the supranuclear, congenital, unilateral "partial" ocular motor paresis.

Cords (1927) attributed the bizarre eye movements of this type to "aberrant" fibers. Bárány (1930) concluded that two destructive processes had taken place— probably due to brain stem hemorrhages occurring during birth — one destroying the nucleus of the left medial rectus muscle, and a second isolating the intact nucleus of the ipsilateral lateral rectus from the cortex as well as from the vestibular area. Bárány also assumed a direct communication between the two abducens nuclei, as a result of which every active impulse to the contralateral abducens area would also lead to an active innervation of the ipsilateral sixth nerve. However, Burian and Cahill (1952) considered it unnecessary to postulate an isolated involvement of the sixth-nerve nucleus. Rather, they assumed that a lesion in the region of the contralateral MLF could account for the supranuclear paralysis of the medial rectus muscle, and that every active impulse destined for the nucleus of the right lateral rectus also reached the left sixth–nerve nucleus through a direct communication between the two nuclei, (as assumed by Bárány). They also thought it possible that the uncrossed fibers from the cortex to the ipsilateral sixth–nerve nucleus (which normally transmit inhibitory impulses) transmitted excitatory impulses, producing the clinical picture observed in the syndrome.

Huber and co-workers (1964) performed EMG examinations on a patient with normal abduction and complete unilateral pseudoparesis of ocular adduction and retraction. They found co-innervation of medial and lateral rectus muscles leading to retraction during attempted adduction but during abduction a normal reciprocal pattern of innervation prevailed. This patient had a congenital adduction palsy but without paradoxical divergence movements.

Another example of a bizarre or "perverted" ocular movement was found in a patient with a partial congenital oculomotor palsy observed by Walsh (Walsh and Hoyt, 1969). In this patient any effort to move the paretic eye downward resulted in marked outward movement of that eye. With the right eye fixing and the eyes directed to the right, the left eye turned straight down. With the right eye fixing and the eyes turned to the left, the left eye turned sharply upward. With the left eye fixing, a mirror image of what has been described was observed.

C. Cyclic oculomotor paralysis; cyclic paranuclear inhibition and excitation

Among the rarest and most fascinating forms of oculomotor palsies is that termed "cyclic oculomotor paralysis." In this condition, some of the extraocular muscles over which the patient has lost all voluntary control contract tonically at more or less regular intervals. The sphincter of the iris and the ciliary muscle contract synchronously with the extraocular muscles although the former is unresponsive to all reflex stimuli.

Over one half the reported cases were congenital or were manifested in the first six months of life. In four adult cases, it was reliably established that the oculomotor paralysis had occurred many years prior to the onset of the cyclic phenomenon. Usually, but not always, the paralysis of the third nerve was complete. The sphincter of the iris and the ciliary muscle were involved in every case; occasionally these intrinsic muscles were solely involved. Next in frequency of involvement was the levator muscle of the upper lid, and occasionally the medial rectus alone took part in the cycles of spasm and inhibition.

In general, in the phase of relaxation, the upper lid hangs slackly over the exotropic globe. The pupil is dilated and accommodation is paralyzed. This phase lasts for one to three minutes. In classical cases, twitching movements of the upper lid occur at the end of this period after which the lid rises suddenly and smoothly to give the lid fissure its normal width. At the same time, the dilated fixed pupil constricts to a diameter of 1 to 3 mm; the eyeball moves to the midline and shows marked spasm of accommodation. This "spastic" phase lasts 30–100 seconds. Then a few twitching movements again appear in the lids, the eye suddenly turns out, the pupil dilates, and the lid drops down.

The classic cases of congenital cyclic oculomotor paralysis of Rampoldi (1884, 1886) are described in the detailed report of Hicks and Hosford (1937). Stevens (1965) reported an acquired case in a woman with a brainstem tumor. Cyclic oculomotor palsy is rarely associated with any other neurological phenomena, although there are isolated cases in the literature associating it with seizures (Petrovic and Tschemolossow, 1931), twitching (Lowenstein and Givner, 1949), or other cranial nerve involvement (Lauber, 1913). While the ocular motor defect is usually unilateral, there have been some occurrences of bilateral nuclear involvement (Stevens, 1965). The physiological mechanism underlying the cyclic activation and inhibition of cells in the oculomotor nucleus is unknown, although several hypotheses have been reviewed by Burian and van Allen (1963).

D. Paradoxical levator excitation and inhibition; congenital and acquired oculopalpebral, mandibulopalpebral, and related synkineses

Anomalies of upper-lid movement have been found to be associated with several congenital paranuclear disorders of eye movement as well as with contraction of a variety of non-ocular muscles. Studies of these lid co-movements provide a unique opportunity to witness anomalous excitation and inhibition of a muscle that performs most of its functions without an antagonist. Except during blinking, lid elevation denotes excitation, and lid lowering, inhibition of levator motoneurons in the oculomotor nucleus. Surprisingly, few studies of supranuclear ocular motor control have taken advantage of this sensitive indicator of pathophysiological activity in the brain stem.

Levator excitation evoked by jaw movement or swallowing. The Marcus Gunn lid phenomenon is so named from a case of Marcus Gunn's in which associated movements of the upper lid and jaw were found (Gunn, 1903). The patient was a 15 year old girl who had congenital ptosis of her left lid; the lid raised when she opened her mouth or when she thrust her jaw to the side. This peculiar lid movement of "jaw winking" had first been observed when she was a nursing infant. As she grew up, the ptosis became less pronounced but the associated movement persisted. The left pupil was slightly smaller than the right.

Recognizing that cases such as this might throw new light on the relationship between the nuclei of the cranial nerves, Gunn's colleagues formed a study committee which concluded that there were abnormal connections between the central mechanism controlling the external pterygoid muscle and the mechanism innervating the levator muscle (Gunn, 1903). More recently, Sano (1959) contributed EMG and other neurophysiological data which support the theory that "jaw winking" is essentially a synkinesis between the pterygoid muscles and the levator palpebrae superioris. He termed the associated movements of lid and jaw a "trigemino-oculomotor" synkinesis, and subdivided them into an external pterygoid–levator synkinesis and an internal pterygoid–levator synkinesis, the former being more common.

Most external pterygoid–levator synkineses are congenital and often familial; in occasional cases a synkinesis first appeared following head injury in childhood (Grant, 1936; Sano, 1959). Ipsilateral congenital elevator palsy is commonly present on the side of the involved lid in congenital cases (Lutz, 1919; Cooper, 1937).

Lid elevation with closure of the mouth or, more exactly, with clenching of the teeth is a rare trigemino-oculomotor synkinesis (Sano, 1959; Papst and Rossmann, 1966). Sano (1959) reported on two patients with levator contraction evoked only by electrical stimulation of the internal pterygoid muscle; stimulation of other muscles of chewing had no effect. He suggested that the rare cases of paradoxical unilateral lid retraction accompanying swallowing movements (e.g., Walsh, 1948) may be examples of this levator synkinesis. Alexander (1949) reported concurrence of ipsilateral facial asymmetry, external ophthalmoplegia and jaw winking.

Surgical attempts to abolish the Marcus Gunn synkinesis by interruption of portions of the fifth nerve have been only partially successful (Grant, 1936; Sano, 1959).

In addition to the pterygoid–levator synkineses, several other levator synkineses have been reported. Unilateral levator excitation is occasionally associated with sternocleidomastoid contraction, representing a spinal accessory–palpebral synkinesis. In some cases the anomalous levator contraction is induced by smiling, or by coughing or other respiratory efforts, as well as by contraction of the neck muscles (Brain, 1933; Parry, 1957; Bradley and Toone, 1967). These cases seem to involve supranuclear (inhibitory) systems regulating and integrating primitive bulbar reflexes.

Paradoxical innervation of the levator muscle may be inhibitory as well as excitatory, as in the case of an oculo-palpebral inhibitory synkinesis. In this form of congenital synkinesis, the affected lid appears normal or only slightly ptotic when the eye is in the primary position of gaze, but when the eye is moved to the side or upward, the lid drops over the pupil. As the patient moves his eye back to center the lid resumes a normal posture. This peculiar pattern of levator contraction and relaxation usually occurs unilaterally, often is associated with a congenital elevator defect, and is evoked by specific ocular rotations (upward rotation, medial rotation, upward and medial rotation, or abduction). Frequently excitement, smiling, or laughing will override synkinetic ptosis and cause irregular jerking retraction of the affected lid (Walsh and Hoyt, 1969; Hepler *et al.,* 1968). Hepler and associates (1968) reported a case of gaze-dependent inhibition of the levator and found a close correlation between EMG data, from the right levator and the left medial rectus, and clinical observation of lid movements.

A rare mandibular inhibitory synkinesis causes associated drooping of a lid during jaw opening, representing a true inverse Marcus Gunn synkinesis (Walsh and Hoyt, 1969).

The pathophysiological mechanisms underlying anomalous synkinesis of the levator with other muscles are not clear, although there are some suggestive observations in the literature. The earliest explanation of the Marcus-Gunn phenomenon proposed an abnormal connection between the central mechanisms for the external pterygoid and the levator muscle, postulating dual innervation of the levator both from the third nucleus and the external pterygoid portion of the fifth nucleus (Gunn, 1903).

More recently Ingraham and Campbell (1941) found that they could evoke the synkinesis by electrical stimulation of the cerebral cortex in an epileptic patient who also had a typical (congenital) Marcus Gunn syndrome. Sano (1959) observed that direct stimulation of the pterygoid muscle could cause lid retraction, suggesting that cortical stimulation may evoke the synkinesis secondarily by causing pterygoid muscle contraction.

In 1948, Wartenberg offered the interpretation that Marcus Gunn synkinesis represents a supranuclear release phenomenon. He proposed that primitive innervational connections between the extraocular muscles and the muscles of mastication are normally "suppressed" by phylogenetically newer mechanisms. He suggested that unspecified peripheral or central dysfunction could alter the newer systems and "release" the primitive systems. The processes Wartenberg termed "suppression" and "release" correspond to the inhibition and excitation that modulates all nervous activity. Neuronal inhibition may be of two types: 1) *post-synaptic,* which has been specifically demonstrated at oculomotor motoneurons by Sasaki (1963), and 2) *pre-synaptic,* which has been shown to be a potent force in regulating sensory input to brain stem and spinal systems (Eccles, 1961).

The levator muscle of the upper eyelid is unique in that its state of inhibition can be observed clinically as lid lowering. The synkinetic inhibition of a lid evoked by gaze can be attributed to anomalous activity in inhibitory interneurons that control the output of cells bordering the midline levator nucleus. Most of these anomalies affect only part of the inhibitory substrate, for the levator muscle usually acts normally during sleep, downward gaze, and periodic or reflex blinking.

Miscellaneous conditions of anomalous levator activity. There are several congenital and acquired paranuclear anomalies of levator innervation in which gaze to the right or left causes reciprocating inhibition of one lid and excitation of the other, i.e., gaze–evoked see–saw lid movements. With Dr. Norman Schatz,one of us (W.F.H.) examined a 4–year–old girl with an anomalous innervation syndrome of remarkable lid movements. She had a partial elevator palsy of the right eye, and upward gaze (with left–eye fixing) evoked oblique movement of the right eye upward and outward. Conjugate (voluntary) gaze to the right caused *unilateral synkinetic levator inhibition* (lid drop) on the right; gaze toward the left evoked the opposite pattern of lid innervation–inhibition of left levator and excitation of the right levator muscle. Alternating right and left lateral gaze produced striking *see–saw movements of the upper lids.* Optokinetic and vestibular stimuli moving toward the left eye evoked a symmetrical ocular response and also unilateral (left–sided) lid nystagmus. Evoked nystagmus with rapid phases to the left caused upward jerking nystagmus of the right lid while the left lid remained inhibited.

The inverse pattern of see–saw synkinesis is, in our experience, more common. In this type, horizontal gaze causes the levator muscle of the abducted eye to contract (lid elevates) and the levator of the adducting eye to be inhibited (lid drops). The congenital form of this gaze–dependent paradoxical movement of the lids can be associated with unilateral elevator palsy, ocular retraction or other signs of anomalous innervation of extraocular muscles. Often there is ipsilateral levator inhibition during gaze upward or medially, and mild ipsilateral ptosis. Patients with the bilateral retraction syndrome frequently show a see–saw lid movement with alternating attempts to look back and forth horizontally. By EMG techniques, Esslen and Papst (1961) demonstrated that the rise and fall of the lids was not merely a mechanical event associated with retraction of the globe.

In some instances see–saw lid movements represent an acquired form of anomalous levator innervation. Usually the lid of the abducting eye is excited and the lid of the adducting eye inhibited. The movement of the two lids during alternating gaze to right and left is not as striking as that occurring with the congenital syndromes. We have observed this levator synkinesis as a sequela of Wernicke's encephalopathy, in a patient whose recovery included a period where he exhibited see–saw lid movements during alternating lateral gaze. A good example of reciprocal excitation and inhibition of the levator muscles of the lids, in some patients with jaw winking, can be evoked by alternate lateral movements of the jaw (as in vigorous chewing).

An unusual case recorded by Spaeth (1947) undoubtedly belonged to the Marcus-Gunn type of mandibulopalpebral synkinesis. The patient had a total congenital elevator "palsy," and particularly when he was animated, there was an asymmetrical see-saw movement of both lids.

Hepler, Hoyt and Loeffler (1968) recorded a mandibulopalpebral see-saw synkinesis electromyographically. Simultaneous recordings obtained from both levator muscles during rapid side-to-side jaw movements showed reciprocal augmentation and inhibition of electrical activity which accurately corresponded to the timing of the see-saw lid movements.

Recordings from the left levator muscle showed definite phasic diminution of tonus during a rapid ipsilateral jaw movement. The mandibulopalpebral synkinesis in this patient invariably overcame any inhibitory synkinesis such as might be developed during gaze in various directions. This excitatory lid synkinesis evoked from jaw movement was not diminished by adaptation or fatigue. These EMG studies showed clearly that the see-saw mandibulopalpebral synkinesis involves inhibitory activity, and is not merely a reciprocal excitation in the motoneurons innervating the two levators of the lids. With each burst of activity from one levator, the other muscle became electrically silent. Additionally, the configuration of the bursts of synkinetic activation of the levator muscles was spindle-shaped since the activation, although relatively rapid, required several milliseconds to reach its maximum amplitude.

A final remarkable example of alternating levator excitation and inhibition occurred in a 50 year old farmer who was examined by Dr. Stanley Thompson (personal communication). The patient had slow onset of *cyclic alternating lid retraction* associated with mild asymmetrical ataxia. One lid would retract for about 15 seconds and then, over an interval of 60 seconds, return to the level of the fellow lid; next the other lid would retract for a 10–15 second interval, etc. This cyclic lid retraction occurred continuously, even during sleep. The patient's ocular movements and pupils were normal. The cause of his unique lid disturbance could not be determined, but the similarity of the cyclic oculomotor phenomenon to cyclic oculomotor palsy is obvious. Cyclic bilateral alternating levator spasm has been described before in rare cases that include cyclic alternating anisocoria, cyclic unilateral palsy, and "spasm" of the extraocular muscles innervated by one third nerve.

Acquired internuclear disorders of excitation and inhibition

The pontine paramedian reticular formation (PPRF), often termed the pontine "center" by clinicians, is the substrate for integration of all ipsilateral versions. Some of the fibers of the median longitudinal fasciculus (MLF) serve to connect the PPRF and ipsilateral abducens nucleus with the contralateral medial rectus subnucleus in the midbrain. Repeated clinico-pathological studies indicate that this crossed excitatory projection from the PPRF to the medial rectus subnucleus decussates before it begins its rostral ascent into the midbrain. The MLF lies adjacent to the midline in the pons and passes more laterally in the midbrain where it skirts the oculomotor nucleus and terminates rostrally in the interstitial nucleus (Crosby *et al.*, 1962). The bundles attain their greatest size between the abducens and the oculomotor nuclei where they are situated immediately dorsal to the paramedian reticular formation. The paired paramedian system of the MLF extends caudally to mid–thoracic levels (Gernandt, 1968).

Unilateral disruption of the MLF at the level of the pons causes "upstream" disconnection of the ipsilateral medial rectus neurons; thus failure of adduction during horizontal versions and normal adduction during vergence is the hallmark of a lesion in the ipsilateral MLF, and is termed clinically an "internuclear ophthalmoplegia" (INO).

There are many causes of MLF lesions (Smith and Cogan, 1959) but in young adults, particularly when signs are bilateral, the etiology is usually multiple sclerosis. In elderly patients, brainstem vascular disease accounts for most MLF lesions and they are usually unilateral. Occasionally the sign indicates the effects of brain stem compression without a structural lesion in the MLF (Madonick, 1951).

Cogan's classification of unilateral MLF syndromes, or INO, into anterior (midbrain) and posterior (pontine) types, rests on preservation or loss of ocular convergence (Cogan, 1956; Smith and Cogan, 1959). Loss of convergence implies a lesion at the level of the oculomotor nucleus (anterior INO) whereas preservation of convergence implies a posterior INO. In 1966, however, there appeared three separate clinico–pathological reports of unilateral MLF lesions with focal disease at the midbrain level causing INO with normal convergence (Harrington *et al.*, 1966; Ross and DeMyer, 1966; Kupfer and Cogan, 1966). These documented cases describe a midbrain INO, a syndrome which cannot be produced experimentally in monkeys (Carpenter and McMasters, 1963). It is evident that retention of convergence can no longer be regarded as crucial in localization of the MLF lesion. Additionally there are many variable factors such as the patient's cooperation, effort and alertness that influence convergence. Also, convergence may be clinically deficient but demonstratable as EMG activity in medial rectus muscles (Orlowski *et al.*, 1965). For these reasons we do not attempt to localize the level of a MLF lesion in a patient with "straight eyes." However, exotropia combined with the clinical signs of INO indicates a lesion in the midbrain involving motor neurons of the paretic medial rectus muscle. Dr. Martin Lubow (personal communication) has termed bilateral medial rectus palsy with exotropia the *WEBINO syndrome* (wall–eyed bilateral internuclear ophthalmoplegia). Most of these syndromes actually represent midline involvements of the oculomotor nucleus.

The adduction paresis of INO is of the same magnitude for either pursuit movements or voluntary saccades. The amplitude of the movement is *never* increased by oculocephalic or caloric stimulation. This confirms experimental studies by Szentágothai (1950) showing that vestibular influences on the oculomotor nuclei are finally mediated through the MLF.

Monocular nystagmus of the abducting eye is associated with the adduction paresis in INO. Whereas adduction weakness is readily explained by the MLF lesion, the mechanism of the "abduction nystagmus" is still unknown. Carpenter's (1963, 1966b) extensive observations of eye movements in animals with experimental MLF lesions are pertinent. Following unilateral lesions at the level of abducens nucleus he noted preterminal degeneration in the opposite abducens nucleus; attributing his finding to disruption of secondary vestibular projections, he speculated that these degenerated fibers were responsible for the abduction nystagmus of INO (Carpenter and McMasters, 1963). However, in later studies Carpenter (1966b) indicated that lesions placed more rostrally in the MLF also were associated with abduction nystagmus, despite a lack of significant preterminal degeneration in the contralateral abducens nucleus. He hypothesized that abduction nystagmus with these more rostral lesions might be due to concomitant interruption of descending fibers in the MLF from the interstitial nucleus of Cajal, although recent work (Carpenter, Chapter 4) showed that discrete lesions in the interstitial nucleus itself do not produce nystagmus of any kind.

An alternative explanation of abducens overactivity secondary to underaction of its yoke muscle is supported by the occurrence of pseudo-internuclear ophthalmoplegia in myasthenia gravis (Glaser, 1966). However, clinical observation indicates that the abduction nystagmus magnitude in INO does not parallel the extent of adductor weakness.

Bilateral brain stem lesions characteristically produce gaze-evoked vertical nystagmus on upward gaze (Bender, 1960); this sign is invariably associated with bilateral INO. Another vertical imbalance occasionally found in patients with INO is skew deviation, usually with a hypotropic abductor (Smith and Cogan, 1959).

Smith and David (1964) recommended use of the optokinetic and the ocular dysmetria signs for diagnosis of minimal or uncertain cases of INO. The *optokinetic* sign of INO depends upon the inability of the "weak" medial rectus to make as large or as rapid a saccade as the lateral rectus of the fellow eye. The eye with the paretic medial rectus will be unable to perform normal optokinetic saccades in comparison to the abducting eye. The *ocular dysmetria sign* of INO is evoked during repetitive refixation saccades in the horizontal plane. The abducting eye consistently overshoots while the adducting eye undershoots. These simple tests can be valuable for demonstration of mild INO in a patient with apparently normal ocular adduction during pursuit movements and questionable abduction nystagmus. Presumably this situation occurs with partial MLF lesions. The medial rectus subnucleus could receive sufficient innervation to perform slow pursuit movements, but not enough for a normal saccade (Loeffler *et al.*, 1966).

Breinin (1958) first used EMG techniques to study patients with INO. He recorded normal levels of tonic activity in the involved medial rectus muscle when the patient's eye was in the primary position. As the patient attempted to adduct the eye, there was no medial rectus facilitation; although the antagonist (lateral rectus muscle) inhibited reciprocally, the eye failed to adduct. Breinin discussed the amount of medial rectus innervation required to overcome orbital resistance to movement and contended that, despite an inhibited antagonist, the medial rectus could not move the eye because it did not display the sudden excitatory burst of unit activity ordinarily associated with the onset of a saccade (Tamler *et al.*, 1959).

Speculation regarding the source of normal resting tonus in the medial rectus in INO was provided by Loeffler *et al.*, (1966) on the basis of their demonstration of inhibitional impairment in the involved medial rectus muscle. During pursuit movements or sustained horizontal gaze the "weak" medial rectus muscle does not display EMG evidence of normal reciprocal inhibition as the eye abducts, even though the eye seems to *abduct* normally. This observation seems limited to pursuit movements, in that a normal pattern of inhibition does appear during saccadic movements in the appropriate direction. Such an inhibitional defect of the medial rectus is not present in all cases of INO (Gonzales and Reuben, 1967). The presence of inhibition in the medial rectus neurons on the side of an MLF lesion depends on several factors; it is favored by chronicity of the lesion, by saccadic innervation of its antagonist, and, importantly, by fixation with the involved eye (Loeffler *et al.*, 1965).

A focal lesion unilaterally affecting an MLF and the ipsilateral PPRF can result in an unusual eye movement; the ipsilateral eye cannot move horizontally in either direction, and the fellow eye can only abduct. This abnormality of eye movement indicates simply a combination of a conjugate lateral gaze palsy and an ipsilateral INO. The sign has been designated the "1½ syndrome" by Fisher (1967).

Lutz' posterior INO: The INO classification proposed by Lutz in 1923 is still used by some authors (Carpenter and McMasters, 1963) and deserves consideration here. This classification refers to a supranuclear failure of adduction as an anterior INO and a supranuclear failure of abduction as a posterior INO. Lutz did not mention how he differentiated his posterior INO from an abducens paresis. Presumably, contraction of the lateral rectus muscle in response to caloric or oculocephalic stimulation would indicate integrity of the final common pathway (the lower motor neuron). Localization of the lesion responsible for the Lutz posterior INO is difficult to conceptualize. Discrete damage between the PPRF and the sixth nucleus would indeed result in a supranuclear paralysis of abduction, but vestibular influences on the abducens neurons require an intact PPRF. The supranuclear process would therefore be identical clinically with a nuclear lesion except for the lack of the usual esotropia that accompanies the latter.

Clinical signs qualifying for a diagnosis of a Lutz posterior INO are exceedingly rare. We have never seen a convincing example of this ocular motor syndrome, nor have Smith and Cogan (1959). Fisher and co-workers (1965) described ipsilateral impairment of ocular abduction during voluntary gaze that was overcome by appropriate caloric stimulation. They referred to this condition as "sixth nerve pseudo-palsy" and stated that it may be seen with acute cerebellar hemorrhage or with hemorrhage in the thalamic-subthalamic area.

Von Kornyey (1959) reported the case of a woman whose eye signs included paralysis of vertical gaze, spastic downward deviation and horizontal voluntary (command) gaze palsy to the left; on gaze to the right, the abducting eye lagged behind. Full tonic ocular deviations were produced by caloric stimulation in either ear. These symptoms followed a sudden right-sided hematoma which extended into the rostral midbrain tegmentum and destroyed the ipsilateral nuclei of Cajal and Darkschewitz. Von Kornyey regarded this type of disproportionate involvement of ocular abduction during attempted lateral gaze as a form of "inverse internuclear palsy." Further, Nashold and Gills (1967) reported two patients with transient ipsilateral paralysis of abduction following stereotactic lesions in the prerubral field of Forel.

Von Kornyey (1959) discussed the possibility that such supranuclear lesions might involve only those descending fibers destined for the sixth nucleus while sparing those to the third (medial rectus sub-nucleus). However, in all of the above three patients the lesions were anterior to the ocular motor decussation, and the abduction pareses were *ipsilateral* to the side of the lesion. We have suggested that *pseudo-abducens paresis* occurring with mesodiencephalic lesions may be the result of convergence effort superimposed upon lateral version movements (see discussion of sylvian aqueduct syndrome).

ACKNOWLEDGEMENT

The authors wish to acknowledge their gratitude to Jane Hyde, Ph.D. for her critical editorial review of the manuscript and to Mrs. Peggy Cumby and Miss Jean Greenan for their patient secretarial help.

REFERENCES

Alessi, D. (1940). Lesioni parenchimatose del cervelleto da carcinoma uterino (Gliosi carcinotossica?). Sintomatologia dissinergico-mioclonica. *Riv. di Pat. nerv. ment.* **55**: 148-174.
Alexander, S. J. (1949). Nuclear aplasia and Marcus Gunn phenomenon. *Amer. J. Ophthal.* 32:711-712.
Altrocchi, P. H. and Menkes, J. H. (1960). Congenital ocular motor apraxia. *Brain.* **83**: 579-588.
Andre-Thomas, Schaefer, H. and Bertrand, F. (1933). Paralysie de l'abaissement du regard, paralysie des inférogyres, hyperponie des supérogyres et des releveurs du regard. *Rev. neurol.* **11**: 535-542.
Appenzeller, O. and Fischer, A. P. (1968). Disturbances of rapid eye movements during sleep in patients with lesions of the nervous system. *Electroenceph. clin. Neurophysiol.* **25**: 29-35.

Aschoff, J. C. (1968). Veränderungen rascher Blickbewegungen (Saccaden) beim Menschen unter Diazepam (Valium). *Arch. Psychiat. Nervenkr.* **211**: 325-332.
Atkin, A. and Bender, M. B. (1964). "Lightning eye movements" (Ocular Myoclonus). *J. Neurol. Sci.* **1**: 2-12.
Balint, R. (1909). Seelenlähmung des "Schauens," optische Ataxie, räumliche Storung der Aufmerksamkeit. *Monat. Psych. Neurol.* **25**: 51-81.
Ealthasar, K. (1966). Uber das anatomische Substrat det vertikalen Blicklähmung. *Proc. Internat. Congress Neurology.* Wein, Vol. II, pp. 213-226.
Balthasar, K. and Hopf, A. (1966). Die Freud–Vogt'sche Herdbildung bei supranuklearer Heberlähmung der Augen mit Lid retraktion. *Dtsch. Z. Nervenheilk.* **189**: 275-296.
Balthasar, K. (1968). Gliomas of the quadrigeminal plate and eye movements. *Ophthalmologica.* **155**: 249-270.
Bárány, R. (1913a). Latente Deviation der Augen und Vorbeizeigen des Kopfes bei Hemiplegie und Epilepsie. *Munch. Med. Wschr.* **60**: *900-905.*
Bárány, R. (1913b). Nystagmus retractorius. *Wiener Klin Wschr.* **26**: 438–440.
Bárány, R. (1930). Ein Fall von monokulärer Lähmung aller seitlichen Blickbewegungen, mit Intakthait der vertikalen Blickbewegungen, mit horizontalem Konvergenz und Divergenznystagmus in Bereich des fur die Willkurbewegungen gelahmten Abducens. *Z. Hals. Nasen. Ohrenheilk.* **26**: 237–244.
Baringer, J. R., Sweeney, V. P., and Winkler, G. F. (1968). An acute syndrome of ocular oscillations and truncal myoclonus. *Brain.* **91**: 473–480.
Behrman, S., Carroll, J. D., Janota, I., and Matthews, W. B. (1969). Progressive supranuclear palsy – Clinical pathological study of four cases. *Brain.* **92**: 663–678.
Bender, M. B. and Savitsky, N. (1940). Paralysis of divergence. *Arch. Ophthal.* **23**: 1946–1051.
Bender, M. B. and Weinstein, E. A. (1953). Functional representation in the oculomotor and trochlear nuclei. *Arch. Neurol. Psychiat.* **49**: 98–106.
Bender, M. B., Postel, D. M., and Krieger, H. P. (1957). Disorders of oculomotor function in lesions of the occipital lobe. *J. Neurol. Neurosurg. Psychiat.* **20**: 139–143.
Bender, M. B. and Shanzer, S. (1960). Effects of brainstem lesions on vertical gaze in monkeys. *Fed. Proc.* **19**: 28.
Bender, M. B. (1960). Comments on the physiology and pathology of eye movements in the vertical plane. *J. Nerv. Ment. Dis.* **130**: 456–466.
Bender, M. B. (1962). Neuroopthalmology. **In**: *Clinical Neurology*, 2nd edn., ed. Baker, A. B., pp. 275–349. New York: Hoeber-Harper.
Bender, M. B. and Shanzer, S. (1964). Oculomotor pathways defined by electric stimulation and lesions in the brainstem of monkey. **In**: *The Oculomotor System,* ed. Bender, M. B., pp. 81–140. New York: Harper and Row.
Bergstedt, M. (1961). Studies of positional nystagmus in the human centrifuge. *Acta Otolaryng. Suppl.,* **165**: 1–144.
Bickford, R. G. and Klass, D. W. (1964). Eye movement and the electroencephalogram. **In**: *The Oculomotor System,* ed. Bender, M. B., pp. 299-302. New York: Harper and Row.
Bielschowsky, A. (1935). Lecture on motor anomalies of the eyes. III Paralysis of conjugate ocular movements of the eye. *Arch. Ophthal.* **13**: 569–583.
Bjerver, K. and Silfverskiöld, B. P. (1968). Lateropulsion and imbalance in Wallenberg's syndrome. *Acta Neurol (Scand.)* **44**: 91–100.
Blackwood, W., McMenemey, W. H., Meyer, A., Norman, R. M., and Russell, D. S. (1963). *Greenfield's Neuropathology,* 2nd edn., Baltimore: Williams and Wilkins Co.
Blodi, F. C., Van Allen, M. W., and Yarbrough, J. C. (1964). Duane's syndrome: a brainstem lesion. *Arch Ophthal.* **72**: 171–177.
Boeder, P. (1961). The co-operation of the extraocular muscles. *Amer. J. Ophthal.* **51**: 469–481.
Bradley, W. G. and Toone, B. K. (1967). Synkinetic movements of the eyelid: a case with some unusual mechanisms of paradoxical lid retraction. *J. Neurol. Neurosurg. Psychiat.* **30**: 578–579.
Brain, W. R. (1933). *Diseases of the Nervous System.* 1st. edn. London: Oxford University Press.
Bray, P. F., Ziter, F. A., Lahey, M. E., and Myers, G. G. (1969). The coincidence of neuroblastoma and acute cerebellar encephalopathy. *Trans. Amer. Neurol. Assoc.,* (In press).
Breinin, G. M. (1957). New aspects of ophthalmoneurologic diagnosis. *Arch. Ophthal.* **58**: 375–388.
Breinin, G. M. (1958). Electromyography — A tool in ocular and neurologic diagnosis. III. Supranuclear Mechanisms. *Arch. Ophth.* **59**: 177–187.
Bremer, J. L. (1921). Recurrent branches of abducens nerve in human embryos. *Amer. J. Anat.* **28**: 371–390.

Brucher, J. M. (1966). The frontal eye field of the monkey. *Int. J. Neurol.* **5**: 262–281.
Brumlik, J. and Means, E. D. (1969). Tremorine–tremor, shivering and acute cerebellar ataxia in the adult and child — a comparative study. *Brain.* **92**: 157–190.
Bucy, P. C. and Weaver, T. A., Jr. (1941). Paralysis of conjugate lateral movement of the eyes in association with cerebellar abcess. *Arch. Surg.* **42**: 839–849.
Bucy, P. C., Keplinger, J. E., and Siqueira, E. B. (1964). Destruction of the "Pyramidal Tract" in man. *J. Neurosurg.* **21**: 385–398.
Burger, A. (1963). Electromyographic aspect of Stilling–Duane's syndrome. *Bull. Soc. Ophth. Fr.* **63**: 554–557.
Burian, H. M. and Cahill, J. E. (1952). Congenital paralysis of medial rectus with unusual synergism of the horizontal muscles. *Trans. Amer. Ophthal. Soc.* **50**: 87–102.
Burian, H. M. and Miller, J. E. (1958). Comitant convergent strabismus with acute onset. *Amer. J. Ophthal.* **45**: 55–64.
Burian, H. M. and Van Allen, M. W. (1963). Cyclic oculomotor paralysis. *Amer. J. Ophth.* **55**: 529–537.
Calne, D. B., Stern, G. M., Laurence, D. R., Sharkey, J., and Armitage, P. (1969). L–Dopa in postencephalitic Parkinsonism. *Lancet.* **1**: 744–747.
Carpenter, M. B. and McMasters, R. E. (1963). Disturbances of conjugate horizontal eye movements in the monkey. II. Physiological effects and anatomical degeneration resulting from lesions in the medial longitudinal fasciculus. *Arch. Neurol.* **8**: 347–368.
Carpenter, M. B. and Strominger, N. L. (1964). Cerebello–oculomotor fibers in the rhesus monkey. *J. Comp. Neurol.* **123**: 221–230.
Carpenter, M. B. (1966a). Brain stem nuclei in studies of experimental dyskinesia. *J. Neuro–surg.* **24**: 185–193.
Carpenter, M. B. (1966b). The ascending vestibular system and its relationship to conjugate horizontal eye movements. **In:** *The Vestibular System and Its Diseases,* ed. Wolfson, R. J., pp. 69–98. Philadelphia: University of Pennsylvania Press.
Cenacchi, V. and Bertoni, G. (1967). Sindrome de Stilling–Türk–Duane. Studio elettro-oculografica. *Riv. Oto–neuro–oftal.* **42**: 101–117.
Chamlin, M. and Davidoff, L. M. (1950). Divergence paralysis and increased intracranial pressure. *J. Neurosurg.* **7**: 539–543.
Cogan, D. G. (1952). A type of congenital ocular motor apraxia presenting jerky head movements. *Trans. Amer. Acad. Ophth. Otol.* **56**: 853–862.
Cogan, D. G. and Adams, R. D. (1953). A type of paralysis of conjugate gaze (ocular motor apraxia). *Arch. Ophth.* **50**: 434–442.
Cogan, D. G. (1954). Ocular dysmetria; flutter–like oscillations of the eyes, and opsoclonus. *Arch. Ophth.* **51**: 318–335.
Cogan, D. G. and Adams, R. D. (1955). Balint's syndrome and ocular motor apraxia. *Arch. Ophth.* **53**: 758.
Cogan, D. G. (1956). *Neurology of the Ocular Muscles.* Springfield: C.P. Thomas.
Cogan, D. G. (1964). Brain lesions and eye movements in man. **In:** *The Oculomotor System,* ed. Bender, M. B., pp. 417–423. New York: Harper and Row.
Cogan, D. G. (1965). Ophthalmic manifestations of bilateral non-occipital cerebral lesions. *Brit. J. Ophth.* **49**: 281–297.
Cogan, D. G. (1966). Congenital ocular motor apraxia. *Canad. J. Ophthal.* **1**: 253–260.
Cogan, D. G. (1968a). Opsoclonus, body tremulousness, and benign encephalitis. *Arch. Ophth.* **79**: 545–551.
Cogan, D. G. (1968b). Down–beat nystagmus. *Arch Ophth.* **80**: 757–768.
Cohen, B., Komatsuzaki, A., and Bender, M. B. (1968). Electrooculographic syndrome in monkeys after pontine reticular formation lesions. *Arch. Neurol.* **18**: 78–92.
Cohen, B. and Feldman, M. (1968). Relationship of the electrical activity in pontine reticular formation and lateral geniculate body to rapid eye movements. *J. Neurophysiol.* **31**: 806–817.
Cooper, E. L. (1937). Jaw–winking phenomenon. Report of a case. *Arch. Ophthal.* **18**: 198–203.
Cords, R. (1927). Ein seltener Fall von Mitbewegungen. *Ber. Deutsch. Ophth. Ges.* **46**: 462–464.
Cords, R. (1929). Zur Pathologie der Fuhrungsbewegungen. *V. Graefes Arciv fur Ophth.* **123**:173-218.
Costenbader, F. D. and Mousel, D. K. (1964). Cyclic esotropia. *Arch. Ophthal.* **71**: 180-181.
Cotte–Rittaud, M. R. and Courjon, J. (1962). Semiological value of adversive epilepsy. *Epilepsia.* **3**: 151-166.
Crosby, E. C., Humphrey, T. and Lauer, E. M. (1962). *Correlative Anatomy of the Nervous System.* New York: Macmillan Company.

Daroff, R. B. and Waldman, A. L. (1965). Ocular bobbing. *J. Neurol. Neurosurg. Psychiat.* **28**: 375-377.

David, M. and Hacaen, H. (1947). Sur certains troubles de la latéralité du regard dans les lésions parietales s'accompagnant de troubles de la somatognosie. *Bull. Soc. D'Ophth. Paris.* **59**: 103-105.

David, N. J., Mackey, E. A., and Smith, J. L. (1968). Further observations in progressive supranuclear palsy. *Neurology.* **18**: 349-356.

Davidoff, R. A., Atkin, A., Anderson, P. J., and Bender, M. B. (1966). Optokinetic nystagmus in cerebral disease. Clinical and pathological study. *Arch. Neurol.* **14**: 73-81.

Davidson, M., Tolentino, Y, and Sapir, S. (1968). Opsoclonus and Neuroblastoma. *New Eng. J. Med.* **279**: 948.

Déjérine, J. (1926). *Sémiologie des Affections du Systeme Nerveux.* 2nd. edn., Paris: Masson et Cie.

DeKleyn, A. and Stenvers, H. W. (1941). Tonic neck-reflexes on the eye-muscles in man. *Proc. Ned. Acad. v. Wetensch., Amsterdam.* **44**: 385-396.

Denny-Brown, D. (1962). *The Basal Ganglia and Their Relation to Disorders of Movement.* pp. 23-26. London: Oxford University Press.

Denny-Brown, D. (1969). Personal Communication.

Dow, R. S. and Moruzzi, G. (1958). *The Physiology and Pathology of the Cerebellum.* Minneapolis: University of Minnesota Press.

Dow, R. S. and Manni, E. (1964). The relationship of the cerebellum to extraocular movements. **In**: *The Oculomotor System.*, ed. Bender, M. B., pp. 280-292. New York: Harper & Row.

Duane, A. (1905). Congenital deficiency of abduction associated with impairment of abduction, retraction movements, contractions of the palpebral fissure and oblique movements of the eye. *Arch. Ophthal.* **34**: 133-159.

Dyken, P. and Kolár, O. (1968). Dancing eyes, dancing feet; infantile polymyoclonia. *Brain.* **91**: 305-320.

Earle, K. M. (1966). Introduction to pathology of extrapyramidal diseases. *J. Neurosurg.* **24**: 247-249.

Eccles, J. C. (1961). Inhibitory pathways to motoneurons. **In**: *Nervous Inhibition*, ed. Florey, E., pp. 47-60. New York: Macmillan Co.

Ellenberger, C., Jr., Campa, J. F. and Netsky, M. G. (1968). Opsoclonus and parenchymatous degeneration of the cerebellum. The cerebellar origin of an abnormal ocular movement. *Neurology.* **18**: 1041-1046.

Elschnig, A. (1913). Nystagmus retractorius, ein cerebrales herd-sympton. *Med. Klin.* **1**: 8-11.

Esslen, E. and Papst, W. (1961). Die Bedeutung den Elektromyographie für die Analyse von Motilitätsstörungen der Augen. *Bibl. Ophthal. Suppl.* **57**: 1-168.

Evarts, E. V. and Thach, W. T. (1969). Motor mechanisms of the CNS: Cerebrocerebellar interrelations. *Annual Review of Physiology.* **31**: 451-498.

Feigenbaum, A. and Kornbleuth, W. (1946). Paralysis of convergence with bilateral ring scotomas following injury to occipital region. *Arch Ophthal.* **35**: 218-226.

Fisher, C. M. (1956). An unusual variant of acute idiopathic polyneuritis (Syndrome of opthalmoplegia, ataxia and areflexia). *New Eng. J. Med.* **255**: 57-65.

Fisher, C. M. (1964). Ocular bobbing. *Arch. Neurol.* **11**: 543-546.

Fisher, C. M. (1967). Some neuro-ophthalmological observations. *J. Neurol. Neurosurg. Psychiat.* **30**: 383-392.

Fisher, C. M., Picard, F. H., Polak, A. *et al.* (1965). Acute hypertensive cerebellar hemorrhage; diagnosis and surgical treatment. *J. Nerv. Ment. Dis.* **140**: 38-57.

Ford, F. R. and Walsh, F. B. (1940). Tonic deviations of eyes produced by movements of head. *Arch. Ophth.* **23**: 1274-1284.

Friedenwald, H. (1896). Notes on congenital motor defects of the eyeballs. Congenital paralysis of the ocular muscles. *Bull Hopkins Hosp.* **7**: 202-203.

Freeman, W. (1922). Paralysis of associated lateral movements of the eyes. A sympton of intrapontile lesion. *Arch. Neurol. Psych.* **7**: 454-487.

Freeman, W., Ammerman, H. H., and Stanley, M. (1943). Syndromes of the pontine tegmentum. Foville's syndrome: Report of three cases. *Arch. Neurol. Psych.* **50**: 462-471.

Freund, C. S. (1913). Zur Klinik und Anatomie der vertikalen Blicklähmung. *Neur. Zbl.* **32**: 1215-1229.

Fuchs, A. F. and Kornhuber, H. H. (1969). Extraocular muscle afferents to the cerebellum of the cat. *J. Physiol.* **200**: 713-722.

Garey, L. J., Jones, E. G. and Powell, T. P. S. (1968). Interrelationships of striate and extra-striate cortex with the primary relay sites of the visual pathway. *J. Neurol. Neurosurg. Psychiat.* **31**: 135-157.

Gassel, M. M. and Williams, D. (1963). Visual function in patients with homonymous hemianopia. Part II. Oculomotor Mechanisms. *Brain.* **86**: 1-36.
Gastaldi, G. (1953). Sulla fisiopathologia del nistagmo vestibolare provocato. *Sist. nerv. Milano.* **5**: 30-65.
Gastaut, H. (1960). Un aspect méconnu des décharges neuroniques occipitales: La Crise Oculo-Clonique Ou "Nystagmus Epileptique." *Les Grandes Activities du Lobe Occipital,* ed. Th. Alajouanine, pp. 169-185, Paris: Masson et Cie.
Gay, A. J., Brodkey, J., and Miller, J. E. (1963). Convergence retraction nystagmus: an electromyographic study. *Arch. Ophthal.,* **70**, 456-461.
Gernandt, B. E. (1968). Functional properties of the descending medial longitudinal fasciculus. *Exp. Neurol.* **22**: 326-342.
Geschwind, N. (1965). Disconnexion syndromes in animals and man. *Brain.* **88**: 237-294, and 585-644.
Gillingham, F. J. (1962). Small localized surgical lesions of the internal capsule in the treatment of the dyskinesias. *Confin. neurol.* **22**: 385-395.
Gillingham, F. J. and Kalyanaraman, S. (1965). The surgical treatment of oculogyric crises. *Confin. neurol.* **19**: 237-245.
Glaser, J. S. (1966). Myasthenic pseudo-internuclear ophthalmoplegia. *Arch. Ophth.* **75**, 363-366.
Goldberg, R. T. and Jampel, R. S. (1963). Flutter-like oscillations of the eyes in cerebellar disease. *Amer. J. Ophth.* **55**: 1229-1233.
Goldstein, J. E. and Cogan, D. G. (1965). Apraxia of lid opening. *Arch. Ophthal.* **73**: 155-159.
Gonzalez, C. and Reuben, R. N. (1967). Ocular electromyography: In the syndrome of the medial longitudinal fasciculus; patterns of inhibition and excitation. *Amer. J. Ophth.* **64**: 916-926.
Goodwin, R. F. and Poser, C. M. (1963). Ophthalmoplegia, ataxia and areflexia. Fisher's syndrome. *JAMA.* **186**: 258-259.
Gowers, W. R. (1879). Note on a reflex mechanism in the fixation of the eyeballs. *Brain.* **2**: 39-41.
Grant, F. C. (1936). The Marcus Gunn phenomenon; report of a case with suggestions as to relief. *Arch. Neurol. Psychiat.* **35**: 487-500.
Grant, G. (1966). Infarction localization in a case of Wallenberg's syndrome: A neuroanatomical investigation with comment on structures responsible for nystagmus, impairment of taste and deglutation. *J. F. Hirnforsch.* **8**: 419-430.
Gunn, R. M. (1903). Congenital ptosis with peculiar associated movements of the affected lid. *Trans Ophthal. Soc. U. K.* **23**: 356-373.
Hall, A. J. (1931). Chronic epidemic encephalitis with special reference to the ocular attacks. *Brit. Med. J.* **2**: 833-837.
Halsey, J. H., Jr., Ceballos, R., and Crosby, E. C. (1967). The supranuclear control of voluntary lateral gaze. Clinical and anatomic correlation in a case of ventral pontine infarction. *Neurology.* **17**: 928-933.
Harrington, R. B., Hollenhorst, R. W., and Sayre, G. P. (1966). Unilateral internuclear ophthalmoplegia. Report of a case including pathology. *Arch. Neurol.* **15**: 29-34.
Harris, H. E., Komatsuzaki, A., and Cohen, B. (1967). Oculomotor deficits after lesion of the mesencephalic reticular formation in monkeys. *Physiologist.* **10**: 195.
Hecaen, H. and deAjuriaguerra, J. (1954). Balint's syndrome (psychic paralysis of visual fixation). *Brain.* **77**: 373-400.
Hensen, V. and Voelkers, C. (1878). Uber den Ursprung der Akkommodationsnerven, nebst Bemerkungen über die Funktion der Wurzeln des Nervus oculomotorius. *Graefes Arch. Ophthal.* **24**, 1-26.
Hepler, R. S., Hoyt, W. F., and Loeffler, J. D. (1968). Paradoxical synkinetic levator inhibition and excitation: an electromyographic study of unilateral oculopalpebral and bilateral mandibulopalpebral (Marcus Gunn) synkinesis in a 74-year-old man. *Arch. Neurol.* **18**: 416-424.
Herman, H. T., Nelson, G. P., Stark, L., and Young, L. R. (Nov. 15, 1962). Effect of pharmacological agents on control of eye movements. *Quart. Prog. Rep. No. 67,* pp. 231-235. Research Laboratory of Electronics, M. I. T.
Hicks, A. M. and Josford, G. N. (1937). Cyclic paralysis of oculomotor nerve. *Arch. Ophthal.* **17**: 213-222.
Higgins, D. C. and Daroff, R. B. (1966). Overshoot and oscillation in ocular dysmetria. *Arch. Ophth.* **75**: 742-745.
Highstein, S., Cohen, B., and Mones, R. (1969). Changes in saccadic eye movements of patients with Parkinson's disease before and after L-Dopa. (In preparation).

Holmes, G. (1917). The symptoms of acute cerebellar injuries due to gunshot injuries. *Brain.* **40**: 461-535.
Holmes, G. (1918a). Disturbances of vision by cerebral lesions. *Brit. J. Ophth.* **2**: 449–468.
Holmes, G. (1918b). Disturbances of visual orientation. *Brit. J. Ophth.* **2**: 506–516.
Holmes, G. and Horrax, G. (1919). Disturbances of spatial orientation and visual attention with loss of stereoscopic vision. *Arch. Neurol. Psych.* **1**: 385-407.
Holmes, G. (1921). Palsies of the conjugate ocular movements. *Brit. J. Ophth.* **5**: 241-250.
Holmes, G. (1930). Spasm of fixation. *Trans. Ophth. Soc. U. K.* **50**: 253-262.
Holmes, G. (1931). Observations on ocular palsies. *Brit. Med. J.* **2**: 1165-1167.
Holmes, G. (1936). Looking and seeing. (Movements and fixation of the eyes.) *Irish J. Med. Sci.* (6th Series). **129**: 565-576.
Holmes, G. (1938). The cerebral integration of the ocular movements. *Brit. Med. J.* **2**: 107-112.
Hood, J. D. (1967). Observations upon the neurological mechanisms of optokinetic nystagmus with especial reference to the contribution of peripheral vision. *Acta Oto-larng.* **63**: 208–215.
Hoyt, W. F. and Nachtigäller, H. (1965). Anomalies of ocular motor nerves: neuroanatomic correlates of paradoxical innervation in Duane's syndrome and related congenital ocular motor disorders. *Amer. J. Ophthal.* **60**: 443–448.
Huber, A. (1961). *Eye Symptoms in Brain Tumors.* St. Louis: C. V. Mosby Company.
Huber, A., Esslen, E., Klöti, R., and Martenet, A. C. (1964). Zum Problem des Duane-Syndrome. *Graefe Arch. Ophthal.* **167**: 169–191.
Ingraham, F. D. and Campbell, J. B. (1941). Marcus Gunn phenomenon. *Arch. Neurol. Psychiat.* **46**: 127-134.
Jampel, R. S. (1959). Representation of the near-response on the cerebral cortex of the Macaque. *Amer. J. Ophth.* **48**: 573-582.
Jampel, R. S. (1962). Extraocular muscle action from brain stimulation in the Macaque. *Invest. Ophthal.* **1**: 565-578.
Jampel, R. S. and Quaglio, N. D. (1964). Eye movements in Tay-Sachs Disease. *Neurology.* **14**: 1013-1019.
Jampel, R. S. and Fells, P. (1968). Monocular elevation paresis caused by a central nervous system lesion. *Arch. Ophthal.* **80**: 45–57.
Jelliffe, S. E. (1929). Oculogyric crises as compulsion phenomena in postencephalitis. Their occurrence, phenomenology and meaning. *J. Nerv. Ment. Dis.* **69**: 59–63; 165-184.
Jung, R. and Kornhuber, H. H. (1964). Results of electronystagmography in man: The value of optokinetic, vestibular, and spontaneous nystagmus for neurologic diagnosis and research. In: *The Oculomotor System*, ed. Bender, M. B. pp. 428–482. New York: Harper and Row.
Kemper, T. L. and Romanul, F. C. A. (1967). State resembling akinetic mutism in basilar artery occlusion. *Neurology.* **17**: 74–80.
Kestenbaum, A. (1961). *Clinical Methods of Neuro-Ophthalmalogic Examination.* 2nd edn. New York: Grune and Stratton.
Khodadoust, A. A. and von Noorden, G. K. (1967). Bilateral vertical retraction syndrome: a family study. *Arch Ophthal.* **78**: 606–612.
Klemme, R. M. (1941). Oculogyric crises. A therapeutic approach. *Amer. J. Ophthal.* **24**: 1000-1004.
Koerber, H. L. (1903). Uber drei Fälle von Retraktionsbewegung des Bulbus. *Ophthal. Klin.* **7**: 65-67.
Kornhuber, H. H. (1966). Physiologie und Klinik des zentralvestibulären Systems (Blickund Stutzmotorik). In: Vol. III, Part 3. *HNO-Handbuch*, eds. Berendes, J., Link, R., and Zollner, F., pp. 2209-2210. Stuttgart: George Thieme.
Kornhuber, H. H. (1968). Neurologie des Kleinhirns. *Zent. f gesamte Neurol.* **191**: 13.
Kornhuber, H. H. (1969). Physiologie und Klinik des Vestibulären Systems. *Arch. Klin. exp. Ohr.-, Kehlk. Heilk.* **194**: 110-148.
Krayenbuhl, H. and Siegfried, J. (1969). La chirurgie stéréotaxique du noyau dentelé dans le traitement des hyperkinésies et des états spastiques. *Neuro-Chirurgie.* (Paris). **15**: 51-58.
Kupfer, C. and Cogan, D. G. (1966). Unilateral internuclear ophthalmoplegia. A clinico-pathological case report. *Arch. Ophth.* **75**: 484-489.
Kyrieleis, W. (1931). Die Augenveränderungen bei entzündlichen Erkrankungen des Zentralnervensystems. In: *Kurzes Handbuch der Ophthalmology*, Vol. 6, ed. Schieck, F. and Bruckner, A. pp. 712-731. Berlin: Julius Springer.
Lauber, H. (1913). Fall von zyklischer Okulomotoriuslähmung. *Wien Klin Wschr.* **26**: 707.
Lebensohn, J. E. (1955). Parinaud's syndrome from obstetrical trauma. *Amer. J. Ophthal.* **40**: 738-740.

Loeffler, J. D., Hoyt, W. F., and Slatt, B. (1966). Motor excitation and inhibition in internuclear palsy. An electromyographic study. *Arch. Neurol.* **15**: 644–671.

Loeffler, J. D., Slatt, B., and Hoyt, W. F. (1966). Motor abnormalities of the eyelids in Parkinson's disease: Electromyographic observations. *Arch Ophthal.* **76**: 178–185.

Lowenstein, O. and Givner, I. (1949). Cyclic oculomotor paralysis: Case report. *Eye, Ear, Nose, Thr. Monthly.* **28**: 274-276.

Lutz, A. (1919). The jaw-winking phenomenon and its explanation. *Arch. Ophthal.* **48**: 144–158.

Lutz, A. (1923). Uber die Bahnen der Blickwendung und deren Dissoziierung (nebst Mitteilung eines Falles von Ophthalmoplegia internuclearis anterior in Vergindung mit Dissoziierung der Bogengange). *Klin. Mbl. Augheilk.* **70**: 213–235.

Lyle, D. J. (1954). Divergence insufficiency. *Arch. Ophthal.* **52**: 858–864.

Madonick, M. J. (1951). Ophthalmoplegia Internuclearis Anterior without a lesion of the posterior longitudinal bundle. *Arch. Neurol. Psych.* **66**: 338–345.

Man, H. X. (1967). A case of unilateral supranuclear elevator muscle palsy. (French). *Bull. Soc. Ophthal. Fr.* **67**: 400–405.

Matiar, H. (1955). Pathophysiology of tonic ocular spasm (oculogyric crises) and its modification by blockade of stellate ganglion (German). *Acta neuroveg.* **12**: 389–404.

Mehler, W. R., Vernier, V. G., and Nauta, W. J. H. (1958). Efferent projections from dentate and interpositus nuclei in primates. *Anat. Record.* **130**: 430–431.

Merwarth, H. R. and Feiring, E. (1939). Modifications of induced nystagmus by acute cerebral lesions. *Brooklyn Hosp. J.* **1**: 99–106.

Meyers, I. L. (1925). Nystagmus: Neuro-Otologic studies concerning its seat of origin. *Amer. J. Med. Sci.* **169**: 742-752.

Meyers, I. L. (1931). Conjugate deviation of the head and eyes. Its value in the diagnosis and localization of abscess of the brain. *Arch. Otol.* **13**: 683–708.

Moberg, A., Preber, L., Silfverskiöld, B. P., and Vallbo, S. (1962). Imbalance, nystagmus and diplopia in Wallenberg's syndrome; clinical analysis of a case and post-mortem examination. *Acta-oto-laryng* (Scand). **55**: 269-282.

Mott, F. W. and Schäfer, E. A. (1890). On associated eye movements produced by cortical faradization of the monkey's brain. *Brain.* **13**: 165–173.

Mowrer, O. H. (1936). A comparison of the reaction mechanisms mediating optokinetic nystagmus in human beings and in pigeons. *Psychological Monographs.* **47**: 294–305.

Nashold, B. S. and Gills, J. P. (1967). Ocular signs from brain stimulation and lesions. *Arch. Ophth.* **77**: 609–618.

Nashold, B. S. and Slaughter, D. G. (1969). Effects of stimulating or destroying the deep cerebellar regions in man. *J. Neurosurg.*, **31**: 172–186.

Nashold, B. S., Slaughter, D. G., and Gills, J. P. (1969). Ocular reactions in man from deep cerebellar stimulation and lesions. *Arch. Ophth.* **81**: 538–543.

Nathanson, M., Bergman, P. S., and Anderson, P. J. (1957). Significance of oculocephalic and caloric responses in the unconscious patient. *Neurology.* **7**: 829–832.

Nauta, W. J. H. (1966). A summary of projections from the lentiform nucleus in the monkey. *J. Neurosurg.* **24**: 196–199.

Nozue, M. and Cohen, B. (Mar.-April, 1968). The median longitudinal fasciculus (MLF) in horizontal eye movements. *Fed. Proc.* **27**: 1313.

Onuaguluchi, G. (1961). Crises in post-encephalitic parkinsonism. *Brain.* **84**: 395–414.

Orlowski, W. J. and Wojtowicz, S. (1962). Is the Stillung-Türk-Duane syndrome an independent pathological entity? I. Electromyographical proof. *Ophthalmologica.* **144**: 199–220.

Orlowski, W. J., Slomski, P., and Wojtowicz, S. (1965). Bielschowsky-Lutz-Cogan syndrome. *Amer. J. Ophth.* **59**: 416–430.

Papst, W. and Esslen, E. (1960). Zur Atiologie der angeborenen Abduzenslähmung. *Klin Mbl. Augenheilk.* **137**: 306-327.

Papst, W. and Rossmann, H. (1966). Die Ptosis des Oberlides: Ihre Atiologie und Therapie unter besonderer Berücksichtigung elektromyographischer Befunde. *Bibl. Ophthal.* **17**: 1–14.

Parinaud, M. H. (1883). Paralysis des mouvements associés des yeux. *Arch. de Neurol.* **5**: 145–172.

Parry, R. (1957). An unusual case of the Marcus Gunn syndrome. *Trans Ophthal Soc. U. K.* **77**: 181–185.

Pasik, P. and Pasik, T. (1964a). Oculomotor functions in monkeys with lesions of the cerebrum and superior colliculi. In: *The Oculomotor System,* ed. Bender, M. B., pp. 40–80, New York: Hoeber Medical Division, Harper and Row Company.

Pasik, T. and Pasik, P. (1964b). Optokinetic nystagmus: an unlearned response altered by section of chiasma and corpus collosum in monkeys. *Nature.* **203**: 609–611.
Pasik, T., Pasik, P., and Bender, M. B. (1966). The superior colliculi and eye movements, and experimental study in the monkey, *Arch. Neurol.* **15**: 420–436.
Pasik, P., Pasik, T., and Bender, M. B. (1969). The pretectal syndrome in monkeys. I. Disturbances of gaze and body posture. *Brain.* **92**: 521–534.
Penfield, W. and Boldrey, E. (1937). Somatic motor and sensory representation in the cerebral cortex of man as studied by electrical stimulation. *Brain.* **60**: 389–443.
Petrović, A. and Tschemolossow, A. (1931). Zur Frage der rhythmischen Angiospasmen in Gebiete der Augenkerne. *Klin Monatsbl. Augenh.* **86**: 491–496.
Plott, S. (1964). Congenital laryngeal abductor paralysis due to nucleus ambiguus dysgenesis in three brothers. *N. E. J. M.* **271**: 593–597.
Plum, F. and Posner, J. B. (1966). *The Diagnosis of Stupor and Coma.* Oxford: Blackwell Scientific Publications.
Poser, C. M. (1969). Disseminated Vasculomyelinopathy. *Acta Neurol. Scand. Supple.* **37**: 1–44.
Raff, N. C. (June 22, 1967). Discussion of case 26–1967, case records of the Mass. General Hosp., *New Eng. J. Med.* **276**: 1432–1439.
Rampoldi, R. (1884). Singolarissimo caso di squilibrio motorio oculo-palpebrale. *Ann.Ottal.* **13**: 463–469.
Rampoldi, R. (1886). Un nuovo caso di congenito squilibrio motorio oculo-palpebrale. *Ann.Ottal.* **15**: 54–56.
Rasmussen, R. and Penfield, W. (1948). Movements of head and eyes from stimulation of the human frontal cortex. *Res. Publ. A. Nerv. & Ment. Dis.* **27**: 346–361.
Reed, H. and Israels, S. (1956). Congenital ocular motor apraxia. A form of horizontal gaze palsy. *Brit. J. Ophth.* **40**: 444–448.
Reese, W. S. and Yaskin, J. C. (1941). Preservation of convergence with paralysis of all lateral movements in a case of intramedullary tumor of the pons. *Amer. J. Opth.* **24**: 544–549.
Regli, F., Filippa, G., and Wiesendanger, M. (1967). Hereditary mirror movements. *Arch. Neurol.* **16**: 620–623.
Richter, C. P. (1968). Clock-mechanism esotropia in children, alternate-day squint. *Johns Hop. Med. J.* **122**: 218–223.
Riley, H. A. (1930). The central nervous system control of the ocular movements and the disturbances of this mechanisms. *Arch. Ophth.* **4**: 885–910.
Robinson, D. A. and Fuchs, A. F. (1969). Eye movements evoked by stimulation of frontal eye fields. *J. Neurophysiol.* **32**: 637–648.
Robles, J. (1966). Congenital ocular motor apraxia in identical twins. *Arch. Ophth.* **75**: 746–749.
Rodin, E. A. (1964). Impaired ocular pursuit movements. *Arch. Neurol.* **10**: 327–330.
Ross, A. T. and DeMyer, W. E. (1966). Isolated syndrome of the medial longitudinal fasciculus in man. Anatomical confirmation. *Arch. Neurol.* **15**: 203–205.
Ross, A. T. and Zeman, W. (1967). Opsoclonus, occult carcinoma, and chemical pathology in dentate nuclei. *Arch. Neurol.* **17**: 546–551.
Salman, S. D. (1969). Positional nystagmus. Critical review and personal experiences. *Arch. Otolaryng.* **90**: 58–63.
Salus, R. (1910). Uber erworbene Retractionsbewegungen der Augen. *Arch. Kinkerheilk.* **47**: 61–76.
Sano, K. (1959). Trigemino-oculomotor synkinesis. *Neurol. Medicochir. (Tokyo).* **1**: 29–51.
Sasaki, K. (1963). Electrophysiological studies on oculomotor neurons of the cat. *Jap. J. Physiol.* **13**: 287–302.
Sato, S. (1960). Electromyographic study on retraction syndrome. *Jap. J. Ophthal.* **4**: 57–66.
Schaller, W. F. (1921). A clinical and anatomic study of a vascular lesion of both cerebellar hemispheres. *Arch. Neurol. Psych.* **5**: 1–19.
Schuster, P. (1921). Zur Pathologie der vertikalen Blicklähmung. *Dtsch. Z. Nervenheilk.* **70**: 97–115.
Segarra, J. M. and Ojeman, R. J. (1961). Convergence nystagmus. *Neurology.* **11**: 883–893.
Shanzer, S. and Bender, M. B. (1959). Oculomotor responses on vestibular stimulation of monkey with lesions of the brain stem. *Brain.* **82**: 669–682.
Shanzer, S., April, R., and Atkins, A. (1965). Seizures induced by eye deviation. *Arch. Neurol.* **13**: 621–626.
Silberpfennig, J. (1939). Contributions to the problem of eye movements. II. Recovery from bilateral gaze paralysis. *Confin. Neurol.* **2**: 15-31.
Silberpfennig, J. (1941). Contributions to the problem of eye movements. III. Disturbances of ocular movements with pseudohemianopsia in frontal lobe tumors. *Confin. Neurol.* **4**: 1–13.

Simon, K. A. and Gay, A. J. (1964). Optokinetic responses in brain stem lesions. *Arch. Ophth.* **71**: 303-307.
Sinclair, W. W. (1895). Abnormal associated movements of the eye lids. *Ophthal. Rev.* **14**: 307-319.
Slatt, B., Loeffler, J. D., and Hoyt, W. F. (1966). Ocular motor disturbances in Parkinson's disease: electromyographic observations. *Canad. J. Ophthal.* **1**: 267-273.
Smith, J. L. and Walsh, F. B. (1957). Syndrome of external opthalmoplegia, ataxia, and areflexia (Fisher). *Arch. Ophth.* **58**: 109-114.
Smith, J. L. and Cogan, D. G. (1959). Internuclear ophthalmoplegia. A review of fifty-eight cases. *Arch. Ophth.* **61**: 687-694.
Smith, J. L., Gay, A. J., and Cogan, D. G. (1959). The spasticity of conjugate gaze phenomenon. *Arch. Ophth.* **62**: 694-696.
Smith, J. L., Zieper, I., Gay, A. J., and Cogan, D. G. (1959). Nystagmus retractorius. *Arch. Ophthal.* **62**: 864-867.
Smith, J. L. and Walsh, F. B. (1960). Opsoclonus-ataxic conjugate movements of the eyes. *Arch. Ophth.* **64**: 244-250.
Smith, J. L. and David, N. J. (1964). Internuclear ophthalmoplegia. Two new clinical signs. *Neurology.* **14**: 307-309.
Smith, J. L., David, N. J. and Klintworth, G. (1964). Skew deviation. *Neurology.* **14**: 96-105.
Sogg, R. L. and Hoyt, W. F. (1962). Intermittant vertical nystagmus in a father and son. *Arch. Ophthal.* **68**: 515-517.
Solomon, G. E. and Chutorian, A. M. (1968). Opsoclonus and occult neuroblastoma. *New Engl. J. Med.* **279**: 475-477.
Spaeth, E. B. (1947). The Marcus Gunn phenomenon. Discussion, presentation of four instances and consideration of its surgical correction. *Amer. J. Ophthal.* **30**: 143-148.
Spiegel, E. A., Wycis, H. T., Szekely, E. G., Soloff, L., Adams, J., Gildenberg, P., and Zanes, C. (1964). Stimulation of Forel's field during stereotaxic operations in the human brain. *Electroenceph. clin. Neurophysiol.* **16**: 537-548.
Spiller, W. G. (July, 1910). Conjugate deviation of the head and eyes in paralysing or irritative lesions of the cerebellum. *Review of Neurology and Psychiatry.* pp. 1-7.
Starr, A. (1967). A disorder of rapid eye movements in Huntington's chorea. *Brain.* **90**: 545-564.
Starr, A. (1969). Personal Communication.
Steele, J. C., Richardson, J. C., and Olszewski, J. (1964). Progressive supranuclear palsy. *Arch. Neurol.* **10**: 333-359.
Stenvers, H. W. (1925). On the optic (optokinetic, opto-motorial) nystagmus. *Acta. Oto-Laryng.* **8**: 545-562.
Stern, F. (1927). Uber psychische Zwangsvorgänge und ihre Entstehung bei encephalitischen Blickkrämpfen, mit Bemerkungen über die Genese der encephalitischen Blickkrämpfe. *Arch. Psychiat. Nervenkr.* **81**: 522-560.
Stern, F. (1928). *Epidemische Encephalitis.* 2nd. edn. Berlin: Julius Springer.
Stevens, H. (1965). Cyclic oculomotor paralysis. *Neurology.* **15**: 556-559.
Stieglmayr, F. S. (Sept. 21, 1967). Balint syndrome. *New Eng. J. Med.* **277**: 660.
Strang, R. R. (1969). "Lid-Drop," a complication of surgery in Parkinsonism. *Dis. Nerv. Sys.* **30**: 117-119.
Szentágothai, J. (1943). Die zentrale Innervation der Augenbewegungen. *Arch. Psychiat. Nervenkr.* **116**: 721-760.
Szentágothai, J. (1950a). Récherches expérimentales sur les voies oculogyres. *Sem Hôp., Paris.* **26**: 2989-2995.
Szentágothai, J. (1950). The elementary vestibulo-ocular reflex arc. *J. Neurophysiol.* **13**: 395-407.
Tamler, E., Marg, E., Jampolsky, A., and Nawratzki, I. (1959). Electromygraphy of human saccadic movements. *Arch. Ophthal.* **62**: 657-661.
Teng, P., Shanzer, S., and Bender, M. B. (1958). Effects of brain stem lesions on optokinetic nystagmus in monkeys. *Neurology.* **8**: 22-26.
Tillack, T. W. and Winer, J. A. (1962). Anomaly of the abducens nerve. *Yale J. Biol. Med.* **34**: 620-624.
Türk, S. (1899). Bemerkungen zu einem Fall von Retraktionsbewegung des Auges. *Zbl. Augenheilk.* **23**: 14-18.
Van Allen, M. W. and MacQueen, J. C. (1964). Ophthalmoplegia, ataxia and the syndrome of Landry-Guillain-Barré. *Trans. Amer. Neurol. Assoc.* **89**: 98-103.
Van Bogaert, L. (1927). Déclenchement des crises toniques du regard au cours du parkinsonisme postencéphalitique par l'épreuve de l'hyperpnée. *J. Neurol. Psychiat.* **27**: 432-436.

Van Gehuchten, P. (1940). Syndrome de Parinaud. *J. belg. neurol.* **40**: 126–137.
Volk, D. and Bruell, J. H. (1956). Eye movements in an adult with cerebral hemispherectomy. *Amer. J. Ophth.* **42**: 319–325.
Von Kornyey, S. (1959). Blickstörungen beivascularen herden des mesodiencephalen Ugerganges-gebietes. *Arch. f. Psych. u. Zeit. f. d. ges. Neurol.* **198**: 535–543.
Von Monakow, C. (1914). Die Lokalisation im Grosshirn und der Abbau der Funktion durch kortikale Herde. Weisbaden: J. F. Bergmann.
Von Noorden, G. K. and Preziosi, T. J. (1966). Eye movement recordings in neurological disorders. *Arch. Ophth.* **76**: 162–171.
Von Noorden, G. K. and Mackensen, G. (1962). Pursuit movements of normal and amblyopic eyes. An electro-ophthalmographic study. I. Physiology of pursuit movements. *Am. J. Ophth.* **53**: 325–336.
Wagshul, A. and Daroff, R. B. (July 12, 1969). L-Dopa for progressive supranuclear palsy. *Lancet.* **2**: 105–106.
Walsh, F. B. (1948). *Clinical Neuro-ophthalmology.* Baltimore: The Williams and Wilkins Co.
Walsh, F. B. and Hoyt, W. F. (1969). *Clinical Neuro-Ophthalmology,* 3rd edn. Baltimore: Williams and Wilkins Co.
Waltz, A. G. (1961). Dyspraxias of Gaze. *Arch. Neurol.* **5**: 638–647.
Wania, J. H. and Walsh, F. B. (1959). Absence of ocular signs with cerebellar ablation in an infant. *Arch. Ophth.* **61**: 655–656.
Wartenberg, R. (1948). Winking-jaw phenomenon. *Arch. Neurol. Psychiat.* **59**: 734–753.
Warwick, R. (1953). Representation of the extraocular muscles in the oculomotor nuclei of the monkey. *J. Comp. Neurol.* **98**: 449–504.
Weber, R. B. and Daroff, R. B. (1970). The metrics of normal human saccadic eye movements. In preparation.
White, J. C. (1969). Familial periodic nystagmus, vertigo, and ataxia. *Arch. Neurol.* **20**: 276–280.
Whitty, C. M. W. (1960). Photic and self-induced epilepsy. *Lancet.* **1**: 1207–1208.
Wilke, G. (1941). Zur Frage des Nystagmus retractorius. *Arch. f. Psychiat.* **113**: 388–404.
Wilson, S. A. K. (1954). *Neurology,* vol. I, 2nd edn. p. 141, London: Butterworth.
Windsor, C. E. and Berg, E. F. (1969). Circadian heterotropia. *Amer. J. Ophthal.* **67**: 565–571.
Winkler, G. F., Baringer, J. R., Sweeney, V. P., and Cogan, D. G. (1966). An acute syndrome of ocular oscillations and truncal ataxia. *Trans. Amer. Neurol. Assoc.* **91**: 96–99.
Wycis, H. T. and Spiegel, E. A. (1958). Parkinsonism with oculogyric crises; stimulation and partial elimination of periaqueductal grey and mesencephalic tegmentum (tegmentotomy). *Confin. neurol.* **18**: 385–393.
Yahr, M. D., Duvoisin, R. C., Schear, M. J., Barrett, R. E., and Hoehn, M. M. (1969). Treatment of Parkinsonism with Levodopa. *Arch. Neurol.* **21**: 343–354.
Yap, C. B., Mayo, C., and Barron, K. (1968). "Ocular Bobbing" in Palatal Myoclonus. *Arch. Neurol.* **18**: 304–310.
Zauberman, H., Magora, A., and Chaco, J. (1967). An electromyographic evaluation of the retraction syndrome. *Amer. J. Ophthal.* **64**: 1103–1108.
Zweifach, P. H., Walton, D. S., and Brown, R. H. (1969). Isolated congenital horizontal gaze paralysis: Occurrence of the near reflex and ocular retraction on attempted lateral gaze. *Arch. Ophthal.* **81**: 345–350.

THE PHARMACOLOGY OF EXTRAOCULAR MUSCLE

KENNETH E. EAKINS and RONALD KATZ

Mammalian extraocular muscle is unusual in that unlike most other mammalian skeletal muscle it possesses two neuromuscular systems. In addition to the twitch system typical of most mammalian skeletal muscle the extraocular muscles also possess a tonic neuromuscular system. This latter system, although unusual in mammals, is commonly found in lower animals and has been studied extensively in the frog.

STRUCTURE AND FUNCTION OF TWITCH AND TONIC NEUROMUSCULAR SYSTEMS IN THE FROG

In 1928 Sommerkamp described two fundamentally different responses of frog striated muscle to acetylcholine: 1) a rapid transient contraction (twitch) seen in the sartorius muscle and 2) a slow maintained contraction seen in the rectus abdominus muscle. This latter type of response occurred in only some of the fibers of other muscles (gastrocnemius, iliofibularis and semitendonosis). It was possible to separate the fibers of the iliofibularis into: 1) a tonic bundle which responded to acetylcholine with a slow maintained tonic contraction, and 2) non-tonic fibers in which acetylcholine produced a twitch response. Subsequent studies by Kruger (1929), Furlinger (1930), and Hess (1960) demonstrated two types of skeletal muscle fibers in the frog. One morphologic type had large, irregular, poorly defined fibrils (Felderstruktur), while the other type of fiber had small, regular, well-defined punctate fibrils (Fibrillenstruktur). The Felderstruktur characteristic of the tonic bundle had numerous small grape-like (en grappe) nerve endings which were derived from small-diameter motor nerves. The Fibrillenstruktur characteristic of the non-tonic or twitch fibers had single large plaque-like (en placque) nerve endings derived from large-diameter motor fibers.

These two distinct morphological systems differ in their electrophysiological and mechanical properties. Stimulation of the small-diameter ventral route nerve fibers results in slow, graded muscle contractions accompanied by non-propagated muscle potentials of small amplitude and long duration. These small nerve fibers are not excited by single shocks but are excited by tetanic rates of stimulation. Stimulation of the large-diameter ventral route

Supported by U.S. Public Health Service Research grants GM 09069 and NB 07079 (now EY 00457) and a Grant-in-Aid (G-303) of the National Council to Combat Blindness, Inc., New York.

fibers produces motor unit twitches accompanied by fast, propagated action potentials. Slow fibers also have a lower resting potential than the twitch fibers. The stimulus thresholds of the small nerve fibers are 3–6 times greater than the most excitable twitch fibers. The peak tension produced by the reflexly activated small nerve system is only 5–15% of the maximal single twitch tension.

TWITCH AND TONIC NEUROMUSCULAR SYSTEMS IN EXTRAOCULAR MUSCLES

Although the twitch and tonic systems described above have been known to exist in frog skeletal muscles since 1928, it is now known that these two neuromuscular systems can be found in the chicken (Hess, 1961), in the snake (Hess, 1963) and among mammalians in the extraocular muscles of guinea pig (Hess, 1961), rabbit (Matyuskin, 1961), cat (Hess and Pilar, 1963) and monkey (Hess, 1962). Recently, it has also been found that the two neuromuscular systems are also present in the extraocular muscles of man (Dietert, 1965).

Hess and Pilar in 1963 described the twitch and tonic types of neuromuscular system in the extraocular muscles of the cat. They found that these two systems were similar to those found in the frog in the arrangement of their fibrils, in their innervation and in their physiological responses. As we have seen before, twitch fibers respond to stimulation of the motor nerve with propagated impulse activity. In contrast slow fibers do not usually exhibit a conducted action potential, but instead undergo a graded development of tension proportional to the degree of membrane depolarization. It should be noted that at least some of these slow multiply–innervated fibers may in fact respond with propagated action potentials (Ginsborg, 1960a and b; Bach-y-Rita and Ito, 1966). However, the degree to which the slow fibers present in the cat extraocular muscles can be made to produce a propagated action potential is currently in question (Pilar, 1967). It is possible that the discrepancies described above can be explained by the studies Dr. Peachey refers to in Chapter 3. He suggests that there are at least five different types of muscle fibers in extraocular muscles. Three of these types are singly innervated and two of these types are multiply–innervated. The different responses seen by Hess and Pilar as compared with Bach-y-Rita and his coworkers may be due to the fact that one group was studying type II fibers while the other group was studying the type V fibers. It should also be pointed out at this time that the different fiber types seen in the extraocular muscles of the cat differ anatomically from the Fibrillenstruktur and Felderstruktur of frog muscle. In view of the multiple types of fibers found in the extraocular muscles, and the anatomical difference as compared with the frog muscle, this raises the question of how to refer to the responses of the extraocular muscles to various pharmacological agents. Since the mechanical response to pharmacological agents is either a twitch or a tonic contraction, we chose to use the terms twitch and tonic to refer to the singly-innervated and multiply–innervated fibers respectively.

One advantage to using the terms twitch and tonic rather than fast and slow is that the latter have been used previously to describe different responses. Twitch muscles have themselves been divided into fast and slow types depending on their speed of contraction. Flexor muscles and superficial extensors (tibialis anterior and gastrocnemius, respectively) are fast-contracting twitch muscles, while deep extensors (soleus) are slow-contracting twitch muscles. The slow-contracting twitch muscles contain more myoglobin than fast muscles which gives them a deeper red color; therefore, these muscles are sometimes termed red muscles as opposed to the paler fast-contracting twitch muscles which are sometimes referred to as white muscles. As a result of this confusing situation, the terms fast and slow are ambiguous while the terms twitch and tonic clearly define the observed responses.

EFFECT OF CHOLINERGIC AGENTS ON EXTRAOCULAR MUSCLE

Duke-Elder and Duke-Elder (1930) showed that choline, acetylcholine and nicotine produce a slow tonic contraction of the extraocular muscles of the dog eye both *in vivo* and *in vitro.* They pointed out that although a similar tonic contraction in response to cholinergic agents had been observed in *denervated* voluntary mammalian muscle, this was the first time that such a response was observed in *normally*-innervated voluntary mammalian muscle. In addition, they drew attention to the fact that the responses of the extraocular muscle to cholinergic agents resembled those seen in amphibian and avian voluntary muscle. It is now clear that the reasons for this are the structural similarities between mammalian extraocular muscles and these avian and amphibian voluntary muscles (see Introduction). Duke-Elder and Duke-Elder also demonstrated that atropine did not block the extraocular muscle responses to cholinergic agents; however, these responses were inhibited by curare. This suggests that the response is not muscarinic but rather can be classified as cholinergic nicotinic.

Intra-arterial or intravenous injection of acetylcholine was also found to contract the extraocular muscles of the decerebrate cat (Brown and Harvey, 1941). This response was later studied by Hess and Pilar (1963), who suggested that the sustained response of the cat superior oblique muscle to acetylcholine *in vitro* resulted from stimulation of the multiply-innervated or tonic fibers. These authors also suggested that some of the initial tension rise was due to stimulation of the twitch fibers.

Kern (1965) showed that in the rabbit's superior rectus muscle it was possible, by careful dissection, to separate the twitch from the tonic fibers. The mechanical responses of the isolated portions of the two muscle types were then studied under identical experimental conditions *in vitro.* Under these circumstances acetylcholine produced an immediate well-maintained contraction of the tonic fibers. In contrast the twitch fibers yielded a smaller, more transient response to acetylcholine (Fig. 1).

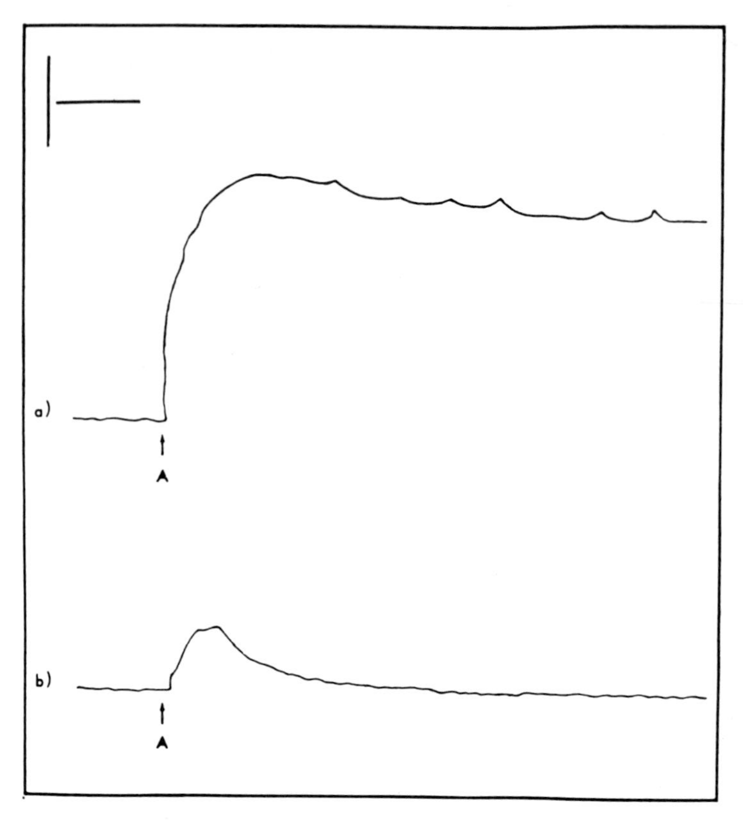

Fig. 1. "Contractures" induced by .05 μg acetylcholine per milliliter bath solution. Calibration: 20 mg, 1 minute. (a) From dissection comprising Feldertype fibers exclusively; weight of muscle piece: 1.1 mg (b) from dissection comprising Fibrillentype fibers with a few Feldertype fibers. Same muscle as 1a; weight of muscle piece: 5.2 mg (*Kern*, 1965).

In an elegant study by Sanghvi and Smith (1969) the actions of a variety of cholinergic agents were studied on the superior oblique muscle of the cat, both *in vivo* and *in vitro.* Acetylcholine, DMPP and nicotine were found to produce a sustained contraction of the extraocular muscles both *in vivo* (Fig. 2) and *in vitro* (Fig. 3). Muscarine, a compound not normally thought to affect skeletal muscles, was unexpectedly found to have a weak stimulant action in these experiments. The effects of various cholinergic blocking agents on these responses of the extraocular muscles were also studied by Sanghvi and Smith. Atropine was found to inhibit the action of muscarine both *in vivo* and *in vitro.* In contrast, it failed to antagonize the responses to acetylcholine, DMPP or nicotine; however, these latter responses were blocked by tubocurarine. The order of potency of these cholinergic drugs together with the blocking action of tubocurarine led Sanghvi and Smith to

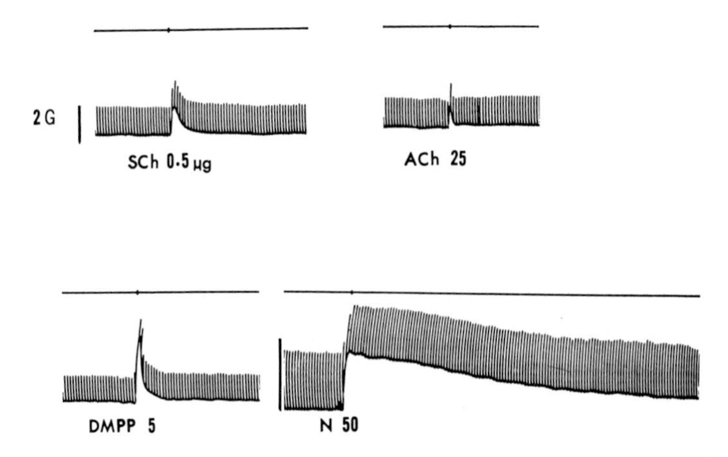

Fig. 2. Effects of cholinomimetics on superior oblique muscle *in vivo.* Upper trace in each pair of records is the time of injection, and the lower trace represents maximal twitches elicited indirectly once every 2 seconds. The vertical bar in the upper left is the 2 g calibration for the muscle twitch tension; for the lower right trace, the gain was increased. At SCh, 0.5 μg of succinylcholine was administered; at ACh, 25 μg of acetylcholine; at DMPP, 5 μg of DMPP and at N, 50 μg of nicotine. The cat weighed 2.2 kg (*Sanghvi and Smith,* 1969).

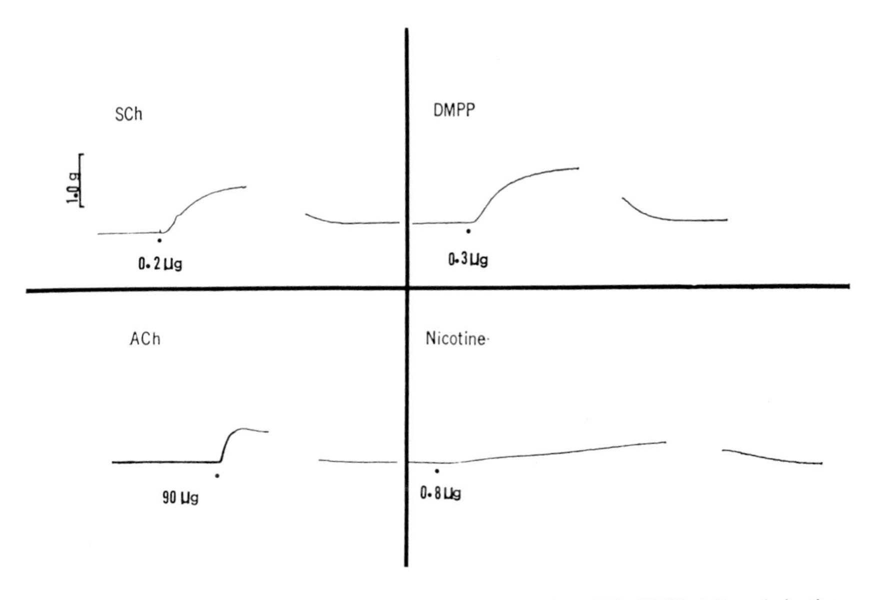

Fig. 3. Contractile response of the isolated superior oblique muscle to SCh, DMPP, ACh and nicotine. During discontinuous trace, drug solution was replaced by fresh bath solution. Dose indicates final concentration in micrograms per milliliter (*Sanghvi and Smith,* 1969).

conclude that the receptors for these agents in cat extraocular muscle are more cholinergic "nicotinic" than "muscarinic." However, their observation of the action of muscarine and the ability of atropine to antagonize the effect of muscarine suggested that some muscarinic receptors may be present in extraocular muscle.

The contractile response of the extraocular muscle to cholinergic drugs has usually been termed a contracture; however, Sanghvi and Smith have referred to these responses as contractions. A contracture differs from a contraction in that a contracture is not associated with propagated electrical activity in the muscle fibers (Gasser, 1930). Sanghvi and Smith preferred the term contraction since they observed "motor unit potentials" during the course of the contracture responses to cholinergic drugs although as the authors themselves pointed out, their extracellular recording techniques did not permit them to determine the site of origin of the electrical activity. Thus, the electrical activity could have come from twitch fibers, presynaptic sites or intrafusal muscle fibers as well as from the tonic fibers. Although this question is not yet settled we use the term tonic contraction to refer to the mechanical response of the extraocular muscles without drawing any conclusions as to the nature of the electrical response.

THE EFFECT OF NEUROMUSCULAR AGENTS ON EXTRAOCULAR MUSCLES

The neuromuscular blocking agents are commonly classified as either 1) depolarizing (non–competitive) or 2) non–depolarizing (competitive). This is based on their effect on the post–junctional membrane of the motor end–plate. The depolarizing agents act by combining with the receptors on the post–junctional membrane and producing a sustained depolarization, so that in a sense, the muscle is refractory to the depolarizing effect of the normal transmitter, namely acetylcholine. Thus, under appropriate circumstances, large doses of acetylcholine itself are capable of producing a neuromuscular block by means of persistent depolarization. This is an over–simplification of the situation, since prolonged application of depolarizing agents can produce another kind of neuromuscular block which has been termed desensitizing blockade (phase 2 or dual block).

The non–depolarizing neuromuscular blocking agents combine with the post–junctional receptor sites but,in contrast to the depolarizing agents, do not produce depolarization of the membrane. The occupation of the receptor site by the non–depolarizing agent prevents acetylcholine from reacting with the receptors, resulting in a block of normal neuromuscular transmission. It is possible to distinguish a depolarizing from a non–depolarizing neuromuscular block by a) the presence or absence of initial transient fasciculations, b) the response to tetanus, and c) the response to cholinesterase inhibitors. With non–depolarizing agents initial fasciculation is not seen, tetanus is poorly sustained, post–tetanic facilitation is present and the block is antagonized by cholinesterase inhibitors. On the other hand, with depolarizing agents initial fasciculation is usually seen, tetanus is well sustained, post–tetanic facilitation is not seen and cholinesterase inhibitors enhance the block. *Neuromuscular depolarizing blocking agents:* Clinically useful depolarizing agents include succinylcholine (Sch), decamethonium (C_{10}) and hexacarbacholine.

Interest in the effects of depolarizing neuromuscular blocking agents on extraocular muscles was aroused by the report of Hofmann and Holzer in 1953, that succinylcholine increased intraocular pressure in man. They made the astute clinical observation that associated with the increase in intraocular pressure, the eyes became divergent and remained fixed. Movement of the eyes returned at the same time that the intraocular pressure decreased. This suggested to them that the increase in intraocular pressure might be associated with, or produced by, the extraocular muscles. Hoffman and Lembeck (1952) demonstrated that succinylcholine contracted extraocular muscle in the anesthetized rabbit. Other workers also found that succinylcholine increased extraocular muscle tension both *in vivo* and *in vitro* (Lincoff *et al.*, 1955, 1957; Dillon *et al.*, 1957; Macri and Grimes, 1957). The mechanism of the contracture responses of the extraocular muscles to the succinylcholine was not known. Eakins and Katz (1965, 1966) attributed the tonic contraction of cat extraocular muscles produced by intravenous succinylcholine to stimulation of the tonic or Felderstruktur systems, which had been shown to be present in the cat extraocular muscle by Hess and Pilar (1963).

Eakins and Katz (1966) found that intravenous succinylcholine produced a dose–dependent increase in extraocular muscle tension (Fig. 4). In these experiments atropine was without effect on the resting tension and did not inhibit the response of the muscle to succinylcholine. However tubocurarine markedly reduced the response to succinylcholine (Fig. 5).

Katz and Eakins (1966a and b) compared and contrasted the effects of various neuromuscular blocking agents on the twitch and tonic systems of the cat's extraocular muscle. This was accomplished by dissecting the superior rectus muscle free of the globe and attaching the cut end to a force

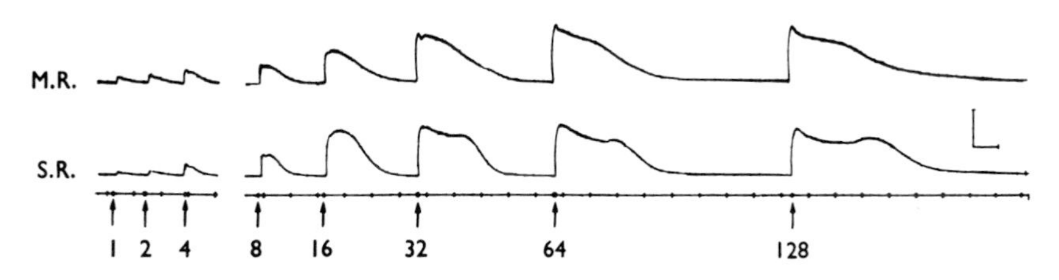

Fig. 4. Cat, 3.7 kg, pentobarbitone anesthesia. Effect of increasing intravenous doses (in μg/kg) of succinylcholine on the tension of the medial rectus muscle (M.R.) and superior rectus muscle (S.R.). Calibrations, 10 g tension and 1 minute (*Eakins and Katz*, 1966).

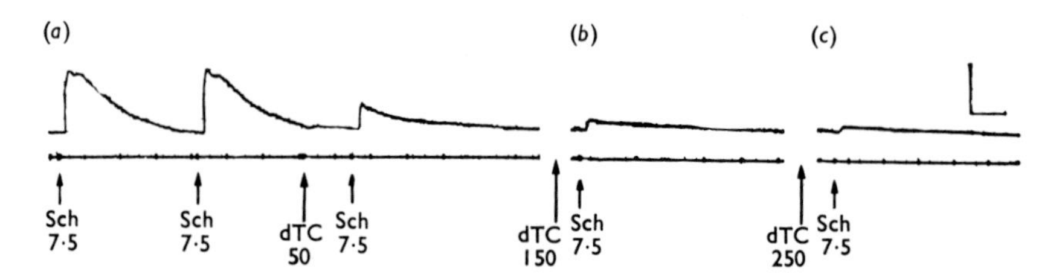

Fig. 5. Cat, 4.0 kg, pentobarbitone anesthesia. Effect of tubocurarine on the response of the medial rectus muscle to succinylcholine. (a) Effect of 50 μg/kg of tubocurarine (dTC) on the response to succinylcholine (SCh); (b) response of the extraocular muscle to succinylcholine after a total dose of 150 μg/kg of tubocurarine; (c) response of the muscle to succinylcholine after a cumulative dose of 250 μg/kg of tubocurarine. All drugs were given intravenously. All doses in μg/kg. Calibrations, 5 g tension and 1 minute (*Eakins and Katz*, 1966).

displacement transducer. Through a parietal craniotomy the third cranial nerve was isolated and periodically stimulated. The effect of intravenous succinylcholine on the evoked twitch and baseline tension was then recorded. Small doses of succinylcholine did not depress the twitch response, but did increase baseline tension (Fig. 6). With larger doses a further increase in baseline tension was seen, while the twitch response was depressed. Thus, succinylcholine depressed the twitch neuromuscular system, while at the same time stimulating the tonic system. Similar results were observed with decamethonium and hexacarbacholine. The duration of the tonic contraction of the extraocular muscle also varied, the action of succinylcholine being shortest and hexacarbacholine the longest. A similar depression of the twitch system and stimulation of the tonic system by depolarizing agents was confirmed by Bach-y-Rita and Ito (1966) and Sanghvi and Smith (1969).

Katz and Eakins (1966a and b) also found that the dose of succinylcholine required to depress the twitch response of the superior rectus muscle was greater than that required to block the twitch response of skeletal muscle (Fig. 7). With decamethonium the difference in sensitivity of the twitch response of the extraocular muscle and leg muscle was present to a smaller degree than with succinylcholine (Fig. 8). Hexacarbacholine occupied an intermediate position between succinylcholine and decamethonium. Thus the extraocular muscles are resistant to the neuromuscular blocking action of all three agents.

NON-DEPOLARIZING NEUROMUSCULAR BLOCKING AGENTS

It has been widely held that mammalian extraocular muscles are more sensitive to the neuromuscular blocking effects of tubocurarine than are other skeletal muscles both in animals and man (Brown and Harvey, 1941; Smith *et al.*, 1947; Drucker *et al.*, 1951; Pelikan *et al.*, 1953; Breinin, 1962; McIntyre, 1965). This concept was challenged by Katz and Eakins (1966a). They compared the effects of tubocurarine on the indirectly stimulated

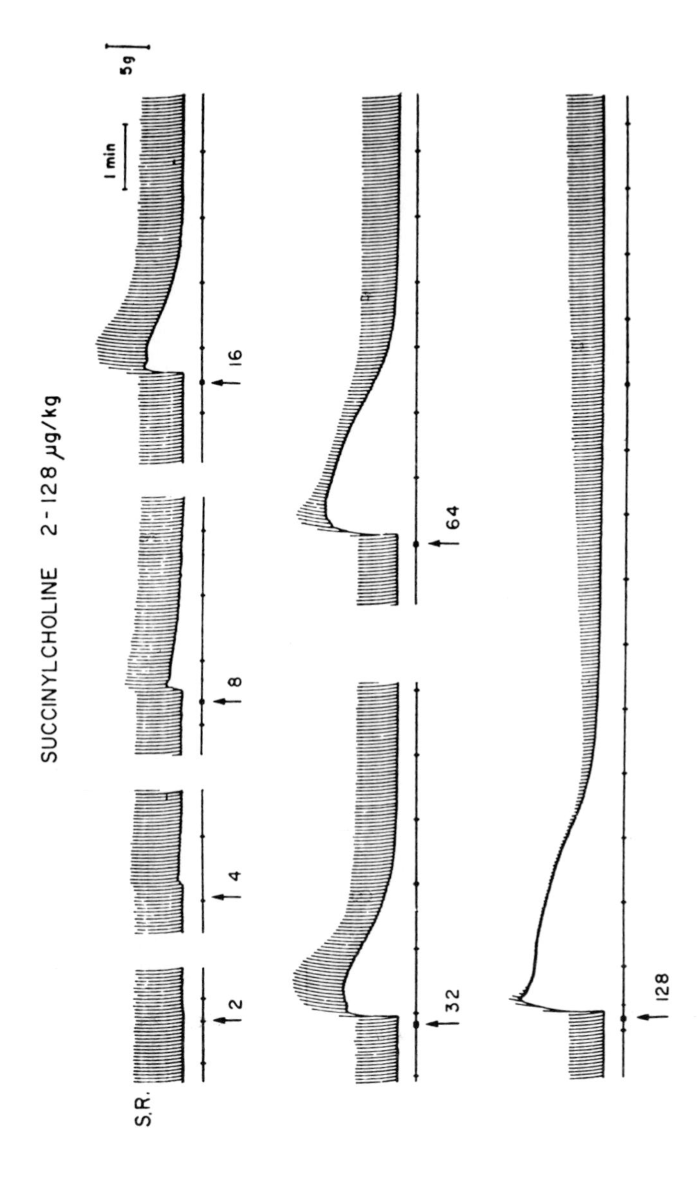

Fig. 6. Effect of increasing doses of succinylcholine on the superior rectus muscle (S. R.) tension and twitch response. Note increase in muscle tension after small doses and depression of muscle twitch only after large doses of succinylcholine. The cat received 36 mg/kg pentobarbital i.p. (*Katz and Eakins*, 1966a).

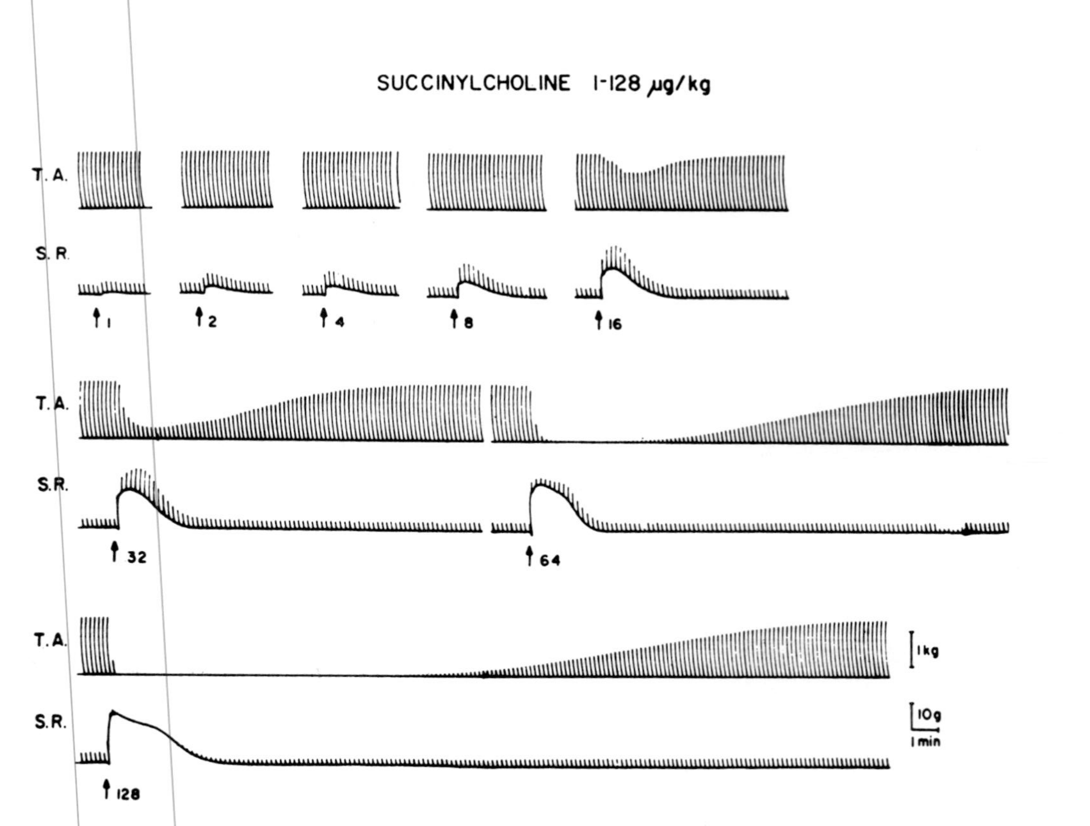

Fig. 7. Cat (under pentobarbital anesthesia). Effect of increasing doses of succinylcholine on the superior rectus muscle (S. R.) tension and twitch response and the tibialis anterior muscle (T. A.) twitch response. Note increase in superior rectus tension after 1 μg/kg, decrease in tibialis twitch after 16 μg/kg and decrease in superior rectus twitch after 128 μg/kg (*Katz and Eakins,* 1966b).

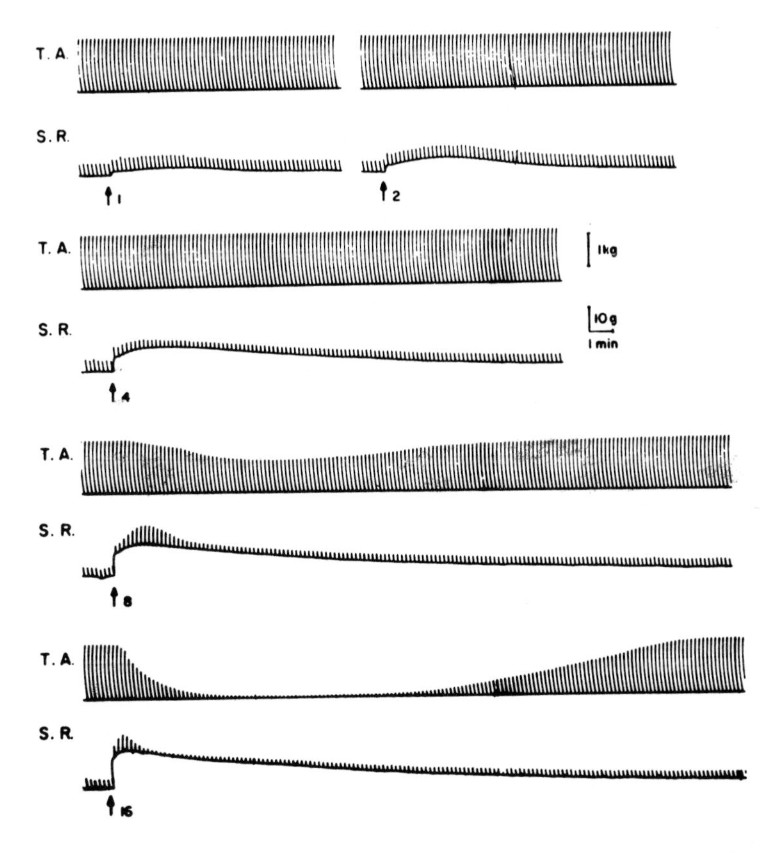

Fig. 8. Cat under pentobarbital anesthesia. Effect of increasing doses of decamethonium on the superior rectus muscle (S. R.) tension and twitch response and the tibialis anterior muscle (T. A.) twitch response. Note increase in superior rectus tension and decrease in both tibialis twitch response and superior rectus twitch response (*Katz and Eakins,* 1966b).

superior rectus and anterior tibialis muscles in the same cat. A dose of tubocurarine which abolished the anterior tibialis twitch response only produced a 50% block in the superior rectus twitch (Fig. 9). These findings were supported by Sanghvi and Smith (1969) using different muscles in the cat. They found that tubocurarine had a greater effect on the gastrocnemius twitch muscle than on the superior oblique muscle. Katz and Eakins (1966b) also studied the differential effects on the tibialis and superior rectus muscles of gallamine and dimethyl tubocurarine. Once again, a greater sensitivity of the extraocular muscle to these two non-depolarizing agents could not be demonstrated (Figs. 10 and 11).

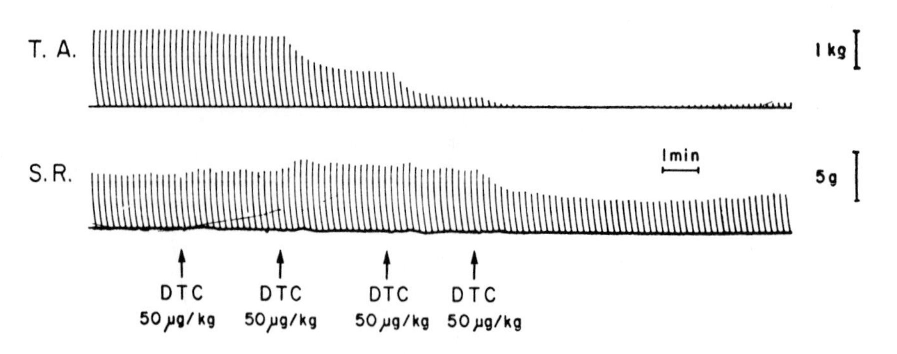

Fig. 9. Effect of d-tubocurarine on the superior rectus muscle (S. R.) and tibialis anterior muscle (T. A.) twitch response. Note greater depression of tibialis anterior muscle twitch response. The cat received 36 mg/kg pentobarbital i.p. (*Katz and Eakins,* 1966a).

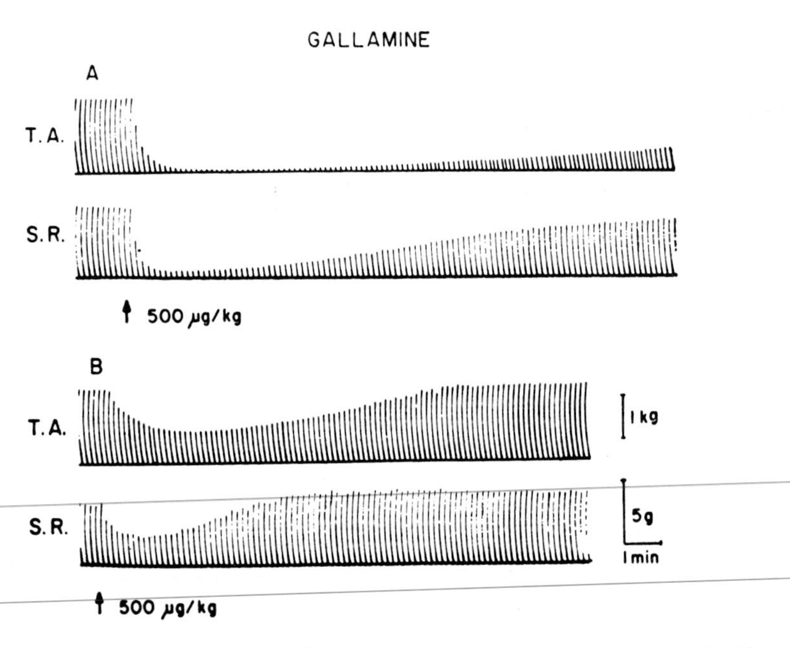

Fig. 10. Cat under pentobarbital anesthesia. Effect of gallamine on the superior rectus muscle (S. R.) and tibialis anterior muscle (T. A.) twitch responses. Note difference in magnitude and duration of block in response of cat shown in panel **A** as compared with that of another cat shown in panel **B**. In each animal the magnitude of block of tibialis and superior rectus muscles was similar, but the duration of action was greater for the tibialis muscle (*Katz and Eakins,* 1966b).

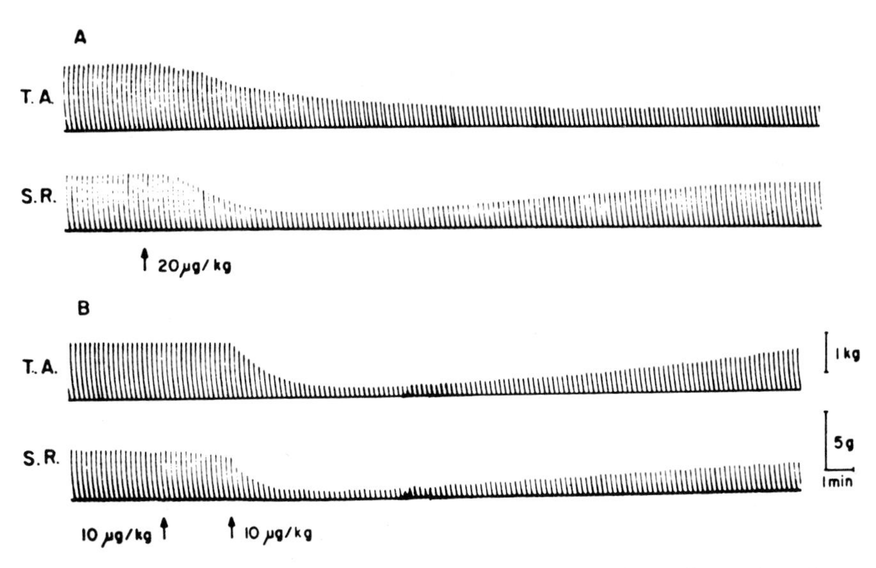

Fig. 11. Cat under pentobarbital anesthesia. Effect of dimethyl tubocurarine on the superior rectus muscle (S. R.) and tibialis muscle (T. A.) twitch responses. (a) Note more rapid onset of block as well as recovery in superior rectus muscle. (b) Note that in this animal the onset and magnitude of block of both muscles were similar, with a more rapid recovery of tibialis muscle (*Katz and Eakins*, 1966b).

Katz and Eakins (1966b) attempted to reconcile their findings of a greater sensitivity of muscles to tubocurarine with those of Brown and Harvey (1941) who found a greater sensitivity of the extraocular muscles. Katz and Eakins pointed out that Brown and Harvey 1) used an impure preparation of tubocurarine (the only one available at that time) and 2) stated that "accurate recording of changes in tension with the ordinary mechanical myograph is impracticable." Furthermore, the comparison made by Brown and Harvey of the dose required to block the tibialis and eye (inferior oblique) muscles was made in different animals. In only one animal (2.6 kg cat) 0.5 mg tubocurarine depressed the inferior oblique twitch response 50% while the tibialis twitch response was unaffected. The results with tubocurarine on the inferior oblique muscle are quite similar to the results of Katz and Eakins on the superior rectus muscle. However, with the dose of tubocurarine used, a profound depression of the tibialis twitch response would be expected.

Concerning man, Sanghvi and Smith (1969) pointed out that human studies used convergence as a test of extraocular muscle function. They suggested that it is not correct to compare vergence,which may be mediated tetanically (Alpern and Wolter, 1956), with the twitch response to single nerve shocks that were studied in the animal experiments. This argument is supported by the observation that the inability to sustain tetanus is a more sensitive index of neuromuscular block than the ability to produce a normal twitch (Katz, 1967).

In summary, we believe that the statement that the extraocular muscles are unusually sensitive to neuromuscular blocking agents is no longer tenable.

A SIMPLE METHOD FOR DETERMINING THE PRESENCE OR ABSENCE OF DEPOLARIZING NEUROMUSCULAR BLOCKADE

Since mammalian extraocular muscles respond to cholinergic drugs with a tonic contraction, they can be used both *in vivo* and *in vitro,* to distinguish between neuromuscular blocking agents which cause depolarization and those which do not. Both types of neuromuscular blocking agents will reduce the twitch contractions produced by motor nerve stimulation, but only depolarizing drugs will also produce a tonic contraction.

THE EFFECT OF CHOLINESTERASE INHIBITORS ON EXTRAOCULAR MUSCLES

The effects of edrophonium and neostigmine *per se* on extraocular muscle and their interaction with succinylcholine were studied in the anesthetized cat (Katz and Eakins, 1966a). Unlike succinylcholine, which depressed the twitch system but stimulated the tonic system, cholinesterase inhibitors were found to stimulate both systems; facilitating the twitch response and increasing baseline tension (Fig. 12). When succinylcholine was injected after the responses to edrophonium had returned to control level, the actions of succinylcholine were enhanced (Fig. 12).

EFFECT OF ADRENERGIC AGENTS ON EXTRAOCULAR MUSCLE

It has long been known that stimulation of sympathetic nerves or administration of sympathetic amines can produce various effects on skeletal muscles (see Bowman and Raper, 1966, 1967 for detailed information on this subject). However, an increase in baseline tension following administration of epinephrine is seen only in chronically denervated skeletal muscle, both *in vivo* (Euler and Gaddum, 1931; Bulbring and Burn,1936, 1959; Bowman and Zaimis, 1961; Bowman and Raper, 1965) and *in vitro* (Montague, 1955; Cambridge, 1961; Bhoola and Schacter, 1961). Bowman and Raper (1965) suggested that the contraction of chronically denervated skeletal muscle produced by epinephrine was due to an action on sympathetic beta-receptors thought to be present in skeletal muscle.

As early as 1930, Duke-Elder and Duke-Elder suggested that mammalian extraocular muscle behaves in many respects like chronically denervated mammalian striated muscle, both yielding tonic contractions to acetylcholine and carbachol. Eakins and Katz (1967) studied the effects of sympathetic

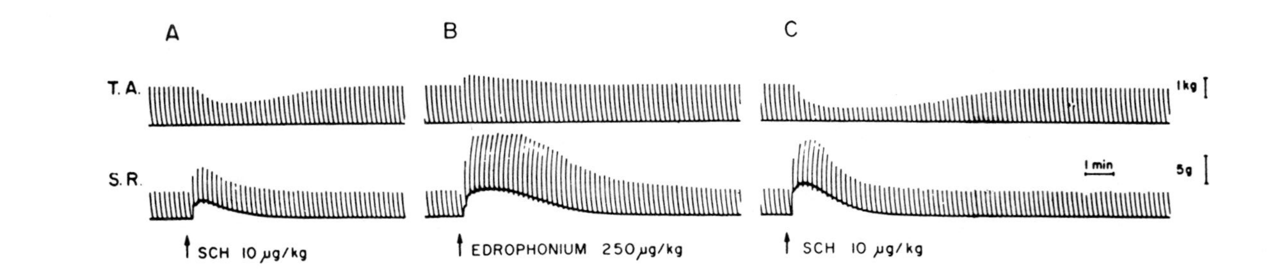

Fig. 12. Effect of edrophonium on the response to succinylcholine (SCh). Panel **A**, control response of superior rectus muscle (S. R.) and tibialis anterior muscle (T. A.) to succinylcholine; panel **B**, effect of edrophonium; panel **C**, note increased magnitude of response to succinylcholine 15 minutes after injection of edrophonium. The cat received 36 mg/kg pentobarbital i.p. (*Katz and Eakins*, 1966a).

stimulation and epinephrine on the superior rectus muscle of the intact cat in order to determine whether the extraocular muscle response was comparable to that seen in chronically denervated skeletal muscle.

Intravenous injections of epinephrine were found to result in a dose-dependent tonic contraction of the superior rectus muscle (Fig. 13). Furthermore, electrical stimulation of the post-ganglionic cervical synpathetic produced a voltage-dependent increase in tension of the superior rectus muscle (Fig. 14). Similar results with epinephrine were obtained *in vivo* on the superior oblique muscle of the cat (Sanghvi, 1967; Sanghvi and Smith, 1969). This response to epinephrine was found to be independent of changes in intraorbital smooth muscle tension or cardiovascular alterations (Eakins and Katz, 1967). It should be noted that the magnitude of the maximal response to epinephrine and sympathetic stimulation is only 1/10th that which can be produced by cholinergic drugs.

The response of the superior rectus muscle to epinephrine was not blocked by the sympathetic beta-receptor blocking agents, pronethalol and propanalol, but was antagonized by the sympathetic alpha-receptor blocking agents, phentolamine and phenoxybenzamine (Figs. 15 and 16). It was therefore concluded that the response of the superior rectus muscle to epinephrine did not correspond to the effects of the amine on chronically denervated mammalian skeletal muscle.

This effect of epinephrine on the superior rectus muscle may be related to its anti–curare action in curare–treated striated muscle (Panella, 1907); Rosenblueth *et al.,* 1936; Wilson and Wright, 1937; Brown *et al.,* 1950). In common with the response of the superior rectus muscle to epinephrine the anti–curare action is blocked by sympathetic alpha–receptor blocking agents (Maddock *et al.,* 1948; Brown *et al.,* 1950; Bowman *et al.,* 1962). This anti-curare effect of epinephrine is thought to be due to an increase in acetyl-

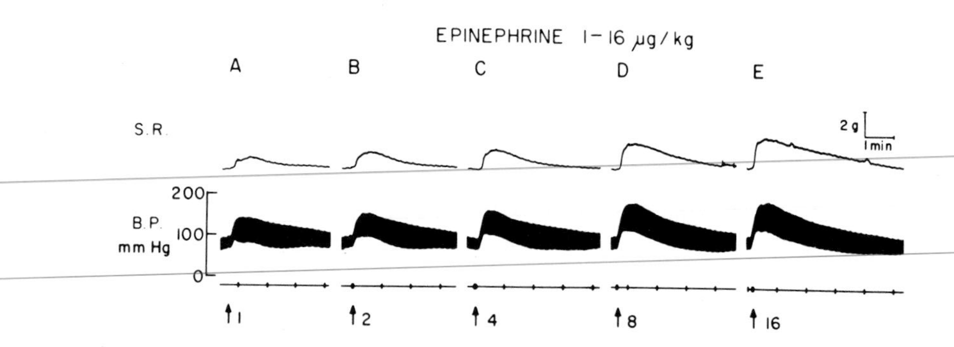

Fig. 13. Effect of epinephrine on the tension of the superior rectus muscle (S.R.) of the cat. Top trace, tension of the superior rectus muscle; bottom trace femoral arterial blood pressure. Intravenous injections of epinephrine were made at arrows; figures represent dose in micrograms per kilogram. Note dose-dependent increase in tension of the extraocular muscle (*Eakins and Katz,* 1967).

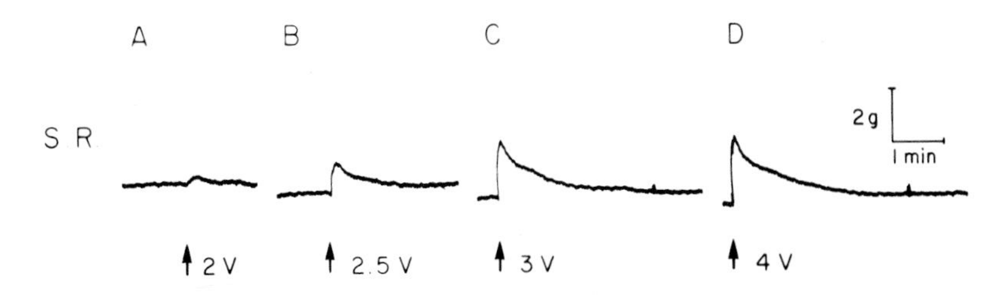

Fig. 14. Response of the superior rectus (S. R.) muscle to post-ganglionic sympathetic stimulation; 20/sec, 3-msec duration, voltage as indicated by arrows, **A–D** (*Eakins and Katz,* 1967).

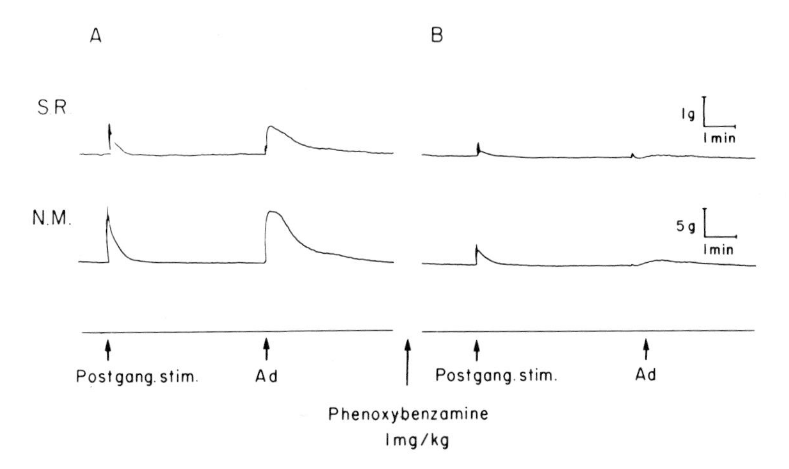

Fig. 15. Antagonism of the responses of the superior rectus muscle (S. R.) and nictitating membrane (N. M.) to sympathetic stimulation (20/sec, 4-msec duration, 4V) and i.v. injection of 7 μg/kg of epinephrine (E) by phenoxybenzamine. **A**, control responses; **B**, responses 15 minutes after i.v. phenoxybenzamine. (I mg/kg) (*Eakins and Katz,* 1967).

choline release resulting from a hyperpolarizing action of epinephrine on motor nerve endings (Krnjevic and Miledi, 1958, 1959).

Another possible explanation of the effect of epinephrine on extraocular muscle was pointed out by Sanghvi (1967). He drew attention to the suggestion made by Kuffler and Vaughan Williams (1953a and b) that frog tonic muscle fibers may have physiological characteristics which lie somewhere between those of smooth muscle and twitch skeletal muscle. In addition, until shown otherwise, we must also bear in mind the possibility that extraocular muscle itself contains some smooth muscle elements. Another possibility, that the epinephrine response may be mediated by one of the multiply-innervated fiber systems present is discussed by Dr. Peachey in another chapter (Chapter 3).

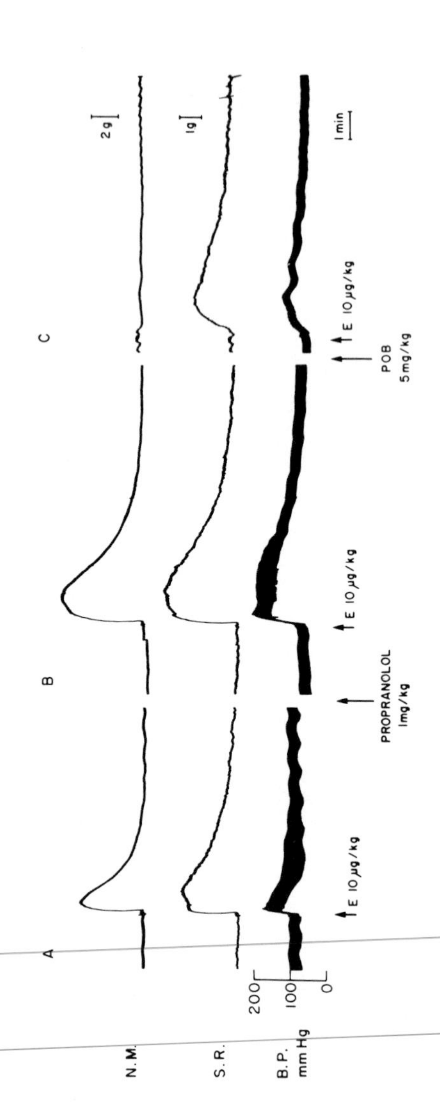

Fig. 16. Effect of propranolol followed by phenoxybenzamine on the response of the nictitating membrane (N.M.) and superior rectus muscle (S.R.) to intravenous epinephrine (E). **A**, control responses; **B**, responses 15 minutes after propranolol (1 mg/kg i.v.); **C**, responses 15 minutes after phenoxybenzamine (POB) (5 mg/kg i.v.). Time elapsed between **A** and **C** was 40 minutes. Note only partial antagonism of the response of S.R. to epinephrine and complete blockade of the nictitating membrane response. B.P., blood pressure (*Eakins and Katz*, 1967).

Another effect of adrenergic agents on *in vitro* preparations of extraocular muscles has recently been described by Kern (1968a and b). He reported that adrenergic agents relaxed acetylcholine-contracted extraocular muscles of the rabbit, cat, and monkey. In the cat and monkey Kern concluded that this effect was mediated mainly by adrenergic beta-receptors, whereas both alpha- and beta-adrenergic receptors were involved in rabbit extraocular muscles.

THE AUTONOMIC NERVOUS SYSTEM AND EXTRAOCULAR MUSCLES

Little work has been carried out in this area. The histological observations of Boeke (1926) and Wolter (1955), indicating that the striated muscle fibers of the extraocular muscles have a double innervation, motor and autonomic, led Alpern and Wolter (1956) to suggest that the slow vergence movements of the eye were under autonomic control. However, little clear-cut evidence is available at the present time to support this view. The study of cholinergic agents on extraocular muscles by Sanghvi and Smith (1969) led them to conclude that the cholinergic receptors present were mainly nicotinic, which appears to rule out the existence of any sizable population of post-ganglionic parasympathetic receptors. Their results with muscarine do indicate the existence of some muscarinic receptors, however; judging from the intensity of the extraocular muscle response to muscarine their importance in normal extraocular muscle function in the cat would be small.

Eakins and Katz (1967) studied the possible role of the sympathetic nervous system in extraocular muscle function. Although they found that stimulation of the superior cervical ganglion produced a contraction of the extraocular muscles, this could not be separated from the simultaneously produced contraction of orbital smooth muscle during superior cervical ganglion stimulation. The inability to separate the extraocular muscle and orbital smooth muscle response to sympathetic stimulation differs from the results observed with epinephrine, where it was possible to dissociate extraocular muscle and orbital smooth muscle responses and thus be sure that epinephrine was affecting the extraocular muscle directly.

REFERENCES

Alpern, M. and Wolter, J. R. (1956). The relation of horizontal saccadic and vergence movements. *A.M.A. Arch. Ophthal.* **56**: 685.

Bach-y-Rita, P. and Ito, F. (1966). *In vivo* studies on fast and slow muscle fibers in cat extraocular muscles. *J. Gen. Physiol.* **49**: 1177–1198.

Bhoola, K. D. and Schacter, M. (1961). Contracture of the denervated rat diaphragm by adrenaline. *J. Physiol.* (Lond.) **157**: 20 P.

Boeke, J. (1926). Die Beziehungen der Nervenfasern zu den Bindegewebselementen und Tastzellen. *Zrschr. mikr.-anat. Forsch.* **4**: 448.

Bowman, W. C. and Zaimis, E. (1961). The action of adrenaline, noradrenaline and isoprenaline on the denervated mammalian muscle. *J. Physiol.* (Lond.). **158**: 24–25 P.

Bowman, W. C., Goldberg, A. A. J., and Raper, C. (1962). A comparison between the effects of a tetanus and the effects of sympathomimetic amines on fast and slow contracting mammalian muscles. *Brit. J. Pharmacol.* **19**: 464–484.
Bowman, W. C. and Raper, C. (1965). The effects of sympathomimetic amines on chronically denervated skeletal muscles. *Brit. J. Pharmacol.* **24**: 98–109.
Bowman, W. C. and Raper, C. (1966). Effects of sympathomimetic amines on neuromuscular transmission. *Brit. J. Pharmacol.* **27**: 313–331.
Bowman, W. C. and Raper, C. (1967). Adrenatropic receptors in skeletal muscle. *Ann. N. Y. Acad. Sci.* **139**: 741–753.
Breinin, G. M. (1962). *The Electrophysiology of Extraocular Muscle.* University of Toronto Press, Toronto. pp. 98–99.
Brown, G. L. and Harvey, A. M. (1941). Neuromuscular transmission in the extrinsic muscles of the eye. *J. Physiol.* (Lond.). **99**: 379–399.
Brown, G. L., Goffart, M., and Vianna Dias, M. (1950). The effect of adrenaline and sympathetic stimulation on the demarcation potential of mammalian skeletal muscle. *J. Physiol.* (Lond.). **111**: 184–194.
Bulbring, E. and Burn, J. H. (1936). The Sherrington phenomenon. *J. Physiol.* (Lond.). **86**: 61–76.
Cambridge, G. W. (1961). Comparison of the properties of denervated rat diaphragm muscle and an invertebrate smooth muscle. *J. Physiol.* (Lond.). **158**: 25–26 P.
Dietert, S. E. (1965). The demonstration of different types of muscle fibers in human extraocular muscle by electron microscopy and cholinesterase staining. *Invest. Ophthal.* **4**: 51–63.
Dillon, J. B., Sabawala, P., Taylor, D. B., and Gunter, R. (1957). Action of succinylcholine on extraocular muscles and intraocular pressure. *Anesthesiology.* **18**: 44–49.
Drucker, A. P., Sadove, M. J., and Unna, K. R. (1951). Ophthalmic studies of curare and curarelike drugs in man. *Amer. J. Ophthal.* **34**: 543–553.
Duke-Elder, W. S. and Duke-Elder, P. M. (1930). Contraction of extrinsic muscles of eye by choline and nicotine. *Proc. R. Soc.* **B107**: 332–343.
Eakins, K. E. and Katz, R. L. (1965). Response of the medial rectus muscle of the cat to syccinylcholine. *Nature* (Lond.). **207**: 1398.
Eakins, K. E. and Katz, R. L. (1966). The action of succinylcholine on the tension of extraocular muscle. *Brit. J. Pharmacol.* **26**: 205–211.
Eakins, K. E. and Katz, R. L. (1967). The effects of sympathetic stimulation and epinephrine on the superior rectus muscle of the cat. *J. Pharmacol.* **157**: 524–531.
Euler, U. S. von and Gaddum, J. H. (1931). Pseudomotor contractures after degeneration of the facial nerve. *J. Physiol.* (Lond.). **73**: 54–66.
Furlinger, F. (1930). Uber einen Zusammenhang Zwischen Struktur und Funktion von Skelettmuskeln bei Rana Temporaria. *Zool. Anz.* **90**: 325–335.
Gasser, H. S. (1930). Contractures of skeletal muscle. *Physiol. Rev.* **10**: 35–109.
Ginsborg, B. L. (1960a). Spontaneous activity in muscle fibers of the chick. *J. Physiol.* (Lond.). **150**: 707–717.
Ginsborg, B. L. (1960b). Some properties of avian skeletal muscle fibers with multiple neuromuscular junctions. *J. Physiol.* (Lond.). **154**: 581–598.
Hess, A. (1960). The structure of extrafusal muscle fibers in the frog and their innervation studied by the cholinesterase technique. *Amer. J. Anat.* **107**: 129–151.
Hess, A. (1961). Structural differences of fast and slow extrafusal muscle fibers and their nerve endings in chickens. *J. Physiol.* (Lond.). **157**: 221–231.
Hess, A. (1962). Further morphological observations of en plaque and en grappe nerve endings on mammalian extrafusal muscle fibers with the cholinesterase technique. *Rev. Canad. Biol.* **21**: 241–248.
Hess, A. (1963). Two kinds of extrafusal muscle fibers and their nerve endings in the garter snake. *Amer. J. Anat.* **113**: 347–352.
Hess, A. and Pilar, G. (1963). Slow fibers in the extraocular muscles of the cat. *J. Physiol.* (Lond.). **169**: 780–789.
Hoffmann, H. and Holzer, H. (1953). Die Wirkung von Muskelrelaxantien auf den intraokularen Druck. *Klin. Monatsbl. Augenheilk.* **123**: 1–16.
Hofmann, H. and Lembeck, F. (1952). The response of the external ocular muscles to curare, decamethonium, and succinylcholine. *Naunyn-Schmiedeberg's Arch. exp. Path. Pharmak.* **216**: 552–557.
Katz, R. L. (1967). Pyridostigmin (Mestinon) as an antagonist of d-tubocurarine. *Anesthesiology.* **28**: 528–534.

Katz, R. L. and Eakins, K. E. (1966a). A comparison of the effects of neuromuscular blocking agents and cholinesterase inhibitors on the tibialis anterior and superior rectus muscles of the cat. *J. Pharmacol. Exp. Therap.* **152**: 304-312.

Katz, R. L. and Eakins, K. E. (1966b). The effects of succinylcholine, decamethonium, hexacarbacholine, gallamine and dimethyl tubocurarine on the twitch and tonic neuromuscular systems of the cat. *J. Pharmacol. Exp. Therap.* **154**: 303-309.

Kern, R. (1965). A comparative pharmacologic-histologic study of slow and twitch fibers in the superior rectus muscle of the rabbit. *Invest. Ophthal.* **4**: 901-910.

Kern, R. (1968a). Uber die adrenergischen Receptoren der extraocularen Muskeln des Rhesusaffen. Eine in vitro Studie. *Albrecht v. Graefes Arch. Klin. exp. Ophthal.* **174**: 278-286.

Kern, R. (1968b). Die adrenergischen Receptoren der extraocularen Muskeln des Kaninchens, der Katze und des Rhesusaffen. II. *Albrecht v. Graefes Arch. Klin. exp. Ophthal.* **175**: 359-374.

Krnjevic, K. and Miledi, R. (1958). Some effects produced by adrenaline upon neuromuscular propagation. *J. Physiol.* (Lond.). **141**: 291-304.

Krnjevic, K. and Miledi, R. (1959). Presynaptic failure of neuromuscular propagation in rats. *J. Physiol.* (Lond.). **149**: 1-22.

Kruger, P. (1929). Uber einen moglichen Zusammenhang Zwischen Struktur, Funktion und Chemischer Beschaffenheit der Muskelin. *Biol. Zbl.* **49**: 616-622.

Kuffler, S. W. and Vaughn Williams, E. M. (1953a). Small nerve junctional potentials. The distribution of small motor nerves to frog skeletal muscle, and the membrane characteristics of the fibers they innervate. *J. Physiol.* **121**: 289-317.

Kuffler, S. W. and Vaughn Williams, E. M. (1953b). Properties of the "slow" skeletal muscle fibers of the frog. *J. Physiol.* **121**: 318-340.

Lincoff, H. A., Ellis, C. H., DeVoe, A. G., DeBeer, E. J., Impastato, D. J., Berg, S., Orkin, L., and Magda, H. (1955). The effect of succinylcholine on intraocular pressure. *Amer. J. Ophthal.* **40**: 501-510.

Lincoff, H. A., Breinin, G. M., and DeVoe, A. G. (1957). The effect of succinylcholine on the extraocular muscles. *Amer. J. Ophthal.* **43**: 440-444.

Luco, J. V. and Sanchez, P. (1959). The effect of adrenaline and noradrenaline on the activity of denervated skeletal muscles. Antagonism between curare and adrenaline like substances. **In**: *Curare and Curare-like Agents,* Elsevier Publishing Co., Amsterdam. pp. 405-408.

Macri, F. J. and Grimes, P. A. (1957). The effects of succinylcholine on the extraocular striate muscles and on the intraocular pressure. *Amer. J. Ophthal.* **44**: 221-230.

Maddock, W. O., Rankin, V. M., and Youmans, W. B. (1948). Prevention of the anti-curare action of epinephrine by dibenamine. *Proc. Soc. Exp. Biol. Med.* **67**: 151-153.

Matyuskin, D. P. (1961). Phasic and tonic neuromotor units in the oculomotor apparatus of the rabbit. *Sechenov Physiol. J. U.S.S.R.* **47**: 65.

McIntyre, A. R. (1965). Curare and related compounds. **In**: *Drill's Pharmacology in Medicine,* ed. by J. R. Di Palma, McGraw-Hill Book Co. New York, pp. 545-558.

Montague, K. A. (1955). On the mechanism of action of adrenaline in skeletal nerve muscle. *J. Physiol.* (Lond.). **128**: 619-628.

Panella, A. (1907). Action du principe actif surrenal sur la fatigue musculaire. *Arch. Ital. Biol.* **48**: 430-463.

Pelikan, E. W., Tether, J. E., and Unna, K. R. (1953). Sensitivity of myasthenia gravis patients to tubocurarine and decamethonium. *Neurology.* **3**: 284-296.

Pilar, G. (1967). Further study of the electrical and mechanical responses of slow fibers in cat extraocular muscle. *J. Gen. Physiol.* **50**: 2289-2300.

Rosenblueth, A. Lindsley, D. B., and Morison, R. S. (1936). A study of some decurarizing substances. *Amer. J. Physiol.* **115**: 53-68.

Sanghvi, I. S. (1967). Effects of cholinergic and adrenergic agents and their antagonists at the neuromuscular junction of the cat extraocular muscles. *Invest. Ophthal.* **6**: 269-276.

Sanghvi, I. S. and Smith, C. M. (1969). Characterization of stimulation of mammalian extraocular muscles by cholinomimetics. *J. Pharmacol. Exp. Therap.* **167**: 351-364.

Smith, S. M., Brown, H. O., Toman, J. E. P., and Goodman, L. S. (1947). Lack of cerebral effects of d-tubocurarine. *Anesthesiology.* **8**: 1-14.

Sommerkamp, H. (1928). Das Substrat der Dauerverkurzung am Froschmuskel. (Physiologische und pharmakologische Sonderstellung bestimmter Muskelfasern). *Arch. exp. Path. Pharmakol.* **128**: 99-115.

Wilson, A. T. and Wright, S. (1937). Anti-curare effect of potassium and some other substances. *Quart. J. Exp. Physiol.* **26**: 127-139.

Wolter, J. R. (1955). Morphology of the sensory nerve apparatus in the striated muscle of the human eye. *A.M.A. Arch. Ophthal.* **53**: 201.

EYE MOVEMENTS AND PERCEPTION

LEON FESTINGER

My task, at the end of the day, seems to be to summarize and explain how eye movements affect the input to the visual system and how these movements affect the use that is made of visual information. In short, what do eye movements have to do with what a person sees?

There are some aspects of this overwhelmingly large question that are almost trivial. Certainly, if the eye is in a position such that a given array of light does not enter through the pupil to reach the retina, there is no input of information and no corresponding visual perception. The eye can be moved to change what does, and, what does not, impinge on the retina. But this function of eye movements is rather unimportant. For a person with a normal binocular field of view it is perhaps surprising how little eye movements alone can shift and extend this field. Head rotations are much more important for this function. But it is perhaps necessary to keep in mind that head and eye movements can substitute for each other in part and that, normally, large rotations are a relatively precise combination of head and eye.

Another obvious function of eye movements is to bring stimulation from the periphery of the retina, where acuity is poor, to the fovea, where acuity is good. These eye movements, saccadic in nature, can be executed with a high degree of precision. How precise the usual saccade is has not been too adequately investigated. There are some indications, however, that frequently they are no more precise than is necessary to obtain the required information.

The best evidence I know of is reported by Leushina. His observers looked at a fixation point until another light appeared in the visual field. This other light always appeared in one of two positions and the observer had to identify whether this light appeared in position A or position B. Leushina (1965) measured, among other things, the latency of the eye movement from the fixation point to the light when it appeared. Position A was always 20° from the fixation point. For a block of trials, position B was also constant and the observer knew what that position was. From one block of trials to another, however, position B was varied so that it was farther away or closer to position A. He reports data on eye movements when the position A light appeared in all conditions so that we are comparing identical situations. The only difference among conditions is where position B was.

His results are straightforward. When the angular separation between positions A and B is 10°, the eye movement latency is about 320 milliseconds. When the angular separation is 5°, this latency increases to about 380 milliseconds. When the separation is only 2°, the latency goes up to almost 480 milliseconds. He further reports on the accuracy of the eye movements, comparing two conditions, one in which the angular separation of positions A and B was 6° and one in which it was 2°. In the latter condition, the standard deviation of the eye movements was less than half of that in the first condition. In short, the finer the discrimination that has to be made, the more precise is the eye movement and the longer is its latency.

It is interesting to note that the more precise the saccade has to be, the longer is the latency of that saccade. It seems as though it takes some time to retrieve, or perhaps formulate, the efferent program for the saccade execution. The sloppier the program, the more quickly it can be put together. The more precise, the longer it takes. We shall have much more to say later about these hypothesized efferent programs. At this point, however, I would just like to point out one other thing. The adult human is primarily able to move his eyes so as to bring stimulation from the periphery to the fovea. Other kinds of eye movements cannot be executed or are executed with great difficulty and rather inaccurately. If one asks an observer, for example, to move his eye from some initial point of fixation to, say, 10 degrees to the left of some other point in the visual field, he finds it very difficult to do. If the two points mentioned are the only distinguishable points in the field, it is well nigh impossible. Regardless of the question of whether these efferent programs are innate or must be learned, only a very small proportion of all possible efferent programs for eye movements exist and are available for use. We will refer to this again later.

EYE MOVEMENTS AND INFORMATION INPUT

Of considerably greater interest, because of its implications for theories about visual information input, is the problem of the relation between perception and the continual small eye movements that are frequently referred to as normal nystagmus. Quite a bit of research has been directed to the question of what happens to visual perception if these small tremors, minor drifts and small saccadic flicks are eliminated. The results of this research are clear and rather unambiguous. If, by means of an optical system, precise correction is made on the retina for any eye movement (thus producing a situation identical on the retina to what would exist if the eye itself were entirely motionless) then the "stabilized image" fades and disappears after a few seconds. Many researchers have reported reappearances and re-disappearances but the presumption, supported by data, is that these reappearances are due to faulty stabilization. If stabilization is perfect one would expect the stabilized image to disappear and never reappear.

One can, of course, make the stabilized image reappear by destroying the stabilization on the retina or, similarly, by moving the physical stimulus itself. One can also cause the stabilized image to reappear by flickering the light source. In other words, it appears from this research that change of stimulation at the retina is necessary for sustained visual perception. If there is no change of stimulation, vision ceases to be an effective source of input after a few seconds.

How are these facts to be understood theoretically? The simplest assumption that suggests itself is that the visual system transmits information only about changes that occur and not about steady states. If a photoreceptor, or group of them, are stimulated by light, information is transmitted briefly to the central nervous system. Following this brief transmission, no more information flows until there is a change in stimulation of those particular photoreceptors. The central nervous system, on the other hand, must receive this one bit of news about something that has happened on the retina, store it, and assume that it remains the same until there is another bit of news. But, for stabilized images to fade and disappear quickly, one must also assume that this central nervous system storage is effective for only a few seconds.

It is consistent with the above view that visual disappearance can be produced in ways other than stabilizing a retinal image. If, for example, the visual field of view were made entirely and completely uniform, then eye movements would be unimportant and irrelevant since these movements would not cause any changes to occur on the retina. And, indeed, under such conditions, color and brightness fade in a few seconds and the entire visual field becomes a foggy "night grey". Some observers report even experiencing "blankout" under these circumstances. That is, they experience complete loss of visual experience altogether. This, of course, occurs regardless of eye movements.

One need not even have a completely contourless field for disappearance to occur. If the contour edges are blurred so that there are only gradual intensity gradients on the retina, and if the observer maintains reasonably steady fixation (eliminating large eye movements but *not* eliminating the normal nystagmus) the image will also disappear. In other words, if the eye movements that occur do not cause appreciable changes in stimulation on the retina, information input is inadequate for maintaining visual perception.

If, indeed, the visual system only transmits information about changes that occur on the retina, this has strong implications for our views of normal visual perception. Let us imagine, for example, an observer who restricts his eye movements to small saccades around the center of a large (perhaps 20 degrees of visual angle) circle that has clear sharp contours. There are, of course, no disappearances under these conditions. Visual perception is adequately maintained. But what we have said above implies that no information is being transmitted from that region of the retina stimulated by the center of the circle. We have implied that information is only transmitted from the area stimulated by the contour edge where small eye movements are sufficient to cause sharp changes of stimulation on various retinal receptors. But, since the middle of the circle does not fade, does not appear dimmer than the area near the contour edge, we must assume that the central nervous system interpolates between the contours and assumes a level of stimulation of uniform intensity between the areas from which information is being received.

Data reported by Yarbus (1967) and confirmed by Gerrits (1967) support this kind of view. Yarbus, in essence, presented to the observer an achromatic, retinally stabilized, small circle on a non-stabilized coloured large square. After a very few seconds the stabilized circle fades and disappears, of course. The interesting question is, however, what is the perception of the observer following this disappearance? The observer does *not* see an empty hole in the colored square. What he sees is simple a uniformly colored square. The stabilized circle that disappeared is filled in with the color of the non-stabilized background. How can this happen? Obviously no information concerning the color is transmitted from that part of the retina on which the stabilized image falls since the stabilized image is achromatic. Also, it is clear that since the contour of the stabilized image has disappeared, that information is no longer transmitted. What must, then, occur is that information is transmitted at the contour edge of the non-stabilized square and that the visual system assumes uniformity between the contour edges. This assumption of uniformity produces the visual perception of a uniformly colored square.

To summarize, we may say that the visual system only transmits information about change of intensity or change of color. If the eyes were immobile (the head and body also being immobile) one would only see things that moved or physically changed in intensity or color. Eye movements are necessary to maintain information input.

INFORMATION ABOUT EYE MOVEMENTS

Thus far we have discussed the importance of eye movements for information input about retinal stimulation. It is also important for visual perception that the central nervous system be provided with information about the eye movements themselves. For example, without information about eye movements, the observer would be sometimes unable to distinguish between movement on the retina produced by an eye movement and retinal change produced by movement in the physical world. Similarly, without information about eye position the observer would be unable to determine the position of an object in the physical world with respect to himself. Since we can, and do, easily perceive both egocentric localization of objects and the difference between movement in the physical world and eye movements, this information is obviously available. The question is what is the nature of this information?

Helmholtz (1962) proposed that there is information directly provided about the efferent output to the extraocular muscles. He based this assertion on several observations. Take a person who, through some accident, suffers a paralysis of, say, the external rectus muscle of the right eye. Occlude the left eye and instruct the person to move his eyes to the right. The person tries to do this but, because of the paralysis, the open eye remains stationary. Under these circumstances the person reports that he perceives the entire visual world to move to the right. In other words, he perceives as if he had moved the open eye and the pattern of retinal stimulation remained unchanged. Helmholtz reasoned that, for this perception to occur, the person must have information about the efference issued to the extraocular muscles.

Similarly, Helmholtz (1962) points out that if the eye moves voluntarily, the visual world remains stationary. If, however, the eye is moved by pressing on the sclera with one's finger, the world is seen to jump. On the other hand, if an after-image is formed on the retina the situation is reversed. Voluntary eye movements produce the perception of movement of the after-image while externally produced eye movements produce the perception of a stationary after-image. The arguments in favor of the Helmholtz proposal seem strong.

Nevertheless, for several decades the James-Sherrington (James, 1950; Sherrington, 1900) view that there was no such information based on efference prevailed. Within the last twenty years, however, the Helmholtz view has been strongly reasserted. Von Holst (1954), for example, argued strongly that the existence of "efference copy" is necessary to distinguish between change produced by self movement and change produced by movement in the physical world. Perhaps the most dramatic demonstration arguing for the existence of information about efference was provided by Brindley and Merton (1960). They anesthetized the eyelids and sclera of their subjects and placed an opaque cap over the cornea. They could then, with plastic forceps, seize hold of the tendon of the medial muscle and move the eye back and forth mechanically. The subject was unaware that his eye was moving. If the eye was mechanically held motionless and the subject was told to move the eye, the subject felt that his eye moved. The conclusion is that there is no conscious information about eye position based on proprioceptive input from the extraocular muscles. Conscious information that does exist must, hence, be due to information about the efferent output.

We need not become involved for our present purposes in the question of whether or not any proprioceptive information about eye position from the extraocular muscles exists at all. If some such information does exist, then we know from Brindley and Merton (1960) that the person is not aware of it. But such information might still exist and be used. It seems clear, however, that there does exist information about efference.

Festinger and Canon (1965) provided additional evidence on this matter. Their study was based on the expectation that the efferent information about an executed saccade would be different from that about an executed smooth tracking motion of the eye. The functional difference between these two kinds of eye movements is well demonstrated by Rashbass (1961). Since a saccade is most likely ballistic in nature, the efferent program necessary to order the execution of the saccade must contain in it the information about where the eye moves to, either in absolute terms or, at least, in terms relative to the prior position of the eye. Hence, information about this efferent program that ordered the saccade provides knowledge about the resulting eye position, at least assuming that the prior eye position was known. Thus, even in the absence of other cues, egocentric localization of a point in space should be good after fixating that point using a saccadic eye movement.

On the other hand, efferent information about a smooth tracking eye movement might contain little information about the end position of the eye. If this tracking motion is, as Rashbass (1961) asserts, a direction and velocity matching movement, then information based on these efferent commands need not contain accurate information about where the eye is. There might be very little information about this or there might be a fair amount but it seems plausible to expect a difference in the accuracy of egocentric localization of a point in space depending on whether the eye fixates it with a smooth tracking or a saccadic eye movement.

The Festinger and Canon (1965) data show this to be the case. If the head is held motionless, observers point more accurately to a target if the eye executed a saccade than if the eye followed the target smoothly to that place. The observer is of course in darkness and without sight of the hand that points. Thus, these data also provide evidence that there is information about eye position based on efference. If, in the above experimental situation the head is free to move, the difference in accuracy of pointing after saccadic or smooth tracking eye movements disappears. Clearly, proprioceptive information about head movements is good enough and accurate enough to substitute for a relative lack of accurate efferent information.

If we accept the proposition that information about eye position based on efferent programs exists, then questions concerning the nature of these programs and the way the retina is calibrated become important. We can only speculate about this. A kind of calibration system that seems simple and plausible was suggested as early as 1852 by Lotze. One can imagine the center of the fovea as a zero point in the calibration system. Each point on the retina can then be represented by two cartesian coordinates. The precision of calibration need only match the precision of eye movements, limiting the number of points which need to be represented. The efferent instruction from the central nervous system need only command the eye to move so that point x_1y_1 is transferred to point zero, zero on the retina. This, when executed, represents a fixation movement of the eye which, as we have previously noted, is the only saccadic movement that is performed with ease.

Thus, the set of efferent programs for eye movements can represent a not too complicated array. It is true that the actual muscle contractions necessary to produce this eye movement will differ depending on the position of the eyeball at the time. One can imagine, however, that this information is computed into the more general efferent instruction at more peripheral levels. We need also not concern ourselves with the question of whether these efferent programs are learned or are inherently built into the organism. If they are learned, it is easy to see how this learning can occur. Under ordinary circumstances, for stationary objects in the physical world, there is a perfect correlation between eye movement and movement of stimulation across the retina. In such a stable world, the learning of the proper efferent programs would not be too difficult.

I have devoted a small amount of time to these speculations about the generality and nature of the efferent programs for eye movements that emanate from the central nervous system, even though it seems remote from the question of perception, because it really is intimately tied into that question. As I will attempt to show in the remainder of this paper, the perception of contour, shape, distance and depth, is probably heavily dependent on the existence of, and activation of, these efferent programs for eye, head and body movements.

EFFERENT PROGRAMS AND PERCEPTION

The impetus for considering the effect of the efferent system on perception came from work on the adaptation of humans to optical distortions of the visual world. In fragmentary form this work goes back quite a way. Helmholtz (1962), for example, reported adapting to the displacement of the visual world produced by looking through a wedge prism. He reports that pointing to an object is initially grossly in error. Very quickly, however, the error is overcome and the person learns to point accurately. He furthermore reports that if this learning is done, say, using the right hand, it transfers to the left hand. Incidentally, it took nearly a century for this to be restudied. Harris (1963) found that Helmholtz was not entirely correct. The adaptation does occur quickly but if the head is held immobile during practice there is little or no transfer to the other hand. As Hamilton (1964) showed, transfer occurs only if the head is free. Helmholtz (1962) made no observations about perception here or about the process of adaptation or about what was adapting. Harris presents highly convincing arguments that the end result of the adaptation process is a change in the felt position of the arm that practiced the pointing. Visual perception, in this case a question of egocentric localization, did not seem to change.

This phenomenon has recently come to be called "visual capture". Perhaps one of the most dramatic examples of such visual capture was first noticed by Gibson (1933) and subsequently by others (Festinger, *et al.*[1967], Harris [1965]). If an observer wears spectacles with wedge prisms in them, bases to the right let us say, physically straight vertical edges appear curved. If the observer, looking at this retinally curved edge, runs his fingers up and down pressing against it, the .hand *feels* that it moves in a curve even though the physical movement is, of necessity, straight. This occurs even though the observer knows that the edge is actually straight. Why and how this occurs is, of course, an interesting and important question to which we shall return.

Another major line of inquiry dates back to Stratton (1897) who was concerned with whether or not one could re-invert an optically inverted visual world. On one occasion he wore such a monocular inverting device (the other eye occluded, of course) for as long as eight days. His reports are somewhat ambiguous but one can reasonably infer that he gradually learned motor adjustments. The visual world, in the sense of visual perception, remained inverted.

ere studies following his that were not of great importance. For ,le, Ewert (1930) had observers wear a binocular inverting optical system 4 to 19 days and reported little significant adaptation at all. Their system, owever, also functioned as a pseudoscope reversing depth and distance cues binocularly, and the lack of adaptation may have been due to the enormous complexity introduced in this manner and the consequent relative lack of physical activity on the part of the wearers.

Erisman and Kohler (reported by Kohler [1964]) gave a new impetus to research on such problems. What provided the impetus was Kohler's report of occasional instances of complete adaptation of perception for persons wearing an inverting optical system and for persons wearing wedge prism spectacles for several days. In Kohler's reports there is no question of whether or not the adaptation was simply motor adaptation. It was clearly a change in visual perception. For example, in connection with the wearing of wedge prism spectacles, he reports that one observer completely adapted to the optically induced curvature and physically straight lines looked straight again. On taking the spectacles off, the visual world was as distorted, for this observer, as it had been when he initially started wearing the spectacles. Kohler also reported instances of conditional adaptation that implied enormous plasticity of visual perception. Perhaps the most startling report of adaptation was made by Taylor (1962), who, for a time, worked with Kohler. He reports that one person wore left-right reversing spectacles part of the time for a few days. During other hours of the day his vision was undistorted. After only a few days, he reports, this observer had developed a perfect conditional adaptation. For example, the claim is made that while riding a bicycle he could put the spectacles on and take them off without interfering with the motor activity and *without altering his visual perception.*

Later workers have not been able to obtain such dramatic results. For example, Pick and May (1964) had nine observers wear wedge prism spectacles for 42 days and found, after that period, only 30% adaptation, on the average, to the prismatically induced curvature. These less dramatic reports are still impressive enough. Certainly they require theoretical explanation. The major theoretical proposals all have elements of similarity among them. The efferent system is important in all.

Held (1961) developed ideas originally proposed by von Holst (1954) concerning the matching of afferent input with efferent copy. When an optical distortion is introduced, the normal correlation of these two is disturbed. The process of adaptation is, for Held (1961), the establishment of new correlations between afference and efferent copy. Testing these ideas experimentally, Held and his coworkers (Held and Freedman, 1963; Held and Rekosh, 1963) have shown that self produced movement is necessary for adaptation to occur. Passive movement does not lead to adaptation to the optical distortion. Others (see Rock, 1966) attempting to repeat these studies, have frequently found some adaptation in their "passive" conditions but usually active movement led to greater adaptation. The demonstration by Howard *et al.* (1965) that adaptation occurs with a passive observer watching a stick move toward him and hit him, leads to a questioning of the concept of what is passive. There is, however, undoubtedly some validity in Held's theory.

Held, however, did not attempt to account for visual perception itself. He only tried to specify some of the conditions that enable the process of adaptation to occur. Taylor (1962) proposed a much more ambitious theory that not only explains adaptation but also attempts to specify the determinants of visual perception. Taylor states that, as a result of learning, engrams are established which essentially consist of the appropriate motor responses for almost any constellation of inputs. In other words, the person has learned a variety of efferent programs and has established a system whereby a given input selects the appropriate efferent program. Taylor further proposes that the totality of engrams brought into play at any moment by the visual input constitutes the conscious experience of visual perception. Visual perception, then, does not consist of some organization of visual input but consists rather of some organization of efferent programs activated by that input.

Festinger, Burnham, Ono and Bamber (1967), elaborated somewhat on the theory proposed by Taylor (1962). The main aspect of this elaboration was to introduce the concept of efferent readiness. Obviously, visual perception cannot be said to depend upon efferent programs actually issued to the motor system since one can perceive contours and shapes, for example, without movement of the eyes, head, limbs or body. If the efferent system determines visual perception in the manner suggested by Taylor (1962), it must be the availability for use of the efferent programs that is important rather than their actual use. The idea, then, is that the visual input acts to bring an appropriate variety of efferent programs into a state of readiness for use. Presumably, visual input corresponding to a curve on the retina would bring into readiness the efferent programs that, if issued, would direct the eye to fixate any part of that contour. In attempting to specify this somewhat, these authors say:

> "Without trying to speculate about the exact physiological mechanisms and arrangements, it seems plausible to imagine that the physical system is limited in the number of sets of stored preprogrammed instructions that can be 'immediately' sent out through the motor pathways. Thus, out of the very large number of sets of efferent instructions that the organism has learned, only some are held in readiness for immediate use. Without intending any precise analogy, we could imagine a jukebox which, at the push of the appropriate button, will immediately play any of a hundred different phonograph records. The owner of the jukebox could also have many thousands of other records available but, obviously, they cannot be played immediately. The owner could, however, with a little bit of work, change the entire set, or part of the set, of the hundred records that are immediately available for playing. One might think of these hundred records as being 'ready for immediate use.'

"If we are to think of the conscious experience of visual perception as being *determined by* these preprogrammed sets of efferent instructions that are activated into readiness by the afferent input, then it is necessary to specify something about the level of generality or specificity of the efferent signals that are issued from the central nervous system. If, using an efference readiness theory of visual perception, we are to be able to have a person perceive a given shape or contour as the same no matter what the eye position is when viewing it, it seems necessary to specify that the efferent instructions issued from the central nervous system must be general in nature, that is, relatively far removed from the final signal that causes the exact muscle twitch. Thus, the efferent signal from the central nervous system could be concerned only with direction and magnitude of deviation from the fovea, and final computation to effectuate the actual muscle contractions could take account of afferent information at more peripheral levels." (p. 12).

It is rather easy to see why the attempt to explain adaptation to optical distortion has led persons in the direction of this kind of efferent readiness theory. To the extent that the adaptation is not simply the learning of new muscular movements but is also accompanied by change in visual perception itself, one must have some way of dealing with it. It is clear from the data that motor activity is important in producing such change in visual perception. Theoretically one is left with a choice between two types of explanations. Let us take the result of one experiemnt to illustrate the point. Cohen (1963) had observers look through wedge prisms at lines that were physically curved so that the retinal image was straight. They of course perceived straight lines. If the head was held motionless, no change in visual perception occurred, that is, no adaptation. If the head was free to move during the inspection period then there was adaptation. The retinally straight line began to look somewhat curved.

Given the necessity for head movements to produce adaptation in this experiment, there are only two main types of explanation that seem possible. In both one must place a major and precise role on information about efference. One can assert that new efferent programs had to be learned to execute accurate head movements and, hence, a change in perception took place. One could alternatively assert that errors of head movement provided information on the basis of which the coding system for the visual input itself was changed. The second alternative is more similar to the Held (1961) theory and the first alternative more in the vein of the Taylor (1962) and Festinger, *et al.* (1967) theories. To the writer the efferent readiness theory seems simpler and has an easier job of explaining the data that exist.

Let us imagine, then, that change in visual perception occurs if there is a change in the efferent programs that are brought into readiness for use by the afferent visual input. Thinking along these lines makes it immediately clear why the amount of visual adaptation to curvature that is generally found is so small. It will be recalled that Pick and Hay (1964) found an average of only 30%

adaptation to prismatically induced curvature for observers who wore prism spectacles continuously for 42 days. It is clear that, when wearing prism spectacles, eye movements to fixate one or another part of the visual field must conform to the retinal image and consequently there is no learning of new efferent programs for eye movements. Body, limb and head movements in this situation must conform to the physical contours in the real world and hence new efferent programs must be formulated for these movements. The change that does occur in the perception of contour depends then on the efferent readiness for bodily movements and not on the efferent readiness for eye movement. Since it is plausible to imagine that efferent programs for eye movements have a lot to do with visual perception, low amounts of adaptation to curvature might be expected.

Taylor (1962), of course, realized this. He reasoned that if the prisms that produced the curvature distortions were mounted on the eyeball itself rather than on the head, then eye movements also would have to correspond to the physical world and not to the retinal image. Under these circumstances large amounts of change in visual perception should occur since new efferent programs for eye movements would also have to be learned. To test this, Taylor had a scleral contact lens specially fitted for his right eye. The contact lens carried a 12 diopter wedge prism. Taylor did not collect data systematically but he reports that, with his left eye occluded, he quickly achieved 100% adaptation to the prismatically induced curvature. The prism used by Taylor produced very little curvature distortion, however, and the report does not constitute strong evidence.

Festinger, Burnham, Ono and Bamber (1967) report on a series of experiments intended to test these theoretical ideas more precisely. They attempted to create experimental conditions in which the afferent input from bodily movement would be constant but which differed in terms of whether or not new efferent programs had to be learned. They reasoned that if efferent readiness were important, changes in the visual perception of contour would occur primarily when new efferent programs were learned and not as a function of the afferent input. They used arm movements rather than eye movements in these experiments but, nevertheless, they are worth reporting on briefly. All these experiments were of the following form. The observer wears prism spectacles and looks at a line oriented so as to yield curvature distortion. The head is immobilized and the only relevant bodily movements are arm movements, that is, the observer moves his arm (or stylus in his hand) along the line. In one condition guidance is provided for the arm so that no new efferent programs need be learned. In another experimental condition the guidance is not provided so that the observer must learn to issue new efferent instructions. That is, he must learn to issue instructions to the arm to move in a straight line, say, when he sees a curve. In both conditions since the arm moves in the same path approximately, the afferent input is the same. In all three experiments that they report, they find adaptation to the prismatically induced curvature distortion primarily in the conditions where new efference had to be learned. The effects are significant although very small. But perhaps only very small effects should be expected on visual perception of contour from a change in efferent readiness for arm movement alone.

The same investigators also repeated Taylor's work with prisms on contact lenses using more systematic measurement and using prisms that produced greater curvature distortion. Specifically, they had 30 diopter prisms on scleral contact lenses fitted for the right eyes of three subjects. The only experience these observers ever had with the prism in their eye (left eye occluded, of course) was with the head immobilized in a biteboard and the entire visual field occupied by a rather uniform white surface with a horizontal line on it (the prisms were all base downward and so curvature distortion existed for horizontal lines). All the subject did was to move his eyes back and forth, scanning the horizontal line. It should be remembered that under these conditions the eye, to maintain fixation on the line, must move in accordance with the objective contour and, hence, new efferent programs must be learned. The results show that after 30 to 40 minutes of such scanning considerable adaptation to the prismatically induced curvature has occurred. If the line is objectively curved to exactly compensate for the prism so that the line is retinally (and apparently) straight, there is about 20% adaptation. If the line is objectively straight and apparently curved, the amount of adaptation after this brief period is more than 40%.

Slotnick (1969) explored this matter further with appropriate experimental comparisons. Recalling the difference between saccadic eye movements and smooth tracking eye movements, he reasoned as follows: If the observer, wearing the prism contact lens, has to scan the line with saccadic eye movements, he must, of course, learn new efferent programs. If, however, he scans the line with a smooth tracking eye movement, there is no necessity for such new learning. Hence, even though in both these conditions the eye movements will cover roughly the same course, there should be large differences in the changes that occur in the visual perception of contour if the efferent readiness theory is valid. His saccadic eye movement condition is quite similar to that reported above. To produce a smooth tracking eye movement condition he provided a small spot that moved back and forth regularly along the lines. The subject was instructed to follow the spot. The results are rather conclusive. Little or no adaptation to the curvature was obtained when the eye engaged in smooth tracking movements. In the saccadic eye movement conditions changes comparable to those reported by Festinger, *et al.* (1967) were found.

The data that exist tend to support an efference readiness theory of the visual perception of contour. The visual input activates a wide variety of efferent programs into a state of readiness for use. The efferent programs involve eye movements, head movements, arm movements and the like. If new efferent programs are learned, and these new, different, programs are brought into readiness by the visual input, then there is a difference in the visual perception.

VISUAL ILLUSIONS

If, indeed, visual perception is determined by the organization of efferent readiness activated by visual input, one immediately raises the question of whether or not this conception is able to deal with the facts of the visual illusions. Presumably these illusions would exist because somehow or other incorrect efferent programs are activated by the visual input. Evidence about this should be obtainable.

We will confine ourselves here to considering the well known Müller-Lyer illusion because more work has been done on it than on others and more is, hence, known about it. There are a number of theories that have been proposed about why the illusion exists, although none of these theories seems entirely adequate by itself. Whatever the correct explanation, if the efferent system is implicated in the existence of the illusion, it should be observable in eye movements that are made. That this is the case has been known for a long time. Judd (1905) measured eye movements of observers who were asked to move their eyes from apex to apex of the illusion figure. The eye movements were too short on the illusory short side and too long on the illusory long side of the figure. This result has been confirmed by Festinger, White and Allyn (1968).

This by itself, of course, does not tell us whether the efferent readiness produces the illusion or whether the illusion produces the incorrect eye movements. There is further evidence, however. It is known that with continued observation there occurs a decrement in the magnitude of the illusion. If the efferent system is involved as we suspect, one could reason that with continued observation the eye movements that are in error tend to be corrected. That is, more correct efferent programs are formulated. This would then lead to a decrement of the illusion. Festinger, White and Allyn (1968) have shown this to be true. With continued observation of the illusion the error in eye movement becomes smaller. McLaughlin, *et al.*(1969) report that they have confirmed this in their laboratory, although they reject the efferent readiness explanation.

Again, of course, the result is not definitive. The illusion could change because of change in eye movements or vice versa. But one can appeal to more data. One can reason that, if the efferent programs must be altered in order to obtain decrement in the magnitude of the illusion, then an observer who fixates one spot on the figure during inspection without moving his eyes should not show decrement in the illusion and the eye movements should not become more accurate. Festinger, White and Allyn (1968) showed this to be the case. Furthermore, one can reason that if the efferent readiness theory is correct, inspection of the illusion with smooth tracking eye movements only should not result in decrement of the illusion. Burnham (1968) has shown this implication also to be correct. It seems likely that eye movements are important in the visual illusions.

SUMMARY

The topic of eye movement and perception covers a very large area and, in this amount of time, one can cover it only superficially. Eye movements serve a variety of functions such as:

1. Acquisition of a source of visual input.
2. Maintaining the flow of information input through the visual system.
3. Providing information about direction and egocentric localization of objects.
4. Providing the basis for the organization that results in visual perception of contours, shape and distance.

REFERENCES

Brindley, G.S. & Merton, P.A. (1960). The absence of position sense in the human eye. *J. Physiol.* **153,** 127-130.

Burnham, C.A. (1968). Decrement of the Müller-Lyer illusion with saccadic and tracking eye movements. *Perception and Psychophysics,* **3,** 424-426.

Cohen, M. (1963). Visual curvature and feedback factors in the production of prismatically induced curved-line after-effects. Paper presented at the Eastern Psychological Association, New York.

Ewert, P.H. (1930). A study of the effect of inverted retinal stimulation upon spatially coordinated behavior. *Genetic Psychology Monographs,* **7,** 177-363.

Festinger, L. Burnham, C.A., Ono, H. & Bamber, D. (1967). Efference and the conscious experience of perception. *J. Exp. Psychol.,* Monograph Supplement **74,** (4, Whole No. 637).

Festinger, L. & Canon, L.K. (1965). Information about spatial location based on knowledge about efference. *Psychol. Rev.* **72,** 373-384.

Festinger, L., White, C.W. & Allyn, M.R. (1968). Eye movements and decrements in the Muller-Lyer illusion. *Perception and Psychophysics,* **3,** 376-382.

Gerrits, H.J.M. (1967). *Observations with Stabilized Retinal Images and their Neural Correlates.* Doctoral dissertation, Catholic University of Nijmegen, Nijmegen, The Netherlands.

Gibson, J.J. (1933). Adaptation, after-effect, and contrast in the perception of curved lines. *J. Exp. Psychol.* **16,** 1-31.

Hamilton, C.R. (1964). Intermanual transfer of adaptation to prisms. *Am. J. Psychol.* **77,** 457-462.

Harris, C.S. (1963). Adaptation to displace vision: visual, motor or proprioceptive change? *Science* **140,** 812-813.

Harris, C.S. (1965). Perceptual adaptation to inverted, reversed, and displaced vision. *Psychol. Rev.* **72,** 419-444.

Held, R. (1961). Exposure-history as a factor in maintaining stability of perception and coordination. *J. Nerv. Ment. Dis.* **132,** 26-32.

Held, R. & Freedman, S.J. (1963). Plasticity in human sensorimotor control. *Science* **142,** 455-462.

Held, R. & Rekosh, J. (1963). Motor-sensory feedback and the geometry of visual space. *Science* **141,** 722-723.

Helmholtz, H. von (1962). *Treatise on Physiological optics.* vol 3. (Trans. by J.P.C. Southall), New York: Dover.

HOLST, E. VON (1954). Relations between the central nervous system and peripheral organs. *Brit. J. Animal Behavior* **2,** 89-94.
HOWARD, I.P., CRASKE, B. & TEMPLETON, W.B. (1965). Visuo-motor adaptation to discordant ex-afferent stimulation. *J. Exp. Psychol.* **70,** 189-191.
JAMES, W. (1950). *Principles of Psychology*. vol. 2. New York: Dover.
JUDD, C.H. (1905). The Muller-Lyer illusion. *Psychol. Rev.* **7,** (Monograph supplement, Whole No. 29). 55-81.
KOHLER, I. (1964). The formation and transformation of the perceptual world. (Trans. by H. Fiss.) *Psychol. Issues,* **3,** (4).
LEUSHINA, L.I. (1965). On estimation of position of photostimulus and eye movements. *Biofizika,* **10,** 130-136.
LOTZE, R.H. (1852). *Medicinische Psychologie oder Physiologie der Seele*. Leipzig: Weidmannische Buchhandlung.
McLAUGHLIN, S.C., DESISTO, M.J. & KELLY, M.J. (1969). Comments on 'Eye movements and decrement in the Müller-Lyer illusion'. *Perception and Psychophysics,* **5,** 288.
PICK, H.L. & HAY, J.C. (1964). Adaptation to prismatic distortion. *Psychonomic Science,* **1,** 199-200.
RASHBASS, C. (1961). The relation between saccadic and smooth tracking eye movements. *J. Physiol.* **159,** 326-338.
ROCK, I. (1966). *The Nature of Perceptual Adaptation*. New York, Basic Books.
SHERRINGTON, C.S. (1960). The muscular sense. **In:** E.A. Schafer (Ed.), *A Textbook of Physiology*. Edinburgh and London: Pentland.
SLOTNICK, R.S. (1969). Adaption to curvature distortion. *J. Exp. Psychol.* **81,** 441-448.
STRATTON, G.M. (1897). Vision without inversion of the retinal image. *Psychol. Rev.* **4,** 341-360; 463-481.
TAYLOR, J.G. (1962). *The Behavioral Basis of Perception*. New Haven: Yale University Press.
YARBUS, A.L. (1967). *Eye Movements and Vision*. (Trans. by B. Haigh). New York: Plenum Press.

PART II

THE HUMAN EYE MOVEMENT CONTROL SYSTEM

INTRODUCTION

GEORGE P. MOORE

No physiological system can surpass the incredible richness in phenomena or elegance of mechanism of the visual system either in its sensory capacities, motor capacities or in the intriguing relations and interdependence between its sensory and motor functions. Nor has research on any other system provided us with so much insight into the functional organization of the brain and its capacities for information processing, communication and control. And in no area of physiology has theoretical and mathematical modeling of system behavior achieved the successes of prediction and inference that we have seen in the study of the visual system.

Of course mathematical modeling is simply a quantitative extension of the normal cycle of hypothesis development, testing, validation and reformulation which is the hallmark of all scientific work (Platt, 1964), but its demands are often far more stringent and exacting than those of other styles of inferential technique. The contributors to this symposium on Modeling of Human Eye Movement Control are all scientists whose work not only meets the test of experimental and descriptive excellence but also has met the more demanding challenges of quantitative theoretical modeling. To many of them we owe a debt of gratitude, therefore, not only for their contributions to the empirical physiological descriptions of the visual system but also for their contributions to the theory of physiological modeling.

Styles in modeling tend to be of two basic types. The first style I will call deductive, the second inductive, in the hopes that this somewhat artificial distinction will serve to clarify the strengths, weaknesses, and contributions of each of the several rather different styles of work which characterize the contributions to this symposium.

The first, or deductive style of mathematical model starts from measurable experimental variables and attempts to formulate a mathematical structure which summarizes the quantitative properties of the experimental results themselves. Frequently this is a formal mathematical expression describing the way in which the system being studied responds to its input. When this expression has sufficient generality it can be used to predict the behavior of the system to any arbitrarily applied input. It is formal in the sense that it quantifies the relation between input and output without necessarily making reference to any physiological properties of the system. When the input and output of the system are both measurable (such an input-output pair of variables might be target position and eye position), and when the mathematical model can predict the one from the other, then its properties are, in this sense, equivalent to the properties of the real system. Such a mathematical expression (frequently in the form of a "transfer function") can then be studied independently to determine other properties which may not be readily apparent from observing the real system which usually exhibits rather restricted behavior in its natural environment. In favorable situations this type of mathematical model may then be used to make inferences about previously unobserved or unexplained physiological phenomena, and in this sense this modeling approach is deductive.

The governing mathematical expressions may be derived in several ways but one technique often used is to determine empirically the frequency-response of the system being studied by measuring the amplitude and phase of its output with respect to a sinusoidally varying input. This standard technique produces a "linear" mathematical model of the real system. The increasing use of this approach is partly a consequence of the fact that some systems appear to behave linearly over a considerable part of their natural dynamic range and partly due to the fact that many experimenters can find ways to linearize the behavior of systems artificially by various experimental techniques or data-processing distortions. Research in the next decade will continue to exploit this technique which, when successful, has enormous power for prediction. When linear models fail, other techniques can be utilized but the end result is still some minimal formal mathematical function which can be used to calculate the response of the system to arbitrarily chosen inputs or stimuli.

Larry Stark's mathematical treatment of the behavior of the pupil in response to light over a decade ago belongs to this style of approach, and indeed, for many of us, this work marks the beginning of the experimental cybernetic approach to living systems (Stark & Sherman, 1957; Stark & Cornsweet, 1958). Not only were these and later experiments brilliant in their conception and choice of system for study, they excited a generation of students who still find in them a model of scientific elegance.

The original linear model was subsequently refined by Stark and others to include non-linear features of the pupillary system so that a tremendous range of behavior of the pupil in response to bizarre forms of stimuli could be predicted. Even more significantly the model itself was then used to predict an unusual physiological property of the pupillary system and the conditions for stimulus-induced hippus were predicted and verified (Stark, 1959; Stark & Baker, 1959). The model itself, by its very nature, did not make any reference to elementary properties of the nervous system, in fact made no direct reference to nerve or muscle.

Several years later I remember my own excitement on discovering that Derek Fender was utilizing the same basic transfer function techniques in the first mathematical studies of eye movement control (Fender & Nye, 1961). What was exciting was not only that he was extending the domain of interest of mathematical techniques to more complicated systems, but also that an integral part of this work dealt with the natural history of eye movement and began to suggest some properties of the component processes which previously had not been considered.

In the environment that pervaded these laboratories it is clear that theory, as always, was structuring and organizing empirical observations.* Without this, it is not possible for me to imagine how any observations of tracking movements of the eye could suggest the possibility that the visual system was acting like a sampling system. But the ideas of control systems theory led Larry Young, then a graduate student of Stark's, to postulate his then arcane Z-transform model of eye motions in response to randomly moving targets. The revolutionary consequence of his observations was a model that postulated a previously unsuspected physiological phenomenon, namely that information about target position is not continuously available to the nervous system for the formulation of motor command signals to the eye, but is only acted upon or "sampled" intermittently (Young & Stark, 1963a,b). I believe this disclosure of a physiological process is an unsurpassed achievement of the deductive style of modeling. Dr. Young contributes a review of the Pursuit System to this volume, while Dr. Albert Fuchs, whose own remarkable experiments (including those on eye movement in monkeys demonstrating their inability to show predictive behavior in tracking periodic targets) are well known (Fuchs, 1967, a,b), discusses the present status of models of saccadic movements.

As final examples of the deductive approach we mention the extension of the transfer function methods to the study of other motions of the eye: first the very beautiful work of Dr. Jacob Meiry (a pupil of Larry Young's and therefore the intellectual grandson of Dr. Stark) concerned with vestibulo-ocular relations (Meiry,1965). That work will be discussed by Dr. Melvill Jones whose contributions to the engineering systems approach to eye movement and the stabilization of the visual field are also well known (Jones, 1965). Secondly, we mention the work of Dr. Bert Zuber who, with Dr. Stark, has extended these methods to the study of vergence movements of the eye (Zuber & Stark, 1968). But in this context we must also acknowledge the vital contributions of Rashbass and Westheimer whose very beautiful earlier studies of these movements (Rashbass, 1961; Rashbass & Westheimer, 1961a,b) served to clarify their basic properties. Both Dr. Westheimer and Dr. Rashbass discuss models of eye movement control in this volume.

*A model of a system need not be correct to be useful. The follow-up servo model (Merton, 1953) of the peripheral neuromuscular system has been a powerful influence in spinal cord research for many years even though it has not been validated.

The second basic style in mathematical modeling, which I have called inductive, takes as its starting point detailed descriptions of component physiological processes, translates these into suitable quantitative statements, often using classical techniques of physics and mechanics, and arrives at a system of equations describing the set of component physiological processes believed to be the basis for an experimental observation. Often these models have the form of a set of simultaneous differential equations, and the coefficients of these equations (each of which may have direct physiological meaning) are either measured directly in an experiment or estimated computationally by minimizing the difference between the behavior of the model and the measurable behavior of the living system. Unlike the deductive approach which exploits experimental data to arrive at a formal mathematical model, this method exploits data to produce formal physiological models.

Carter Collins' work has this style, and this kind of model has great potential for clinicians because starting from these models, computer techniques are available which can proceed from some overall patient performance data to estimate detailed values of critical physiological variables, such as extraocular muscle stiffness, without recourse to direct measurements. The work of Dr. Collins and Dr. Alan Scott (Collins *et al.* 1969; Robinson *et al.* 1969) who both contribute to this volume, is of the utmost importance because it brings together the skill of the clinician (whose techniques can validate these models) with the skill of the physicist (whose techniques create models valid for future patients).

In this regard we again owe a great deal to the earlier work of Westheimer (1954, 1958) and others on orbital and muscular mechanics. David Robinson's earlier work is also of this character although, again subjectively, my excitement about his work results not only from his contributions to the mathematical modeling of component behavior of the extraocular muscles but also to the fact that when I first read his papers on the mechanics of eye movement (Robinson 1964, 1965) I realized I had never fully understood neuromuscular physiology and I became aware of the terrible fact that physiologists had intellectually separated muscles from nerves decades before modern neurophysiology emerged.*

I know of no other general area in physiology in which quantitative modeling has had such success as in the visual motor systems. Paradoxically, this has been achieved almost wholly without the use of computers which, because they liberate the theoretician from the burden of finding mathematical solutions to his model equations, have been the primary catalyst in the recent expansion of theoretical biology. The unique result is that these mathematical models have stimulated a whole group of neurophysiologists to search directly for sub-processes in the brain which underly or participate in the overall

*This would correspond to the distinction between real muscle physiology and the more widely practiced meat science.

processes such as sampling and saccadic suppression which have been predicted by the models. The experimental difficulties alone are enormous; but in addition we must also realize that since deductive models may make no reference to specific neuronal processes they may also give no clue as to what might be encountered at the neuronal level; and inductive models refer to the average behavior of a postulated neuronal group without necessarily implying that a single neuron would ever exhibit this behavior.

Indeed, I believe that some difficult experimental and theoretical problems will arise when we attempt to search for component behavior at the neuron level which has properties attributable to the system as a whole. For in fact the neurons of a performing network may never exhibit, singly, properties that would even suggest that they are part of a network of known functions, and our almost total ignorance of network physiology may lead us to discard observations on neurons that are part of system of interest. Conversely, I suppose it is also likely that we will become obsessed with other neurons whose responses are exactly what we hoped to find but which turn out to be irrelevant to the system being studied. Dr. Robinson explores some aspects of this problem in his contribution to this symposium.

In the limit, then, we come to the area in which many mathematical models of physiological systems---cardiorespiratory, endocrine, renal---abandon the struggle: in the neuronal networks of the brain which we are unable to model at a detailed physiological level because there is no physiology of nerve networks to base such a model on. But here, in this symposium volume, we can enjoy the rich results of that happy union of skilled experimentation and sophisticated theorizing that characterizes work of such outstanding quality that we can look to the future with optimism.

REFERENCES

Collins, C.C., Scott, A.B. and O'Meara, D.M. (1969). Elements of the peripheral oculomotor apparatus. *Amer. J. Optom.* **46,** 510-515.

Fender, D.H. and Nye, P.W. (1961). An investigation of the mechanisms of eye movement control. *Kybernetic* **1,** 81-88.

Fuchs, A.F. (1967). Saccadic and smooth pursuit eye movements in the monkey. *J. Physiol.* **191,** 609-631.

Fuchs, A.F. (1967). Periodic eye tracking in the monkey. *J. Physiol.* **193,** 161-171.

Jones, G.M. and Milsum, J.H. (1965). Spatial and dynamic aspects of visual fixation. *IEEE Transactions on Bio-Medical Engineering.* **BME-12,** 54-62.

Meiry J.L. (1965). *The Vestibular System and Human Dynamic Space Orientation.* Sc.D. Thesis, MIT.

Merton, P.A. (1953). Speculations on the servo-control of movement. **In:** *The Spinal Cord,* ed. Wolstenholme, G.E.W., 247-255, London, Churchill.

Platt, J.R. (1964). Strong inference. *Science* **146,** 347-353.

Rashbass, C. (1961). The relationship between saccadic and smooth tracking eye movements. *J. Physiol.* **159,** 326-338.

Rashbass, C. and Westheimer, G. (1961). Disjunctive eye movements. *J. Physiol.* **159,** 339-360.

RASHBASS, C. and WESTHEIMER, G. (1961). Independence of conjugate and disjunctive eye movements. *J. Physiol.* **159,** 361-364.

ROBINSON, D.A. (1964). The mechanics of human saccadic eye movement. *J. Physiol.* **174,** 245-264.

ROBINSON, D.A. (1965). The mechanics of human smooth pursuit eye movement. *J. Physiol.* **180,** 569-691.

ROBINSON, D.A., O'MEARA, D.M., SCOTT, A.B., and COLLINS, C.C. (1969). The mechanical components of human eye movements. *J. Appl. Physiol.* **26,** 548-553.

STARK, L. (1959). Stability, oscillations, and noise in the human pupil servomechanism. *Proceedings of the IRE* **47,** 1925-1939.

STARK, L. and BAKER, F. (1959). Stability and oscillations in a neurological servomechanism. *J. Neurophysiol.* **22,** 156-164.

STARK, L. and CORNSWEET, T.N. (1958). Testing a servoanalytic hypothesis for pupil oscillations. *Science* **127,** 588.

STARK, L. and SHERMAN, P.M. (1957). A servoanalytic study of consensual pupil reflex to light. *J. Neurophysiol.* **20,** 17-26.

YOUNG, L.R. and STARK, L. (1963). A discrete model for eye tracking movements. *IEEE Trans. on Military Electronics* **7,** 133-115.

YOUNG, L.R. and STARK, L. (1963). Variable feedback experiments testing a sampled data model for eye tracking movements. *IEEE Trans. on Human Factors in Electronics,* **HFE-4,** 38-51.

WESTHEIMER, G. (1954). Mechanism of saccadic eye movements. *A.M.A. Arch. Ophthal.* **52,** 710-724.

WESTHEIMER, G. (1958). A note on the response characteristics of the extraocular muscle system, *Bull. Math. Biophys.* **20,** 149-153.

ZUBER, B.L. and STARK, L. (1968). Dynamic characteristics of the fusional vergence eye-movement system. *IEEE Trans. Sys. Sci. Cyber.* **SSC-4,** 72-79.

ORBITAL MECHANICS

CARTER C. COLLINS

In recent years there have been a number of approaches to the study of the control of eye movements, as witnessed by the variety of topics covered in the first half of this volume. For the present study, the word "control" is used to imply a neuronal input system which has adapted to the viscoelastic properties of the oculomotor plant, that is, to the mechanical system supported and rotated within the orbit.

At the present time, our comprehension of orbital mechanics is rather fragmentary. The MUD (mechanical underlying determinants) restraining ocular motion must be probed more deeply in order to better understand the interactions of the biophysical forces mediating the control of eye movements.

Surprisingly few physiological studies aimed at determining the mechanical properties of isolated oculorotary muscle and globe restraining tissue have been performed. When this information has been needed for eye movement modeling purposes it has often been borrowed from the classic examinations of skeletal muscles. Inasmuch as these experiments serve as excellent prototypes for the needed orbital mechanical studies, a few are mentioned here:

Fick (1871) determined the coefficient of elasticity of muscle, which he reported changed with stimulation. Blix (1892) first determined the length–tension characteristics of skeletal muscle. Dynamic, quick-stretch experiments were performed by Schenck (1895). Gasser and Hill (1924) devised a viscoelastic model of active muscle, and determined that both the coefficients of viscosity and elasticity increased during stimulation. Levin and Wyman (1927) organized the active components of muscle as we know them today into a viscoelastic contractile element with an undamped series elastic element. Buchthal and Kaiser (1951) determined the dynamic elastic and viscous stiffness of isolated fibers, and described the contractile process as a shortening of long chain polymeric molecules.

A number of studies of the mechanics of the intact eye have been performed in recent years, notably by Westheimer (1954), Hyde (1959), Vossius (1960), Boeder (1961), Fender and Nye (1961), Young and Stark (1963),

These investigations were supported by Public Health Service Research Grant 5 RO1 EY 00498 and Program Project Grant PO1 EY 00299 from the National Eye Institute, and Contract N0014-70-C-0141 from the Office of Naval Research.

Robinson (1964), Stone, Thomas and Zakian (1965), Cook and Stark (1967), and Zuber (1968). However, biophysical studies of the orbit, i.e., isolated oculorotary muscle and globe restraining tissues, have been more limited. Robinson *et al.*, (1969) and Collins, Scott, and O'Meara (1969) have reported observations on the static properties of human oculorotary muscles. We are now in a position to report some preliminary dynamic studies of isolated oculorotary muscles and globe restraining tissues, primarily carried out on cats but with some observations on humans.

The first section of this chapter thus treats the static and dynamic mechanical properties of the orbital elements of the cat under conditions of graded stimulation. These preliminary investigations have resulted in a conceptual model of the mechanical part of the oculomotor system from which we will base further investigations of the human oculomotor plant.

The second section of this chapter deals with measurements of the mechanical characteristics of the human eye movement control system. Although these measurements are less complete than those of the animal investigations, nevertheless, insights derived from the mechanical measurements and calculations of the oculomotor system of the cat permit us to guide our further research and interpretations of mechanical parameters of the human oculomotor system which may be of clinical significance.

Inasmuch as 20 to 40 percent of strabismus cases require reoperation (Costenbader, 1961), there is an evident need to improve our knowledge of the relations between the mechanical defects of strabismus and the mechanical surgery applied to overcome them. It is hoped that numerical evaluation and a conceptual and analytic description of orbital mechanics will contribute a better quantitative understanding of both the neural and the mechanical deviations from normality found in strabismus.

MECHANICAL CHARACTERISTICS OF CAT OCULOMOTOR APPARATUS

The static and dynamic mechanical characteristics of orbital tissue in the cat were studied with the experimental apparatus shown in Fig. 1. The electromechanical tissue dynamometer applies a predetermined displacement and measures force and displacement in the tissue being studied. In different experiments described below, sine, ramp or step functions of length have been imposed upon the tissue, while recording the concomitant tensile force as a function of tissue length. From these recordings appropriate calculations result in values for the mechanical properties of elasticity and viscocity for each type of tissue studied. The first portion of results analyses the mechanical characteristics of the globe restraining tissues, leading to a mechanical model (Fig. 2-7); then the characteristics of passive elements of the muscles will be described (Figs. 8-14); thirdly, determinations of the viscoelastic properties of the active contractile element of oculorotary muscles will be presented (Figs. 15-24). The combinations of these various components of the cat oculomotor plant will result in the models of Figs. 25 and 26.

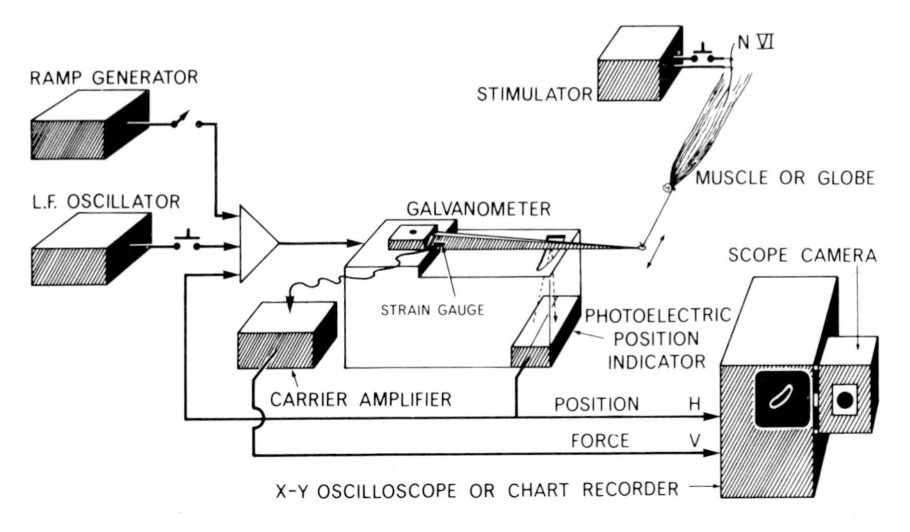

Fig. 1. Apparatus for measuring the dynamic mechanical properties of orbital tissues. Force and displacement are applied and measured by an electromechanical tissue dynamometer consisting of a galvanometer penmotor driven by a power amplifier with arbitrary input functions. For these investigations sine, ramp and step functions have been imposed upon the length of the tissue studied and the concomitant tensile force has been continuously recorded by means of a four-arm foil strain gauge force transducer bridge mounted at the base of the tissue lever (galvanometer pen). The position of the moving end of the tissue lever is detected by means of a photoelectric position indicator utilizing a lightweight front surface mirror (made of a microscope cover slip) attached to the underside of the arm. The mirror reflects collimated light through a wedge-shaped slit to a photocell whose output is proportional to lever arm position. This instantaneous tissue length measurement is recorded simultaneously with tissue tension by means of an x-y oscilloscope to produce dynamic length-tension curves or tension-time records. N VI stimulus is independently programmed to occur at the required times during the automatically controlled experiment.

Globe restraining tissues

The length–tension characteristics of the cat globe restraining tissues were obtained by slowly rotating the globe of an anesthetized cat at a constant low velocity of tissue extension (5 deg/sec). A ramp function of displacement was imposed upon the tissues being measured while the force required to extend the tissues was concomitantly measured by means of the strain gauge force transducer bridge affixed to the base of the galvanometer motor driven force lever. Fig. 2a shows the results of rotating the intact globe (with passive oculorotary muscles attached) and Fig. 2b depicts the length–tension characteristics of the isolated cat globe restraining tissues (horizontal rectus muscles detached from the globe). In the second case the magnitudes of the forces and elasticities are somewhat smaller, since the parallel mechanical impedance of the horizontal oculorotary muscles has now been removed. Superimposed upon this static length–tension curve, a small amplitude (less than 1 mm peak to peak) high velocity, periodic tissue

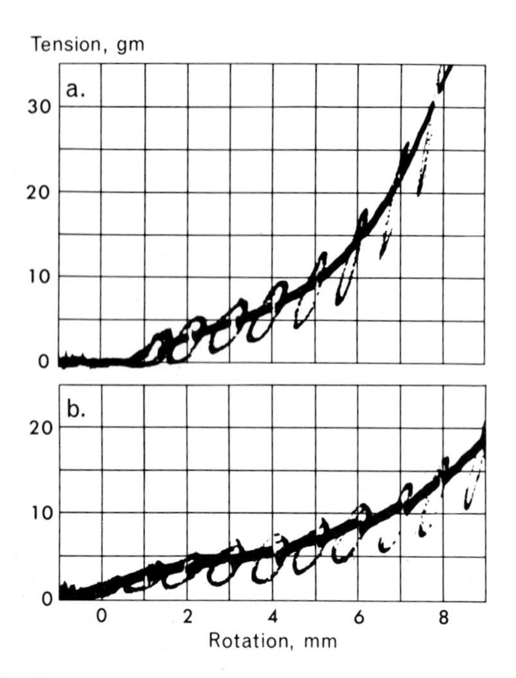

Fig. 2. Length-tension characteristics of the passive tissues restraining motion of the globe in a cat. These curves were obtained by rotating the globe in the horizontal plane by means of a suture firmly attached to the limbus, wrapped slightly over the cornea and pulled tangentially by the tissue dynamometer at a constant rate of five degrees per second. a) Upper curve: intact globe with all muscles attached. b) Lower curve: horizontally isolated globe with medial and lateral rectus muscles surgically detached from their insertions on the globe. Calibrations: horizontal: 1 mm per cm; vertical: 5 gm per cm. Primary position of the eye is about 1 square from left edge of graph. The ellipses were produced by short bursts of small 20 Hz sine wave displacement of the globe, and show the dynamic response characteristics superimposed on the static length-tension curves. Note that the dynamic slope (or stiffness) is considerably greater than the static slope in all cases.

oscillation was applied in the form of a sine wave of displacement of the arm at a fixed mechanical frequency of 20 Hz. The amplitude of the oscillation corresponded to a peak velocity in the neighborhood of 300 to 600 deg/sec., within the saccadic realm of eye movement velocities. It can be seen from these measurements that the elasticity and stiffness is higher for the high velocity movements. During these experiments it was noted that the stiffness or steepness of the slope did not significantly increase as the mechanical frequency or velocity of pull was increased beyond the equivalent of 600 deg/sec. (20 Hz). Consequently, the steepest slope (the slope of the major axis of the ellipse) should correspond to the elasticity of the elastic element which is not encumbered by a large parallel viscous element. The flatter slope, on the other hand, represents the steady state elasticity measured at or near the point of temporal equilibrium of forces. This steady state elasticity represents the series addition of the elasticities of all elastic elements constituting the equivalent mechanical model of the tissues measured. The mechanical dissection of the magnitudes of each of the elements comprising the model will be treated later. Suffice it here to note that both the static and dynamic elasticity of these tissues increases with tension and extension of the tissue. From Fig. 2b it is also possible to derive a measurement of the viscosity of the globe restraining tissues by measuring the minor axes of the ellipses or by measurement of the area included within the ellipse. The minor axis (or more exactly, the vertical or force displacement between points of maximum velocity) is an indication of the force required to displace the tissues at the maximum difference of velocity inherent in sine wave displacement. This velocity difference is proportional to 2π fL, where f is the frequency of the mechanical displacement in Hz, L is the maximal displacement of the sinusoidal motion in mm, and $\pi = 3.14$. The area contained within an ellipse on the length–tension diagram is a measurement of the energy dissipated per cycle of sinusoidal oscillation due to the viscous resistance of the tissue.

Fig. 3 shows the result of a step function of force applied to the isolated cat globe. This is an isotonic experiment (0 applied force) in which the isolated cat globe was pulled to 25° from the primary position and then suddenly released. Under these conditions, a constant (0) force was applied to the globe and the time course of displacement recovery towards the primary position was measured by means of a photoelectric eye position indicator (O'Meara, 1966). In this recording, it will be noted that the displacement recovery occurs in more than one step. This recovery can be approximated by two exponential functions, one high velocity recovery segment with approximately a ten millisecond time constant followed by a much longer time constant recovery of approximately eight hundred milliseconds.

It can also be noted, in the isotonic displacement recovery of the isolated globe shown in Fig. 3, that the excursion amplitudes of the slow and fast phases are different. From them we can calculate the ratio of stiffness of K_{1G} and K_{2G}, the elastic components associated with the fast and slow

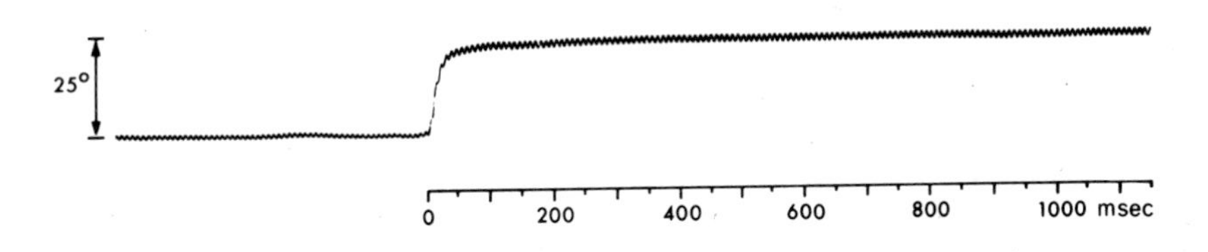

Fig. 3. Dynamic mechanical response of a horizontally isolated cat globe to quick release from a lateral displacement of 4 mm (25 deg). The vertical axis represents eye position recorded with a photoelectric limbus sensing device and is plotted as a function of time. It may be seen that the medial return of the eye toward primary position occurs with fast and slow time constants of approximately 10 and 800 milliseconds respectively. These characteristics are ascribed to the viscoelasticity of the passive tissues restraining motion of the globe (not including passive muscle elements).

time constants of the globe restraining tissues. These calculations are corroborated by the values from the data of Fig. 2 (with low and high velocity ramp and sinusoidal displacements).

These measurements made on the isolated cat globe all indicate that there is more than one elasticity associated with these tissues. When the component elasticities are calculated as being effectively in series with one another, we can relate the magnitude of the elasticities by the following expression:

$$K_{CG} = \frac{K_{1G} \quad K_{2G}}{K_{1G} + K_{2G}}$$

Now, since we have measured K_{CG} (the steady state combined elasticity of K_{1G} and K_{2G} in series), and we have measured K_{1G} (the fast responding elastic element), we can calculate K_{2G} as:

$$K_{2G} = \frac{K_{1G} \quad K_{CG}}{K_{1G} - K_{CG}}$$

The process of ferreting out individual elasticities by calculation might be called mechanical dissection of the tissues.

The measured and derived values of elasticity or stiffness are plotted in Fig. 4, as a function of tension of the globe restraining tissues. Note that the values of all of these coefficients of elasticity are not constant, but vary linearly with the tension in the tissue being measured. It will be seen later that the relation of these elasticities to tissue length is non-linear.

The data contained in Fig. 3 allow us to calculate the viscosity (B) of the tissues from the time constants of isotonic recovery. This is done in the following manner. Since we know the values of K, we can calculate the values of B at any point on the recovery curve: $B = K\tau$, where τ is a time constant. These calculated values are substantiated by those derived from sine wave analysis. The value of the coefficient of viscosity, B, is not constant, but (like the value of the coefficient of elasticity, K) varies linearly with tension in the tissue.

The values of K and B derived from sine wave analysis are plotted as functions of tissue length in Fig. 5 and 6. In each case we clearly see the non-linear relationship between these coefficients and eye rotation. Since linear relationships are more easily dealt with both analytically and conceptually, we will make use of the coefficients K and B as (linear) functions of tissue tension, T.

These elasticities and viscosities can be arranged in a mechanical model or analogue of the cat globe restraining tissues, as shown in Fig. 7. Since both the K's and B's vary linearly with T, and since $\tau = B/K$, the values of the mechanical time constants τ_{1G} and τ_{2G} remain essentially fixed with changes of tissue tension.

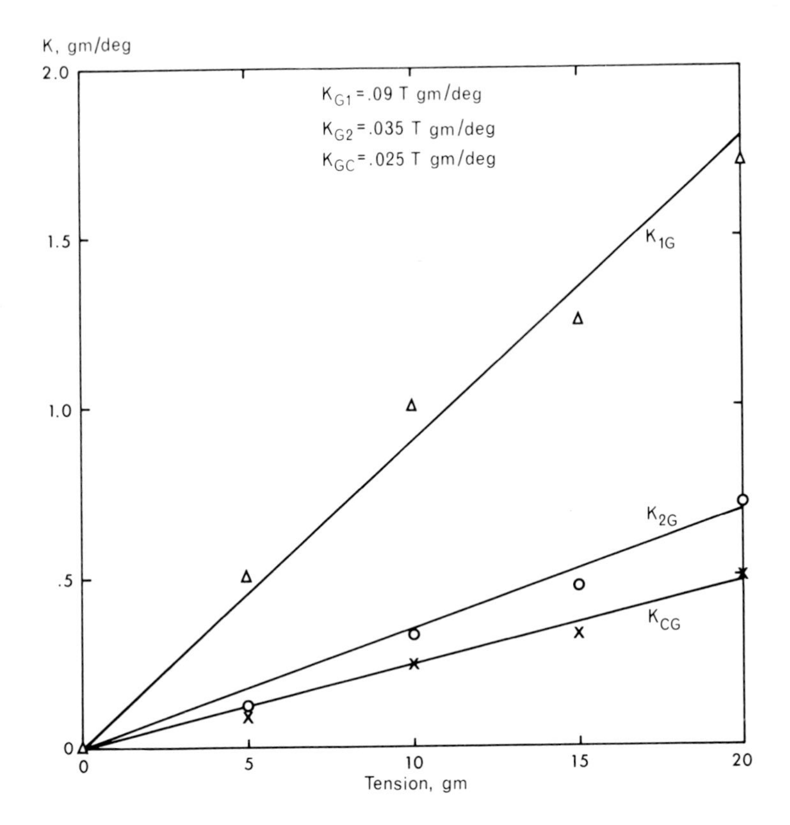

Fig. 4. Mechanical dissection of the values of the elasticities of the fast and slow elements of the passive tissues restraining motion of the globe.

K_{CG}, the combined series elasticity measured at or near steady-state conditions, is obtained from the slopes of smooth curves such as shown in Fig. 2b.

K_{1G}, the elastic component associated with the fast time constant of the globe restraining tissues, is calculated from transient or dynamic measurements such as step (quick release, Fig. 3) or sine functions (as in Fig. 2b).

K_{2G}, the elasticity in parallel with the high viscosity, slow responding element of globe restraint, is calculated as:

$K_{2G} = K_{1G}K_{CG}/K_{1G}-K_{CG}$

It will be noted that none of these elasticities remain constant, but vary with eye position or tension in the tissue. The variation of elasticity appears to be linearly related to the tension of the globe restraining tissue, and is plotted as such here with the analytic expressions for the various elasticities.

Passive element of cat oculorotary muscle

If we attach the tissue dynamometer (Fig. 1) to an oculorotary muscle of an anesthetized cat without stimulating the nerve to this muscle, we can measure the mechanical properties of the passive elements of the muscle.

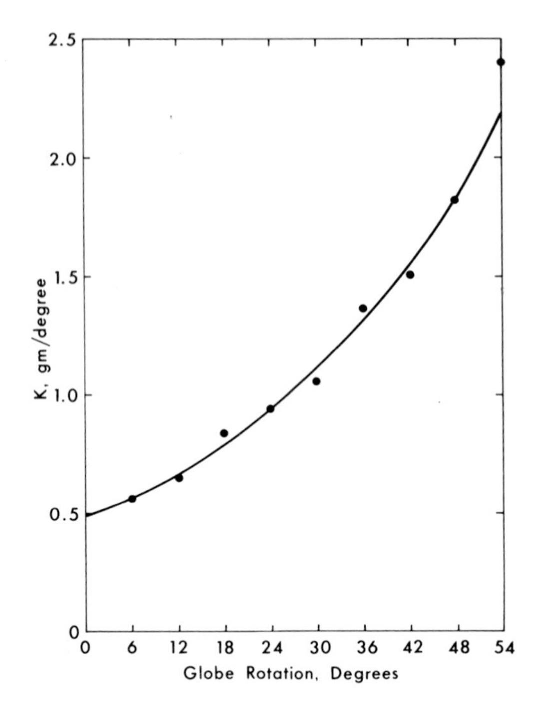

Fig. 5. The dynamic elasticity of the cat globe restraining tissues, K, varies non-linearly with eye position as plotted here. These values were taken from the slopes of the major axes of the length-tension ellipses of Fig. 2b, which were obtained by driving the eye with relatively high velocity sine waves (20 Hz, 300 degrees per second eye movement) with 5 degrees or less peak to peak displacement. The normal range of rotation of the cat globe from primary position is probably not over 35 degrees (*Richardson and Davis,* 1960).

We have performed measurements similar to those of Fig. 2 in order to evaluate the various components of the passive muscle. Fig. 8 shows the results of an experiment in which the rate of extension of a cat right lateral rectus muscle was varied between the limits of 0.2 mm/sec and 100 mm/sec, the latter corresponding to some 600 deg/sec (saccadic velocity). The lowest rate of movement indicates the static or steady state length–tension characteristics of passive muscle since lower rates resulted in the same length–tension curve. The slope of this length–tension curve permits estimation of the static elasticity. This represents the series combination of the series elastic and parallel elastic elements of the passive component of oculorotary muscle. As the rate of pull is increased, we measure a component of force due to the viscous element of passive muscle.

Both the viscous and elastic elements of passive muscle can also be calculated from experiments in which a step function of displacement is applied to the passive muscle, as shown in Fig. 9. This figure illustrates the isometric

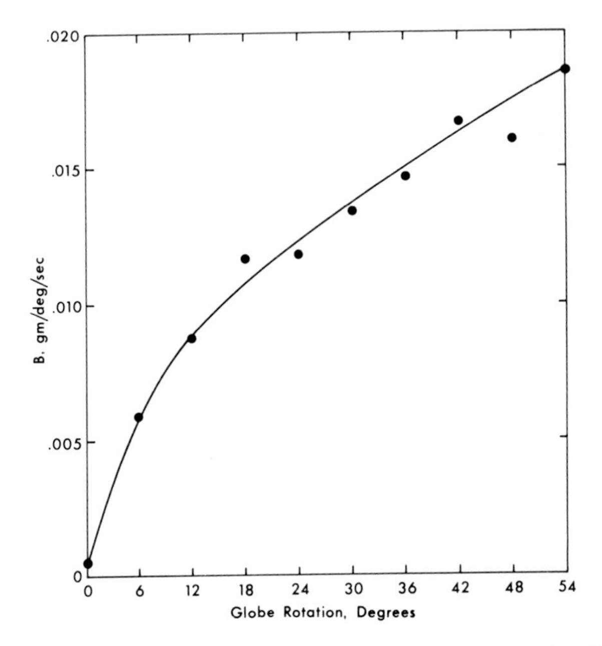

Fig. 6. The viscous resistance of the cat globe restraining tissues, B, as calculated from 20 Hz sine wave measurements similar to those of Fig. 2b. Because of the great disparity in magnitudes of B_{1G} and B_{2G} (Fig. 7) we can estimate B_{1G} as the force component 90° out of phase with a high frequency sinusoidal displacement of the tissue.

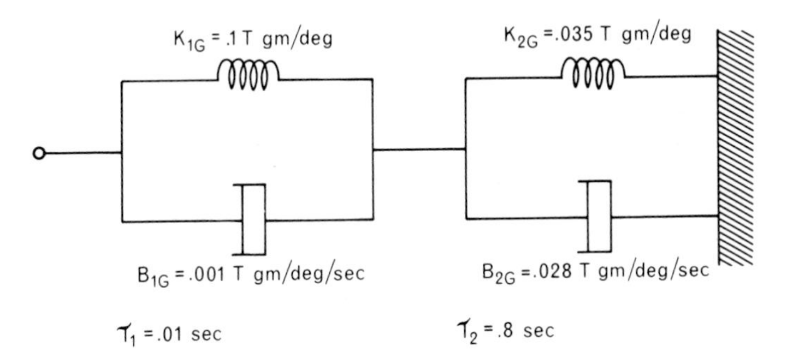

Fig. 7. A mechanical model of the globe restraining tissues of the cat combining the values for the elasticities, K, derived as previously discussed. The fast and slow time constants, τ_{1G} and τ_{2G} can be measured directly from quick release data. The values of viscosity B_{1G} and B_{2G} can also be obtained as $B = K\tau$.

Note that although both B and K vary, they do so in a parallel fashion such that the time constant $\tau = B/K$ remains essentially fixed in value.

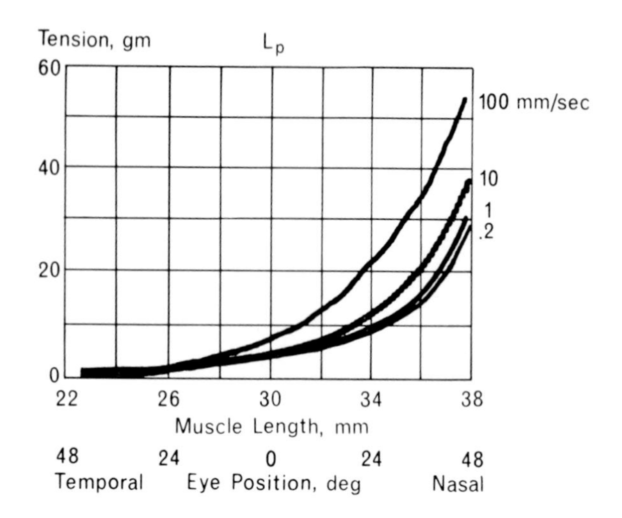

Fig. 8. Cat lateral rectus muscle length–tension records made under passive conditions at various constant velocities of muscle pull (ramp data). The tension required to extend a muscle at higher velocities is greater due to the viscosity of the passive muscle.

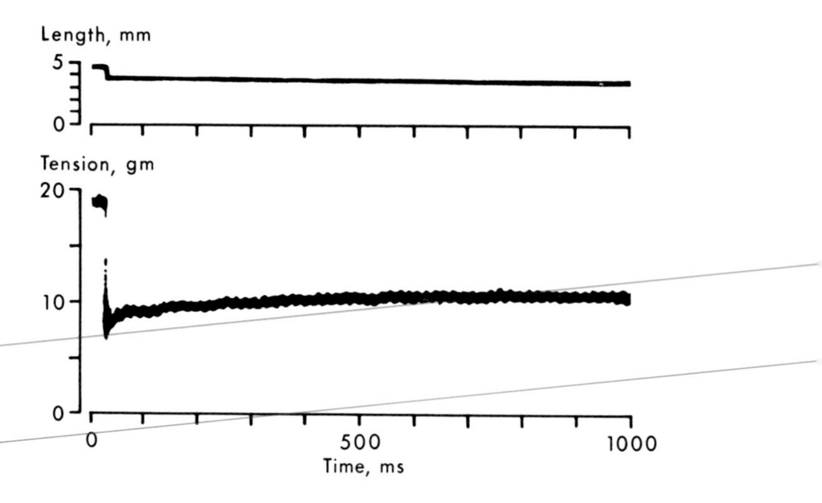

Fig. 9. Tension recording from the passive lateral rectus muscle of the cat initially stretched 5 mm (about 30 degrees) beyond primary length and quickly released 1 mm (to Lp + 4 mm). The isometric tension recovery time course shows a time constant of about 100 ms. The initial and final tension differences permit calculation of the coefficients of elasticity of the series and parallel elastic elements (Fig. 10).

tension recovery time course following a one mm step decrease in muscle length. The same methods as employed in the previous section are applicable to the data of Figures 8 and 9, in order to evaluate both the elastic and viscous components of passive muscle. Measurements and calculations from both these forms of data tend to match one another.

The results of these determinations are shown in Fig. 10, illustrating the dependence of the various elastic components of passive muscle upon the tension in the muscle. Note that, as in the case of the globe restraining tissues,

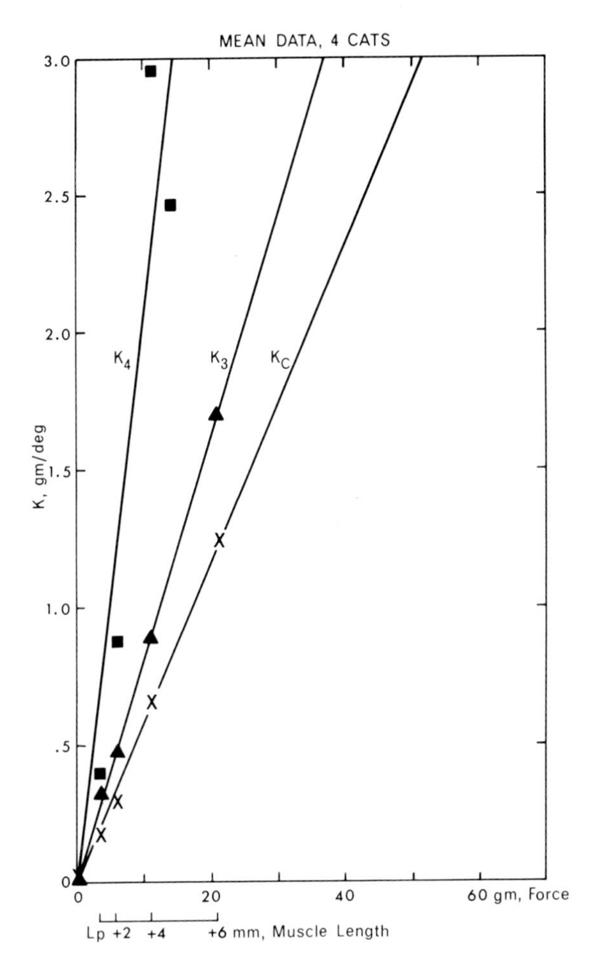

Fig. 10. The values of the coefficients of elasticity (K) of the various passive muscle components of the cat were obtained from quick-release data such as in Fig. 9. These figures increase linearly and quite rapidly with tension in the passive muscle.

the elasticities vary linearly with muscle tension. Also observe here the extreme steepness of the slopes of the coefficients of elasticity as functions of muscle tension.

Separate measurements at low (following) velocities of eye movement have yielded the data shown in Fig. 11, in which viscous force is plotted as a function of velocity of extension with muscle length as a parameter. It is seen here that the force velocity relationship is linear, indicating that at given muscle length and at low velocities, the viscosity of passive muscle is Newtonian, that is, the viscous force is proportional to velocity of movement up to 30 deg/sec. This indicates that there is a constant coefficient of viscosity; $B = T\dot{\theta}$, under these conditions, where T is tension and $\dot{\theta}$ is velocity (Collins, Meltzer, O'Meara and Scott, 1969).

The family of different slopes indicate the coefficient of viscosity is a function of muscle length. As with elasticity, viscosity varies linearly with the tension in the muscle. This is shown in Fig. 12, which was computed from the time constants of recovery of quick-release step data (similar to those of Fig. 9). Note the steep slope of the coefficient of viscosity of the passive muscle component as a function of muscle tension.

Both the elastic and viscous components of passive muscle can be plotted as functions of muscle length. As shown in Fig. 13, they are then

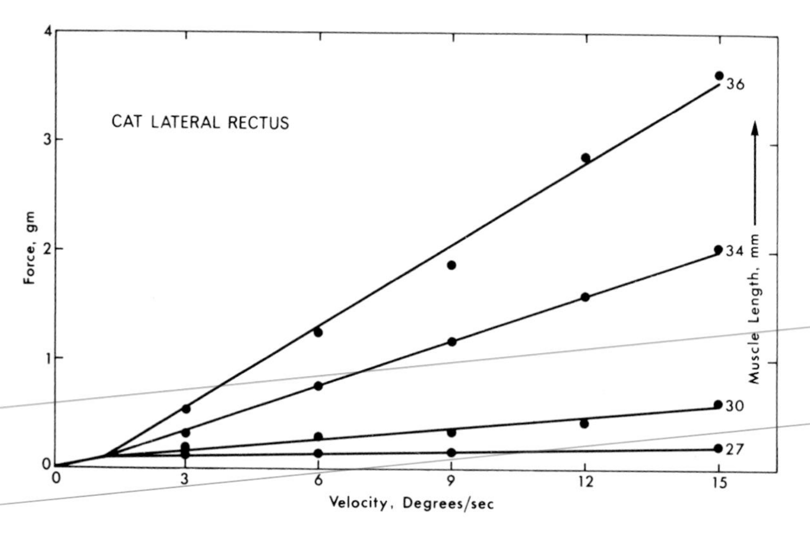

Fig. 11. Viscous force varies linearly with velocity of extension of a passive muscle at rates up to the velocity of following movements. This graph was plotted from ramp data (constant velocity of pull) at lower velocities than those of Fig. 8. The viscous force plotted here was obtained by subtracting the static elastic force from the total muscle force at a given velocity (and at various muscle lengths). The linear relationship seen at these low velocities indicates that viscosity is Newtonian in this region (i.e., there is a constant coefficient of viscosity).

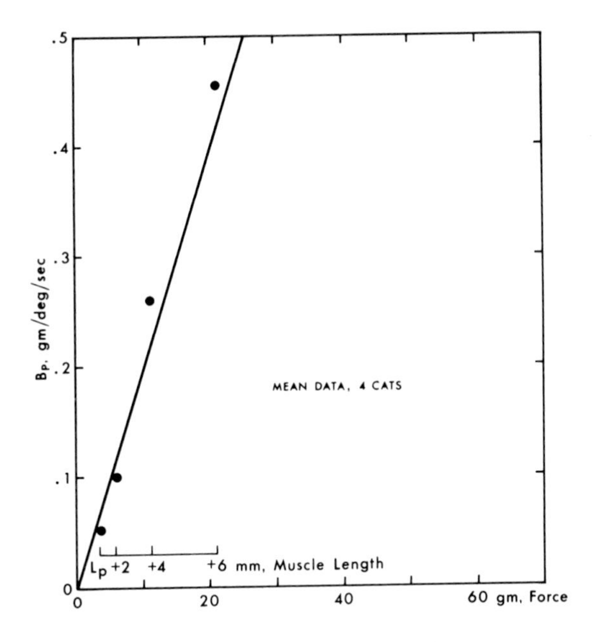

Fig. 12. The coefficient of viscosity, B_p, of the passive component of an oculorotary muscle of the cat can be seen to vary linearly with tension in the passive muscle. Tension was varied by fixing the muscle at various lengths. Following a quick-release the isometric force recovery time course exhibited an essentially fixed time constant, τ_p, regardless of the large variation in B_p. The coefficient of viscosity, B_p, was calculated from this time constant and the coefficients of elasticity at the same tension: $B_p = (K_3 + K_4)\,\tau_p$.

found to be nonlinear. Consequently, as mentioned, we will endeavor to express elasticity and viscosity in terms of muscle tension rather than of muscle length. This will permit linear analytic descriptions of the mechanics of passive muscle, as was done in the case of the globe restraining tissues. Fig. 14 illustrates a simple mechanical model of the passive muscle component with values for elasticity and viscosity as derived above.

Contractile element of cat oculorotary muscle

The lateral rectus muscle of 16 anesthetized cats was attached by a 000 surgical silk suture to the pre-calibrated arm of the tissue dynamometer with the eye in primary position. The muscle was then severed from its insertion. The globe was subsequently removed, carefully preserving the muscle sheath and blood supply. The sixth nerve was dissected out and severed or crushed rostrally after being placed across a pair of platinum stimulating electrodes. The preparation was kept under oil at approximately body temperature and remained viable (with essentially unchanging response characteristics to

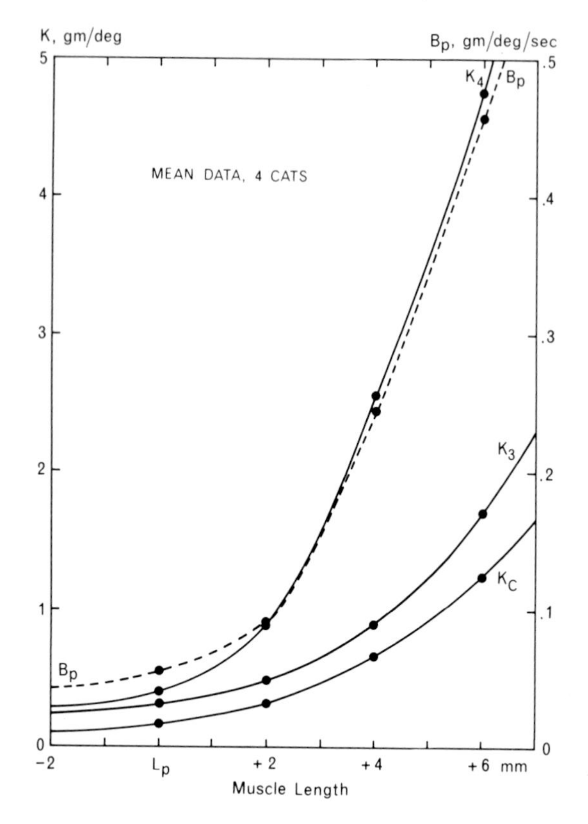

Fig. 13. The coefficients of viscosity (B) and elasticity (K) of passive oculorotary muscle are nonlinear functions of muscle length. Consequently it is more expedient to express these coefficients analytically in linear terms of tension in the passive component of cat oculorotary muscle, as was seen in Figs. 10 and 12.

stimulation) for periods up to three hours; however, most of the experimental results were obtained within an hour and a half after the preparation had been completed.

Both the muscle length (arm position) and muscle tension were recorded on a Beckman RB multi-channel pen recorder and on a storage oscilloscope, Tektronix Model 564, with a polaroid oscilloscope camera attachment.

For stimulating the sixth nerve, a pulse width of 0.2 msec was employed. The required stimulus voltage for maximal muscle response was established and found generally to lie below 3 volts. In these experiments supramaximal voltage levels were employed; a level one and a half times the maximum for each preparation was used. The frequency of stimulus pulses

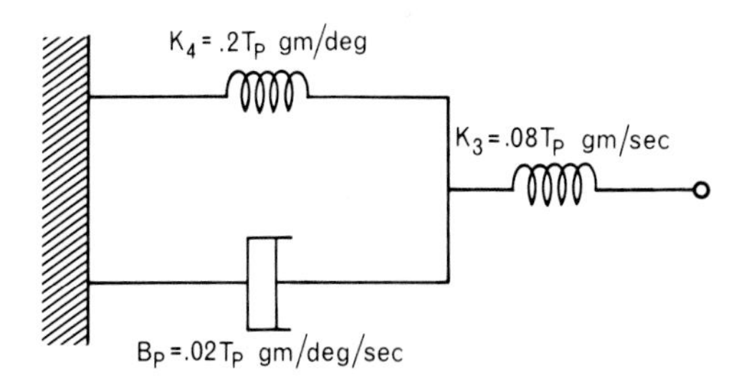

Fig. 14. A mechanical model of the passive component of the lateral rectus muscle of a cat can be formulated from the results of ramp and step function experiments such as shown in Figs. 8 and 9. The values of the coefficients in the model are seen to vary with passive muscle tension as plotted in Figs. 10 and 12.

Since both the coefficients of viscosity (B) and elasticity (K) vary linearly with passive muscle element tension, the mechanical time constant remains fixed as $\tau = B/K$.

was varied as a parameter to establish graded levels of stimulation of the muscle. Generally levels of 0, 25, 50, 100, 150, and 200 pulses per second were used.

Three types of measurements were made. Firstly, to obtain the steady state length-tension relationship of the muscles, ramp functions of muscle extension were employed. In each instance, the suture running from the muscle to the tissue dynamometer arm was co-linear with the long axis of the muscle. The results are shown in Fig. 15. The lateral rectus muscle of the cat was pulled at a rate of 1 mm/sec, and stimulus pulses were applied at the points indicated on the curve for periods of approximately one half second to allow the build up of maximal developed tension by the muscle. The frequencies of graded stimulation are indicated on the figure.

The second procedure was designed to measure the elasticity of the series elastic element as a function of graded innervation of the muscle. In this experiment the muscle was held at its primary length and a sinusoidal mechanical oscillation in the length of the muscle was imposed by the tissue dynamometer. The amplitude of this oscillation was approximately 1 mm peak to peak excursion, and its frequency was 20 Hz. It was noted that at this frequency (corresponding to saccadic velocities of approximately 600 deg/sec) the slope of the dynamic length-tension curve had reached its maximum. That is, increasing the frequency further did not tend to increase the slope significantly. Figure 16 shows the results of this type of experiment in which the only parameter varied was that of stimulus frequency to the sixth nerve. (Due to the compliance of the tissue dynamometer, as the series elastic stiffness increased with muscle stimulation the excursion of the dynamometer decreased. This resulted in a maximum velocity of approximately 300 deg/sec at the highest levels of stimulation without resetting the external drive of the tissue dynamometer). It will be noted from these measurements that the stiffness increases as a function of stimulus frequency or innervation.

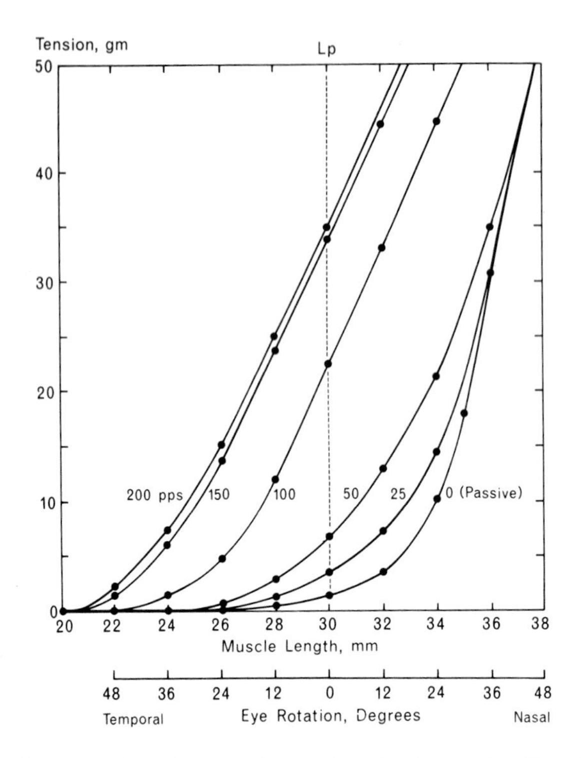

Fig. 15. Family of static length-tension curves for a cat lateral rectus muscle, with graded innervation as the parameter. Each curve represents the force necessary to extend the muscle with a fixed frequency (pps) of supramaximal stimulation of the sixth nerve. Muscle extension is given in millimeters (upper scale) and the equivalent eye rotation in degrees (bottom scale) taken as 6 deg/mm for an average measured cat globe diameter of 19 mm. The primary muscle length averaged approximately 30 mm.

In these measurements the viscosity of the active component of the muscle is also seen to increase with muscle stimulation. This is noted as an increase in the area within the ellipse, or as an increase in the minor axis dimensions (or more properly the vertical displacement at the center of the ellipse due to forces generated only by viscosity). Viscosity was also determined by measurements of the tension increments required to extend the stimulated lateral rectus muscle at constant velocities from 0.2 mm/sec through 100 mm/sec.

In the third procedure the tissue dynamometer was programmed to apply a step change of length to the stimulated muscle, constituting the conventional quick release experiment. The stimulated muscle was initially held at a pre-determined length. It was then suddenly decreased in length by one mm, and held rigidly at this length. An example of the isometric tension

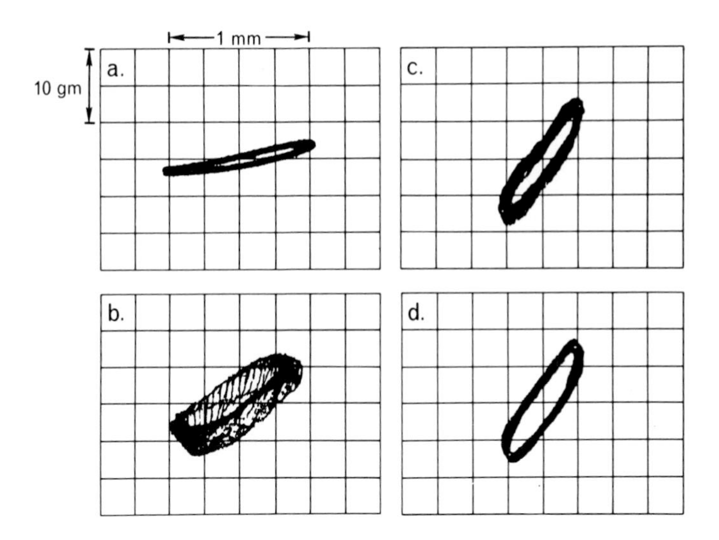

Fig. 16. A group of dynamic length-tension curves for the cat lateral rectus muscle measured with 20 Hz sinusoidal length oscillations of less than 0.5 mm peak centered around the primary muscle length. Peak muscle velocity was 300–600 deg/sec (saccadic region). The experimental procedure followed was: Application of the mechanical oscillation; 200 ms later, supramaximal stimulus applied to N VI; 100 ms later, camera shutter opened for ½ sec. The N VI stimulus conditions shown are: **a** - 0 pps (passive); **b** - 50 pps; **c** - 100 pps; **d** - 200 pps (maximal tension). Comparing Figs. 15 and 16a it can be seen that the dynamic elasticity (L-T slope) of passive muscle is an order of magnitude greater than its static elasticity. Upon maximal stimulation the dynamic elasticity increases still another order of magnitude. The viscosity can also be seen to increase with stimulation (i.e., the area of the ellipse increases).

recovery time course is shown in Fig. 17. Note here that the initial tension of 42 grams dropped to 28 grams and slowly recovered to a steady state value of approximately 34 grams in a period of some 250 msec. This indicates a mechanical recovery time constant in the neighborhood of 50 msec for the contractile element under these conditions. In actual fact there is a spectrum of time constants, ranging from 10 to 100 msec, with 50 msec predominating.

The quick release procedure permits evaluation of the coefficient of elasticity of the series elastic element at a given tension. In the above case it can be calculated from the initial drop of 14 grams, divided by 6 deg. (1 mm) of displacement to give 2.3 gm/deg. The series combination of the series elastic element and the parallel elastic element results in the final value of tension difference, or 8 gm divided by 6 deg. final displacement, giving 1.3 gm/deg. From these two values of series spring constants the parallel elastic element can be calculated as described previously for the globe restraining tissues and passive muscle component.

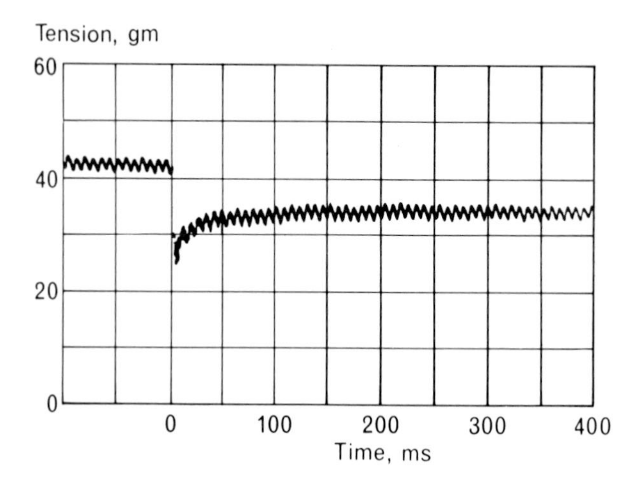

Fig. 17. Step function measurement of cat lateral rectus muscle, initially held at 34 mm and, at time 0, quickly released by one mm to 33 mm, held isometrically. N VI was stimulated continuously, from 100 msec prior to quick release throughout experiment (supramaximal stimulation of 0.2 msec., 5 V, at 150 pps). Isometric tension recovery permits calculation of coefficients of elasticity, K_C, K_1, and K_2, as outlined in Fig. 4, after subtracting passive muscle tension contributions. The results of measurements at primary muscle length are displayed in Fig. 18.

The values of elasticity computed by the three methods tend to corroborate one another. Fig. 18 presents elasticities of the contractile element as a function of tension. Tension in the active element was developed by stimulating the sixth nerve at the frequencies indicated in the diagram with the muscle held at primary length. It can be seen that the slopes of the curves of muscle stiffness versus muscle tension pass through the origin, indicating zero stiffness at zero muscle tension, which corresponds to actual observations.

A comparison of the slopes of the active element elasticities as a function of muscle force (Fig. 18) and those of the passive component elasticities (plotted to the same scale in Fig. 10) reveals that the latter are considerably steeper. This dichotomy clearly indicates the mechanical difference between the active and passive components of muscle. It is the basis for modelling the oculorotary muscle with two separate components, as will be seen below.

From measurements such as those illustrated in Figs. 16 and 17 the viscosity, B, of the active muscle element can be computed. Viscosity is shown in Fig. 19 as a function of muscle force, calculated from quick release data similar to those of Fig. 17. One notes that the viscosity varies linearly with muscle tension and is observed to be zero at zero muscle tension. The viscosity computed from changes in velocity of pull of the muscle, as well as from the area or force-velocity differences with applied mechanical sine waves, corroborates the data shown in Fig. 19. It can now be seen that since both the elasticity and viscosity of the active element increase linearly with

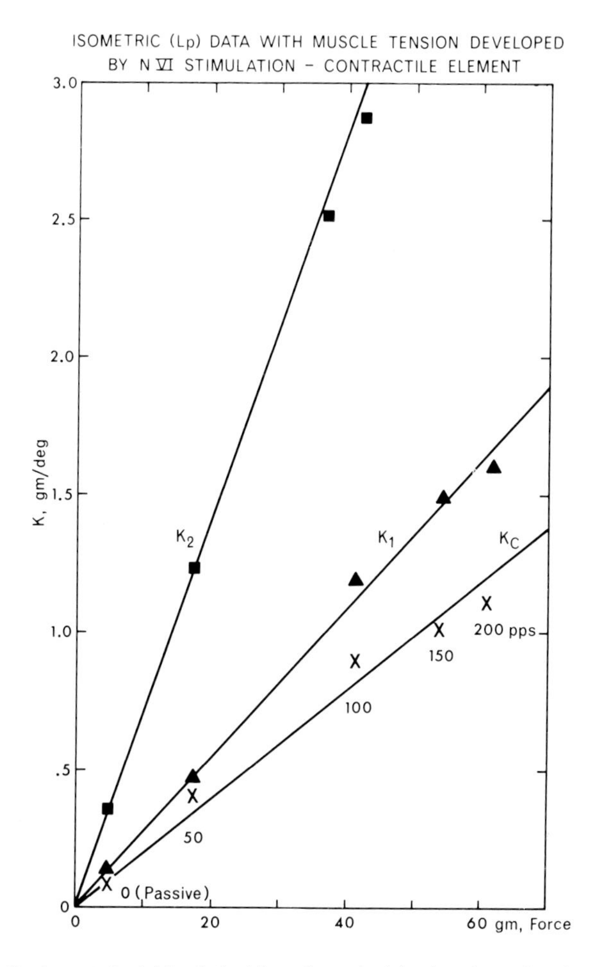

Fig. 18. Contractile element elasticities derived from 1 mm (quick-release) step function and tension recovery (similar to Fig. 17) by mechanical dissection at primary muscle length.

K_C = combined elasticity of K_1 and K_2 in series (as indicated by steady-state length tension measurement).

K_1 = elasticity of series elastic element (as measured from initial transient force decrease).

K_2 = elasticity of elastic element in parallel with viscosity (calculated as $K_2 = K_1 K_C/K_1 - K_C$). The elasticities were determined over a range of muscle tensions by grading the N VI stimulus (shown on the graph as pps). Figs. 10 (passive elements) and 18 (contractile elements) are plotted on the same scale to facilitate direct comparison. Note the dichotomy between contractile and passive elements as clearly evidenced by the much smaller (1/3 X) tension-elasticity slopes of the contractile element.

muscle tension, the mechanical time constant of the contractile element (ratio of viscosity to elasticity) remains essentially fixed with changes of

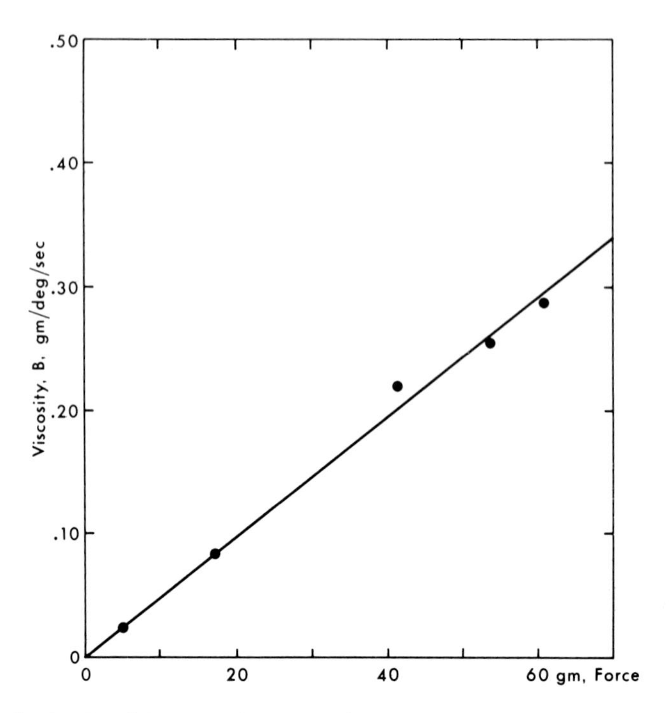

Fig. 19. B_a, the viscosity of the contractile element of cat lateral rectus muscle, is calculated from elasticities (K_1 and K_2) and the isometric recovery time constants, τ_a, measured at various tensions developed by N VI stimulation. Since K_1 and K_2 are in parallel with respect to B_a, $B_a = \tau_a (K_1 + K_2)$.

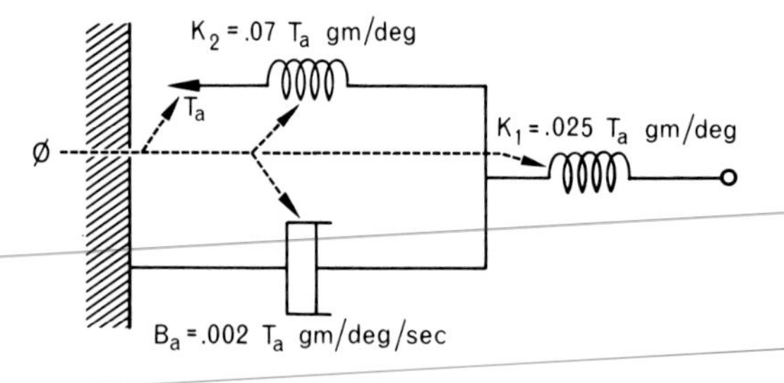

Fig. 20. A mechanical model of the active component of the cat oculorotary muscle takes the form of a Voigt element (parallel spring and dashpot), and a series elastic element. The magnitudes of the visco-elastic coefficients (K_1, K_2, B_a) are not constant but vary linearly with the active state tension, T_a. The isometric active state tension itself varies approximately as the square of the innervation frequency, ϕ, over a wide range as shown in Fig. 21. It is not clear at this time whether the dependence of the viscoelastic coefficients on tension is an inherent mechanical property of contractile element tissue or whether the coefficients are under the direct control of innervation, as is shown for convenience in this model.

tension and length of the muscle, even though the individual mechanical viscosities and elasticities are varying with muscle tension and length.

A mechanical model of the active component of cat oculorotary muscle is shown in Fig. 20. The magnitude of each mechanical element is shown as a function of tension in the contractile element. It can be clearly seen that this model, although similar in basic configuration to that of the passive muscle element of Fig. 14, has values only one third those of the model for the passive component.

Muscle tension as a function of stimulus frequency was determined isometrically at the primary muscle length, and is plotted in Fig. 21. This innervation-force transfer function resembles that of the human (which will be seen later, in Fig. 31). The relationship between innervation and muscle force is fundamental in the control of eye movements. It appears in the analog mechanical model, corresponding to $\phi \rightarrow T_a$ in Fig. 20.

Not only does the force generated by the muscle vary with stimulus frequency, but also the stiffness and viscosity of the muscle, as determined by

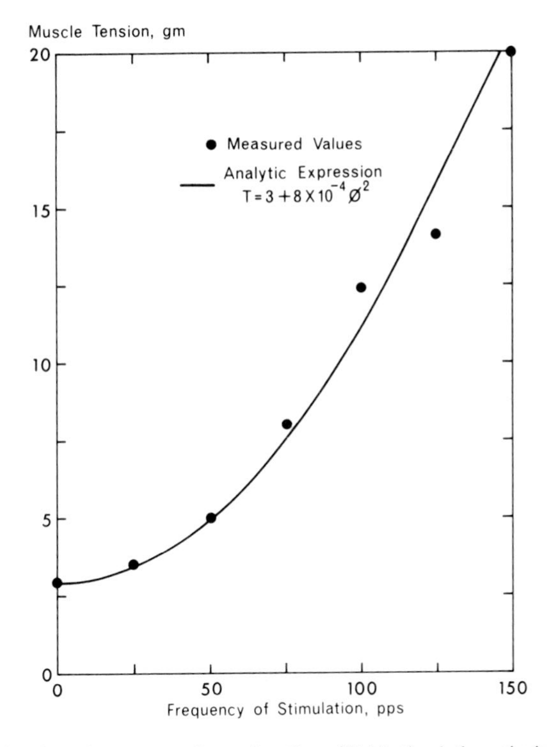

Fig. 21. Tension of cat lateral rectus muscle as a function of N VI stimulation: the innervation-force transfer function at primary muscle length. Isometric muscle tension tends to vary as the square of stimulus magnitude over a wide range.

quick stretch experiments. Stiffness (elasticity) is plotted in Fig. 22, and viscosity in Fig. 23, both as functions of stimulus frequency.

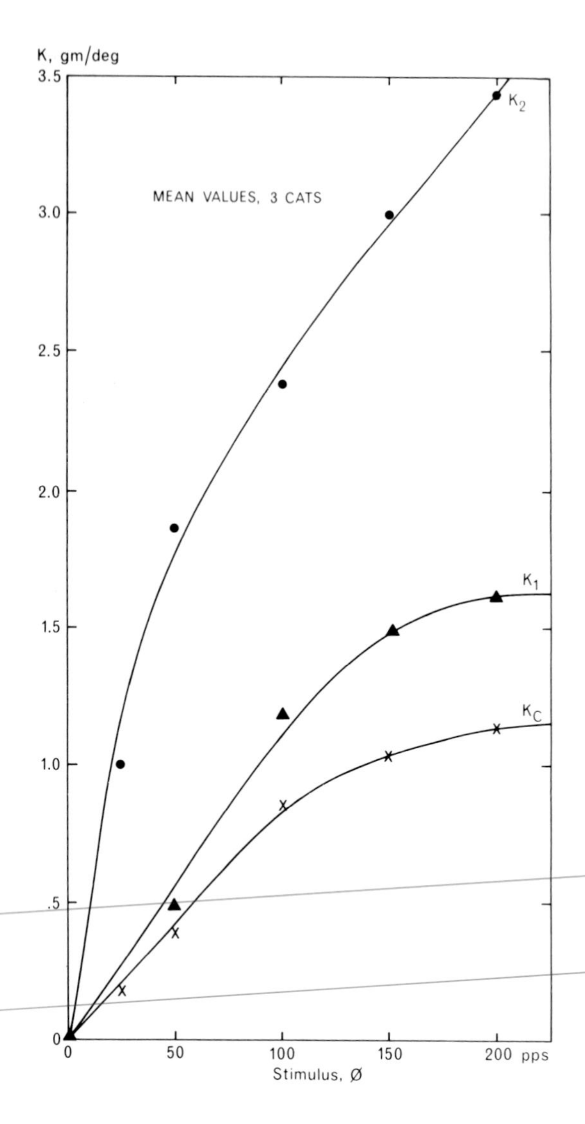

Fig. 22. The elasticity (K) of the contractile element of the cat lateral rectus muscle increases with stimulation of N VI, but tends to level off to a saturation value beyond stimulation at 150 pps. From isometric determinations with muscle at primary length.

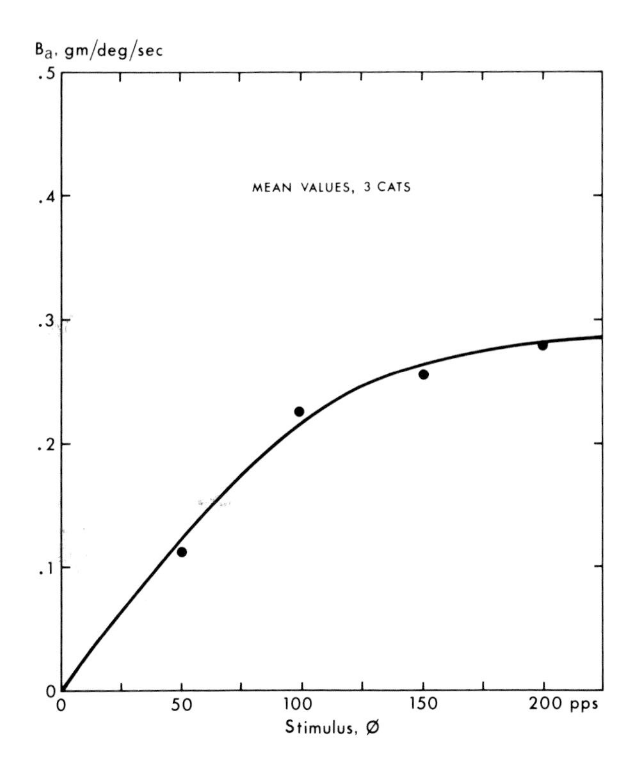

Fig. 23. The viscosity (B_a) of the contractile element of the cat lateral rectus muscle increases upon stimulation of N VI but levels off above 100 pps.

Muscle length–tension characteristics were plotted with velocity of muscle pull as a parameter for given fixed stimulus frequencies. By a series of such experiments at various levels of stimulation, the viscosity was determined and plotted as a function of velocity of pull as seen in Fig. 24. The results of these experiments are similar to those of Fig. 8, where the vertical distance between members of the family of curves is due to the viscosity of the muscle. Fig. 24 shows that the viscosity remains essentially constant at a given level of stimulation up to about 30 deg/sec (corresponding to the velocity of following movements). Beyond this point the viscosity tends to fall off with increasing velocity. At the higher stimulus frequencies viscosity drops an order of magnitude for velocities at 600 degrees per second. Oculomotor viscosity thus appears to be thixotropic. This must result in a concomitant facilitation of fast movements with an increase in efficiency and reduction of effort achieved in the production of high velocity saccadic eye movements.

The observations which we have made to date allow us to construct a mechanical model of the oculorotary muscle of the cat, as shown in Fig. 25.

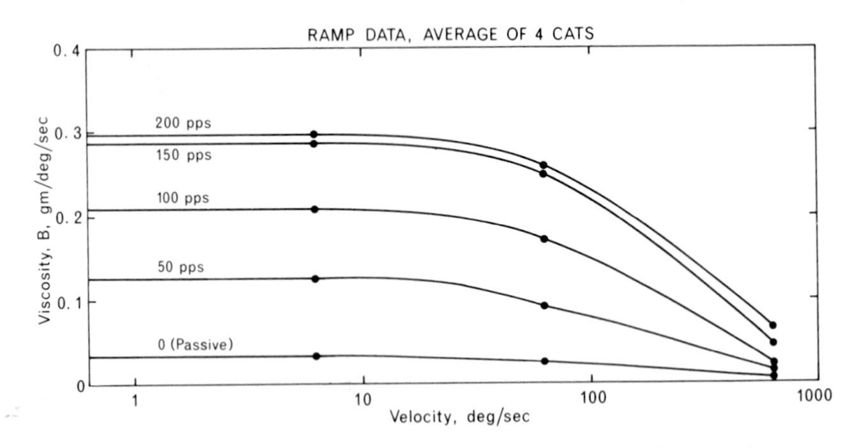

Fig. 24. The viscosity, B, of the cat oculorotary muscle contractile element is a function of innervation, and is independent of velocity in the region of following movements (up to 30 deg/sec). However, above this velocity the coefficient of viscosity decreases progressively. At 600 deg/sec, (saccadic velocity) the coefficient of viscosity has fallen to 20% of its static value. This thixotropic phenomenon reduces the effort required of a muscle to make saccadic eye movements.

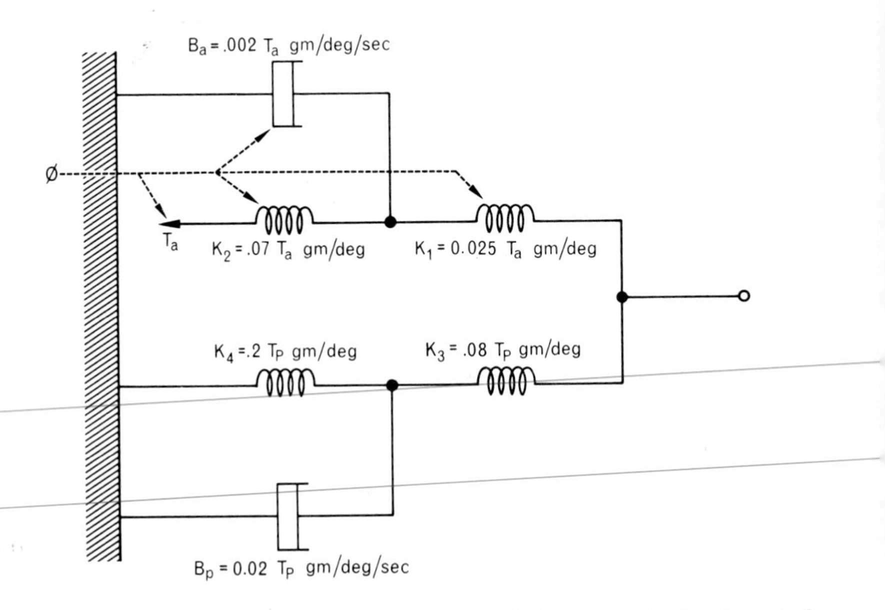

Fig. 25. A mechanical model of the cat oculorotary muscle combining passive and active elements of Figs. 14 and 20. Note that the values of the various viscoelastic coefficients are dependent upon the parallel but generally unequal division of total muscle tension between the contractile and passive elements.

Here there is a distinct mechanical dichotomy between active (contractile) and passive elements of the muscle. Since the magnitudes of stiffness (K) and viscosity (B) for the stimulated contractile element (Fig. 20) appear to be smaller than those for the passive element (Fig. 14), it is concluded that there are two discrete entities which constitute the complete muscle. These two elements are shown connected in parallel.

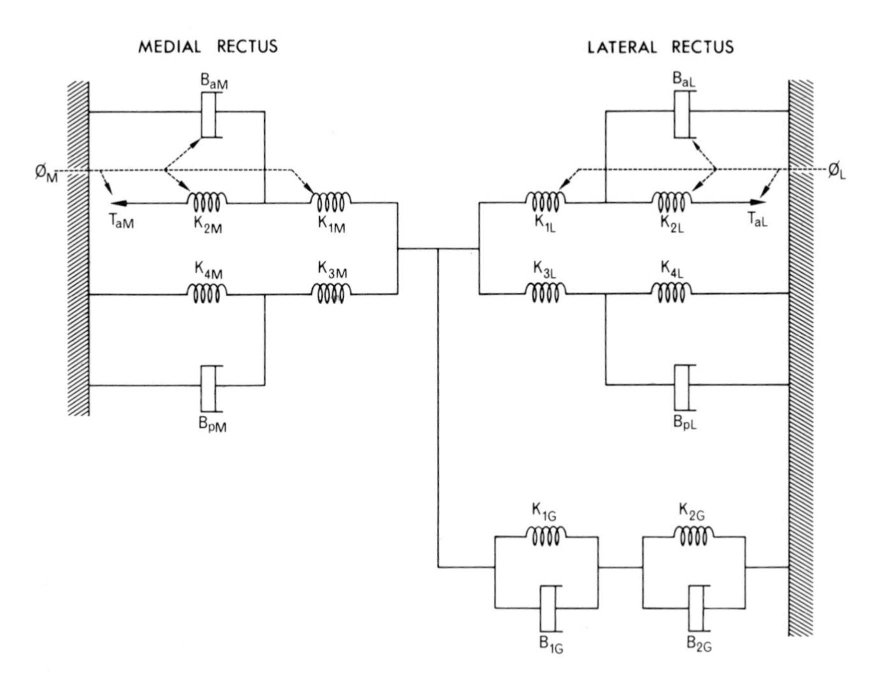

Fig. 26. Mechanical model of cat oculomotor plant.
M, L, (subscripts): medial rectus, lateral rectus
$B_a = 0.002\,T$ gm/deg/sec, coefficient of viscosity of contractile element
$B_p = 0.02\,T$ gm/deg/sec, coefficient of viscosity of passive element
$K_1 = 0.025\,T$ gm/deg, coefficient of elasticity of contractile series elastic element
$K_2 = 0.07\,T_a$ gm/deg, coefficient of elasticity of contractile parallel elastic element
$K_3 = 0.08\,T_p$ gm/deg, coefficient of elasticity of passive series elastic element
$K_4 = 0.2\,T_p$ gm/deg, coefficient of elasticity of passive parallel elastic element
$B_{1G} = 0.001\,T$ gm/deg/sec, coefficient of viscosity of fast globe Voigt element
$B_{2G} = 0.028\,T$ gm/deg/sec, coefficient of viscosity of slow globe Voigt element
$K_{1G} = 0.1\,T$ gm/deg, coefficient of elasticity of fast globe Voigt element
$K_{2G} = 0.035\,T$ gm/deg, coefficient of elasticity of slow globe Voigt element
$T_a = A\theta^2$ = Tension in (active) contractile element
T_p = Tension in passive element
T = Tension in non-muscular tissue restraining movement of the globe
ϕ = innervation, or control signal (average frequency of firing in nerve supplying oculorotary muscle).

In general it is difficult to determine the division of tension between the active and passive elements. However, by use of the passive length–tension relationship, it should be possible to determine the contribution of the passive element if the muscle length is known. Consequently, the difference between this and the total tension should be that developed by the contractile element. Although this model is somewhat more complicated than those previously suggested, it better fits the physiological measurements which we have been able to make in some detail. By means of anatomical and mechanical dissections we have been able to obtain further experimental data permitting more precise definition of the elements of the model.

Fig. 26 shows the overall mechanical model of the oculomotor plant for the cat in terms of elasticities, viscosities, tension and innervation. This model permits determination of the individual contributions of the antagonist muscles and the globe restraining tissues. Since we now know the length–tension relationships of the oculorotary muscles at various levels of innervation it appears that we have most of the needed information for modelling the oculomotor plant. It is hoped that this model will help fill the gap in the information needed to deal with both the peripheral and central mechanisms of oculomotor control.

MECHANICAL CHARACTERISTICS OF HUMAN OCULOMOTOR APPARATUS

Human globe restraining tissues

The data presented here were gathered from sixteen informed and consenting patients during the course of required strabismus surgery. The investigative setup for these measurements is shown in Fig. 1 of the next chapter by Alan Scott (Chapt. 11). A force measuring strain gauge was attached to a micromanipulator to permit controlled displacement of the strain gauge and tissue under study. The displacement was transduced by a potentiometer attached by means of a gear train to the micromanipulator drive mechanism. Hence, direct length–tension recordings could be made electrically on an X-Y recorder or X-Y oscilloscope. A 000 suture was attached to either the stump of the detached muscle insertion on the isolated globe or to a medial or lateral rectus muscle to investigate the static length–tension characteristics of these tissues. The appropriate angle of pull of the globe or the oculorotary muscles was established by clamping the apparatus to a frame attached to the operating table as shown in Fig. 1 of Dr. Scott's chapter.

The length–tension characteristics of the orbital restraining tissues of two isolated human globes are shown in Fig. 27. Each of the patients measured exhibited a 40 prism diopter exotropia. While not proven, it is suspected that the observed asymmetry in the length–tension characteristic for abduction versus adduction of the globes of these patients bears a causal relationship to their exotropia. We have not yet had the opportunity to make such measurements on normal subjects. In these records the elasticity of the orbital restraining tissues for nasal (adduction) movement of the globe is approxi-

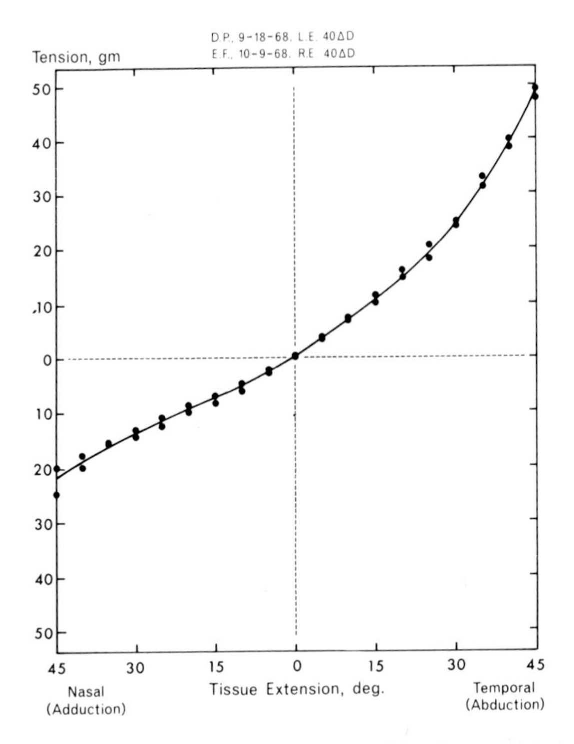

Fig. 27. Static length tension relationship of human globe restraining tissues with both medial and lateral rectus muscles detached. Note twice as much force required to rotate these eyes temporally as nasally; data obtained from two patients, both of whom exhibited 40 prism diopters intermittent exotropia.

mately 0.5 grams per degree, and the stiffness in the temporal quadrant rises to more than twice this value. These measured values of elasticity should permit us to determine the division of forces between the agonist and antagonist muscles and the supporting tissues restraining rotation of the globe. It is hoped that this kind of information may become useful in the diagnosis and correction of oculomotor pathology.

Fig. 28 shows the isotonic displacement recovery time course to the step function input of quick release of the isolated human globe. This type of dynamic record permits us to calculate the viscosity of the globe restraining elements as well as corroborate the elasticity measurements of the globe shown in Fig. 27. It can be clearly seen that the displacement recovery occurs in two phases, fast and slow. This record was produced by pulling the globe to a position 45 degrees left of primary position and cutting the suture abruptly, allowing the eye to travel back towards the primary position. The time course of eye movement was recorded by means of a photoelectric eye

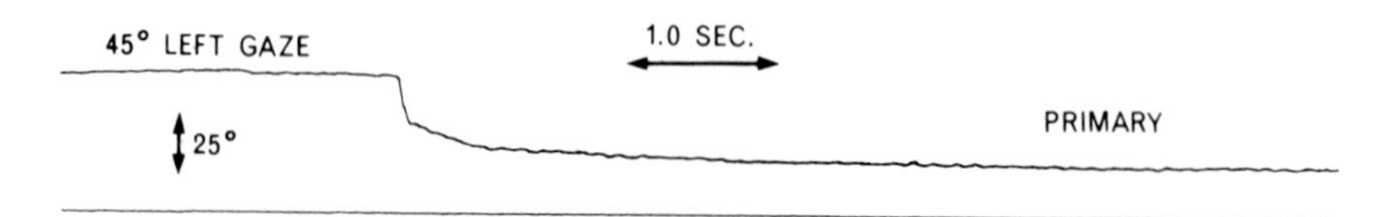

Fig. 28. Isotonic displacement time course of a human globe with both medial and lateral rectus muscles detached. The eyeball was pulled to the 45 degree temporal gaze position and quickly released. Note that recovery of the globe to primary position occurs in two steps, with a fast time constant (0.02 second) followed by a slower, 1 second time constant.

position transducer which tracked the limbus of the moving eye (O'Meara, 1966). From records such as this the time constants of recovery of the fast and slow elements of the restraining tissues of the globe can be directly determined. With knowledge of these time constants (τ) and the associated elasticities (K), the corresponding viscosities (B), can be computed as:

$$B = K\tau$$

The values of elasticity and viscosity so derived are arranged in the form of a mechanical model of the human globe restraining tissues in Fig. 29. The values given are taken at the primary position of the globe. It is appreciated that these values should be functions of the tension existing in the globe restraining tissues, as has been observed with the cat. However, insufficient measurements at this time preclude our analytical description of the variation of elasticity and viscosity of these tissues with tension. We plan further human investigations to describe more completely the variation of these mechanical parameters. As it stands, this model of the human globe restraining tissues may give us a start in the partitioning of the forces involved in the human oculomotor process.

Human oculorotary muscle

In these studies information was derived from measurements on the oculorotary muscles during various states of graded voluntary innervation. Studies were made on 6 adult patients under topical anesthesia during the course of corrective surgery for intermittent exotropia. Each patient was supine on the operating table and his head was supported by a vacuum sand bag which molded to the contours of the head, holding it rigidly in position. The horizontal rectus muscles were detached from the globe. Before corrective reattachment, the lateral rectus was attached by a 000 surgical silk suture to the micromanipulator-mounted strain gauge. Muscle tension was recorded as a function of muscle length on an X-Y recorder and both were recorded as functions of time on a six-channel chart recorder and a magnetic tape recorder with a bandwidth of 625 cycles per second.

The degree of innervation of an oculorotary muscle was determined by requesting the patient to fix given target lamps with the normal eye such

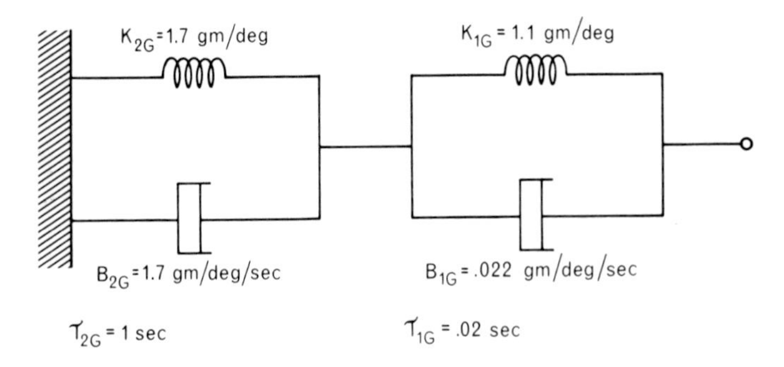

Fig. 29. Mechanical model of the human globe restraining tissues with values taken at primary position. This model is derived in large part from the isotonic results of Fig. 28. Two Voigt elements in series adequately duplicate the observed results. The form of this model is consistent with that of the cat globe restraining tissues, Fig. 7. K (coefficient of elasticity or stiffness), B (coefficient of viscosity) and τ (time constant) are presented for both fast (1G) and slow (2G) components of the globe restraining tissues. The values of the coefficients are derived as follows:

τ_{1G} = .02 sec from direct observation of Fig. 28.
K_{1G} = 1.1 gm/deg since 30 gm globe restraining force resulted in 27 deg of fast eye movement.
B_{1G} = .022 gm/deg/sec = $K_{1G}\,\tau_{1G}$
τ_{2G} = 1 sec, from Fig. 28
K_{2G} = 1.7 g/deg since 30 gm globe restraining force resulted in 18 deg of slower eye movement.
B_{2G} = 1.7 gm/deg/sec = $K_{2G}\,\tau_{2G}$

$$K_C = \frac{K_1 K_2}{K_1 + K_2} = .67 \text{ gm/deg}$$

which checks with the observed value of K_C at 5 deg temporal rotation in Fig. 27.

that the operated eye would assume positions of 0, ±15, ±30, and ±45 degrees. The operated eye was occluded and the muscle to be tested was adjusted to its primary length from whence known displacement variations could be made.

To measure the passive length–tension curve, the patient was requested to fixate a lamp maximally out of the field of action of the muscle being studied, i.e., 45° left for the right lateral rectus. The length–tension relationships of this relaxed muscle compared well with the same procedure repeated on six other patients under general anesthesia (q.v. Fig. 2, Chapter 11).

The steady state length–tension characteristics of the right lateral rectus muscle for a representative patient are seen in Fig. 30. This family of static length–tension curves was derived with various levels of innervation as the parameter. Each curve represents a separate constant conjugate effort of the right lateral rectus muscle while the unoperated left eye remained fixed in gaze on one of the designated targets.

It is of interest to note that the slopes of these length–tension curves are essentially constant, forming parallel straight lines particularly above 15 or 20 grams muscle tension. Below this value, the muscle starts to go slack and the curves bend towards zero tension. We also note that the tension in

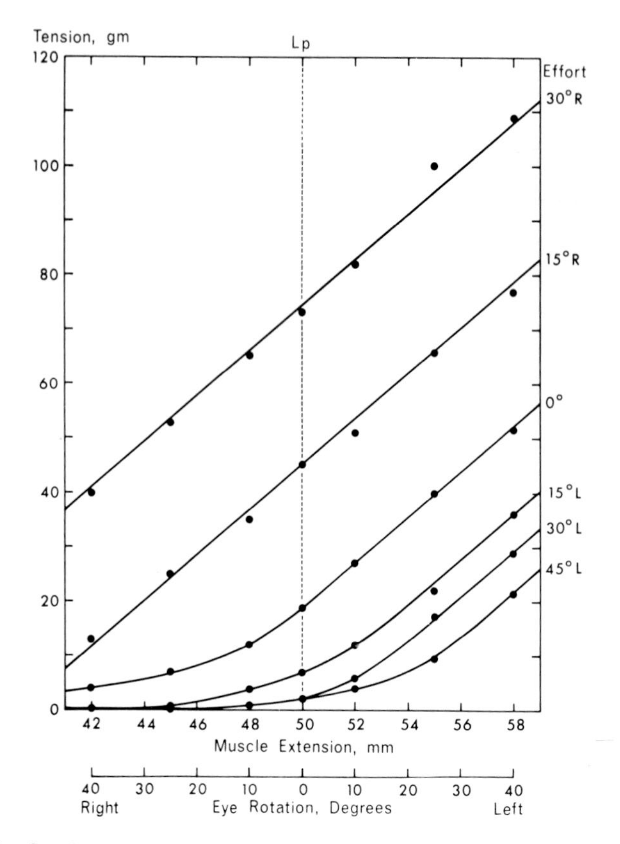

Fig. 30. Family of static length–tension curves for a human right lateral rectus muscle. Each curve represents a separate constant conjugate effort of the right eye muscle under study, (R) right, (L) left effort from primary position (0°). For each curve the unoperated left eye remained fixed in gaze on a designated target indicated on the right ordinate. At 45° left rotational effort the innervation to the right lateral rectus muscle is essentially zero. (This is confirmed by the observation that the same passive length–tension curve is measured under anesthesia). Below the graph, muscle extension is given in millimeters (upper scale) and the equivalent eye rotation in degrees (lower scale), taken as 5 degrees per millimeter for an assumed globe diameter of approximately 24 mm. The primary muscle length, L, for the human lateral rectus muscle is taken as approximately 50 mm from the dissection data of Volkmann (1869).

a waking patient fixing in primary position is some 15 to 20 grams. Consequently, the steady state tension in a human oculorotary muscle never falls below a level which would put the operating characteristics in a nonlinear region of the length–tension relationship.

It has been difficult to determine whether this linear length–tension relationship for human oculorotary muscle is an inherent property of the muscle or whether it is a manifestation of neural feedback mediated by tension receptors in the muscle or tendon. Professor Granit (personal communication) has suggested that the parallel tension extension curves of an extrinsic eye muscle in man may be evidence for an alpha-gamma linkage or neuromechanical feedback system responsible for the linearity of the measured length–tension relationships of the human oculorotary muscles. As Dr. Granit points out, such "parallel curves are a definite sign of proprioceptive control, probably executed jointly by spindles and tendon organs on the alpha motor neurons, the former excitatory, the latter inhibitory" (Granit, Chapter 1).

Fender (personal communication) believes that these parallel linear length–tension curves strongly suggest a tension servo system with feedback from a tension measuring element. These explanations are most persuasive. Indeed, the absence of parallel linear length–tension relationships at low innervation levels in the cat tends to support the proprioceptive hypothesis. However, in our animal experiments with the sixth nerve cut or crushed, eliminating the possibility of proprioceptive feedback, the length–tension characteristics at high levels of innervation reveal a parallel linear relationship (Fig. 15). These experiments would suggest that, at least for high innervation levels, another basis for the linear length–tension characteristics may be found in the intrinsic properties of the muscle itself.

From the human oculorotary muscle length–tension characteristics under steps of graded innervation we can derive a transfer function relating muscle innervation to force generated by the muscle. In Fig. 30 the vertical line at the primary muscle length passes through points indicating the force or tension generated at various levels of stimulation (effort). These points are plotted in Fig. 31 for a medial rectus muscle to provide an isometric innervation–force transfer function. The upper scale on the abscissa shows the eye position in degrees of temporal or nasal rotation. The bottom scale indicates the percentage maximal excitation of that muscle on a linear effort scale. When the eye is rotated completely out of the field of action of a given muscle, the innervation to that muscle is essentially zero. The passive length–tension characteristics measured at surgery under anesthesia agree with the length–tension characteristics derived under these minimally innervated conditions of the muscle.

In attempting to fit a smooth curve to the experimental data points of Fig. 31, we find that a simple analytic expression fits the observations quite well. Thus in this particular case, we can use the parabolic expression:

$$T = 93\ E^2 \text{ grams.}$$

It is interesting to note that a parabolic relationship is also observed upon stimulating the sixth nerve of the cat in equal increments of frequency of stimulus (Fig. 21). This suggests that the degree of innervation for holding the eye at any fixed position of lateral gaze is a linear function of the angle of gaze, even though the force developed appears as the square of the average frequency of innervation. This square law effort-tension relationship has

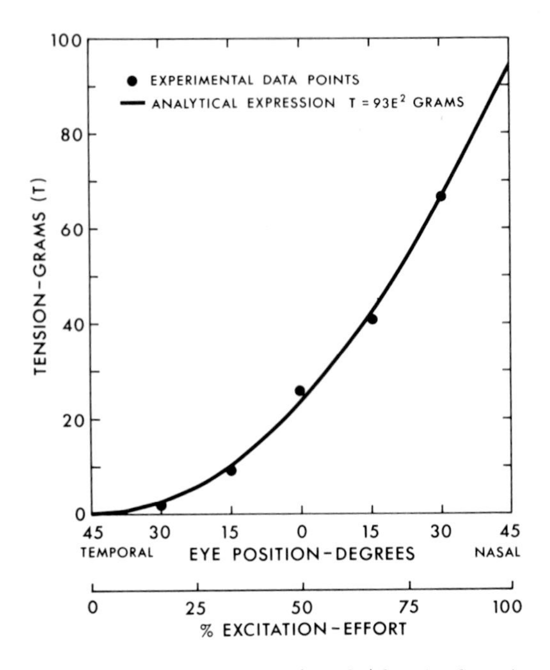

Fig. 31. Innervation–tension diagram or input–output (transfer) function for an isometric human medial rectus neuromuscular unit. Note that equal increments of innervational effort result in progressively increasing increments of tension. The resulting square law relationship is shown on the diagram with T = muscle tension and E = rotational effort in % maximum. This parabolic relationship is also seen in the cat oculorotary muscle, Fig. 21.

been observed for the half dozen conscious patients we have been able to measure thus far.

The seemingly disparate observation of linear innervation producing a square law (neuromechanically generated) force which in turn results in linear positioning of the eye may be more readily acceptable on the following hypothesis. The oculomotor system appears to constitute a so-called "push–pull" output system. It employs "class A" operation in fixation and tracking, both of which increase the fidelity of response, (i.e., reduce the harmonic or nonlinear distortion). In contrast, the highest speed (saccadic) eye movements are controlled by "class B" or "class C" operation which has the inherent advantage of higher power output and consequently greater speed of operation. The concomitant loss of output fidelity is displayed in ballistic, non-tracking eye movements. There are a number of reasons for fidelity of the "class A" operation. Feedback is continuous; "class A" operation does not shut off at any time; it removes the length–tension nonlinearities when the muscle goes "slack", and the square law relationship of one muscle is balanced off by the inverse square law relationship of the opposed antagonist operating in a reciprocally innervated situation.

From the fixed-step graded innervation length-tension characteristics shown in Fig. 30 we can derive information relative to the forces required to hold the globe at any angle of eccentric fixation. Fig. 32 shows the "static locus" or the physiological values of tension employed to hold the eye at various angles of deviation. This curve was derived by marking points of corresponding eye position (horizontal axis) on the fixed innervation-tension curve required to hold the eye in this position (innervation being indicated at the upper right end of the diagonal length-tension lines). The intersection of each innervated length-tension curve with the corresponding eye position must indicate the tension employed to hold the eye at this position under steady state conditions. The curve joining each of these points is the steady state fixation tension locus or "static locus", and the tension is described in this case by the analytic expression:

$$T = 0.017\,(\theta - 15)^2 + 16 \text{ gm},$$

where θ represents eye position in degrees from primary position.

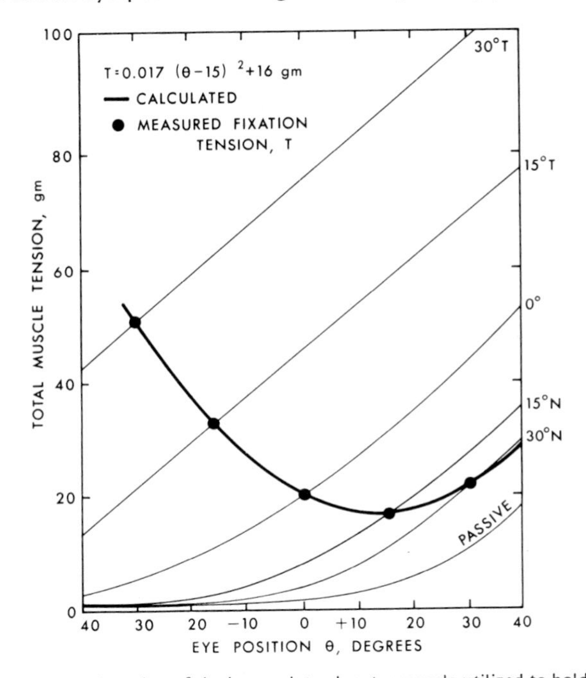

Fig. 32. The measured total tension of the human lateral rectus muscle utilized to hold the eye at various angles of lateral gaze. The points represent the naturally innervated tension of the agonist which balances the opposing tensions of the antagonist muscle and the orbital supporting tissues restraining movement of the globe. This "static locus" or fixation tension curve is shown as the heavy parabolic arc with an analytic expression which fits the measured data points. The light lines depict the length-tension curves of the muscle as shown in Fig. 30.

We intend to further investigate this concept of a static fixation tension locus in human oculorotary muscles by means of miniature implanted force transducers during fixation in various positions of lateral gaze. A photograph of one of these miniature strain gauge transducers, developed in the author's laboratory, is shown in Fig. 33. It has been tested in animals with encouraging results. We plan further application of these implanted gauges to determine the actual forces exerted by human oculorotary muscles during eye movements and fixation. The existence of a static fixation tension locus for conjugate eye movements (Fig. 32) suggests that there may be a different static locus for disjunctive eye movements. This hypothesis will also be tested in our laboratory with the miniature implanted strain gauges.

From the static length–tension characteristics for human oculorotary muscle (Fig. 30) we can derive the elasticity of the isometric human lateral rectus muscle. Fig. 34 presents the mean values for three cooperating patients. The elasticity of the passive element (Kp), of course, remains constant

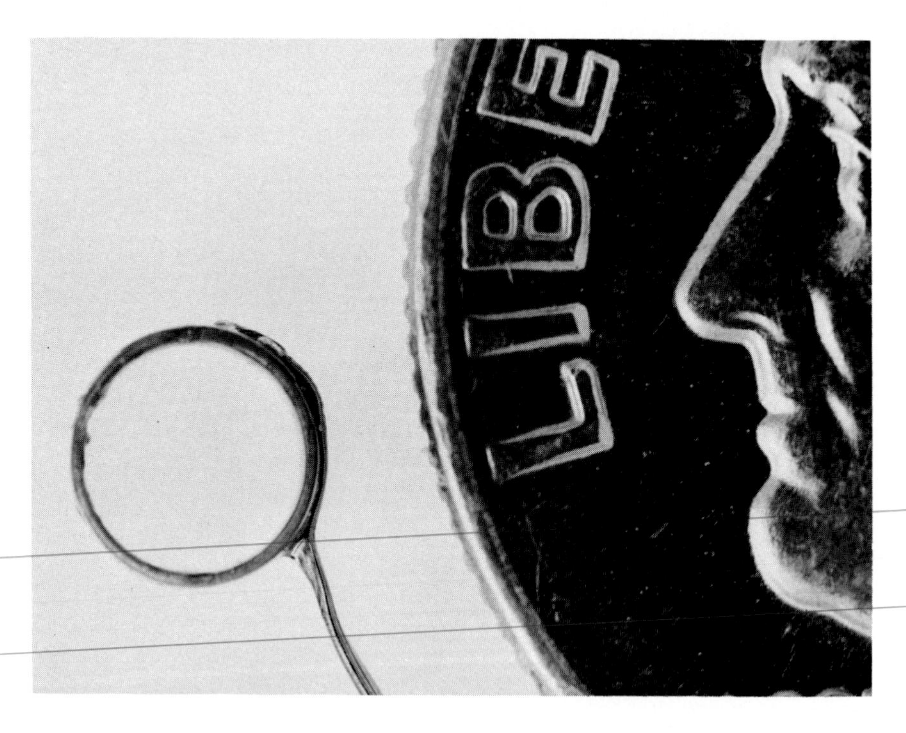

Fig. 33. A miniature ring strain gauge shown in comparison with a dime. The metal foil strain sensing element is cemented to a stainless steel ring (diameter 2.5 mm; wall thickness 0.25 mm). These miniature force transducers have been implanted in series with the tendons of oculorotary muscles of the cat to provide continuous measurement of the muscle tension during eye movements.

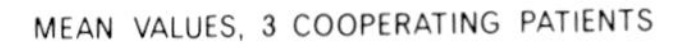

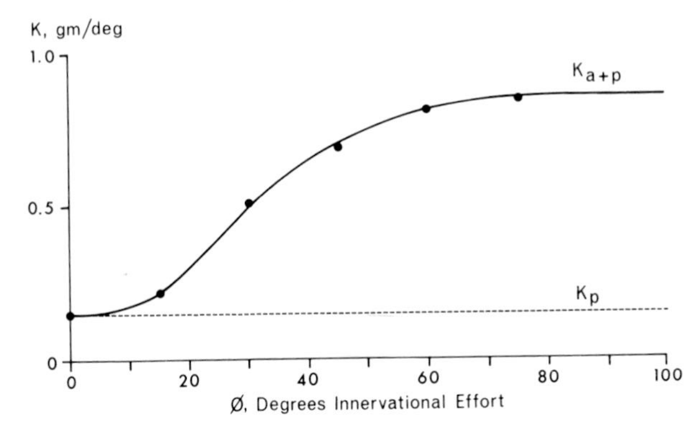

Fig. 34. Coefficient of elasticity of the isometric human lateral rectus muscle as a function of natural innervation. Note that isometric elasticity increases up to about 50% innervational effort and then remains essentially constant above this level. These values were obtained from the slopes of length-tension curves similar to Fig. 30. K_a and K_p are the active and passive elasticities respectively.

at any given length. However, the increase of isometric elasticity with innervation of the contractile element can be seen to change the elasticity of the oculorotary muscle by a factor of four. At some level above fifty or sixty percent innervation, the elasticity of the active element reaches a saturation point and levels off to an essentially constant value. These measurements are corroborated by those in the anesthetized cat, in which we find the elasticity to be a function of innervation, as expected from the recruiting of more active fibers. The reader may wish to compare Fig. 34 with Fig. 22 derived from cat oculorotary muscle.

Elasticity of the passive and contractile elements of human oculorotary muscles can be measured under steady state physiological fixation conditions, if the eye is permitted to move in a normal physiological manner and to find its resting point of fixation at any degree of eccentric gaze. Fig. 35 presents such values of elasticity derived from Fig. 32, the steady state fixation tension locus. Under these conditions innervation shortens the agonist, and consequently the stiffness of the passive element decreases (in this case, from a value of 1.3 grams per degree to 0 at a point just beyond 50 percent innervational effort). On the other hand, the stiffness of the active element starts from a 0 value at 0 innervation and increases linearly up to the 50 percent innervation level; at this point the stiffness tends to saturate and become constant at a level of approximately 0.8 grams per degree. If the total stiffness, that is, the sum of the passive and active elements, is plotted, we get the third curve, the stiffness of the total muscle, which is represented in Fig. 35 as Kp + a. Now, we see that the stiffness of the total muscle appears

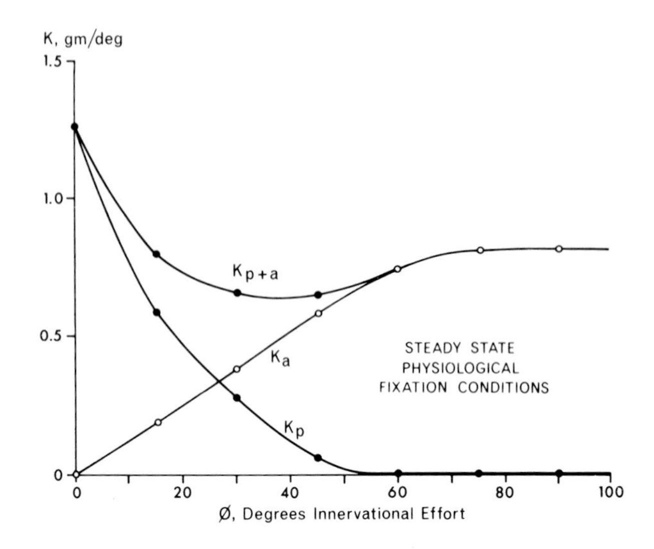

Fig. 35. Coefficient of elasticity of human lateral rectus muscle under physiological conditions of eye fixation, as the muscle shortens to rotate the eye against the load of the antagonist muscle and the globe restraining tissues. The elasticities of the passive element, K_p, the active element, K_a, and their parallel combination, the total muscle $K_p + K_a$ are shown as functions of the percentage innervational effort, θ, of the lateral rectus muscle.

These values were taken as the slopes of the appropriate length-tension curves and the fixation tension locus of Fig. 32. Muscle elasticity is roughly constant over a wide range of eye rotations, providing insight into the parallel family of length-tension curves (Fig. 30).

nearly constant over the entire range of innervation above 5 or 10 percent innervational effort.

Hopefully, these observations may provide deeper insight into the mechanisms responsible for the mechanical characteristics of human oculorotary muscles, and allow us to gaze deeper into the MUD (mechanical underlying determinants) impeding ocular motion.

Let us now study the dynamic nature of the innervation and concomitant forces developed by the muscle to move the eyes. We can make isometric measurements of the tension developed by a muscle under conditions of natural innervation which produce conjugate saccadic movements. Fig. 36 shows the isometric muscle tension developed in a human right lateral rectus muscle during a 30 degree saccade of the left eye. Note the very definite overshoot of tension followed by an approximately exponential decay to a final steady state value of holding tension (which is the tension indicated on the static fixation tension locus of Fig. 32). Teleologically, we can argue that this overshoot of tension hastens movement of the eye by producing additional acceleration required to overcome the various viscous resistive forces. The final value of steady state tension then adjusts itself to the level required by the elasticities of the opposing tissues. A further confirmation of this

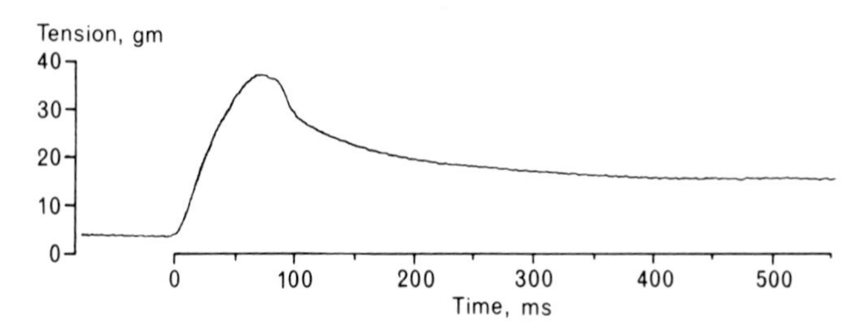

Fig. 36. The isometric tension developed by a human right lateral rectus muscle during a 30 degree right saccade to primary position (by the left eye) while the measured muscle was held at primary length. Note the tension overshoot which overcomes the large viscosity of the oculomotor plant to produce a fast saccadic eye movement with no overshoot.

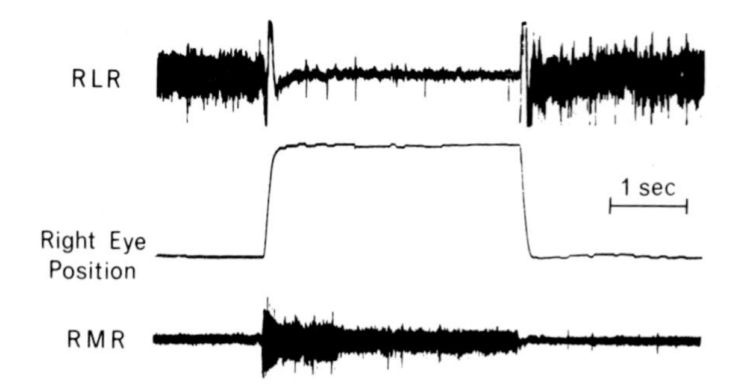

Fig. 37. Simultaneous electromyographic and eye movement data for a 20° saccade to the left of primary. One sees total inhibition of the antagonist (right lateral rectus) during the actual eye movement. Also note small changes of fixation of right eye as it apparently searches over a 1° wide target. These small movements are each accompanied by a single large EMG spike in only the muscle appropriate to the direction of movement. (*Record reproduced by courtesy of Professor Arthur Jampolsky, M.D.*)

overshoot in muscle activity is shown in Fig. 37. This electromyographic recording is of a saccadic refixation from 0 to 20 degrees. Note that the right medial rectus muscle, which is brought into play to move the eye, shows an overshoot in the electromyogram. This indicates that the tension shown in Fig. 36 was indeed produced by an overshoot of innervation. We also note that there is *no* overshoot in eye position. Thus, as Robinson has pointed out, the oculomotor control system has adapted its control output signal to match the viscous and elastic characteristics of the oculomotor plant in such manner as to produce fast and accurate control of eye movements, that is, with no overshoot or oscillation.

Note in Fig. 37 that as the subject fixated the target, which was approximately 1 degree wide, he apparently looked from edge to edge of the target.

This is seen in the eye position record, which shows a number of deviations of approximately one degree. It is striking to see that for each small saccade, there is a corresponding burst of EMG activity in the muscle which produces movement in that direction.

Differential forced duction evaluation of muscle and orbital tissue characteristics

We have performed a series of differential forced duction measurements, both pre- and post- operatively, on consenting strabismus patients who have had oculorotary muscle length–tension determinations made during surgery. A suction cup scleral contact lens has been used for measuring the passive tangential force required to rotate the intact globe and muscles through a predetermined arc, with a method similar to that employed by Stephens and Reinecke (1967). Fig. 38 shows the experimental setup, with a motor driven force transducer used to make the differential forced duction measurements described below. The suction contact lens permits mechanical attachment to the intact globe and neuromuscular system, as the patient fixates a series of distant targets with the unencumbered eye (the measured eye is occluded).

The procedure is based on the findings of our human oculorotary muscle length–tension data shown in Fig. 30. From this figure it can be seen that for nasal rotational efforts, and with the muscle simultaneously shortened to the twenty degree lateral position, the lateral rectus muscle goes slack, i.e., exhibits zero elasticity. The same effect is seen for the medial rectus during temporal rotational efforts. Hence, we can measure the combined elasticity

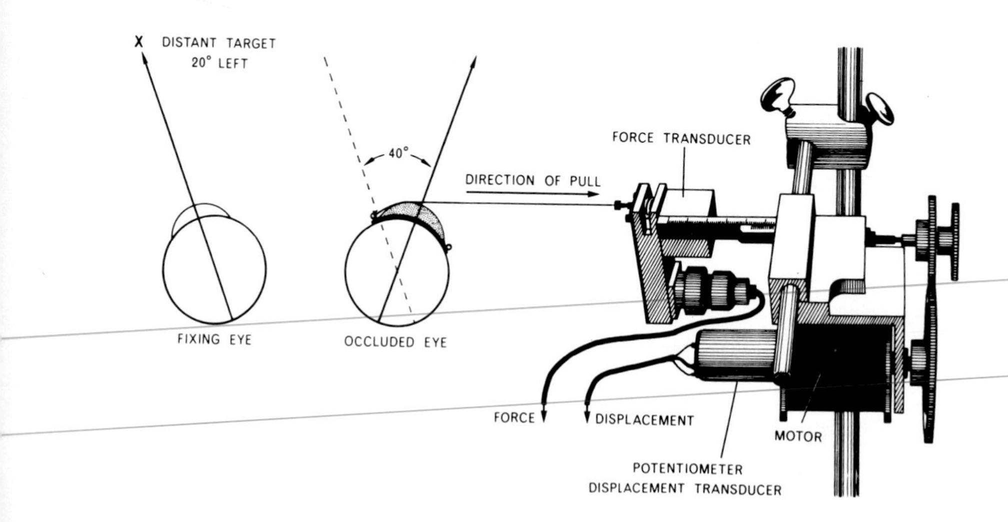

Fig. 38. Motor driven strain gauge force transducer mounted on a micromanipulator to determine the length–tension characteristics of human oculorotary muscles and globe restraining tissues during differential forced duction measurements. Procedure 2 of the protocol is being carried out on the right eye (see Table I).

TABLE I

PROTOCOL OF DIFFERENTIAL FORCED DUCTION MEASUREMENTS

1. a) Subject looks right with free eye to a point constraining measured eye to assume 20° right position.
Observer pulls measured eye to 20° left position with suction contact lens and records tension versus position on X-Y plotter.
The resulting slope $\Delta T/\Delta\Theta$ represents the sum of $K_L + K_O$ if right eye is measured, as shown in Fig. 40 (or $K_M + K_O$ if left eye is measured).

b) With measured eye pulled to 20° left position, subject fixates targets which previously resulted in the measured eye assuming 0°, 15°, and 30° right positions and steady state tensions are recorded.
The higher tensions are due almost exclusively to T_L, lateral rectus developed tension of right eye (T_M of left eye).

2. Subject looks left with free eye to a point constraining measured eye to assume 20° left position.
Observer pulls measured eye to 40° left position measuring tension versus position.
The slope $\Delta T/\Delta\Theta$ in this position represents the sum of $K_L + K_M + K_O$ in left gaze.

3. a) Subject looks left with free eye to a point constraining measured eye to assume 20° left position.
Observer pulls measured eye to 20° right position recording tension versus position.
The slope $\Delta T/\Delta\Theta$ in this position represents the sum of $K_M + K_O$ of right eye (or $K_L + K_O$ of measured left eye).

b) With measured eye pulled to 20° right position, subject fixates targets which previously resulted in the measured eye assuming 0°, 15°, and 30° left positions and steady tensions are recorded.
The higher tensions are due almost exclusively to T_M of right eye (T_L of left eye).

4. Subject looks right with free eye to a position resulting in measured eye fixing at 20° right.
Observer pulls measured eye to 40° right position measuring tension versus position.
The slope $\Delta T/\Delta\Theta$in this position represents the sum of $K_L + K_M + K_O$ in right gaze.

Now evaluate parameters separately from above measurements:

$K_L + K_M + K_O - (K_L + K_O) = K_M$, the stiffness of the medial rectus

$K_L + K_M + K_O - (K_M + K_O) = K_L$, the stiffness of the lateral rectus

$K_L + K_O - K_L = K_O$, the stiffness of the globe restraining tissues

$K_M + K_O - K_M = K_O$, the stiffness of the globe restraining tissues

One can then calculate the eye position for a given combination of muscle forces, T_L and T_M, or conversely the muscle force imbalance responsible for an observed deviation:

$$\Theta = (T_L - T_M) \;/\; K_L + K_M + K_O$$

Also, a significant part of the static length-tension diagram can be constructed for both medial and lateral rectus muscles of the measured eye (q.v. Fig. 30).

of the globe and of only one muscle. This value can be subtracted from a measurement including the elasticity of both muscles and the globe, to yield a value for elasticity of the other muscle alone. Thus, three appropriate measurements allow calculation of the three individual and independent elasticities associated with the restraining tissues of the globe, the lateral rectus muscle, and the medial rectus muscle. The method of performing these measurements is summarized in Table I, a protocol for differential forced duction measurements.

A typical record obtained by our forced duction technique is shown in Fig. 39, and indicates that there is a considerable region in which the length-tension characteristic is essentially linear. It is this linear slope which we use in calculation of the values of the elements of a clinical static oculomotor

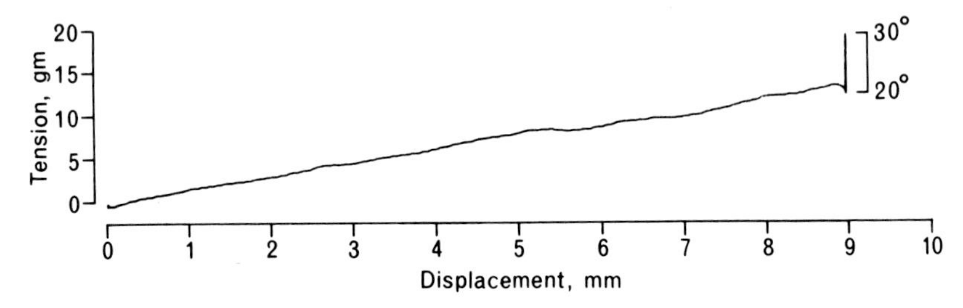

Fig. 39. Typical results of procedure 2 of the differential forced duction measurement with the free left eye fixed at 20° left rotation while the tension required to pull the right eye temporally through a 40 degree arc is continuously recorded as a function of eye rotation in mm. This record measures the elasticity of the right medial rectus muscle and the globe restraining tissues. (These raw tension values must be multiplied by a factor greater than one to correct for the thickness and resulting greater radius of curvature at the suction-held contact lens).

model for each patient studied. The values of elasticity calculated from the forced duction measurements compare well with those measured directly during surgery, tending to establish the validity of the indirect forced duction methods.

Fig. 40 presents a simplified linear model of the innervated human peripheral oculomotor apparatus. In this model the spring constants of each muscle can be evaluated, as can those of the passive orbital tissue restraining motion of the globe. In addition, the contributions of the contractile elements can also be calculated. It is by this means that we hope to be able to distinguish between muscular and tissue elasticity anomalies or deviations from the normal balance of reciprocal innervation interplaying upon the medial and lateral rectus muscles producing normal eye movements.

CONCLUSIONS

The physiological measurements performed in these studies have provided detailed evaluations of the various elements of the oculomotor plant. Their interrelationships have permitted more precise analytic descriptions of orbital mechanics. From these preliminary studies it is clear that the oculo-

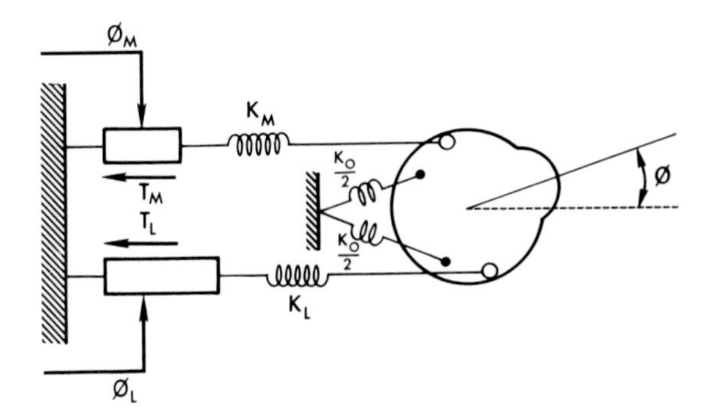

Fig. 40. A simplified linear model of the peripheral oculomotor apparatus. Each K represents a spring constant of $\Delta T/\Delta L$, X represents the hypothetical length of a contractile element which is set by its magnitude of innervation, ϕ, resulting in a muscle tension, T. Ocular deviation or position is shown as θ. The five parameters of this clinical model, K_O, K_L, K_M, X_L and X_M can be evaluated for an individual patient by five differential forced duction measurements (see text and Table I).

Equations of ocular fixation for this model can be given as:
$T_M = (X_M + r\theta)K_M$; $T_L = (X_L - r\theta)K_L$; $T_O = r\theta K_O$ at equilibrium,
$T_M + T_{O(lat.)} = T_L + T_{O(med.)}$, and by substitution,
$\theta = (X_L K_L - X_M K_M)/r(K_L + K_M + K_O)$

motor neuromechanical plant is basically quite nonlinear and that further work will be required to elucidate its exact nature.

The model evolved here resembles that due to Robinson (1968); however, the magnitude of each of the elements is not constant. Our results confirm Cook and Stark's hypothesis (1967) of proportionality between viscosity (B) and tension which was assumed from the original work of Hill (1938). In addition, the elasticity (K) is also proportional to tension, as was first surmised by Fick (1871). Linearity of each of the individual components of the oculomotor model can be assumed only over a small segment of eye rotation. The magnitudes of the viscoelastic elements change not only with tension due to muscle length, but also due to isometric developed tension changes. This observation that the values of the viscoelastic elements vary directly with tissue tension may be of fundamental utility. It indicates that tissue tension should vary exponentially with muscle length, that is:

$$\text{If } K = dT/dL = mT$$

then

$$T = e^{mL}$$

The general form of the mechanical impedance of all tissues measured appears quite similar. Two series viscoelastic Voigt elements with the magnitude of each element varying directly with tension appears to adequately model each tissue element. The increase of viscoelasticity with length performs a natural snubbing or shock-absorbing action, that is, an increasing resistance and reactance to over-stretch. However, at very high velocities viscous resistance (damping) decreases which facilitates rapid saccadic movements with less energy expenditure.

It will also be noted from the length–tension curves that as the muscle is lengthened the stiffness of the active element apparently remains constant up to approximately primary length and then falls with the inverse function of the stiffness–length characteristic of the passive element. Thus, the elasticity of the total stimulated muscle remains constant over nearly the entire range of eye movements, particularly at high levels of stimulation. This results in linear, parallel length–tension curves over the greater range of eye movements and innervations.

This observed linearity permits us to describe the peripheral oculomotor plant in the static state in terms of a simple linear clinical model which can be evaluated for individual patients by means of a differential forced duction technique.

Although the isometric tension of the contractile element increases as the square of innervation, eye position varies linearly with innervation. This occurs because the muscle is loaded by the square law characteristic of its antagonist. The oculorotary muscles work together in reciprocally innervated push–pull opposition to cancel the large nonlinearities in each.

Although orbital viscosity and elasticity vary widely over the normal range of eye movements the mechanical time constants of the oculomotor system appear essentially fixed. These are the time constants to which the oculomotor control system has become adapted. The most rapid saccadic eye movements are produced by a burst of maximal oculorotary muscle tension so well modulated that no eye movement overshoot occurs. Robinson (personal communication) has found separate control signals in the oculomotor nuclei which are each proportional to the viscosity (B) and elasticity (K) of the oculomotor plant. These control signals occur in the ratio of $B/K = \tau$, the major time constant of the peripheral oculomotor system.

We have found evidence for, and will pursue further, the appearance of a small viscosity in parallel with the series elastic component of the contractile element, resulting in a time constant somewhat less than 5 milliseconds. Also in our model there may be a time constant of the order of 10 milliseconds associated with the series elastic component of the passive element, which will be further studied. The disparity in values of K_{2G} between the cat and the human must be resolved by more definitive measurements which we can now undertake in the human.

Dynamically the complete oculomotor plant appears as a first order second degree system. Certain approximations may permit lumping and linearization of constants to reduce the complexity, but the system remains inherently grossly nonlinear over a large range of eye movements. Insights derived from the dynamic mechanical measurements and calculations of the oculomotor system of the cat should permit us to better guide further research and interpretation of the mechanical parameters of the human oculomotor system which may be of clinical significance.

ACKNOWLEDGEMENT

The author gratefully acknowledges the collaboration of Dr. Alan Scott, Dr. Arthur Jampolsky, Dr. Gerald Meltzer, and Mr. David O'Meara in collecting the data from which the reported results have been derived.

REFERENCES

Blix, M. (1892). Die Länge und die Spannung des Muskels. *Skand. Arch. Physiol.* **3**, 295–318.
Boeder, P. (1961). The cooperation of extraocular muscles. *Amer. J. Ophthal.* **51**, 469–481.
Buchthal, F. and Kaiser, E. (1951). The rheology of the cross striated muscle fiber. *Dan. Biol. Medd.* **21**, 6-318.
Collins, C. C., Scott, A. B., and O'Meara, D. (1969). Elements of the peripheral oculomotor apparatus. *Amer. J. Optom.* **46**, 510–515.
Collins, C. C., Meltzer, G. O'Meara, D., and Scott, A. B. (1969). Viscoelasticity of oculorotary muscle of the cat (abstract). *Invest. Ophthal.* **8**, 650.
Cook, G. and Stark, L. (1967). Derivation of a model for the human eye-positioning mechanism. *Bull. Math. Biophys.* **29**, 153–174.
Costenbader, F. D. (1961). Infantile esotropia. *Trans. Am. Ophthal. Soc.* **59**, 397–429.
Fender, D. H. and Nye, P. W. (1961). An investigation of the mechanisms of eye movement control. *Kybernetik.* **1** 81–88.
Fick, A. (1871). Über die Änderung der Elasticität des Muskels während der Zuckung. *Arch. für die Ges. Physiologie.* **4**, 301-315.
Gasser, H. S. and Hill, A. V. (1924). The dynamics of muscular contraction. *Proc. Roy. Soc. B.* **96**, 398–437.
Hyde, J. E. (1959). Some characteristics of voluntary human ocular movements in the horizontal plane. *Am. J. Ophthal.* **48**, 85–94.
Levin, A. and Wyman, J. (1927). The viscous elastic properties of muscle. *Proc. Roy. Soc. B.* **150**, 218–243.
O'Meara, D. (1966). Photoelectric eye movement detector. *Proc. 19th Conf. Engineer. Med. & Biol.* p. 241.
Robinson, D. A. (1964). The mechanics of human saccadic eye movement. *J. Physiol.* **174**, 245–264.
Robinson, D. A., O'Meara, D., Scott, A. B., and Collins, C. C. (1969). The mechanical components of human eye movements. *J. Appl. Physiol.* **26**, 548–553.
Schenck, F. R. (1895). Weitere Untersuchungen über den Einfluss der Spannung auf den Zuckungsverlauf. *Arch. für die Ges. Physiologie.* **61**, 77–105.
Stephens, K. F. and Reinecke, R. D. (1967). Quantitative forced duction. *Trans. Am. Acad. Ophthal.* **71**, 324.
Stone, S. L., Thomas, J. G., and Zakian, V. (1965). The passive rotatory characteristics of the dog's eye and its attachments. *J. Physiol.* **181**, 337-349.
Volkman, A. W. (1869). Zur mechanik der augenmuskeln. *Trans. Leipzig Soc. Sci.* **21**, 28–70.
Vossius, G. (1960). Das System der Augenbewegung (I). *Z. Biol.* **112**, 27.
Westheimer, G. (1954). Mechanism of saccadic eye movements. *A. M. A. Arch. Ophthal.* **52**, 710–724.
Young, L. R. and Stark, L. (1963). Variable feedback experiments testing a sampled data model for eye tracking. *IEEE Trans. Profession Tech. Group on Human Factors in Electronics.* HFE-**4**, 38.
Zuber, B. L. (1968). Eye movement dynamics in the cat: the final motor pathway. *Exptl. Neurol.* **20**, 255-260.

EXTRAOCULAR MUSCLE FORCES IN STRABISMUS

ALAN B. SCOTT

The motor aspects of strabismus are tested by binocular alignment in the primary position, by alignment in eccentric gaze (versions), by assessing the boundaries of rotation ability (ductions, overactions, underactions), and by assessing the resistance to passive rotation (traction test, forced duction test). Deriving from our studies of the mechanical properties in strabismus, there are additional tests which are helpful in understanding, diagnosis, and treatment. This chapter reviews some pertinent data on the passive and active forces giving horizontal alignment, shows that a quantitative approach to the forced duction test yields useful information, and describes how to assess the active force which the muscle gives during fixation or while the eye tries to move (force generation tests). We will deal first with the static forces which balance one another during steady fixation. Then we shall show how one can get useful information from the *dynamic* behavior of the eye as it moves or tries to move with inputs from the various motor systems of the general oculomotor apparatus.

STATICS - PASSIVE FORCES

In deep anesthesia or in death the eyes of normal persons point nearly straight ahead (Cogan, 1956). The "common knowledge" on this point still presumes the eyes are substantially outward and upward when tonus is removed. Observation on the positions of eyes of normal anesthetized persons, or

These investigations were supported by Public Health Service Research Grant 5 RO1 EY 00498 and Program Project Grant PO1 EY 00299 from the National Eye Institute, and Contract N0014-70-C-0141 from the Office of Naval Research.

in removing some dozens of eyes post-mortem for corneal grafts will confirm the generality that the passive position is about straight. The passive forces holding the eye are obviously balanced for this to be so. These forces are divisible into: 1) passive muscle tension 2) passive globe tension (provided by the suspensory tissues in the orbit, Tenon's fascia, etc.) 3) a third force is the orbit tissue pressure, which moves the eye forward about 3 mm when rectus muscle tension is removed. When rotary motions are restricted active forces are often translated along this axis, causing retraction or protrusion of the eye. This is resisted by the orbit elasticity which is about 20 grams per mm (Duke-Elder, 1952).

Passive Muscle Elasticity

In 8 strabismus patients under general anesthesia the detached lateral rectus muscle of eyes previously unoperated was connected via a 3-0 silk suture to a strain gauge (Fig. 1). As one pulled out the muscle there were increasing increments of tension with each millimeter of pull (Fig. 2). (Collins, *et al.,* 1969; Esslen and Huber, 1967.) In angular measurement this is about 0.2 grams per

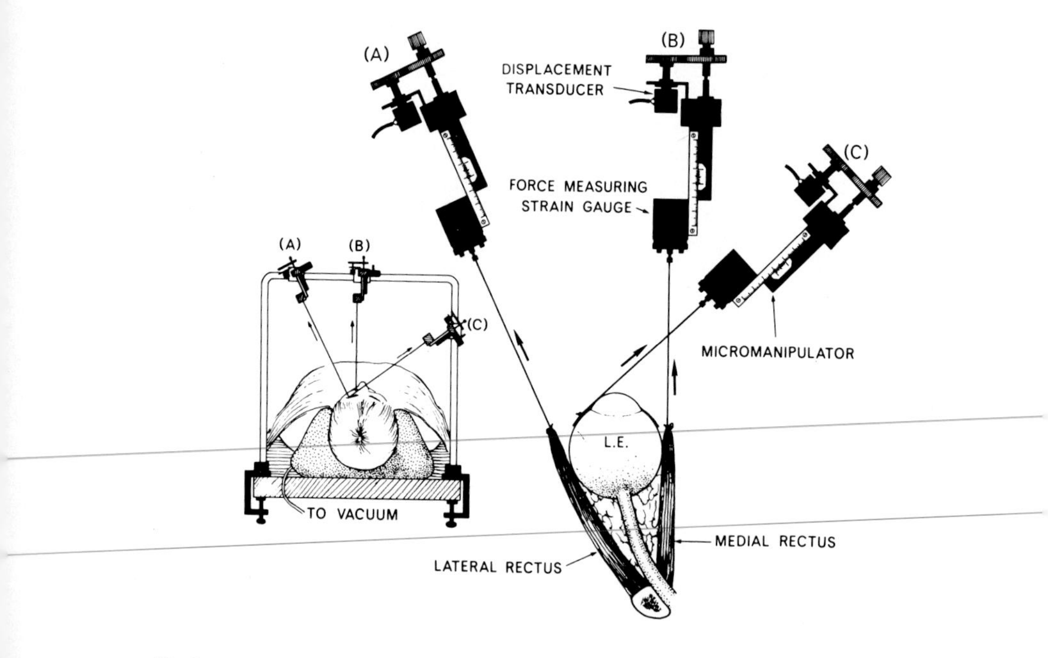

Fig. 1. Scheme of the experiment at surgery. At times a perimeter is placed above the patient to provide accurate fixation positions.

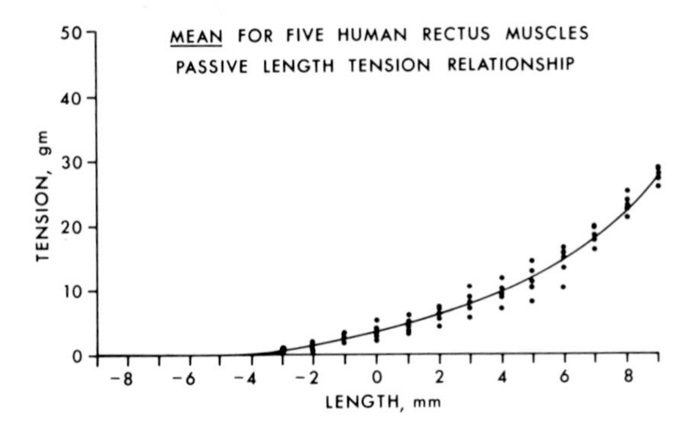

Fig. 2. Elasticity of the passive muscle under deep general anesthesia. A similar curve is obtained in alert patients if the muscle is inhibited by gaze away from its field of activity.

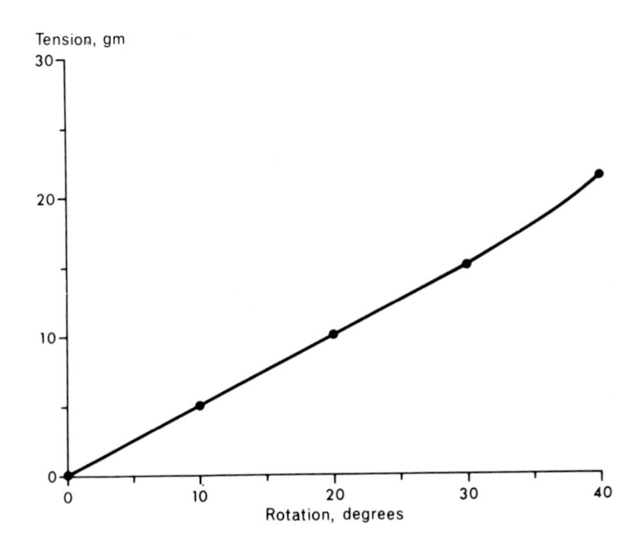

Fig. 3. Elasticity of the globe and attached tissues after removing horizontal muscles (patient anesthetized). It is not yet established that there is the same elasticity for adduction and abduction in normal persons, as the figure indicates.

degree in the primary position. It is important to note that the elasticity of these various muscles was similar even although the patients differed, having surgery for esotropia (2), exotropia (5), and enucleation (1). The variation between individuals increased at the limits of pull. This same curve is obtained in awake patients by pulling on a muscle whose action is inhibited by gaze to the opposite side. Thus a muscle may be construed as passive under such conditions.

Passive Globe and Orbit Tissues

When one pulls the globe and its attached tissues, the result is about equal increments of tension, a nearly linear line with a slope of 0.5 grams per degree over a 30 degree range (Fig. 3).

Contracture

It was long recognized that restrictions to rotation may occur in the various tissues making up these passive elastic components. (Duane, 1896, for

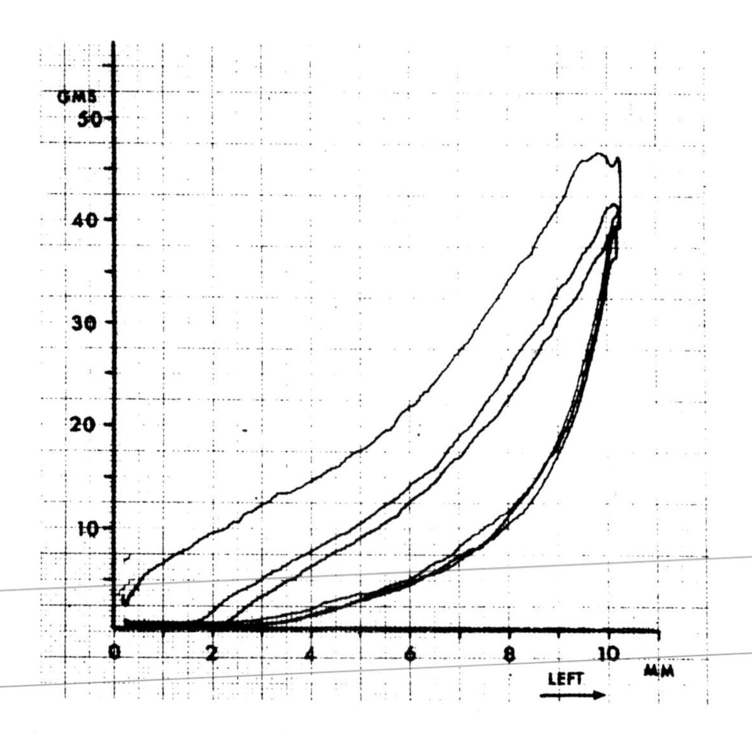

Fig. 4. Stiffness of "contracted" lateral rectus. Notice that the muscle is extended easily and in about linear fashion initially (0.56 gm/degree). The linear range, however, is much shortened and at about 6 mm. the "second part" of the muscle, the shortened stiff collagen sheath tissues, begin to be stretched (1.5 gm/degree).

example). This is the *clinical* meaning of contracture not the tetanic contraction implied in the physiologists' use of the word. In practical surgical technique such restrictions are assessed by the surgeon rotating the eye with its attached tissues and muscles. On the average this requires a force through the primary position of about 1.2 grams per degree under anesthesia. This rises slightly as one approaches the boundaries of rotation. Immediately after recession of a muscle this curve is spread out and displaced and the stiffness in the primary position is less when one pulls against the recessed muscle. When contracture occurs, however, we see a change in the position of the rising portion of the curve, that is, a narrowing of the boundary of rotation. Fig. 4 shows the altered stiffness of a lateral rectus muscle found recessed 10 mm and contracted. For 5 to 6 mm it was stretched normally (0.56 gm/degree), then it reached the end of its elastic limit and became extremely stiff and restricting (1.5 gm/degree). A similar curve is seen from the contracted medial rectus following a lateral rectus palsy (Fig. 5). Here the eye can easily be moved with no excessive stiffness even through the primary position. However, shortly beyond that point the stiffness suddenly rises. Similar types of restriction to movement are seen in Duane's retraction syndrome and in endocrine exophthalmos. This tells us that there is a range of motility wherein the elasticity of the orbital tissues is normal and not greatly restricting to movement. This is important for we can assess *active* muscle forces in this normal range (see below). There is therefore not a constant increase in stiffness in "contracture" but only a narrowing of the

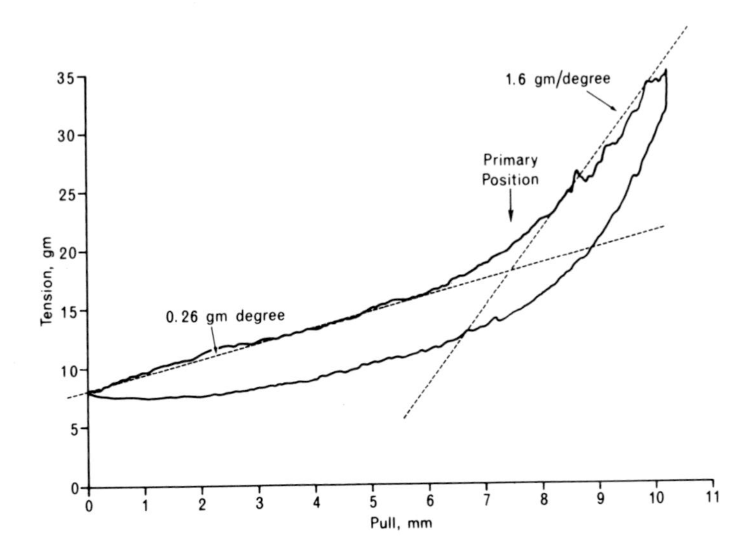

Fig. 5. "Contracture" of the medial rectus muscle. As in Figure 4 notice the restriction of the range of normal elasticity.

range of normal elasticity due to the "leash" effect of muscle and sheath tissues. After intravenous succinylcholine in two humans stiffness did increase over the whole range of motility, returning to normal in 10 to 20 minutes, depending on the dose. This alteration of actual *muscle stiffness* has a different "feel" than the *collagenous tissue shortening* which gives rise to the "leash effect" of contracture.

Surgical Considerations

At the end of surgery passive muscle forces should be balanced around a zero point coincident with the primary position. Schillinger (1966) had the notion that the balance of these forces should extend an equal distance each side of the primary position. When pulled by a force of a few grams in one direction the eye should move the same distance as a similar force in the opposite direction. However, active forces are added to these passive forces when the patient wakens. If one knew beforehand that these would also be exactly balanced, then a balancing of the passive forces would be a valuable technique. In comitant strabismus the active forces (20 grams for each horizontal rectus muscle in the primary position) are several times more than the passive elastic rotary forces (4 grams near the primary position). Thus the passive orbit forces are of significance when they reach boundary limits, but the variation of elasticity through the primary position has a relatively small part to play in alignment in comitant strabismus. In paralytic and in incomitant strabismus where contracture exists passive forces may predominate. In marked contracture the stiffness may rise such that over 100 gms are required to pull an eye to the primary position, far outweighing active fixation forces.

STATICS - ACTIVE FORCES

In the normal person the eyes which were about straight under anesthesia are also aligned when alert. This requires about equal force in the medial rectus and lateral rectus (MR and LR). The muscle forces in the primary position are about 20 grams in the LR in our patients measured under topical pontocaine anesthesia at the time of strabismus surgery (Robinson, *et al.*, 1969). It is important to point out the necessary conclusion that the net horizontal vector of the combined vertical rectus and oblique muscles must be zero for this to occur. That is, the vertical muscles do not, taken all together, contribute significantly to the horizontal balance in the primary position (Tschermak-Seysenegg, 1952). Further evidence of this normal medial-lateral equality is that when both horizontal muscles are inactive (for example, when the LR is paralyzed and the antagonist MR fully inhibited by gaze into the paralyzed side) the eye moves to the midline. This is true also in third nerve paralysis, (Cogan, 1956).

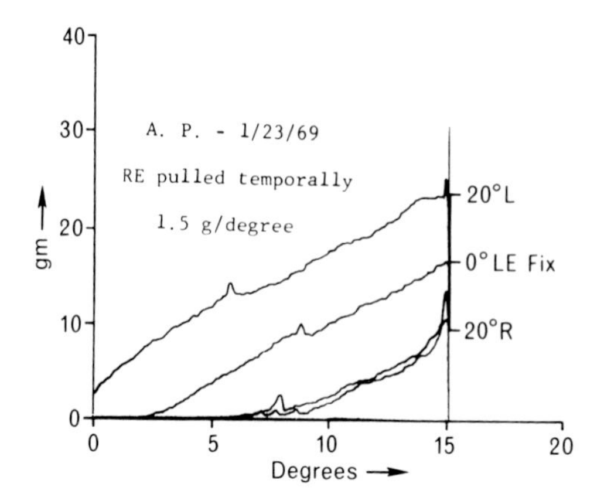

Fig. 6. Elasticity of the globe and muscles in an alert human with normal motility. Each curve is obtained as the fellow eye maintains fixation in a different position.

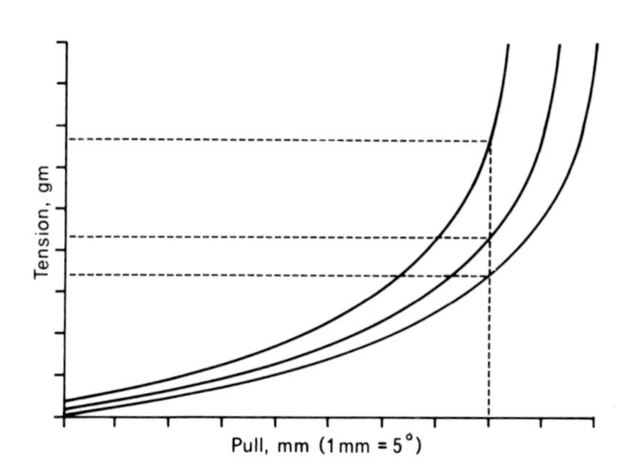

Fig. 7. Hypothetical scheme of the variation in elastic limits which might explain the variability of elasticity found by Stephens and Reinecke. If one passively stretches a muscle a set distance near its boundary of linear elasticity, the force required to move this distance will vary greatly with only small variations in the position of this boundary (indicated by the 3 identical curves). An initial and a final force reading would indicate much variation in stiffness - whereas the actual stiffness near the primary position is exactly the same in these curves.

STATICS - COMBINED ACTIVE AND PASSIVE FORCES

If one passively rotates a normal eye as its fellow fixes steadily, the rotation follows the increase in force in linear fashion through 30 degrees of rotation. This is a fully different situation than pulling on the passive muscle alone where a curve was obtained. This elasticity is about 1.82 grams per degree and is much the same in persons we have studied and is similar whether fixation is in the midline or to the right or left (Fig. 6). It becomes non-linear and begins to increase rapidly around 40 degrees. In an important earlier series of experiments, Stephens and Reinecke (1967) passively abducted eyes 5 mm with a suction-contact lens attached to the anterior portion of the eye to hold the globe. They found the elasticity in normals to vary greatly if they compared the beginning tension with the final position. To reconcile this variability in their data with the similarity of our patient data, we presume that the boundary of linear elasticity varies from among persons. One might find 5 mm of pull placed very high on the force curve of one patient, whereas in another 5mm of pull might still be on the beginning of the steep rise. The slope in the primary position could still be very nearly the same for each patient (Fig. 7). In this regard, Velez (1969) found that the limits of voluntary abduction varied from 8 to 11 mm, 40 to 55 degrees. This *variation* of boundary limits would also be in keeping with the above analysis and help to reconcile these experiments to our own.

From the linear nature of Fig. 6 it would be predicted that moderate recession of a non-contracted muscle would give about similar amounts of correction in the primary position for each mm of recession surgery. This is our empirical experience also (Fig. 8). It would similarly follow that the proportion of recession or resection within this linear range is not of great importance for the primary position alignment since one works with equal effects by recessing one muscle or resecting its antagonist. This also conforms to our experience in 40 exotropic patients where recess-resect procedures were done. This is by no means to say that these procedures have equal effects in other regards. Recession procedures are usually done on stiff muscles and therefore such operations will have greater effect by relaxation of such a tightness. Also, the slack in the system created by recession tends to be taken up in varying proportions by the antagonist and the operated muscle and by anterior-posterior translation of the globe. Perhaps this is what causes the greater *uncertainty* of the results of recession surgery as compared to the situation where the antagonist is resected a somewhat similar amount, taking up the slack (Fig. 9). Surgical procedures on horizontal muscles, with a few exceptions, are done on the very stiff tendon part of the horizontal muscles, so that the muscle elasticity is very rarely changed by shortening at surgery.

Active Forces

The actual force generated by the extraocular muscles can be assessed in a number of ways.

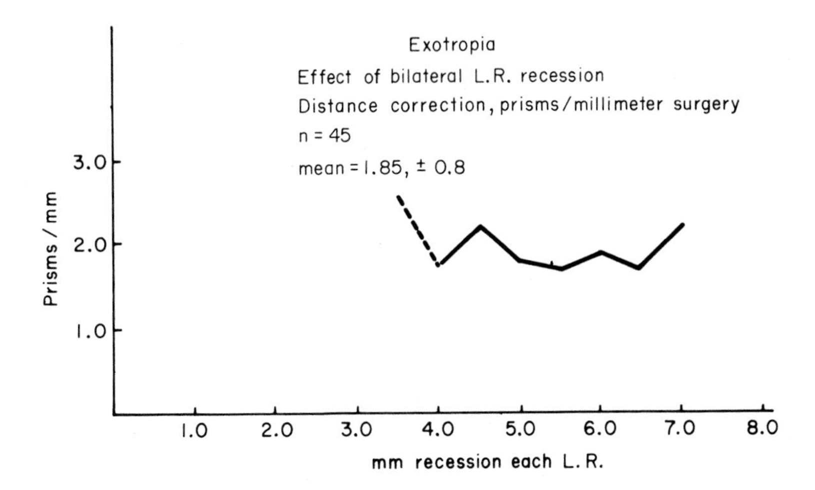

Fig. 8. Data from patients with intermittent exotropia, taken a minimum of one year after surgery. Fixation at distance in the primary position. There is a constant increment of alignment change for each unit of muscle length change.

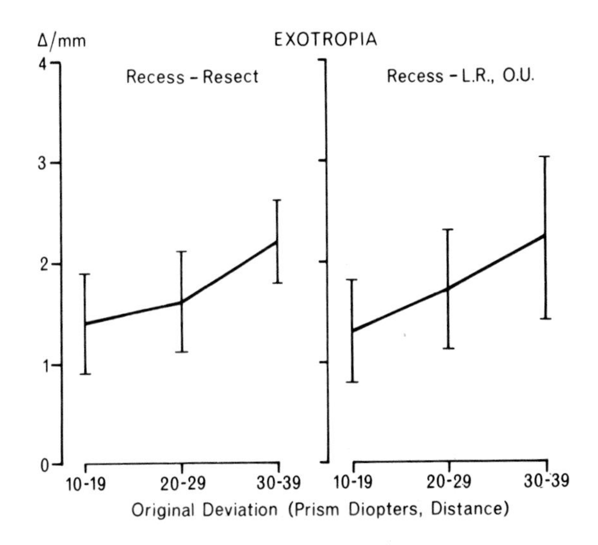

Fig. 9. Data from patients with exotropia. Notice the greater standard deviation of results in recession (lengthening) operations, as compared to recession of one muscle combined with shortening of its antagonist. Ordinate shows the correction effect in prism diopters for each mm of surgery.

Alignment, altered by paralysis or weakness of the muscle, is immediately reflected in the deviation of the eye to the opposite side. In a complete paralysis of a lateral rectus there is esotropia in the primary position due to loss of the 15 - 20 grams tension in the normal circumstance. The unbalanced medial recuts pulls the eye inward. The eye achieves a position where the tension of the medial rectus now equals the combined tension of the stretched passive lateral rectus (0.2-0.3 grams per degree) and the stretched lateral orbital tissues (0.5 grams per degree). With reference to these rotatory forces; a succession of approximations from Fig. 32 of Collins (Chapter 10) shows that one will arrive at about 12 degrees of esotropia for the new position of the palsied eye when the good eye is fixing in the primary position. This is quite accurately the position clinically observed in acute lateral rectus palsy. At this position of the palsied eye the tension of the medial rectus is about 8 grams. Since passive forces are quite significant in the circumstance of a *weak muscle,* it will never be clear from alignment alone what the proportion of forces is in the agonist and antagonist in paralytic strabismus.

Ocular rotations

Restriction of motility occurs immediately upon paralysis. Later, the narrowed range of rotation can be the consequence of the paralysis, or alternatively, can be the result of contracture of the antagonist muscle. Active force can be inferred in this circumstance if the passive forces are known to be normal. Thus, if the patient is unable to rotate the eye temporally, but the elasticity of the tissues is tested and found not to abnormally restrain temporal rotation, one can accurately infer that the generated force is abnormally low. However, if a contracture exists, one cannot then be sure if active force is weak or not.

Pursuit movements and generated force

As the eyes follow a target moving with velocities less than 30 degrees a second, or as they fix in eccentric gaze, activity in the agonist muscle rises to balance the elastic restraining forces which resist movement. (The effect of inertia is small, and the effect of viscosity at low velocities is small). From abundant electromyographic measurements we know the coordinated relaxation of the antagonist during following movements to be quite exact. If one *holds* an eye which is innervated to move as its fellow follows a target, he will measure relaxation of antagonist tension together with the active pull of the agonist muscle. To obviate this contamination of the measurement of active tension, one must rotate the eye to slack the antagonist. Thus, if a left lateral rectus palsy exists in uncertain degree and one wishes to know the active generated tension in the left lateral rectus, he should rotate and hold the left eye far nasally (Fig. 10). This will then slacken the innervated left medial rectus and medial tissues. Further relaxation of them as the eye is later asked

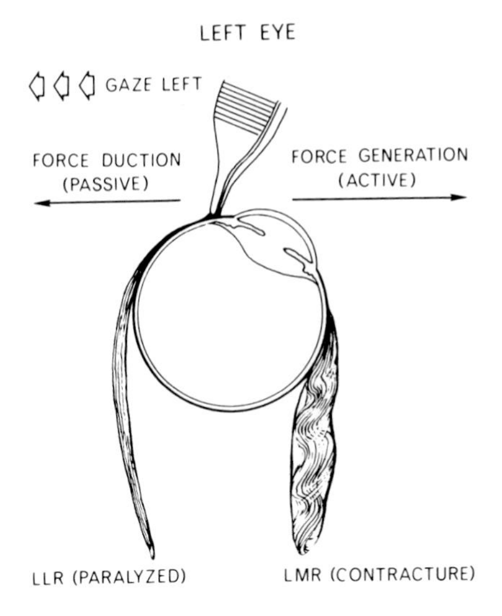

Fig. 10. Active force test. To tell the active force, hold the eye against the direction of gaze.

to move temporally will not be sensed. Only active lateral rectus pull will be felt. The increase of active pull for following movements on fixation at 45 degrees is to about 40 grams. When paralysis is marked but not complete it is difficult to sense small variations in "following" forces by holding the eye with forceps. These are readily appreciated by turning to the large *pulsatile* driving force seen in *saccadic* movements, however.

Saccadic movements and generated force

It is well established that saccadic movements are produced by a large pulse of activity in the agonist and relatively complete inhibition in the antagonist for a brief interval (Tamler *et al.,* 1959). Some of our electromyographs from human subjects show the same motor units at work in saccadic, following, and vergence movements. It is not altogether certain that all units are active for all activities (Bach-y-Rita, 1967). Probably some units, rarely if ever used otherwise, are called into play to generate the high forces of over 100 grams seen only with large saccadic movements. However, I believe moderate saccadic contraction tests the function of "usual" motor units adequately. This pulse of activity is readily appreciated by an examiner, holding the eye, because of its suddenness as well as because of its high magnitude (Fig. 11). The *absence* of this "pulse" is readily perceived if only antagonist relaxation occurs (Fig. 12).

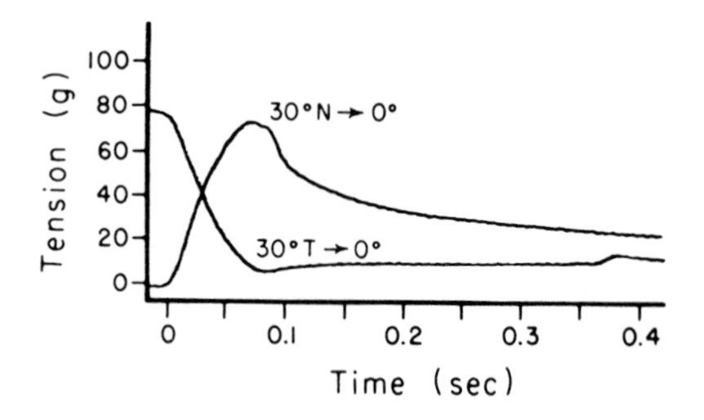

Fig. 11. 30 degree saccadic eye movement. The ordinate reflects the isometric tension of the agonist, which increases to very high levels in a brief time.

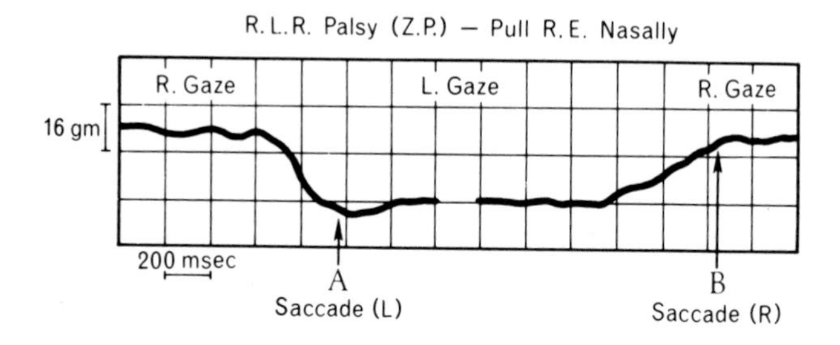

Fig. 12. Right lateral rectus palsy. The eye is passively rotated nasally while the fellow eye fixes straight ahead. A saccade of the good eye (at "A") 20 degrees, to the left, relaxes the pull needed. A return saccade shows only the relaxation.

Dynamic behavior - saccadic velocity and duration in paralysis

The situation in paralysis of one muscle is especially instructive. If a saccadic movement of 15 degrees to the left is made by the normal right eye in a left lateral rectus palsy, there is a sudden turning off of the left medial rectus. The paralyzed LLR, however, does nothing. The temporal passive orbital tissues which had been stretched nasally now gradually take up this slack and the eye "floats" temporally. We have measured the time constant of these passive movements in patients under anesthesia (Fig. 13). The remarkably similar movement of the paralyzed left eye in Fig. 14 should be compared with this. This slow "floating" movement is readily perceived when compared to

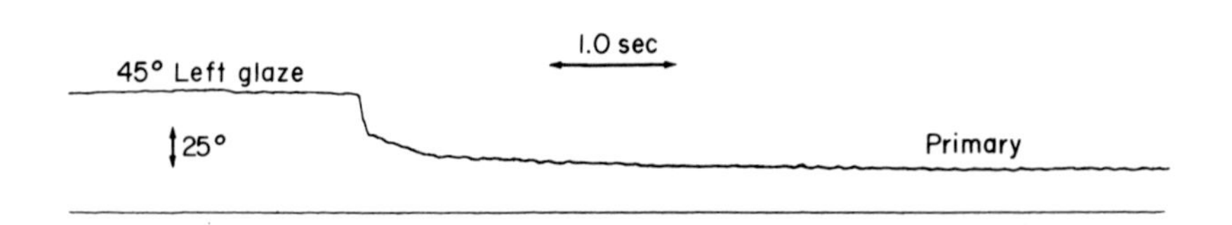

Fig. 13. The eye was pulled 10 mm from its position of rest under general anesthesia. It was then suddenly released. Notice the initial rapid and the subsequent slow time course of return to the position of rest.

the sudden return saccadic movement which the left eye will make as the right eye jumps 15° back to the original target. The LMR is now innvervated with no restraint from the paralyzed LLR which would ordinarily constitute much of its load. Thus the LMR creates a brisk movement of the eye nasally, whereas the movement temporally is the "off response" of the LMR and the "floating" of the eye outward because of passive tissue forces (Fig. 14).

This saccadic test is one of the *time* course of movement, not the *amount* of movement. If a restriction exists without paresis, the pulse of active forces still carries the movement to completion in a relatively normal time. It is possible, of course, to ask a paretic eye to move in a span where restriction prevents motion - but as discussed above, one can typically find an area with normal elasticity of passive tissues. The good eye makes saccades back and

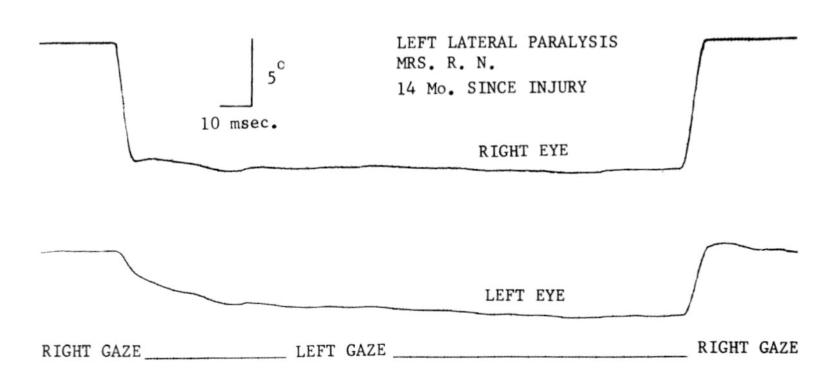

Fig. 14. Time course of saccadic eye movements in normal right eye (upper trace) and in left eye with palsy of lateral rectus. As the normal eye changes fixation to left gaze, the paralyzed eye "floats" slowly leftward. As the normal eye moves back to the right, the left eye moves rapidly, and even overshoots somewhat.

forth in this range while the observer watches the "paretic" eye for its floating behavior. O'Meara *et al.* (1969) have noted the frequent overshoot of nasalward saccades of the paretic eye in LR paresis as the good MR muscle pulls suddenly without the restraining viscosity normally present in the LR. The tension of the relaxing antagonist normally takes some 20 msec to diminish to 1/3 its value. Lack of this restraint allows the eye to over-accelerate, and thus overshoot and fall back at the end of the nasal saccade (Fig. 14).

Electromyography is not fully reliable to test paresis. In several cases we have seen disparity between a good electrical recovery of the muscle and faulty mechanical capacity which has regenerated. It is thus essential to assess the forces involved.

These tests of the generated forces are useful in other conditions as well. In Duane's syndrome there is often an abnormal pattern of innervations whereby the lateral rectus ceases its activity in attempted abduction. One can tell by passive traction test whether abduction is being restricted by stiff medial tissues. But surgery to release this restriction will have little effect unless the lateral rectus is actively contracting. This can be tested by the force generation tests of holding the eye as it attempts to move out, and by observing whether the attempted movement temporally is an abrupt one (even though it does not go very far) or whether it is a "float" movement from a nasal position (Fig. 15). Similarly, with certain gaze or elevator paralyses there is no passive restriction of upward motility but, on the contrary, no contraction of the muscle is felt to pull the eyes superiorly. One sees the eye make a brisk downward movement; while attempting upward movement the eye "floats". It is interesting

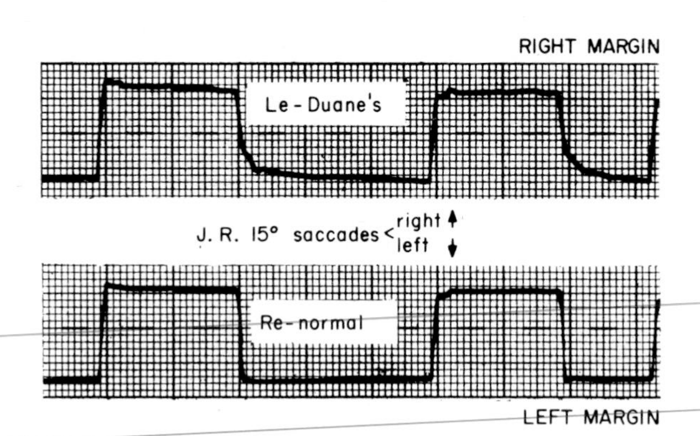

Fig. 15. Saccadic eye movements in Duane's syndrome. In this case EMG showed that the lateral rectus ceased activity with left gaze. The medial rectus had been recessed, so no restriction to abduction of the left eye was present. Notice the "square wave" nature of the rapid saccades of the normal RE (lower trace). Compare this to the slow "floating" movement of the LE as it moves to the left. Calibration is not the same for the RE and LE amplitudes of movement.

that in some cases this lack of elevation in the eye occurs mainly when the upward gaze is attempted with the involved eye in the adducted position, with relatively normal elevation in the abducted position. This kind of case looks very much like the tendon sheath syndrome of Brown where actual restriction to upward movement exists. In the "gaze palsy," however, one could move the eye upward, normally, could see the upward float movement, and could hold the eye and feel that there is no activity of the elevators with attempted upgaze. A similar application is orbit floor fracture. Force generation and saccadic tests can tell paresis of the inferior rectus due to nerve injury which can happen with or without restriction.

SUMMARY

For the horizontal system, passive medial-lateral and active medial-lateral forces in the human are approximately balanced. This gives alignment in the primary position. In normal active muscle a linear relationship exists between length and force. This implies that muscle surgery in comitant strabismus should have effects proportional to amount of surgery which we confirm empirically. Similar reasoning and empirical evidence supports the notion that the proportion of recess-resect is not important over the range 1/1 to 2/1. Design of surgery is strongly influenced by whether the active generated forces are unbalanced or by whether there is abnormal elasticity restricting movement. If elasticity is abnormal and can be released then motility will be enhanced. If the active generating force in one direction is paralyzed, however, then it needs to be balanced by a similar amount of weakening of the antagonist, or by the provision of force vectors through transplantation of other muscles. Alterations of the passive orbital tissue and muscle tissue elasticity are measured by forcibly rotating the eye under anesthesia or during maintained fixation, the classic forced duction test. The notion of "contracture" is shown to be mainly an alteration of the boundary of elasticity, not a stiffening of the tissues at all lengths. Lack of rotation when no passive restriction exists is a clear indication of paralysis. Actual generated muscle force is assessed directly by restraining the eye as it attempts to move during following and saccadic movements, the active force generation test. An indirect but most useful guide to generated force is the comparison of velocity and duration of saccadic movements toward and away from the suspected muscle, the saccadic test. We anticipate eventually to measure complete alignment and rotation forces for individual cases to guide treatment. Already, however, general notions such as the saccadic and force generation tests, the documentation of contracture as a leash effect, and the linear length-tension relationship for active muscle have practical clinical application and have enhanced our quality of care and our understanding of strabismus.

REFERENCES

BACH-Y-RITA, P. (1967). Neurophysiology of extraocular muscles. *Invest. Ophthal.* **6,** 229-237.

COGAN, D.G. (1956). *Neurology of Extraocular Muscles.* p. 20; 61. C. Thomas Company, Springfield.

COLLINS, C.C., SCOTT, A.B., O'MEARA, D. (1969). Elements of the peripheral oculomotor apparatus. *Amer. J. Optom.* **46,** 510-515.

DUANE, A. (1897). A new classification of the motor anomalies of the eye, based upon physiologic principles. *Annals of Ophthal.* **6,** 84-122.

DUKE-ELDER, S. (1952). *Textbook of Ophthalmology.* Volume V. Ocular Adnexa. C.V. Mosby Company, St. Louis.

ESSLEN, E. und D. & HUBER, A. (1967). Elektromographische Innervationsanalyse des Strabismus concomitans. Uber die beim Strabismus concomitans wirksamen Muskelkrafte. *Ophthalmologica,* **154,** 189-200.

O'MEARA, D.M., METZ, H.S., STEWART, H. L., and SCOTT, A.B. (1969). Eye movement patterns in strabismus. (abstract) *Invest. Ophthal.* **8,** 651.

ROBINSON, D.A., O'MEARA, D., SCOTT, A.B., and COLLINS, C.C. (1969). The mechanical components of human eye movements. *J. Appl. Physiol.* **26,** 548-553.

SCHILLINGER, R.J. (1966). The prevention of over-correction and under-correction in horizontal strabismus surgery. *J. Pediat. Ophthal.,* **3,** 38-41.

STEPHENS, K.F. & REINECKE, R.D. (1967). Quantitative forced duction. *Trans. Amer. Acad. Ophthal. & Otolaryng.* **71,** 324-329.

TAMLER, E., MARG, E., JAMPOLSKY, A., & NAWRATSKI, I. (1959). Electromyography of human saccadic eye movements. *Arch. Ophthal.* **62,** 657-661.

TSCHERMAK-SEYENEGG, A. (1951). *Introduction to Physiological Optics.* Translated by Paul Boeder, C. Thomas Company, Springfield. p. 251.

VELEZ, G. (1969). Calibrated measurement of eye movements. *J. Pediat. Ophthal.,* **6,** 19-21.

THE SACCADIC SYSTEM

ALBERT F. FUCHS

Only one model has been proposed which simulates the behavior of the saccadic control system and which, with slight modifications, has survived since its original presentation in 1962. Before this model is described and evaluated, some pertinent saccadic properties which must be satisfied by the model are reviewed. In conclusion, some of the oculomotor pathways and areas believed to be concerned with the saccade are discussed.

CHARACTERISTICS OF THE SACCADE AND ITS CONTROL SYSTEM

A saccade is the most rapid movement of which the oculomotor system is capable. Its object is to redirect the eyes from one target in the visual field to another in the shortest possible time. Seeing is not important during the saccade; in fact, visual functions (perception of a light flash ((Latour, 1962; Volkmann, 1962; Zuber & Stark, 1966)) or various target orientations ((Volkmann, 1962)) and movements ((Beeler, 1967; Gross, Vaughan & Valenstein, 1967))) seem to be suppressed. Saccades of equal magnitude and direction in the visual field are made simultaneously by both eyes.

Saccades can be elicited by a number of stimuli. If an object of interest appears eccentric to the fovea, one makes a voluntary saccade to position the object on the fovea. The movements made in examining a picture (Jeannerod, Gerin & Pernier, 1968; Yarbus, 1967) or reading a line of print (Trinker, 1958) are composed of a series of such saccades. Rashbass (1961) has shown that saccades are responsive to target displacement only and that displacements of less than 0.3 deg do not result in a saccade. Young (1966) arrived at the same size dead zone by demonstrating greatly increased response times to target jumps of less than 0.3 degrees. Once the object has been located on the fovea, the involuntary miniature movements of fixation (physiological nystagmus) take

Supported by Grant Number FR 00166 from the National Institutes of Health.

over to prevent the image of the object from fading. One of the three types of miniature movements is the microsaccades which have been believed to reposition the object on the most sensitive part of the fovea after drifts had created an intrafoveal position error (Cornsweet, 1956). Therefore, one could imagine a fine positional error control system operating within the dead zone of a system concerned with large errors.* Such a concept over-simplifies the situation, however, since it has recently been shown that 15% of the microsaccades do not correct for positional errors caused by drift (Boyce, 1967) and furthermore, that in the absence of saccades, the eyes do not drift off the target but seem to correct themselves with smooth pursuit-like movements (Steinman, Cunitz & Timberlake, 1967).

The rapid eye movements of optokinetic and vestibular nystagmus are a third example of saccadic movements. Optokinetic nystagmus results when the visual environment rotates about a stationary observer (*e.g.*, the view from the window of a moving train). The eyes automatically follow a passing object for a time and then make a rapid movement in the opposite direction to acquire a new object. This sequence of movements repeats itself and yields a sawtooth-like record of eye movements. Mackensen and Schumacher (1960) have shown that these rapid movements have the characteristics of voluntary saccades. Vestibular nystagmus occurs when the head is turned within a stationary visual environment. The vestibular apparatus is excited to drive the eyes in a direction counter to the head rotation in order to stabilize the image of the environment on the fovea. This slow eye movement is interrupted by rapid eye movements which allow compensation to continue as new visual surroundings are brought into view by continued head rotation. The stimulus which initiates the saccades of either type of nystagmus is unknown, but the old notion that rapid movements reset the eye after it has been rotated to its physical limit is probably not true (Robinson, 1968).

Because it is easy to control, the voluntary saccade has received the greatest attention and its characteristics will now be considered. A target, stepping suddenly in a random direction off the fovea, produces a saccadic eye movement after a characteristic time interval called the reaction time. The reaction time increases with saccadic magnitude so that the average latency to a 5 deg saccade is 200 msec; to a 40 deg saccade, about 250 msec (Bartz, 1962; Saslow, 1967; White & Eason, 1962). When a simple target step is one of several more difficult movements, the average latency for a 6 deg saccade increases to 230 msec (Wheeless, Boynton & Cohen, 1966). If the position of the target jump is predictable, *e.g.*, a periodic square wave, subjects gradually improve their tracking performance until they are able to move their eyes in step with the target and even anticipate it (Dallos & Jones, 1963; Stark, Vossius & Young, 1962).

*In the discussion, T. Cornsweet stated his belief that a functional foveal dead zone does not exist and that microsaccades behave as though they are merely the low amplitude extension of a continuous spectrum of saccades.

The trajectory and velocity of the saccades of alert subjects are not influenced by voluntary effort or practice, although fatigue, sedatives and alcohol reduce saccadic velocity (Becker & Fuchs, 1969). Hence, normal saccades are sterotyped movements with predictable characteristics. Figure 1 shows a family of representative eye movements ranging from 5 to 40 degrees. For magnitudes between 5 and 15 deg, the eye accelerates rapidly, reaching a maximum velocity about midway to the target. The eye decelerates onto the target with little overshoot and no oscillation, yielding an overall trajectory which is roughly symmetrical about its midpoint. Yarbus (1965) has even shown that the saccadic trajectory can be matched with a sine wave. Vossius (1960) described five different ways in which the saccadic eye movement trajectory approaches its final position. The most common responses resemble those of Fig. 1, but he also observes overshooting and oscillatory saccades. While a small overshoot may exist in the saccadic trajectory (Fuchs (1967) found a constant 0.5 deg. 15 msec overshoot for angles larger than 25 deg in the monkey), oscillations appear to be very rare. In response to target displacements greater than 15 deg, the eye usually falls short of the target and requires a second saccade to reach its objective. Large saccades become noticeably asymmetric, reaching their peak velocities early in the trajectory and exhibiting a long deceleration phase (Hyde, 1959). As seen from Fig. 1 and the experiments of Becker and Fuchs (1969), the delay between the end of the first saccade and the onset of the second is about 130 msec and is independent of saccadic magnitude.

The duration and maximum velocity of a saccade increase with its magnitude (Fig. 2). A 5 deg human saccade lasts about 30 msec with each additional degree increase in magnitude requiring about another 2.0 msec (Cook, 1965; Dodge & Cline, 1901; Hyde, 1959; Robinson, 1964). This linear relation between duration and magnitude holds for movements up to 80 degrees (Hyde, 1959). The

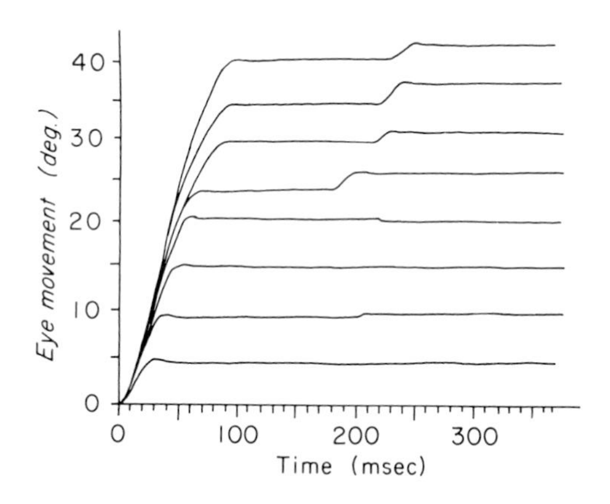

Fig. 1. Superimposed tracings of saccadic eye movements in eight steps from 5° to 40° (after Robinson, 1964).

maximum velocity reached during a saccade is an increasing function of magnitude for movements between 5 and about 20 deg, after which a velocity saturation tends to occur at approximately 700 deg/sec. Zuber and Stark (1965) showed that the microsaccades of fixation (several minutes of arc) have maximum velocities which also lie on the velocity characteristic of Fig. 2B and suggested that a common physiological system produces or limits the dynamics of all saccade types. Furthermore, the microsaccades possess durations on the order of 20 msec, indicating that the duration curve may also be extended to its "Y" intercept.

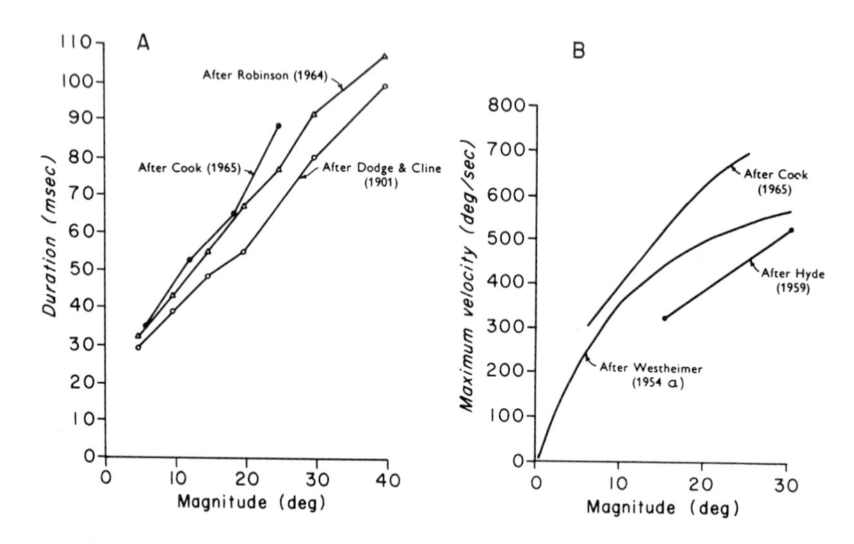

Fig. 2. Saccadic duration (A) and maximum velocity (B) as a function of magnitude.

The saccadic system has several non-linear properties. It has already been mentioned that the saccadic reaction time increases with magnitude. The most important nonlinearity is revealed in Fig. 2, which shows that the response time of the system, its duration, is a function of saccade size. Zuber, Semmlow & Stark (1968) have demonstrated that this nonlinearity reduces the saccadic system bandwidth from 16 Hz for a 5 deg movement to 10 Hz for a 20 deg movement. In addition, the maximum saccadic velocity in humans is limited to about 700 deg/second. Horizontal saccades also appear to be direction-sensitive. Both Dodge and Cline (1901) and Robinson (1964) have observed that saccades in a temporal direction are faster than those in a nasal direction. Travis (1936), on the other hand, claimed that temporal saccades are quicker. To further complicate matters, Hyde (1959) found no clear difference between rightward and leftward saccades, and Cook (1965) recorded faster saccades toward the primary position of gaze than away from it.

One of the striking characteristics of the saccadic system is that, presented with an interesting target moving eccentric to the fovea, it will execute a series of saccades spaced at fairly regular intervals of about 0.2 sec until the error between eye and target has been reduced to less than 0.3 degrees. In 1954 (b), Westheimer caused a target to step to one side off the fovea and return to its original position in 40 msec. The eye responded with a saccade after a reaction time of about 150 msec, despite the fact that any response at all was wholly inappropriate at that time. Furthermore, the eye remained deviated for 200 msec before returning to the correct target location. This phenomenon led Young and Stark (1962) to propose a discrete control system which sampled the error created by a target step and then became refractory to any subsequent target behavior for 200 msec, after which it executed a movement appropriate to the error that existed 200 msec previously. This saccadic response clearly cannot be modelled by a continuous system possessing simply a 200 msec delay, since such a system would predict that in the above example the eye would return after 40 and not 200 msec.

Additional evidence in support of a sampled-data model with 200 msec sampling intervals results from observing the saccadic response under conditions of altered visual feedback and from measuring the system frequency response. The saccadic system is a closed-loop servo with a unity negative feedback from eye position to target position since every eye movement results in an equal-but-opposite movement of the target image on the retina. This intrinsic feedback loop can be modified externally by controlling target position with a signal proportional to eye position (Fender & Nye, 1961). If the external feedback signal is precisely equal but of opposite sign to the eye position, the intrinsic feedback is cancelled, so that the system is operating under open loop conditions. In other words, an eye movement results in no relative displacement of the target image on the retina, and the system is always driven by a constant, noncorrectable error. In response to an initial target step, the eye executes a series of saccades in an attempt to catch the ever-receding target. The saccades occur only at 200 msec intervals, giving the staircase response seen in Fig. 3A.

Fleming, Vossius, Bowman & Johnson (1969) opened the loop pharmacologically by a unilateral, retrobulbar injection of Xylocaine which paralyzed the extraocular muscles. They also found that the mobile eye exhibited a staircase walk-away to an initial target displacement. If the target was returned to its starting position, thereby reducing the error to zero, the eye remained displaced. Only when the target then stepped to the other side did the eye return to center and execute a series of saccades in the opposite direction. The external loop may also be adjusted so that the net feedback, rather than being zero, is −2, and the target will move an amount equal to, but in the opposite direction of, the eye movement. If the eyes faithfully pursue the elusive target, oscillations will result (Fig. 3B). Once again the saccades are spaced at regular intervals of 200 to 250 msec. Finally, when subjects are asked to track continuous, unpredictable targets, Young and Stark (1963) find a peak in the gain frequency response curve

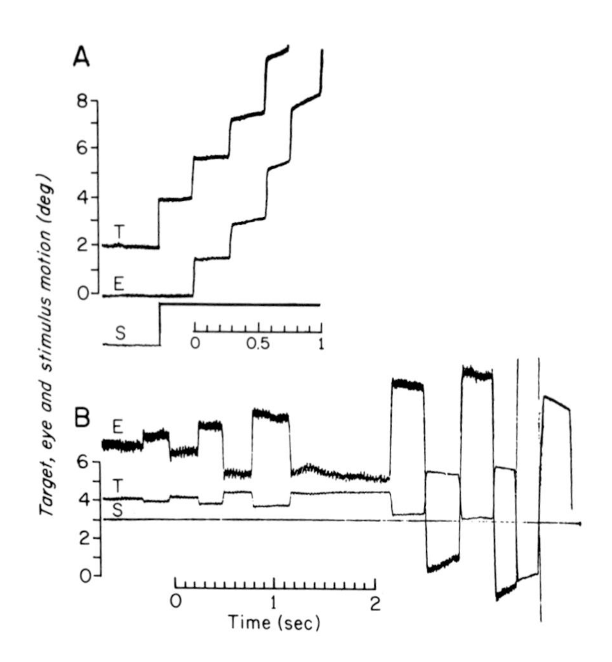

Fig. 3. Responses of the saccadic system to conditions of variable visual feedback. A, open loop conditions; B, an overall feedback of -5. In both cases, E is horizontal eye position; T, horizontal target position and S the initial target stimulus (after Robinson, 1965).

at 2.5 Hz consistent with a sampled-data system operating at a sampling period of 0.2 seconds. Also, if at low frequencies the target is suddenly extinguished, the eye will continue to move smoothly for about 200 msec before the first saccade occurs.

SACCADIC SYSTEM MODELS

The sampled data model

The possibility of a sampled-data model for saccadic eye movements was first mentioned by Vossius in 1961. The first actual circuit diagram was presented a year later by Young and Stark (1962) and analysed in detail in Young's doctoral dissertation (1962). Figure 4 shows their original model which described both saccadic and pursuit eye movements in response to unpredictable target signals. Miniature fixation movements and the involuntary movements of nystagmus were considered as disturbances. Only the saccadic branch is considered here.

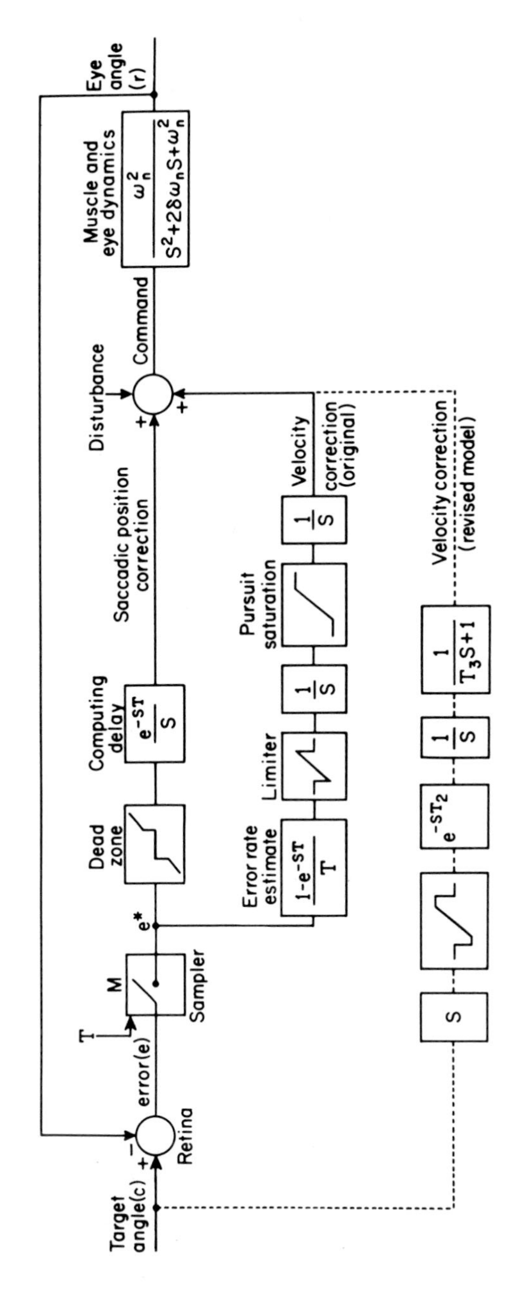

Fig. 4. The sampled-data model for voluntary eye tracking. The latest (revised) model replaces the original sampled smooth pursuit path by a continuous path with no feedback. Both models have a sampled path for saccadic eye movements.

The error between the desired angle of gaze (c) and the actual eye position (r) is sensed at the retina. This error is sampled by an impulse modulator, M, at sampling intervals, T, of 200 msec, the refractory period of saccadic movements. The synchronization of the demodulator coincides with the onset of target motion, provided that the eye has not made a saccade within the previous 200 msec. A nonlinear dead zone element accounts for the afore-mentioned lack of saccadic responses to very small target displacements. Each error impulse is delayed by one refractory period and integrated to give a step command which, when filtered through the muscle and eye dynamics, yields that saccade appropriate to swing the eye onto the angular position occupied by the target 200 msec earlier. The muscle and eye dynamics are represented by the second-order model of Westheimer (1954a).

Young and Stark applied the Z transform to describe the input-output relationships of their sampled-data model. It is possible to shortcut some of the mathematics (the reader is referred to Young (1962) for a detailed description) by using the results of Ragazzini and Zadeh (1952) who demonstrated that the output R(S) of a simple sampled data system with a single sampler in the forward path and unity negative feedback may be written as:

$$R(S) = C^*(S) \frac{G(S)}{1 + G^*(S)}$$

where G(S) is the forward loop transfer function, G*(S) the sampled transfer function, and C*(S) the sampled input function. In Fig. 4, considering only the saccadic path with the dead zone and eye dynamics neglected

$$G(S) = \frac{e^{-ST}}{S}$$

Allowing, according to Young, $e^{-ST} = Z$ and referring to Ragazzini and Franklin (1958) for the appropriate transforms, the saccadic transfer function may be written as:

$$\frac{R(S)}{C^*(S)} = \frac{\frac{Z}{S}}{1 + \frac{Z}{(1-Z)}} = \frac{Z(1-Z)}{S}$$

If a step target displacement [C(S) = 1/S or C*(S) = 1/(1 − Z)] is applied to the system, its response is simply R(S) = Z/S or the step input delayed by one sampling interval (Fig. 5A).

The sampled data model is at its best when predicting the saccadic response under conditions of altered visual feedback. If K is the net negative feedback around the system (i.e., the intrinsic unity feedback plus any added feedback),

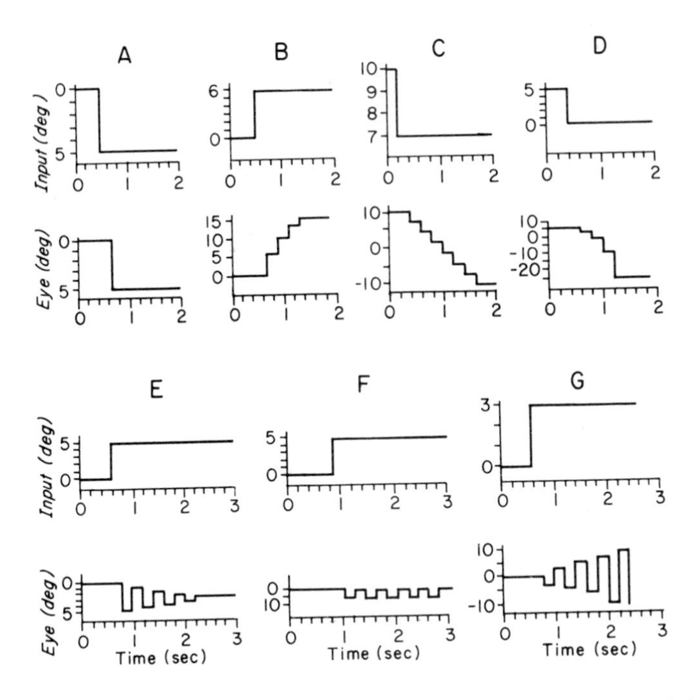

Fig. 5. Model step responses under variable feedback. (A) k = 1.0 (B) k = 0.3 (C) k = 0.0 (D) k = −1.0 (i.e., positive feedback) (E) k = 1.75 (F) k = 2.0 (G) k = 2.3 (after Young and Stark 1963).

Young and Stark (1963) show that the error-to-input sampled transfer function is

$$\frac{E(Z)}{C(Z)} = \frac{1-Z}{1-(1-K)Z}$$

Since the transformation $Z = e^{-ST}$ maps the left half S–plane into the region exterior to the unit circle in the Z–plane, the condition for a stable system in general is that $|Z| > 1$ and for the saccadic system in particular, $|1/(1-K)| > 1$. Therefore, the limits of stability are $0<K<2$. For $K=0$, the model, operating open loop, correctly predicts that the eye will walk away on a series of equally-spaced steps (compare the model response of Fig. 5C with the actual eye movement in Fig. 3A). For $K<0$, the poles of error-to-input function lie inside the unit circle on the positive real axis, yielding a response which walks away on a staircase of ever-increasing steps (Fig. 5D). A net negative feedback of $K=2$ places the poles on the unit circle so that the model breaks into sustained oscillations (Fig. 5F). If $K>2$, the poles reside inside the unit circle on the negative real axis and result in growing oscillations (Fig. 5G). Contrary to the results of

Young and Stark (1963), other investigators cannot elicit sustained oscillations at net feedback of -2. Vossius and Werner (1969) reported that naive subjects are able to stabilize their oscillations when subjected to a net feedback of -4. The conditions for system stability, i.e., zero error, are realized by inserting into the forward path an adaptable gain element whose amplification, $r_i = 1/(1 - r_a)$ where r_a is the amount of external feedback. Robinson (1965) found a net feedback as high as -5 necessary to yield sustained oscillations, since even inexperienced subjects often simply stop tracking, thereby suppressing their oscillations (Fig. 3B). He speculated that subjects actually begin predicting their own oscillations and shift into a predictive tracking mode which requires a greater feedback to become unstable. This hypothesis is probably true, since, for the monkey who exhibits no predictive tracking behavior (Fuchs, 1967b), it has been shown (Fuchs, 1967a) that sustained, machine like oscillations will occur at an overall feedback of -2.3, a value in close agreement with the theoretical one predicted by the sampled-data model.

Although the model performs well when only saccadic movements are required, it occasionally predicts an incorrect saccadic response when the saccade is made in conjunction with a smooth pursuit movement. For example, Rashbass (1961) observed that if the target steps to one side before moving at a constant velocity in the opposite direction and recrosses its original position in about one reaction time (Fig. 6A), no saccadic response at all occurs (Fig. 6B). The model, however, predicts the response seen in Fig. 6C. Therefore, Young and his coworkers (1968) have revised the original model to provide a sample whose occurrence is stochastically related to the target movement. In addition, several investigators had demonstrated the continuous nature of the smooth pursuit system (see the next paper in this symposium by Young), so Young *et al.* (1968) replaced the sampled pursuit path of the original model but retained the excellent saccadic response characteristic of a sampled data system (Fig. 4, dashed velocity correction branch). Although both a target-synchronized and non-synchronized sampler control logic were evaluated, most of their evidence favored the former. In that case, after the target has moved, a stochastically distributed delay elapses before the sample is taken. The sample is followed by a constant processing delay of 150 msec (reduced from the 200 msec of the original model) before the eye can move. Successive samples have a minimum 200 msec separation. By adjusting the occurrence of the samples, the model will correctly predict many classes of eye movement, (e.g., the model yields the response of Fig. 6D if the samples occur at the arrows in Fig. 6A).

Limitations of the sampled-data model

One important response that cannot be predicted is the correct answer to a pulse-step target. Wheeless *et al.* (1966) presented a spot which first stepped 6 deg to one side for T msec, after which it jumped 12 deg in the opposite direction (see insert Fig. 7). For T = 100 msec, 77% of the responses ignored the initial target displacement and made just a single saccade to the final target position.

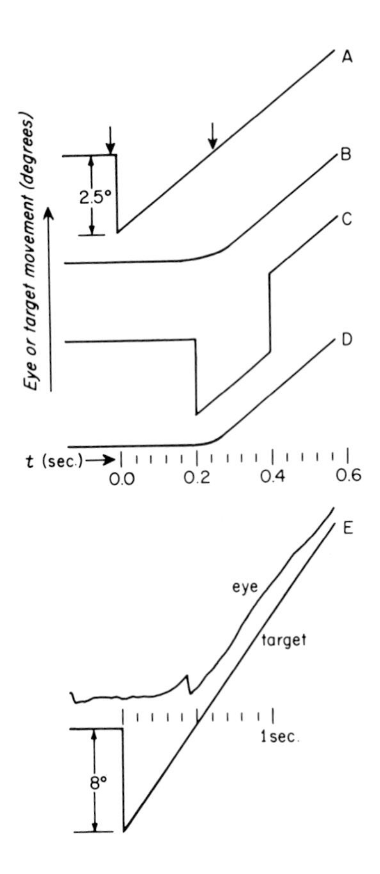

Fig. 6. Saccadic responses to targets with ramp components. A. The Rashbass step-ramp target. B. The actual eye movement response to A. C. The original sampled data model response to A. D. The revised sampled-data model response to A. E. A monkey eye response to a step-ramp. The error between target and eye is never as small as the resulting saccade, demonstrating that the saccadic system also uses error *rate* to determine saccadic magnitude.

In fact, their data show that the eye has a 32% chance of correctly responding to target displacements occurring just 85 msec before the ensuing saccade. Several authors (Becker & Fuchs, 1969; Robinson, 1968) interpret the Wheeless data as suggesting that the sample actually has a finite time width rather than the infinitesimal width of an impulse sample. A finite interval error signal, however, would require an extensive revision of the remainder of the Young model. A second possibility would be to retain the impulse sampler but to distribute its time of occurrence stochastically according to Fig. 7. These data, taken from Wheeless

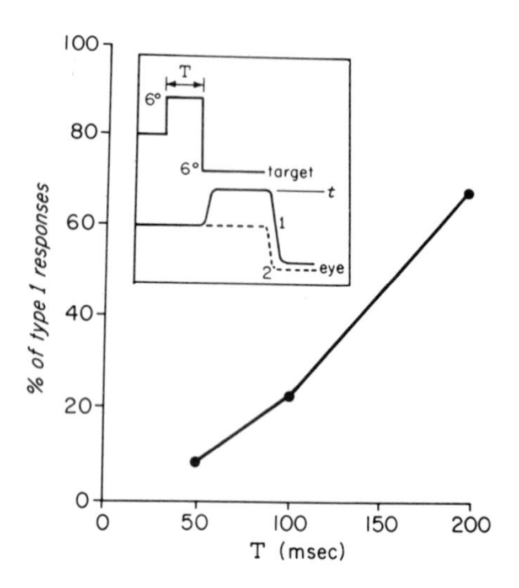

Fig. 7. The pulse-step experiment of Wheeless *et al.*, (1966). Insert shows the target motion and the two possible resulting eye responses. Plotted is the percentage of Type 1 responses for various values of T.

et al. (1966), show the percentage of eye movements that responded to both target steps (Type 1, Fig. 7 insert). A double saccade response would result if the time of occurrence of an impulse sample t_s, were less than T. Hence, Fig. 7 also shows the probability of a sample's having already occurred T msec after a target movement (i.e., p $[t_s < T]$). Since there is at least a 30% chance that the sample will occur after T=200 msec, the constant processing delay must now be reduced to about 50 msec.

The spacing of successive saccades is also influenced by the target input. For target displacements greater than about 15 deg, the eye usually makes a large initial saccade covering about 90% of the distance followed in only about 130 msec by a second saccade which puts the eye on target (Becker & Fuchs, 1969; Johnson & Fleming, 1963). By causing the target to move in the interval between the first and second saccades, Becker and Fuchs (1969) showed that 50% of the second saccades respond to target changes occurring 70 msec after the end of the first. Since Wheeless *et al.* (see Fig. 7) demonstrated that 50% of the first saccades responded to target changes occurring 150 msec after an initial target displacement, Becker and Fuchs concluded that the error was sampled for a finite time and that the error sample width for the second saccade was about half that of the first. They suggested that for large angles the response is prepackaged as two movements; the shorter sample width (and hence the shorter time between saccades) is possible since less information is required for the second saccade whose direction and approximate amplitude are predetermined. Another suggestion offered by Johnson and Fleming (1963) is that the innervation patterns to the eye muscles also go to a feedback element which has transfer characteristics of the eye mechanical system. The output of this eye plant model is immediately compared with the original error and if a discrepancy still exists, a second saccade can be executed after a very brief latency. Also in response to ramp target trajectories moving at velocities greater than 20 deg/sec, both man (Johnson, 1963) and monkey (Fuchs, 1967a) often make a sequence of saccades spaced as closely as 80 msec apart. Therefore, when the error or rate of change of error is large the saccadic system increases its sampling rate (and also decreases the sample width) to minimize the pursuit time required before the eye acquires the target. A fixed interval sampler then is an oversimplification.

Another weak point of the revised model is synchronizing the sampling instants with the target motion to yield responses appropriate to a variety of target inputs. Contrary to the claims of the authors, the relative frequencies of occurrence of various actual eye movement responses to identical stimuli do not agree with the percentages predicted by *uniformly* varying the synchronization of the model sampling instants to the input. For example, in response to a 10 deg/sec ramp, the revised model predicts 20% of the eye movements will be composed of 2 saccades when actually 41% have two saccades (Robinson, 1965). In response to the step ramp of Fig. 6A, a uniform variation of sampling instants predicts a very low incidence of the model response in Fig. 6D, whereas if the target recrosses its initial position in about 250 msec, the percentage of actual eye movement responses with no saccade is considerable (56% in the monkey tracking a 10 deg/sec target after a 2.5 deg offset). Therefore, the distribution of sampling instants is biased in favor of certain responses depending upon the form of the input target trajectory. Such a nonlinearity would greatly complicate the model.

Finally, it seems rather tenuous to try to account for the absence of a saccade in the response of Fig. 6B by the fortuitous occurrence of samples at times of zero error (i.e., at the arrows). Another possibility would be that the saccade size is determined not only by the error but by the rate of change of error as well. Fig. 6E shows a monkey response to an 18 deg/sec ramp, offset by an 8 deg step. The saccadic correction of 1.5 deg gets the eye on target, although at no time between the initial target step and the saccade was the error signal as small as 1.5 degrees. Therefore, the saccadic magnitude could not be based on the error alone but was actually predicted with the help of error rate information. Lauringson and Shchedrovitskii (1965) came to the same conclusion after presenting the step-ramp to humans. Similar phenomena were also observed by Zuber (1965) who presented subjects with a ramp to the left-step to the right-ramp to the left target in which the slope of the second ramp was randomly varied between 2 and 10 deg/sec. As the slope of the second ramp increased, the magnitude of the saccade decreased, again showing that the saccade size is at least partially determined by the error rate.

One scheme for making the saccade rate sensitive is seen in Fig. 8 (block A). Fig. 6E shows that if the error and rate of change of error have opposite signs, the saccade is smaller than predicted on the basis of an error sample alone.

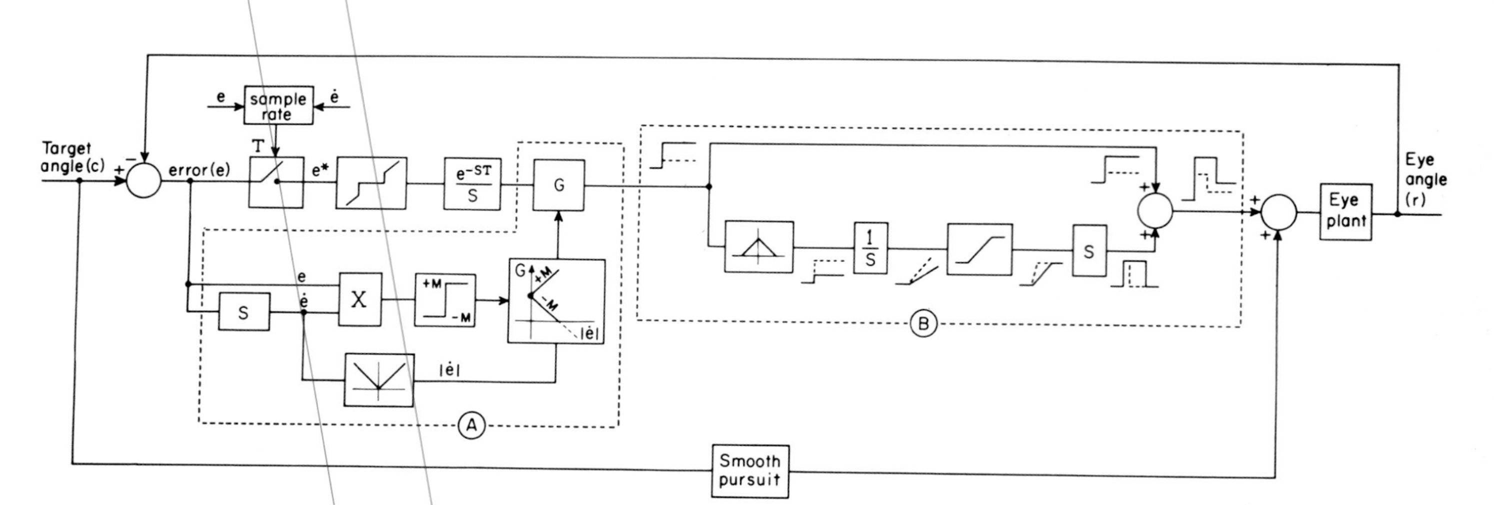

Fig. 8. A model for the saccadic system. Two additional blocks (enclosed by dashes) are added to the basic sampled-data model so that it will correctly respond to a larger variety of target inputs.

Similarly, for an error and rate of change of error of the same sign, we may expect larger saccades. Therefore, e is multiplied by $\dot{e}$ so that $+M$ results for e and e of the same sign and M results for e and $\dot{e}$ of opposite signs. The sign of M determines which branch of the gain characteristic is applicable so that as the error rate increases, the gain factor in the saccadic branch is either greater or less than 1. Exactly how the gain varies with $\dot{e}$ is unknown and much more data is necessary to quantify the role of error rate on saccadic magnitude.

Models of the saccadic plant

Young and Stark simplified the eye dynamics by using the plant (muscle and eye dynamics) model of Westheimer (1954a) who suggested that a saccade-like trajectory results when a step function is applied to a second order linear system. Robinson (1964) has since demonstrated that actually a burst of force is applied to the extraocular muscles during a saccade and that the plant input more nearly resembles a pulse superimposed upon a step. The magnitude of the burst of excess force is essentially constant for saccades up to 40 deg and the width of the pulse determines the magnitude of the saccade. Robinson suggested the existence of a functionally separate group of all-or-nothing motor neurons which only are called upon during the saccade. This hypothesis can be incorporated into the Young model by taking the step saccadic position correction and feeding it to two parallel paths (Fig. 8, block B). One path with a unity gain passes the step unchanged; the second converts the step into a pulse whose width is proportional to the magnitude of the step. The fate of a large (solid) or small (dashed) input step to block B is shown. The two path outputs are added to form a command which drives the muscle and eye dynamics.

Vossius (1960) has suggested that the saccadic trajectory may be controlled by a local proprioceptive loop around the extraocular muscle. He proposed a proportional plus integral feedback which has a loop delay of about 6 msec and would therefore affect primarily the terminal portions of the saccade. Although stretch receptors have been identified histologically in both man and monkey and neurophysiologically in the cat, the evidence for a change of neural activity in the oculomotor nuclei or the extraocular muscles upon stretch of the eye muscles is equivocal.

Conclusion

On the basis of the limitations discussed above, saccadic eye movements cannot be subserved by a fixed interval-impulse sampled control system. The original model of Young and Stark was an excellent example of the application of servo analysis techniques to a biological system and at the time predicted many of the known eye movement responses. However, to retain the sampler in light of the more recent experiments, one must postulate a finite width sample whose synchronization with the target is an extremely complicated function of the target characteristics. It may be more appropriate, therefore, to discard the notion of a sampler and to describe the system only as discontinuous.

Further attempts to patch up the sampled-data model to provide responses to a large variety of different target inputs rapidly leads to a very complicated system with essentially no neurophysiological basis (e.g., Fig. 8). The nature of the discontinuity must still be clarified and can be attacked from without by observing eye responses to various target inputs. Questions regarding saccadic and smooth pursuit interaction and the nonlinear effects of target amplitude on saccade characteristics are also amenable to similar external approaches. However, the real future for the control systems engineer involves plunging *into* the oculomotor system to try to locate and quantify some of the black boxes proposed in Fig. 8. The following section briefly discusses some of the more recent oculomotor research dealing with rapid eye movements and points up how little is as yet known about the innards of the saccadic control system.

NEUROPHYSIOLOGY OF THE SACCADIC SYSTEM

The classically cited pathway for the execution of voluntary saccadic eye movement has been as follows: 1) Signals due to passage of the target image over the retina are led via the optic nerve to the lateral geniculate body and thence to area 17 of the occipital lobe. 2) Association fibers from area 17 communicate with areas 18 and 19, where the error signal is probably formed. 3) The error signal somehow reaches the frontal eye fields (Brodmann's cortical area 8) where it is processed to form the saccadic motor command signal. 4) The command signal descends via the corticobulbar tract to the mesencephalic-pontine reticular formation and then to the appropriate oculomotor nuclei.

The visual cortex

Ablation and stimulation studies have shed little light on the role of the visual cortex in the saccadic pathway. Stimulation of the occipital lobe in the monkey does yield long latency (70 msec) saccadic eye movements as part of a complex response involving body movements (Robinson and Fuchs, unpublished observations); however, an exhaustive study of the responses has not been made. A recent single unit study in area 17 (Wurtz, 1968) shows that the activity of at least some visually-excited cortical cells is inhibited during a saccade. However, no neurons discharging prior to the saccade were observed.

The frontal eye fields

The notion that the frontal eye fields are the cortical motor area for saccadic eye movements stems primarily from observations by Holmes (1938) who reported that humans with damage to Area 8 or its projection fibers were unable to execute rapid eye movements. Robinson and Fuchs (1969) have shown that stimulation of Area 8 in the monkey yields saccadic eye movements after latencies as short as 15 msec. By using stimuli near threshold, they determined that saccades of a particular size and direction are represented by localized areas within the fields. Contrary to their results is the single unit work of Bizzi (1968) in which two cell types, one of which fires during, but not preceding, the saccade, are described. Furthermore, most of the cells firing during voluntary saccades could not be antidromically activated by stimulation of the cerebral peduncle. Hence, the stimulation study suggests that the frontal eye fields are primary motor areas, whereas the single unit study discovers no efferent neurons discharging before the eye movement.

The reticular formation

The pontine and mesencephalic reticular formations receive inputs from probably every oculomotor-related area of the brain. It is here that the burst of neural activity necessary for the saccade is thought to be created, since many lower animal forms with no cortex display optokinetic and vestibular nystagmus with its attendant fast (saccadic) phase. Since the reticular area in question (the saccade of vestibular nystagmus depends only on the integrity of the brain stem between the oculomotor and vestibular nuclei ((Robinson, 1968))) is composed of a relatively homogeneous distribution of neurons, it would be difficult to pick out a target for a neurophysiological study. Komatsuzaki, Harris & Cohen (1967) have been able to produce saccadic eye movements in the monkey by stimulating the median zone of the pontine reticular formation. Subsequent recording in the same area with gross electrodes revealed a slow potential which began 10-20 msec before each saccade (Cohen & Feldman, 1968). A microelectrode study would now be in order to study the role of individual units in creating the signal that enters the oculomotor nuclei.

The oculomotor nuclei

The oculomotor nuclei, as the final common pathway for all eye movements, are a logical place to begin a study of the oculomotor system and they are presently receiving the most attention. The burst of force applied to the eyeball is the result of a burst of neural activity clearly seen in the electromyogram (Miller, 1958). Schaefer (1965) finds this burst of activity in single units of the abducens nucleus in rabbits undergoing vestibular nystagmus. The firing pattern of his cells is qualitatively what would be expected if the force applied to the eyeball (i.e., approximately a pulse added to a step) were encoded as spike frequency. Reinhardt and Zuber (1968), approaching the problem from the opposite direction, have stimulated the abducens nerve with a modulated train of pulses to find that a saccade-like trajectory will result only if the stimulus contains a burst of pulses. Several investigators are currently working on the problems of single unit recording from the oculomotor nuclei of alert monkeys.*

Other saccadic areas

Saccade-like responses can be elicited by stimulating the cerebellum of the alert cat (Cohen, Goto, Shanzer & Weiss, 1965). In humans, Kornhuber (1968) has observed that the eyes of patients with cerebellar atrophy often travel large angular distances by a series of saccades rather than one large saccade followed by a small second correction. The cerebellum also receives an input from the extraocular muscles (Fuchs & Kornhuber, 1969). Hence, although Dow and Manni (1964) feel the cerebellum is a non-essential part of the oculomotor system, it does seem to have a modifying influence on saccadic eye movements.

Finally, although many brain lesions selectively abolish smooth pursuit movements, few affect only saccades.** Starr (1967) has recently found that in three of nine patients with Huntington's chorea, a disease causing degeneration of the caudate nucleus, all rapid eye movements were absent, although smooth pursuit movements were unaffected. Therefore, the caudate nucleus has emerged as a hitherto-unsuspected oculomotor area concerned specifically with saccadic eye movement.

*Two such studies were presented at this conference. Based on unit recordings from the oculomotor nucleus, D.A. Robinson suggested that oculomotor neurons are driven by separate inputs concerned with saccades, smooth pursuit movements and fixation. G. Melvill Jones showed that the firing rate of vestibular and oculomotor neurons is a function of head velocity in the cat.

**Based on an extensive survey of many neurological cases reported elsewhere in this symposium, Hoyt and Daroff conclude that the saccadic mode is involved as often if not more often than the smooth pursuit mode.

REFERENCES

Bartz, A. (1962). Eye movement latency, duration and response time as a function of angular displacement. *J. exp. Psychol.* **64,** 318-324.

Becker, W. & Fuchs, A. (1969). Further properties of the human saccadic system: eye movements and correction saccades with and without visual fixation points. *Vision Res.* **9,** 1247-1258.

Beeler, G. (1967). Visual threshold changes resulting from spontaneous saccadic eye movements. *Vision Res.* **7,** 769-775.

Bizzi, E. (1968). Discharge of frontal eye field neurons during saccadic and following eye movements in unanesthetized monkeys. *Exp. Brain Res.* **6,** 69-80.

Boyce, P. (1967). Monocular fixation in human eye movement. *Proc. Roy. Soc.* **B167,** 243-315.

Cohen, B. & Feldman, M. (1968). Relationship of electrical activity in pontine reticular formation and lateral geniculate body to rapid eye movements. *J. Neurophysiol.* **31,** 806-817.

Cohen, B., Goto, K., Shanzer, S. & Weiss, A. (1965). Eye movements induced by electrical stimulation of the cerebellum in the alert cat. *Exp. Neurol.* **13,** 145-162.

Cook, G. (1965). *Control Systems Study of the Saccadic Eye-Movement Mechanism.* Sc.D. Thesis. M.I.T., Cambridge, Mass.

Cornsweet, T. (1956). Determination of the stimuli for involuntary drifts and saccadic eye movements. *J. Opt. Soc. Amer.* **46,** 987-993.

Dallos, P. & Jones, R. (1963). Learning behavior of the eye fixation control system. *IEEE Trans. automatic Control* **AC8,** 218-227.

Dodge, R. & Cline, T. (1901). The angle velocity of eye movements. *Psychol. Rev.* **8,** 125-157.

Dow, R. & Manni, E. (1964). The relationship of the cerebellum to extraocular movements. **In** *The Oculomotor System,* ed. Bender, M. New York: Harper & Row.

Fender, D. & Nye, P. (1961). An investigation of the mechanisms of eye movement control. *Kybernetik* **1,** 81-88.

Fleming, D., Vossius, G., Bowman, G. & Johnson, E. (1969). Adaptive properties of the eye-tracking system as revealed by moving-head and open-loop studies. *Ann. N.Y. Acad. Sci.* **156,** 825-850.

Fuchs, A. (1967a). Saccadic and smooth pursuit eye movements in the monkey. *J. Physiol.* **191,** 609-631.

Fuchs, A. (1967b). Periodic eye tracking in the monkey. *J. Physiol.* **193,** 161-171.

Fuchs, A. & Kornhuber, H. (1969). Extraocular muscle afferents to the cerebellum of the cat. *J. Physiol.* **200,** 713-723.

Gross, E., Vaughan, H., Jr. & Valenstein, E. (1967). Inhibition of visual evoked responses to patterned stimuli during voluntary eye movements. *Electroenceph. clin. Neurophysiol.* **22,** 204-209.

Holmes, G. (1938). The cerebral integration of the ocular movements. *Brit. med. J.* **2,** 107-112.

Hyde, J. (1959). Some characteristics of voluntary human ocular movements in the horizontal plane. *Am. J. Ophthal.* **48,** 85-94.

Jeannerod, M., Gerin, P. & Pernier, J. (1968). Déplacements et fixations du regard dans l'exploration libre d'une scène visuelle. *Vision Res.* **8,** 81-97.

Johnson, L., Jr., (1963). Human eye tracking of aperiodic target functions. 37-B-63-8, Systems Research Center, Case Institute of Technology, Cleveland, Ohio.

Johnson, L. & Fleming, D. (1963). A model of model feedback control for saccadic eye movement. *Proc. 16th Ann. Conf. Eng. Med. Biol., Balt.* **5,** 76-77.

Komatsuzaki, A., Harris, H. & Cohen, B. (1967). Characteristics of the final common pathway for horizontal gaze. *Proc. 20th Ann. Conf. Eng. Med. Biol., Boston.*

Kornhuber, H. (1928) Neurologie des Kleinhirns. *Zentbl. Neurol.* **191,** 13.

Latour, P. (1962). Visual threshold during eye movements. *Vision Res.* **2,** 261-262.

Lauringson, A. & Shchedrovitskii, L. (1965). Certain information on the system of tracking of the eye. *Biofizika* **10,** 137-140.

Mackensen, G. & Schumacher, J. (1960). Die Geschwindigkeit der raschen Phase des optokinetischen Nystagmus. *Graefes Arch. Ophthal.* **162** 400-415.

Miller, J. (1958). Electromyographic pattern of saccadic eye movements. *Am. J. Ophthal.* **46,** 183-186.

Ragazzini, J. & Franklin, G. (1958). *Sampled-data Control Systems.* New York: McGraw Hill.

Ragazzini, J. & Zadeh, L. (1952). The analysis of sampled data systems. *Trans. A.I.E.E.* **71,** 225-234.

Rashbass, C. (1961). The relationship between saccadic and smooth tracking eye movements. *J. Physiol.* **159,** 326-338.

Reinhardt, R. & Zuber, B. (1968). Control of eye position by the lateral rectus muscle in the cat. Proc. 21st Ann. Conf. Eng. Med. Biol., Houston.

Robinson, D. (1964). The mechanics of human saccadic eye movement. *J. Physiol.* **174,** 245-264.

Robinson, D. (1965). The mechanics of human smooth pursuit eye movement. *J. Physiol.* **180,** 569-591.

ROBINSON, D. (1968). The oculomotor control system: a review. *Proc. IEEE* **56,** 1032-1049.
ROBINSON, D. & FUCHS, A. (1969). Eye movements evoked by stimulation of frontal eye fields. *J. Neurophysiol.* **32,** 637-648.
SASLOW, M. (1967). Latency for saccadic eye movement. *J. opt. Soc. Amer.* **57,** 1030-1033.
SCHAEFER, K.P. (1965). Die Erregungsmuster einzelner Neurone des Abducenskernes beim Kaninchen. *Pflüg. Arch.* **284,** 31-52.
STARK, L., VOSSIUS, G. & YOUNG, L. (1962). Predictive control of eye tracking movements *IRE Trans.* **HFE3,** 52-57.
STARR, A. (1967). A disorder of rapid eye movements in Huntington's chorea. *Brain* **90,** 545-564.
STEINMAN, R., CUNITZ, R. & TIMBERLAKE, G. (1967). Voluntary control of microsaccades during maintained monocular fixation. *Science* **255,** 1577-1579.
TRAVIS, R. (1936). The latency and velocity of the eye in saccadic movements. *Psychol. Monogr.* **48,** 242-249.
TRINKER, M. (1958). Recent studies of eye movements in reading. *Psychol. Bull.* **55,** 215-231.
VOLKMANN, F. (1962). Vision during voluntary saccadic eye movements. *J. opt. Soc. Amer.* **52,** 571-578.
VOSSIUS, G. (1960). Das System der Augenbewegung. *Z. Biol.* **112,** 27-57.
VOSSIUS, G. (1961). Die Regelbewegung des Auges. **In** *Aufnahme und Verarbeitung von Nachrichten durch Organismen,* ed. VDE. Stuttgart.
VOSSIUS, G. & WERNER, J. (1969). The functional control of the eye-tracking system and its digital simulation. 4th Int. Fed. Automatic Control Congress, Warsaw.
WESTHEIMER, G. (1954a). Mechanism of saccadic eye movements. *Arch. Ophthal.* **52,** 710-724.
WESTHEIMER, G. (1954b). Eye movement responses to a horizontally moving visual stimulus. *Arch. Ophthal.* **52,** 932-941.
WHEELES, L., Jr., BOYNTON, R. & COHEN, G. (1966). Eye-movement responses to step and pulse-step stimuli. *J. opt. Soc. Amer.* **56,** 956-960.
WHITE, C. & EASON, R. (1962). Latency and duration of eye movements in the horizontal plane. *J. opt. Soc. Amer.* **52,** 210-213.
WURTZ, R. (1968). Visual cortex neurons: response to stimuli during rapid eye movements. *Science* **162,** 1148-1150.
YARBUS, A. (1956). The motion of the eye in the process of changing points of fixation. *Biofizika* **1,** 76-78.
YARBUS, A. (1967). Eye movements during perception of complex objects. **In** *Eye Movements and Vision.* New York: Plenum Press.
YOUNG, L. (1962). *A Sampled Data Model for Eye Tracking Movements.* Sc.D. Dissertation M.I.T., Cambridge, Mass.
YOUNG, L. (1966). The dead zone to saccadic eye movements. *Proc. Symp. Biomed. Eng., Milwaukee* **1,** 360-362.
YOUNG, L. & STARK, L. (1962). A sampled-data model for eye-tracking movements. *Quart. Progr. Rep. Res. Lab. Electr. M.I.T.* **66,** 370-384.
YOUNG, L. & STARK, L. (1963). Variable feedback experiments testing a sampled data model for eye tracking movements. *IEEE Trans.* **HFE 1,** 38-51.
YOUNG, L., FORSTER, J. & VAN HOUTTE, N. (1968). A revised stochastic sampled data model for eye tracking movements. 4th Ann. NASA-Univ. Conf. Manual Control, University of Michigan, Ann Arbor.
ZUBER, B. (1965). *Physiological Control of Eye Movements in Humans.* Ph.D. Dissertation, M.I.T., Cambridge, Mass.
ZUBER, B. & STARK, L. (1965). Microsaccades and the velocity-amplitude relationship for saccadic eye movements. *Science,* **150,** 1459-1460.
ZUBER, B. & STARK, L. (1966). Saccadic suppression: elevation of visual threshold associated with saccadic eye movements. *Exp. Neurol.* **16,** 65-79.
ZUBER, B., SEMMLOW, J. & STARK, L. (1968). Frequency characteristics of the saccadic eye movement. *Biophys. J.* **8,** 1288-1298.

THE CONTROL SYSTEM FOR VERSIONAL EYE MOVEMENTS

LAWRENCE STARK

The purpose of this review of the control system for versional eye movements is to expose the current state of knowledge as the complex situation it really is: two well formulated models under attack by their very success in generating critical new experiments; a few less refined models encompassing behavior we as yet do not understand; some quantitative descriptions without adequate underlying formulation; and many qualitative descriptions of complex phenomena, pursuit of which may lead to further crystallizations as new models. Because of this heterogenous state of our knowledge, the presentation is divided into four sections each devoted to a somewhat separable major physiological process of the versional system.

I. Dual mode control;

II. Intermittency;

III. Plant dynamics;

IV. Prediction and pattern recognition;

and within each of the above sections are collected models and quantitative descriptions that are related to each one of these four control phenomena.

Partial support is acknowledged from ONR Contract No. N00014-67-A-0114-0022, Bioengineering Experiments on Human Visual Motor Coordination System, and from NIH Grant No. 7 R01 NB08546-01, Neurophysiological Information Coding.

DUAL MODE

Schematic vs Tracking eye movements

The dual mode, the intermittent motion, the saccadic trajectory, and the predictive operator all must be considered in any interpretation of experimental data. The classical experiments of Dodge (Dodge and Cline, 1901) and others have described two types of versional eye movements: the position controlling saccades and the velocity controlling smooth-pursuit movements. An old finding, easy to demonstrate, is that voluntary or schematic eye movements only consist of saccades. Figure 1 shows such a classical experiment wherein the subject is asked to track a target moving in a regular to and fro fashion. He is told that when the target light is turned off, he should attempt voluntarily to move his eyes in a manner as similar to the previous tracking movement as possible. During the period that the target light is turned off, the subject's eye movements consist only of a sequence of saccades which make a rough first order approximation to the unseen target motion. When the light is turned on again, the control system for smooth-pursuit movements is re-established and the eye approximation to target movement is much closer. In the experiment of Figure 1, the target moved at a 45° angle to the horizontal so that both vertical and horizontal components of the single 45° eye tracking movement were required; these were separately measured and recorded. It is clear that these orthogonal components are almost identical; a bit later we shall show some subtle, although important, differences between these components.

Optokinetic nystagmus

Optokinetic nystagmus (OKN) will next be discussed as a further example of the dual mode of operation of the eye movement control system. There are two types of OKN which depend upon the mental set of the subject; the first type occurs when he is instructed to follow the moving stripes. In this case the subject makes relatively rapid smooth following movements (the slow phase) interrupted by large saccades (the fast phase) in the opposite direction. As seen in Figure 2, the velocity of the slow phase is very close to the velocity of the stripes up to approximately 30°/sec.

A second type of OKN called staring or fixated OKN occurs when the subject is instructed not to follow the stripes but to stare straight ahead. Additionally, he may be provided with a fixation point to help in maintaining a relatively fixed gaze in the straight ahead or staring position. As seen in Figure 2 the amplitude of the slow phase of staring of OKN is very small, less than 5°/sec. and is not a strong function of stripe velocity. The amplitude of fixated OKN is even smaller, due to the opposing action of the fixation point.

If one studies fixated OKN as shown in Figure 3, one finds that the amplitudes of both the fast phases and the slow phases are irregular and noisy but

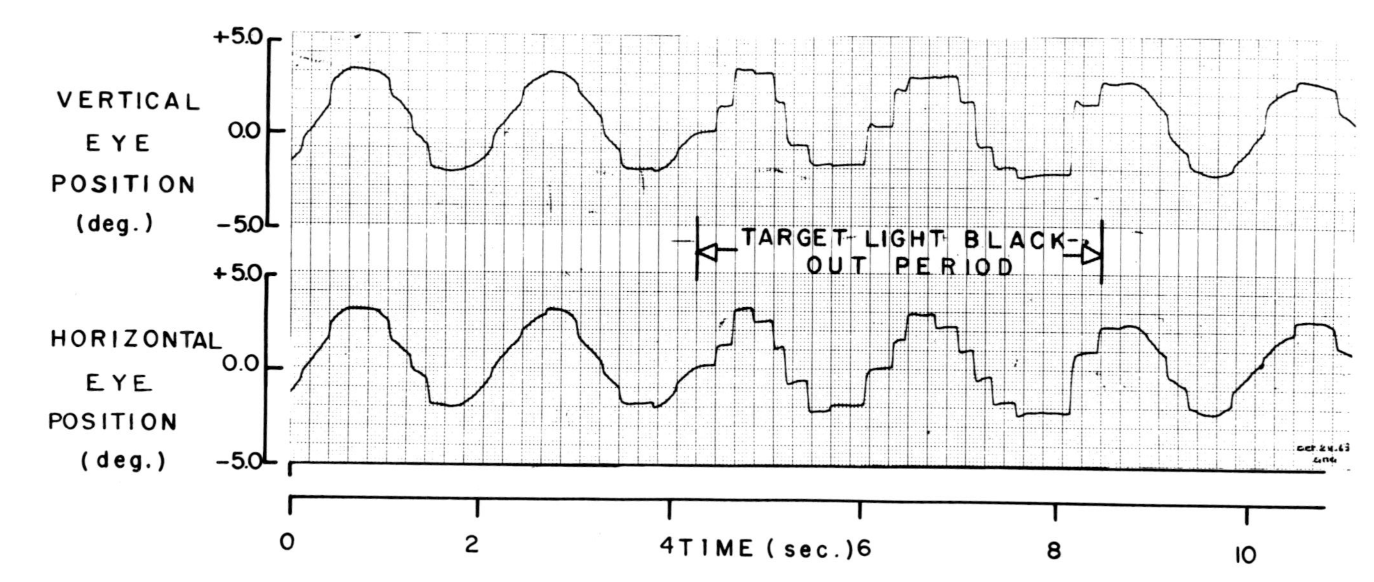

Fig. 1. Schematic saccades vs dual mode tracking. Horizontal and vertical components of tracking eye movements following visible target which makes a regular sequence of alternating ramps, contrasted with voluntary schematic eye movements during the period when the target illumination was turned off and no retinal image was available to drive the smooth pursuit system as well. Subject voluntarily approximating unseen target motion. *(Gauthier, Noton, Schor and Stark,* unpublished experiment).

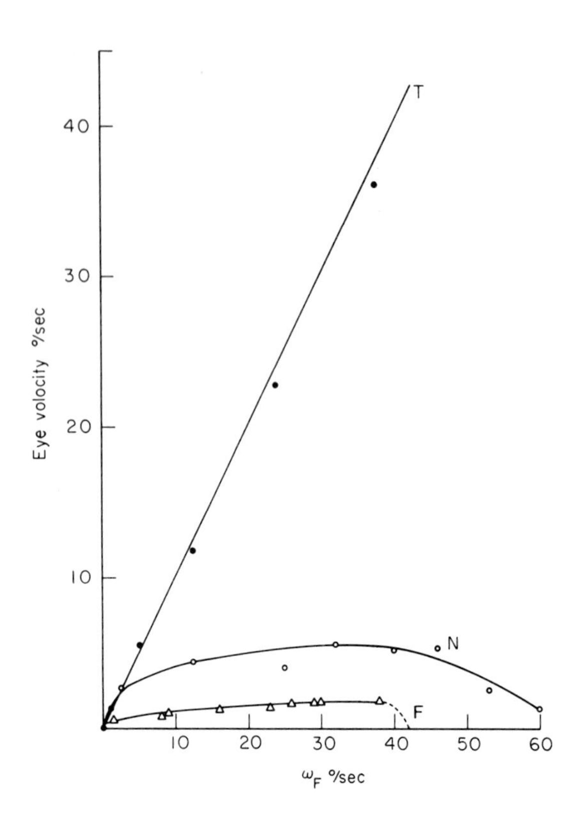

Fig. 2. Following vs staring optokinetic nystagmus. Three curves are for following (T), staring (N) and fixated (F) OKN respectively, and show dependence of slow phase of OKN on stripe velocity, operating conditions, and especially "mental set" or instructions to the subject. *(Nelson and Stark,* 1962).

show almost identical microstructure in each eye. These random variations in the amplitudes of the slow phase and the fast phase can be plotted as quantitative measurements in scattergrams such as those of Figure 4. These demonstrate that the amplitude of the slow phase is highly correlated ($0.86, p<0.005$) with the preceding fast phase and is thus correcting some position error variable randomly disturbed by the preceding fast phase. In contrast, the fast phase is practically uncorrelated ($0.14, p<0.005$) with the preceding slow phase, thus contradicting a commonly accepted view that fast phase actively corrects retinal error introduced by the preceding slow drift, which slow drift was in turn induced by the target stripe velocity.

It is important to obtain an indication of how precisely the subject is able to fixate during fixation OKN. This problem led to the experiments shown in

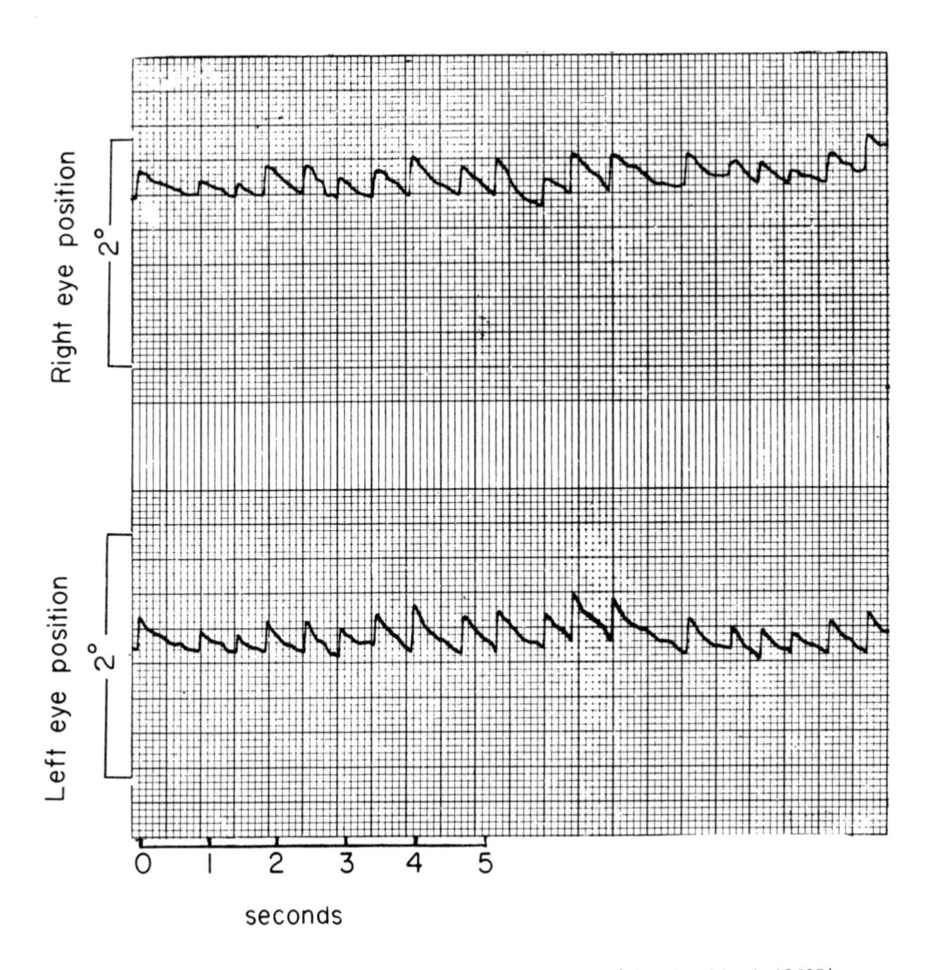

Fig. 3. Fixated OKN. Note bilateral correlation: Hering's Law. (*Merrill and Stark,* 1963B).

Figures 5 and 6. First we examined the precision of tracking relatively small amplitude ramps. We see that the subject is able to track utilizing mainly smooth pursuit movements but with an occasional saccadic correction occurring especially at the turn-around points. The movements are almost identical in the two eyes, in agreement with Hering's Law. However, when we superimpose fixated OKN on top of this ramp tracking task, we see a rather striking pattern of complex eye movements. First the moving fixation point is able to produce rather regular tracking patterns which, if one disregards the superimposed discontinuities due to OKN, can be seen on the average to be rather precise

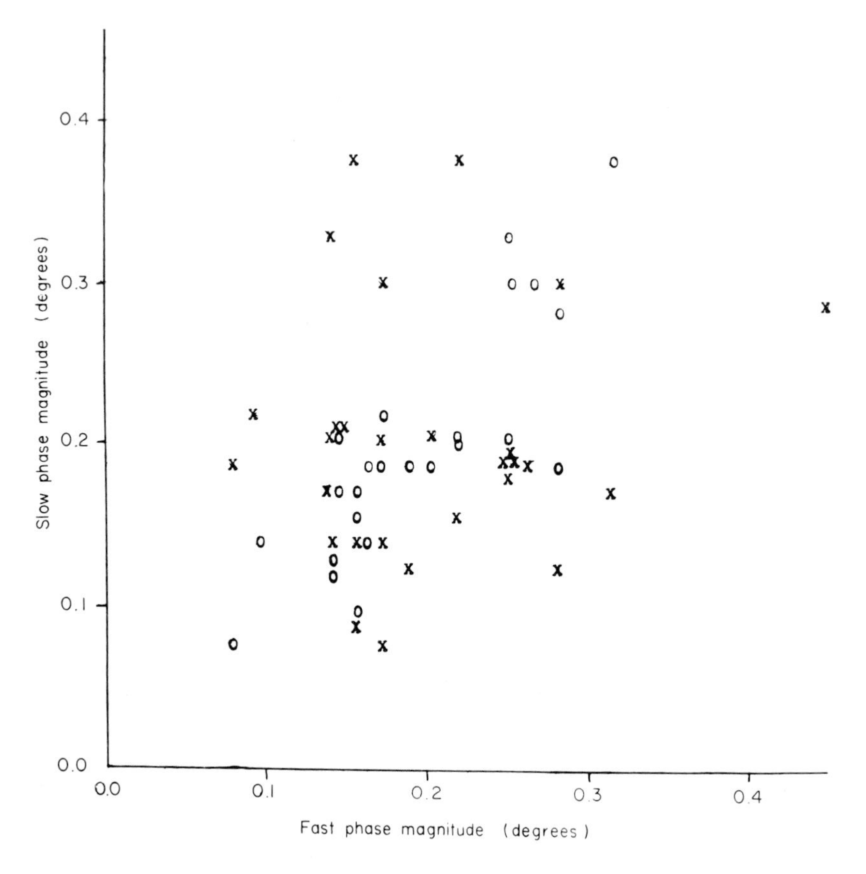

Fig. 4. Two scattergrams relating slow and fast phase amplitudes. Circles show the strong correlation (0.86) between a slow phase and preceding fast phase; x's show the absence of correlation (0.14) between a fast phase and preceding slow phase. *(Merrill and Stark,* 1963B).

following movements and thus provides evidence for the accuracy of fixation during fixated OKN. Second, the OKN, although continually superimposed, is quite different depending on whether the fixation target is moving in the same or opposite direction to the target stripes producing the OKN. The velocity of tracking the ramp fixation point is plus or minus 0.76°/sec. The average velocity for the smooth movements where OKN and tracking are in opposite directions is 0.19°/sec; the average velocity for the smooth movement in the other half cycle is plus 1.76/sec. The difference between the tracking velocity with and without OKN is approximately 0.93 and 1.02°/sec. which corresponds

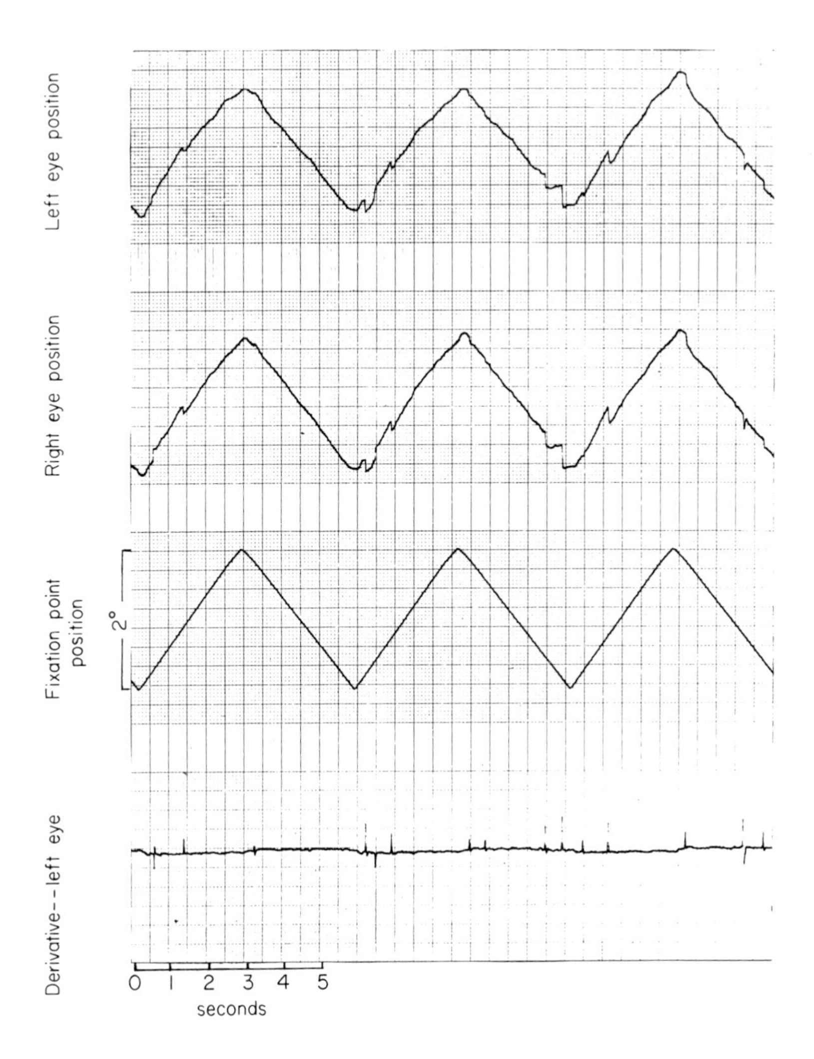

Fig. 5. Versional ramp tracking. Shows dual mode control for each eye; note derivative trace for left eye. *(Merrill and Stark,* 1963B).

to other velocities of the smooth phase of fixated OKN. Thus we see that a tracking input plus an OKN input results in linear superposition of responses to within the precision of the experiment.

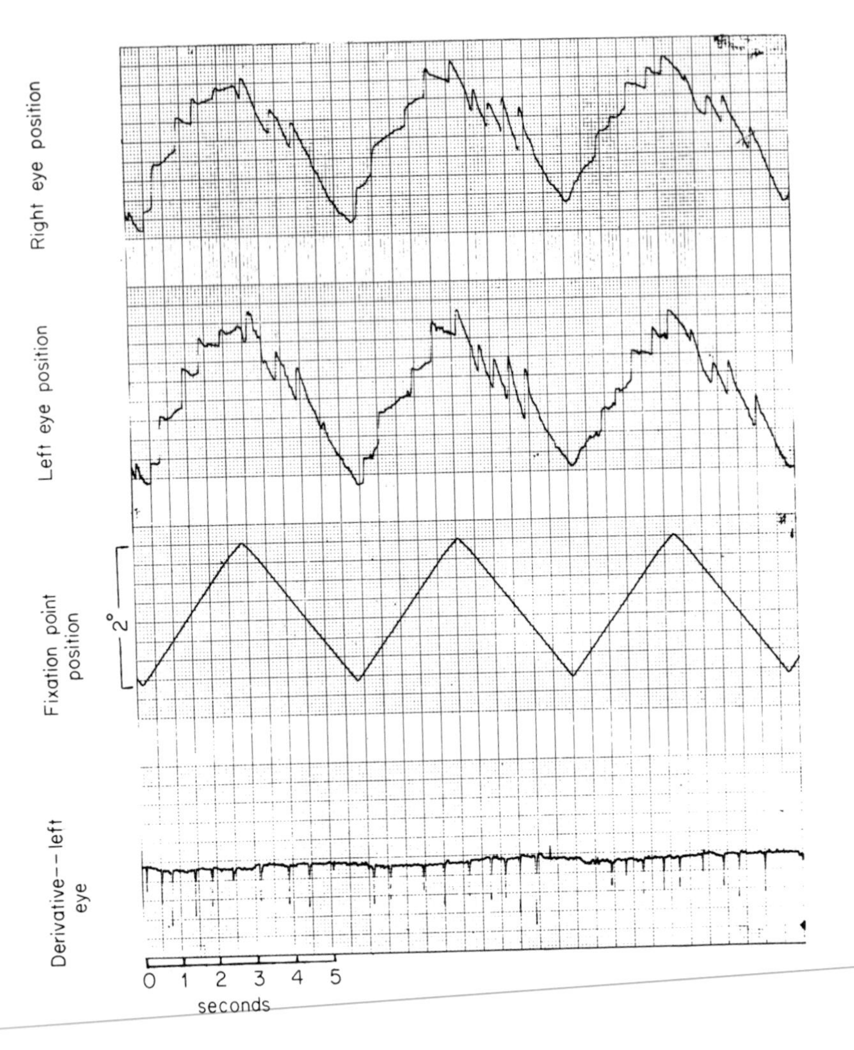

Fig. 6. Versional ramp tracking with superimposed fixated OKN. Shows algebraic summation of slow phases possibly secondary to fast phase effect. *(Merrill and Stark,* 1963B).

On the other hand, if we superimpose two patterns of stripes moving in opposite directions the subject shows, as seen in Figure 7, alternation in the direction of OKN. By cutting out the fast or saccadic phases from the record

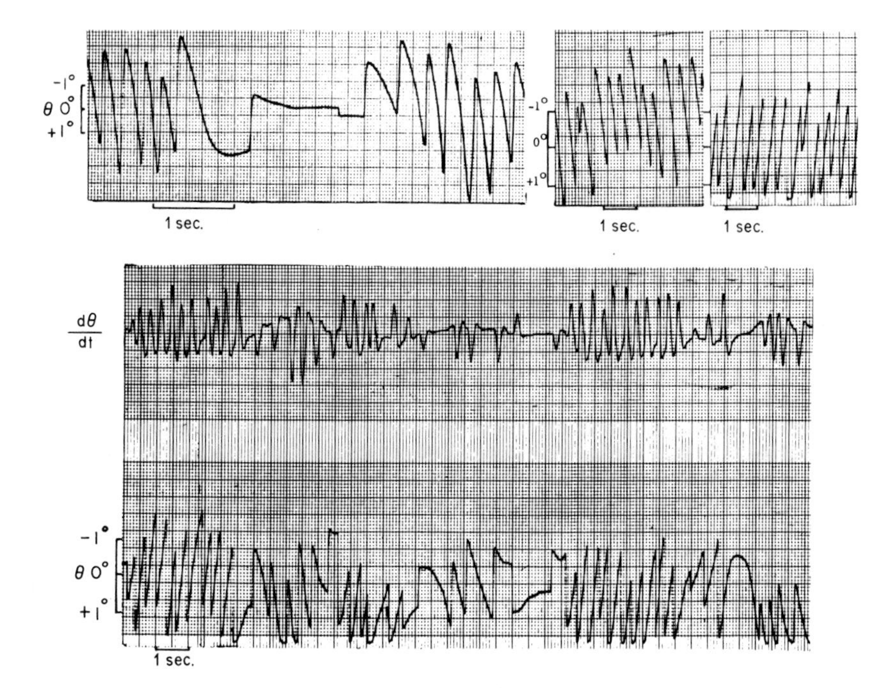

Fig. 7. Records of OKN. Shows upper left, spontaneous deceleration and reacceleration of slow phases, upper right, two symmetrical and opposite responses to opposite target directions, below, smooth accelerations and decelerations as *simultaneously* presented opposite target stripe velocities compete for control. *(Merrill and Stark,* 1963A).

and piecing together the slow phases we obtain the constructed sequences as shown in Figure 8. Here we see the slow phase velocity continuously varying with a rough oscillation period of about two seconds.

The constructed sequence of slow phases can be analyzed by means of autocorrelation function computations and shown to have significant correlation up to a period of approximately one second, after which the autocorrelation is relatively small. This defines the period of coherence of the slow phase in the situation where there is a rivalry between stripes moving in opposite directions, and as such may indicate the time constants for retinal and/or visual cortical reorganization.

In the constructed sequences it is clearly seen that the two smooth phases of the two OKN responses do not summate linearly but rather interact and compete with one another. When we recall that the normal smooth tracking movement summated linearly with the slow phase of OKN we see that this is evidence suggesting that the smooth pursuit movement is not the same in versional tracking and in fixated OKN. However, under both conditions the

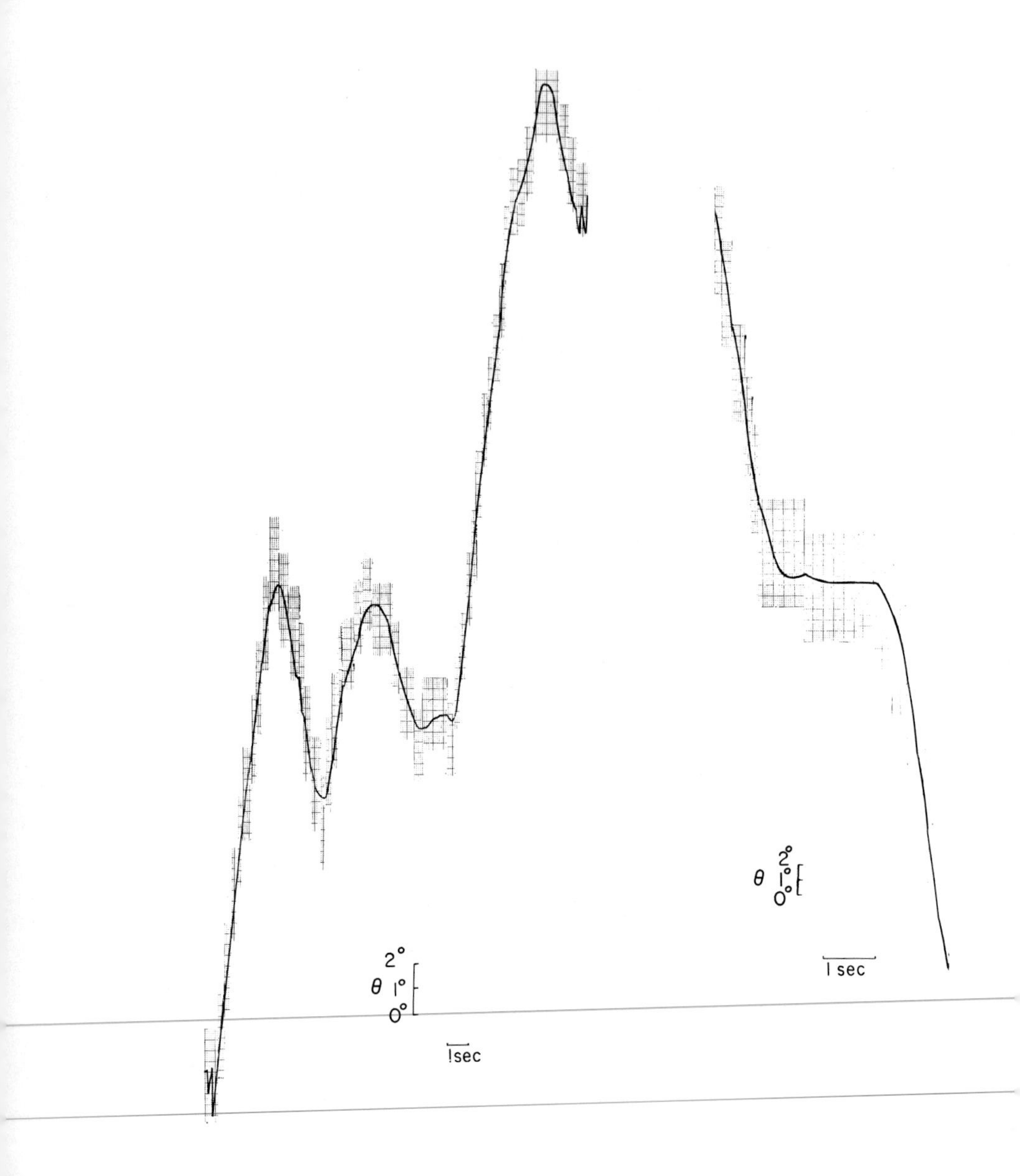

Fig. 8. Constructed sequences of slow phases. These are taken from records shown in preceding Fig. 7, and are obtained by cutting out the fast or saccadic phases from the record and piecing together the slow phases. *(Merrill and Stark,* 1963A).

dual mode of saccades and smooth pursuit is the dominant one of eye movement control. Additional experiments indicated that the fovea was not necessary for these OKN responses. Also interactions were similar when the stimuli were injected separately one into each eye rather than both superimposed onto one eye. This again is evidence for nonlinearity in the response to the two OKN inputs.

A final series of experiments on fixated OKN turns our attention to the initial and final periods when the moving stripe target is instantly turned on or instantly turned off respectively; this is performed by means of a mirror galvanometer directing the stimulus generator into the visual field. As seen in Figure 9 the response begins with a fast phase in a direction away from the fixation point and toward the direction from which the stripes are coming. Thus, this saccadic movement is not a corrective one in terms of correcting for position error introduced by the slow phase, but in itself introduces a position error with respect to straight ahead gaze and the fixation point. It seems more similar to the saccades in voluntary "schematic" eye movements or to tracking saccades seeking to acquire a target, rather than to corrective saccades bringing the eye back onto the fixation point.

The response time of the first saccade is approximately 300 milliseconds. There is a suggestion of an initial slow phase of small amplitude beginning with a response time of 200 milliseconds. However, the fast phase is not compensating for the small initial slow phase; this rather suggests that, just as in dual mode tracking movements, the smooth pursuit component has a somewhat shorter delay time.

After the stimulus stripes have instantaneously ended, fixated OKN continues only as a slow phase bringing the eye back to the gaze or fixation position. Occasionally a fast phase will occur immediately after the ending of stripes; in these rare occasions it is clear that the command signals had already been given and the latent period, during which the saccadic anticipatory signal sets off the "frame of reference" computation with its accompanying saccadic suppression, is occurring. Although there is no nystagmus which persists after the stimulus ceases, there is seen some low amplitude drifting of the eye both before and after the stimulus, which should be compared to the very early pursuit responses.

Thus we see that fixated OKN is a curious and special type of eye movement with dual mode control and almost independent action of slow and fast phases; their main link seeming to be the strong correlation between the amplitude of the slow phase variations and the amplitude of the preceding fast phase as shown in Figure 4. The saccadic phase is not positionally corrective but rather represents a searching response in the direction from which the moving stripes come. The slow phase returns the eyes toward the fixation or staring position; there again it is different from the smooth pursuit movement with which it shows linear superposition when the fixation point is moved in rampwise during fixated OKN.

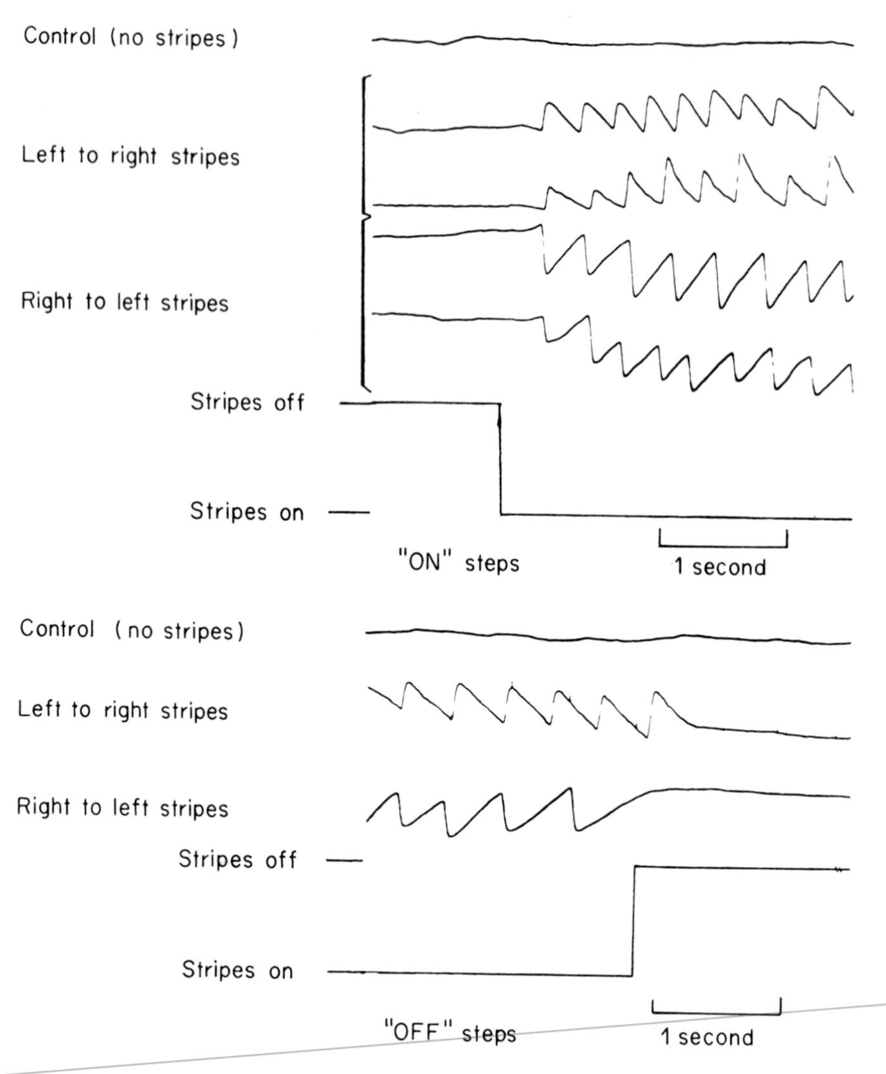

Fig. 9. OKN: Step experiment. Shows on and off periods of OKN with instantaneous starting and stopping of stimulus stripes. Note initial fast phase and final slow phases. *(Merrill and Stark,* 1963A).

Vergence correction for aberrant non-yoked saccades

In searching for interactions between the two components, the saccadic and the pursuit phase, we happened across certain interactions between saccadic and vergence eye movement. These occurred while tracking versional targets under conditions when the subject was fatigued, and could be observed since both eyes were monitored. Examples of such recordings are striking in that they show a complete breakdown of Hering's Law. In Figure 10, we note that the initial saccade is missing or very attenuated in the right eye and thus produces an asymmetrical divergence disparity. Both eyes then exhibit symmetrical vergence movements to a position midway between the two targets.

Figure 11 shows a similar violation of Hering's Law during the return saccade in response to a wide pulse change in target position. In this case, we have an asymmetrical vergence movement correcting only that eye in which the abnormally small versional saccade occurred. By careful inspection of the derivative trace for the abnormal eye movement, the presence of the small initial saccade can be confirmed. It should be compared with both the earlier normal saccade seen just a second before and the small secondary corrective saccade, as well as with the slower vergence correction. Figure 12 shows another example; this time the initial abnormal saccade occurs with reduced latency and is shortly followed by a large corrective saccade; the convergence continues throughout this second saccade.

One wonders how often movements of this type could be noted in patients with latent or clinical strabismus or, indeed, as in this case with a normal subject (L.S.) who was 'fatigued'. Professor Jampolsky, of the Smith-Kettlewell Institute of Visual Sciences, has noted interactions between blinking and eye position of patients with intermittent exotropia, a related phenomenon. In any case, we see here the occurrence of a disparity. This disparity then stimulates vergence movements during versional saccades which do not obey Hering's Law. Certainly this is an interesting interaction between the saccadic phase of dual mode control of versional eye movements and the slow eye movement for vergence control of retinal disparity, which is, of course, quite different from versional smooth pursuit movements.

Absence of smooth pursuit mode in hand movement

The dual mode nature of the eye movement control system has an interesting counter-example in terms of hand control as recently reviewed (Stark, 1968). The hand and eye systems are similar in many ways, the predictive operator and the intermittency control being important features of both. However, in Figure 13, from Navas and Stark (1963, 1968), can be seen an intermittent response of hand rotation to unpredictable ramp inputs. The particular point to emphasize, in conjunction with the present paper on eye movement, is the absence of the smooth pursuit component in hand tracking. This experiment on hand movement has to be carefully designed since limiting dynamical loads can easily smooth out intermittent hand movement trajectories, thus making it difficult to obtain as clear records as in eye movements. In the latter, plant dynamics do not so limit and the intermittent controller signals are rather faithfully recorded as saccadic eye movements.

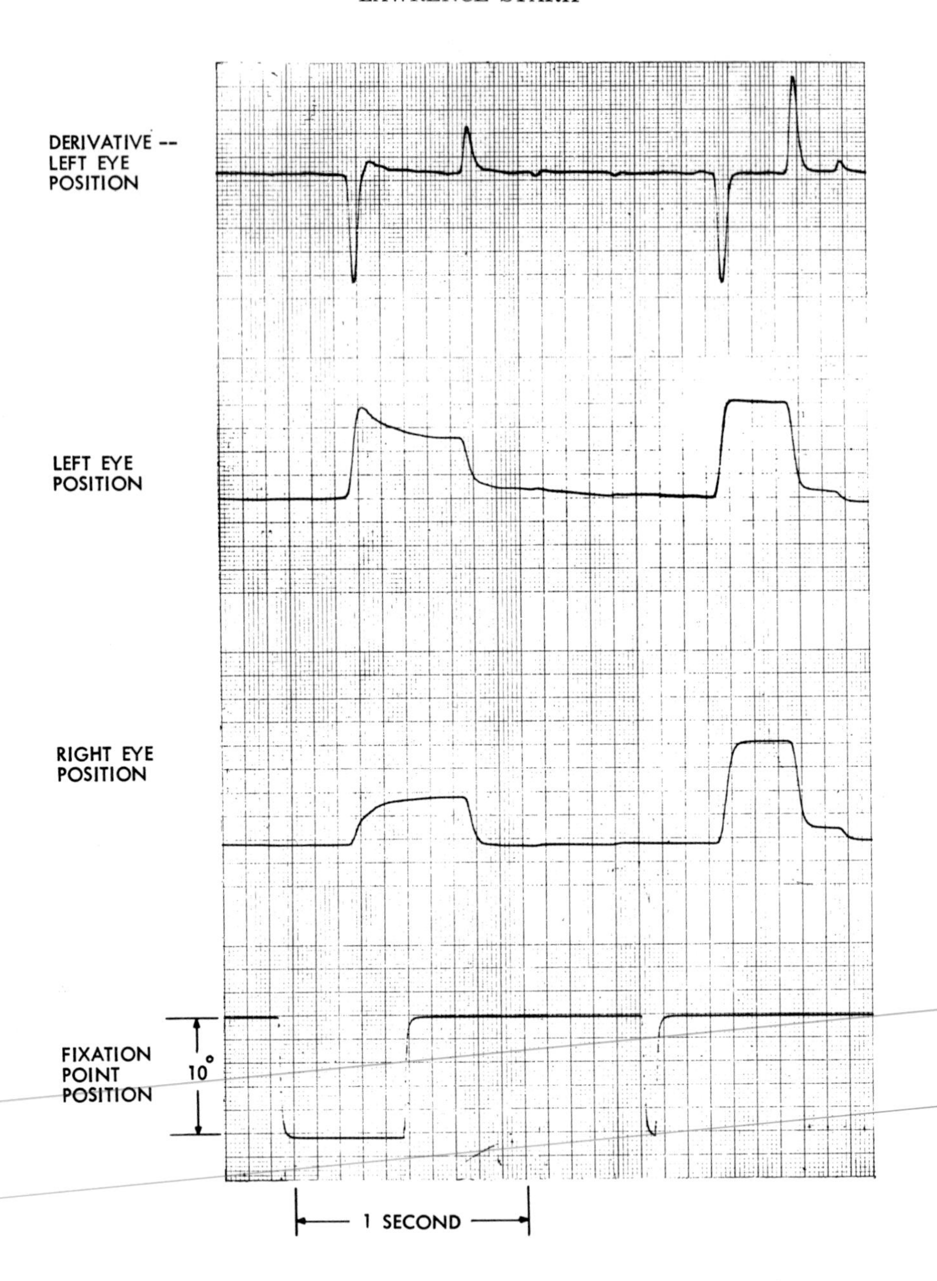

Fig. 10. Version and vergence eye movements. Record of versional saccade not obeying Hering's Law and causing a divergence disparity; note symmetrical corrective movement, to center. Left upward for both eyes. (Unpublished experiment of the author).

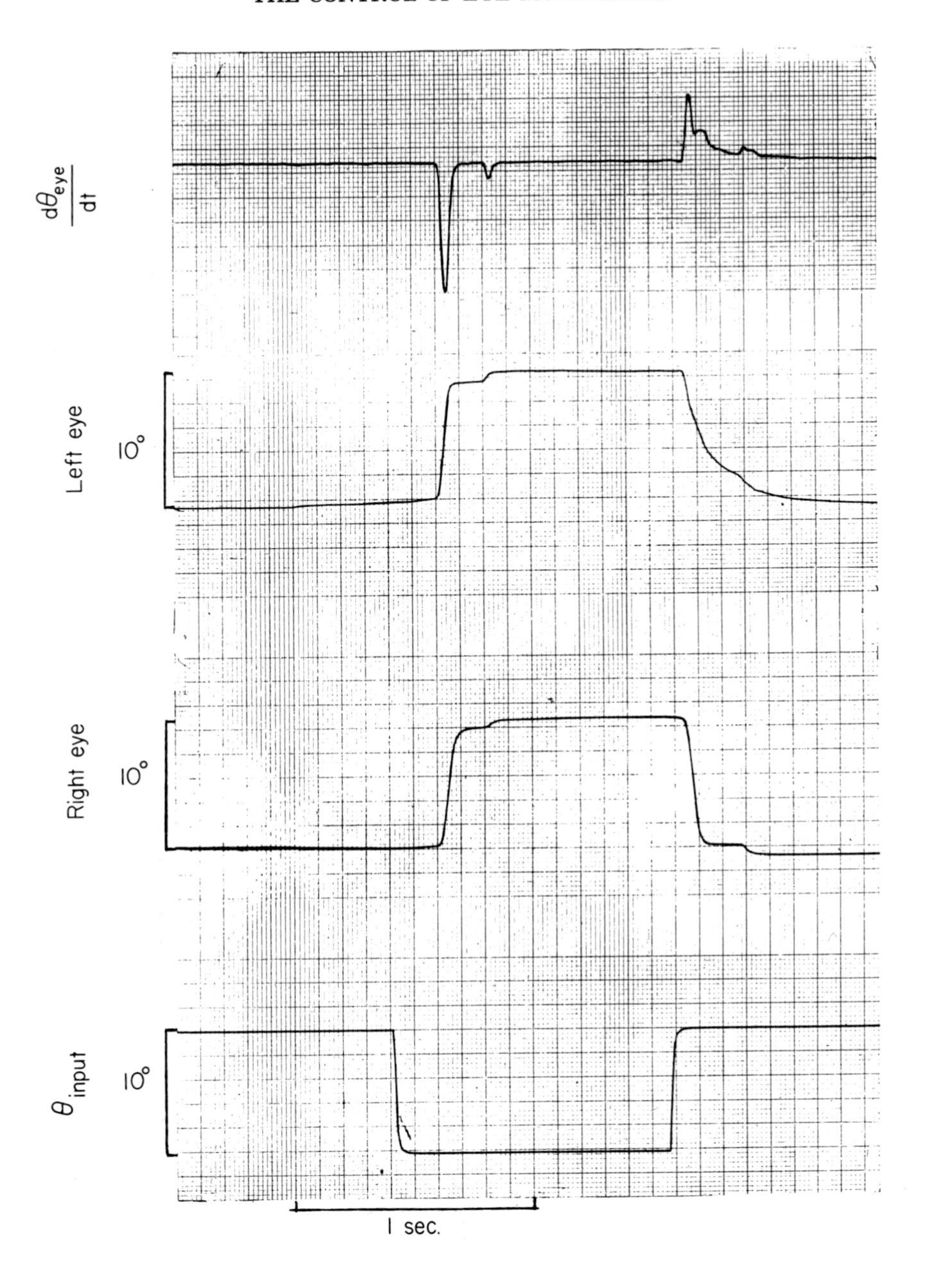

Fig. 11. Version and vergence eye movements. Record of saccades not obeying Hering's Law; again causing a divergence disparity; note asymmetrical convergence correction, and also derivative trace showing abnormal movement. (Unpublished experiment of the author).

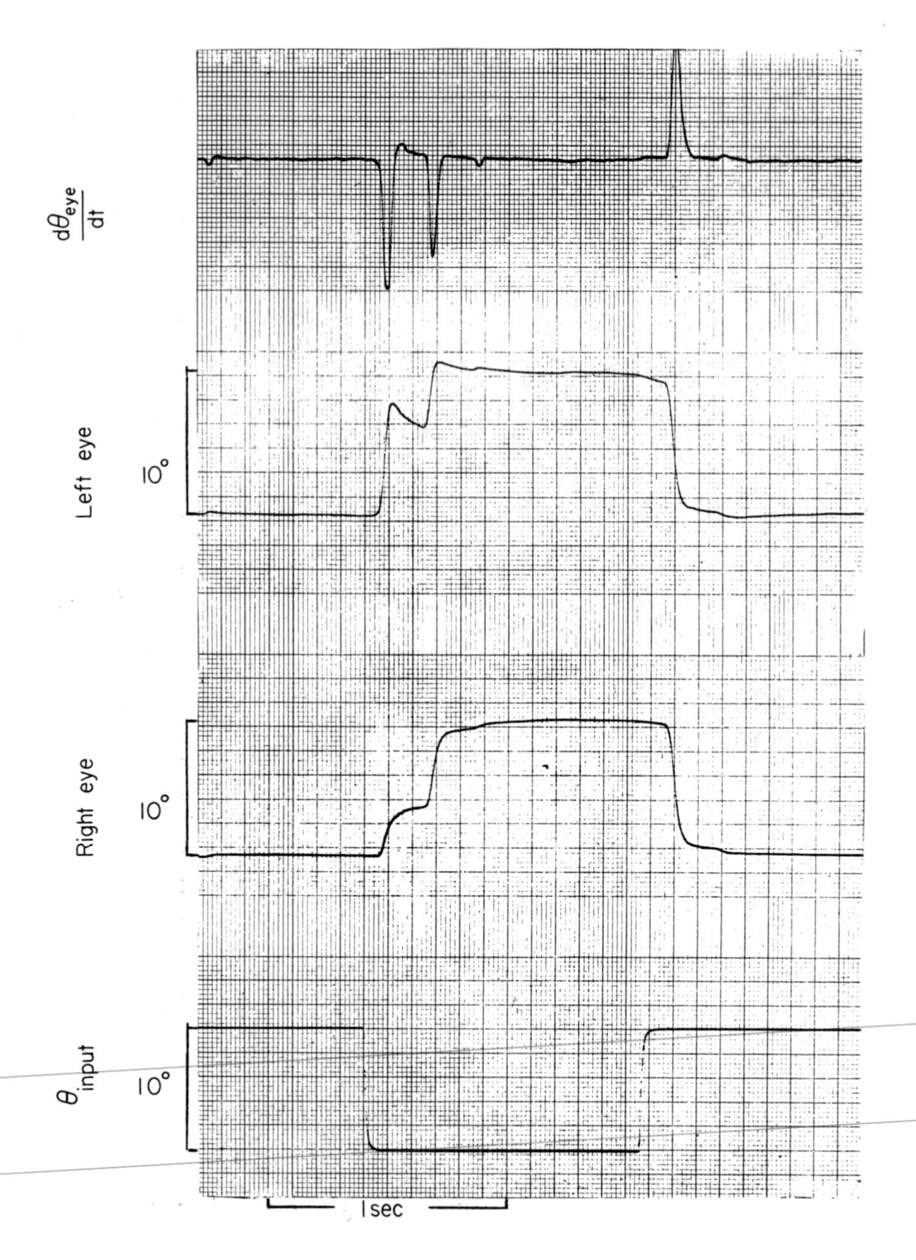

Fig. 12. Version and vergence eye movements. Record of saccades not obeying Hering's Law; note slow symmetrical vergence corrective movement, as well as a large secondary corrective saccade occurring 200 milliseconds later, while the convergence continues. (Unpublished experiment of the author).

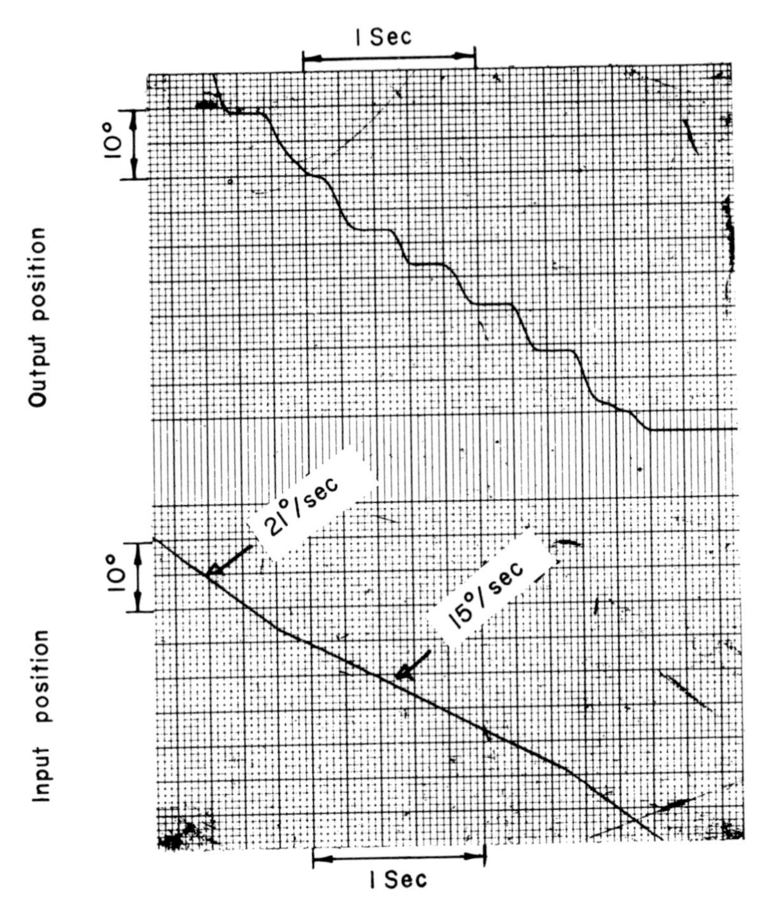

Fig. 13. Intermittent responses of hand control system. Responses to random ramp target motion showing intermittent position corrections, and absence of analog to smooth pursuit eye movement. Compare with schematic eye movements, and contrast with dual mode eye tracking; both shown in Fig. 1. *(Navas and Stark,* 1963, 1968).

Differences in dual mode control in horizontal and vertical eye movements

Another dimension of eye movement control comes into play when we consider the vertical and horizontal components of the versional dual mode eye movement control system. Recently this has been studied by Gauthier, Noton, Schor and myself (unpublished), using several different arrangements of reflective eye movement monitors (Stark, Vossius and Young, 1962). Vertical movements are more difficult to measure because of the absence of sclera

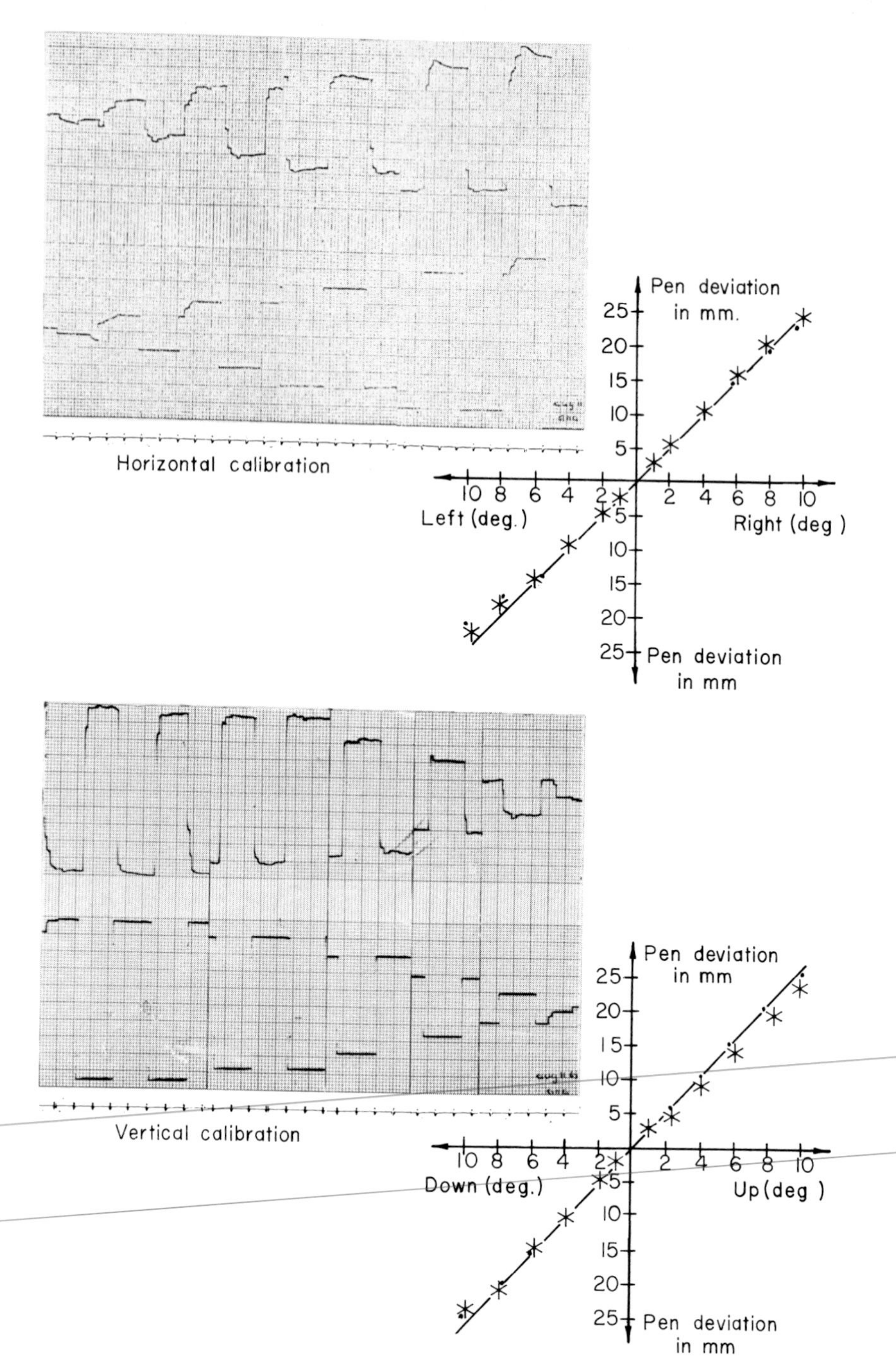

Fig. 14. Measurement of horizontal and vertical eye movements. Calibration in both horizontal and vertical directions of recording eye movement monitors. *(Gauthier, Noton, Schor and Stark,* unpublished data).

above and below the iris for balanced reflectivity; it is however possible to make such measurements with considerable precision, as shown in the calibrations of Figure 14. The essential features of the experimental set-up are an experienced subject who can view the position of the photosensors in a mirror and the ability to quickly and carefully calibrate the photosensing devices as a function of eye position in two dimensions. It is also important to ascertain the interaction or "contamination" of vertical eye movement signal on the horizontal eye movement signal, and horizontal on the vertical, so that these erroneous components can be minimized or eliminated. Continued practice using trained observers, continual recheck of calibrations and nonorthogonal "contamination" by supposed orthogonal components, have led to consistent and reliable observations over a period of three years, using a variety of different configurations of photosensors in different experiments. Indeed, these observations have recently been completely rechecked using a procedure somewhat uncomfortable for the subject, of pulling both the upper and lower eyelids away from the eyeball with tape!

Both horizontal and vertical movements show the dual mode control system as indicated in the classical experiment shown in Figure 1; when examined in detail, however, they show quite interesting differences.

During fixation, horizontal eye position is maintained under excellent control mainly by means of fast microsaccadic movements as shown in Figure 15; although smooth movements are also present, their amplitudes and velocities are rather minimal. Vertical eye position, on the other hand, shows a much greater range of drift, correction by smooth pursuit movement, and a relative absence of microsaccades in controlling fixation. It should be emphasized that these measurements are made simultaneously on the same eyeball and merely indicate the orthogonal components of control of eyeball fixation. We have also noted changes in these parameters under different operating conditions, such as DC position of the fixated target, subject fatigue, and with intersubject variation. These results should be considered as related to observations by Nachmias (1959), Yarbus (1967) and St. Cyr and Fender (1969), who showed dependence of such movements on target shape and also showed intersubject variation.

We initially expected that microsaccades correct position-error and the smooth pursuit movements velocity-error. Indeed a simplifying assumption might be that the saccades would be able also to correct position error caused by drift of the eyeball due to lack of tight control by the velocity servomechanism. That this may be true in some subjects under certain experimental conditions may have led Cornsweet (1958) to the apparently erroneous conclusion that only microsaccades were corrective in fixation. However, the smooth pursuit system here corrects vertical position errors and maintains fixation (Figure 15).

The interactions between the two phases of the dual mode system are complex. In tracking tasks we know, of course, that the smooth pursuit system does not attempt to compensate for velocity changes produced during a saccadic correction (Young and Stark, 1963a and 1963b; Stark, 1968). Also, during

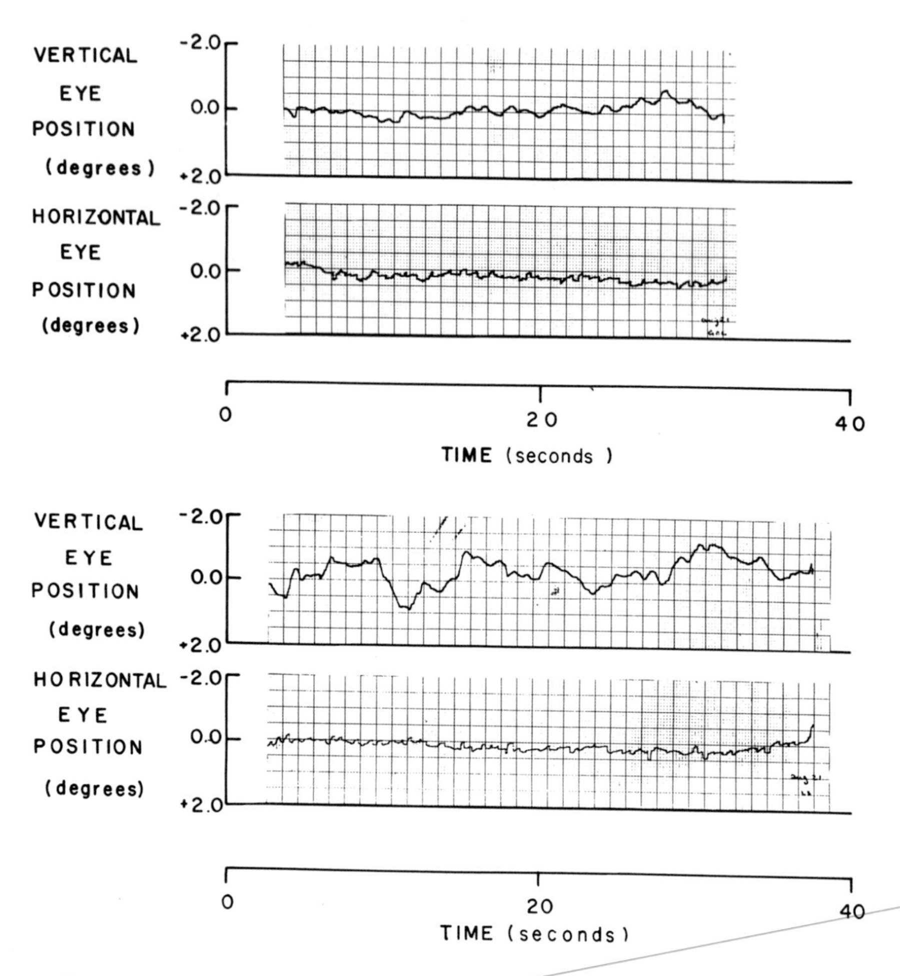

Fig. 15. Comparison of horizontal and vertical eye movements. Two examples of horizontal and vertical components of eye position during maintained fixation. Note stability of horizontal eye movements, mainly multiple microsaccades; and contrast instability of vertical eye position, mainly smooth pursuit movements in this case. *(Gauthier, Noton, Schor and Stark,* unpublished data).

a saccade it is easier for the smooth pursuit system to accelerate from one continuously maintained velocity to another (see Young, Chapter 14 in this volume). This latter fact led Young and myself to propose a sampled data model which included sampling for pursuit, the continuous nature of which will be discussed in the next section.

Differences in detailed behavior of horizontal and vertical components of the dual mode versional movement are seen again when the eye is engaged in a tracking task. In Figure 16 we see two fairly rapid sinusoidal target motions in the vertical and horizontal directions and the eye tracking responses to each one. The horizontal movement seen in the upper part of the figure shows rather moderate-sized undershooting saccades during the high velocity portion of the sinusoidal tracking movement, and rather regular smooth pursuit movements during the lower velocity portions of the quasi-sinusoidal motion.

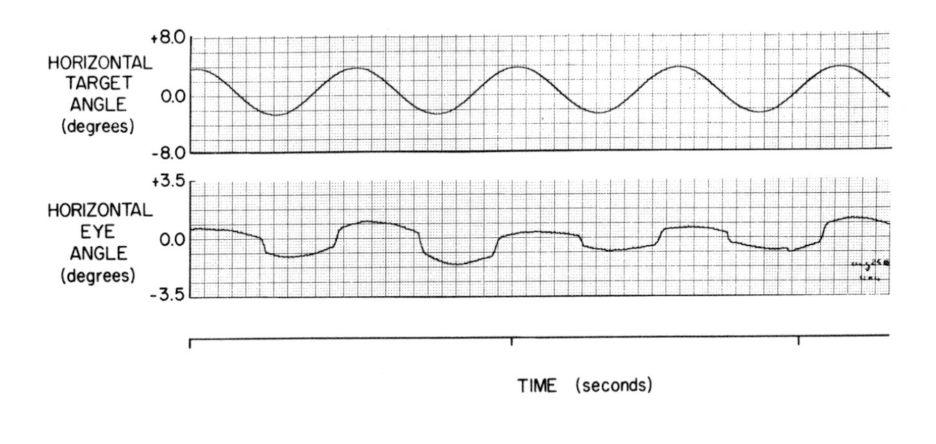

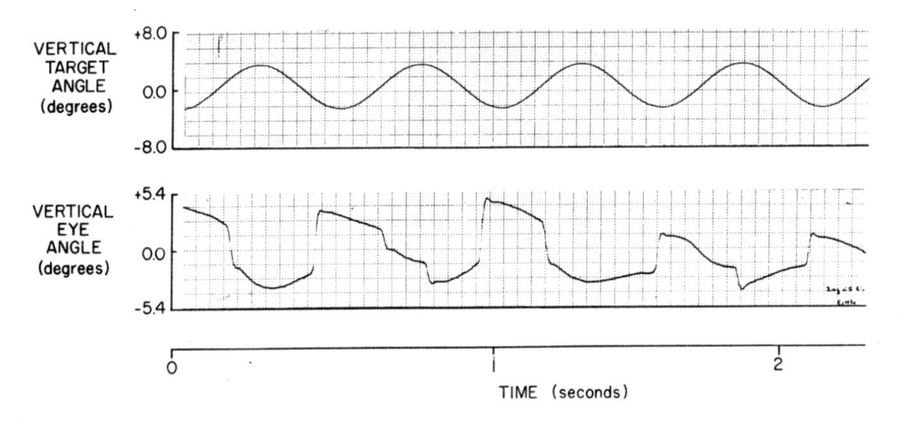

Fig. 16. Comparison of horizontal and vertical eye movements. Versional eye tracking of horizontal and vertical target motions showing differences in response characteristics; however, in both cases dual-mode control behavior is clearly seen. (*Gauthier and Stark,* unpublished).

The gain of the system is less than unity. In contrast, the vertical eye response to vertical target motion shows large irregular overshooting saccadic movements joined by less regular smooth pursuit movement trajectories. Some of the vertical smooth pursuit movements are similar to the horizontal pursuit movements, but others are monotonic. The rapid acceleration phase of these vertical smooth pursuit movements is seen to be concentrated during saccadic movements, an important interaction between the two modes of the dual-mode control system. The gain of this vertical response is greater than one.

From a number of experimental results, such as seen in Figure 16, Bode diagrams of the frequency response of vertical and horizontal eye movements could be obtained as shown in Figure 17. Here we see the increased peaking at approximately 2 Hz in the vertical eye movement responses for low amplitude inputs.

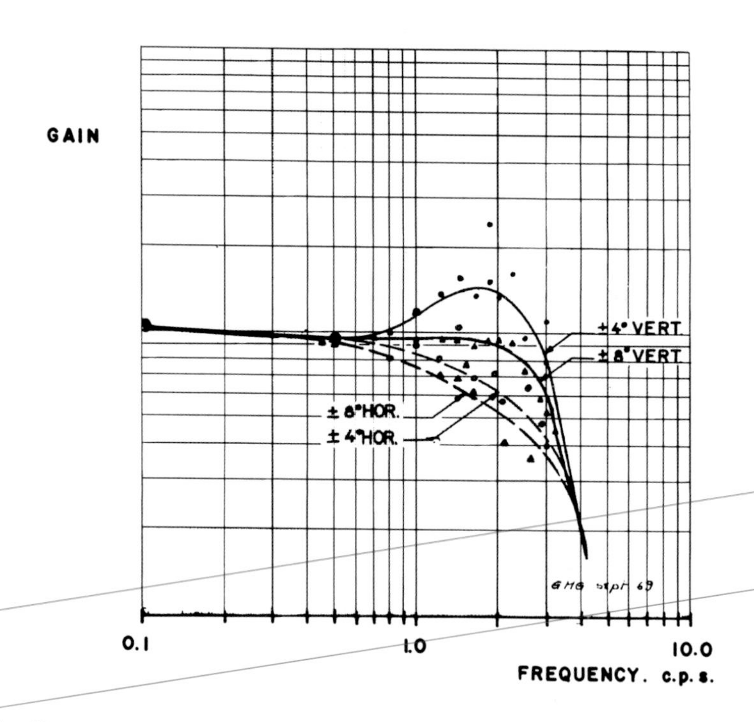

Fig. 17. Comparison of horizontal and vertical eye movements. Amplitude portion of Bode diagram showing peaking of frequency response curve of small amplitude, ±4° vertical eye movements tracking as contrasted with larger amplitude, ±8° vertical; and both large and small amplitude horizontal tracking. *(Gauthier, Noton, Schor and Stark,* unpublished).

One could thus predict from the preceding tracking responses that the vertical control system should be less stable. By using the variable feedback technique (Young and Stark, 1963b), we were able to produce instability in either the horizontal or vertical eye movements (Gauthier and Stark, unpublished observations). The needed additional gain was approximately 0.9 for the vertical movements and 1.1 for the horizontal movements in order to produce conditions of relatively continuous oscillations composed of successive saccades as shown in Figure 18. Although not directly relevant, it should be remembered here that it is known from horizontal eye movement experiments by Robinson (1965) and Brodkey and Stark (1968) that the smooth pursuit system is more stable, i.e. has a lower gain than the saccadic system.

The decreased stability margin of the vertical movements in the artificially increased feedback operating conditions of Figure 18, the overshooting saccades seen in the vertical tracking of small sinusoids of Figure 16, and the peaking of frequency response of Figure 17 are all directly related; we must look to some other behavioral characteristics for possible or probable causal factors. Of interest in this regard is the absence of different frequency response characteristics for horizontal and vertical tracking for unpredictable target motions (Stark, Vossius and Young, 1962). Is it that vertical eye movements, when quite small, have a less accurate predictor operator and this results in overshooting saccades and less curvilinear smooth pursuit segments (Figure 16)? Attempts using distribution functions of delayed and predictive response times to show differences between the predictor apparatus for vertical and horizontal movements have produced slight but not statistically significant tendencies for less prediction for vertical movement; these studies are still in progress (Gauthier and Stark, unpublished observations).

INTERMITTENCY

Current modifications of the Young-Stark sampled data model

Intermittency was initially approached in a quantitatively controlled theoretic manner with the Young-Stark model (Young and Stark, 1963 a&b; Stark, 1968). One of the historical background areas of this model comes from ideas relating to the psychological refractory period which goes back at least to work in the early thirties such as the interesting paper by Telford (1931), and sampling was mentioned by Rashbass (1961) and Vossius (1961). The advantage of control theory, as in the sampled data model, lies in its ability to make quantitative predictions that can be tested experimentally. The original model had sampled data feed-forward paths for both saccadic and smooth pursuit movements; however, evidence suggesting a modification was put forward by Robinson (1965) and Brodkey and Stark (1968).

The smooth pursuit system *can* change its velocity in a continuous fashion; this had been shown before by many early observers, but in the original sampled data model the continuous change of the smooth pursuit system was attributed to the prediction operator. It should be recalled that

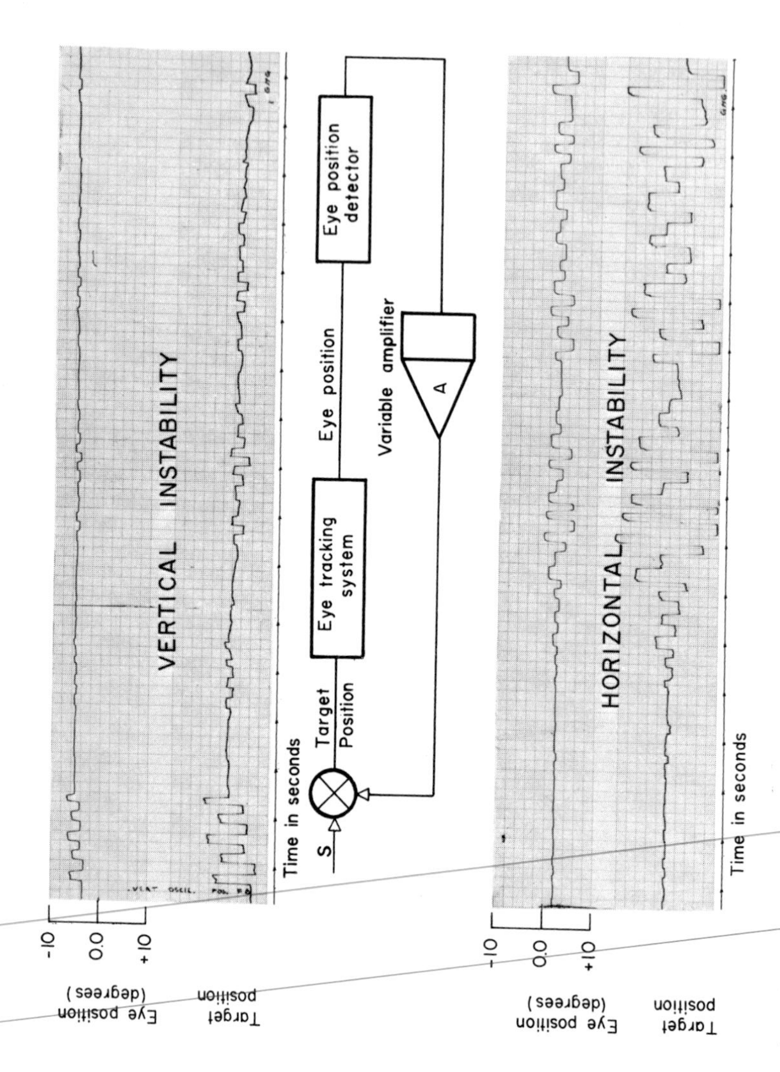

Fig. 18. Comparison of horizontal and vertical eye movements shows variable feedback experiments wherein external gain is increased as shown in inset to produce instability. Gain was increased less to obtain vertical instability than necessary for horizontal eye instability. Frequency but *not* amplitude of the oscillations is predictable from the analytical Young-Stark sampled-data model. (*Gauthier and Stark, unpublished*).

the sampled data model was limited to tracking of nonpredictable stimuli. However, even in these cases Stark, Vossius and Young (1962) showed that continuous changes of smooth pursuit movement could occur (see, for example, their Figure 11). Also, data on OKN such as shown in Figures 8 and 9 above, demonstrated that smooth pursuit movement could change continuously.

Another line of evidence concerning the continuous nature of the smooth pursuit system came from variable feedback experiments wherein the saccadic component was removed either by nonlinear filtering, as in Robinson's (1965) experiments or by linear filtering as in Brodkey and Stark's (1968) experiment. Under these conditions and with the increased variable feedback gain that the lower gain smooth pursuit system requires, continuous instability oscillations could be achieved.

A further line of evidence was rather difficult to obtain because of the requirement for highly sensitive but low noise sensors measuring eye movement velocity. Once these were achieved, the velocity of eye movement responses could be studied under special unpredictable tracking conditions such as rapid successive changes in target velocity, i.e. a brief pulse in velocity. The most consistent results, as shown in Figure 19, indicated the absence of a refractory period for these successive changes in smooth pursuit eye movements. This then is a crucial experiment suggesting the continuous nature of the smooth pursuit forward path. However, the above evidence should be considered with respect to the strong tendency for accelerations in the pursuit mode to occur simultaneously with saccades, as seen in Figure 16 above, and as discussed by Professor Young in Chapter 14.

Two similar modifications of the original Young-Stark sampled data model, shown in Figure 20A, were proposed by Murthy and Deekshatulu (1967) and by Foster, (1968), a student of Young's. The new models both indicate, as shown in Figure 20B and 20C, a continuous pursuit control system with an unsubstantiated input from target position, rather than from error in eye rate. These new models do not purport to be "homeomorphic"; that is, they do not claim a one-to-one correspondence between elements of the mathematical expression and elements of the physical or physiological system; their only aim is to predict input-output behavior.

Further evidence concerning the block in flow of information in control of saccadic movements

The actual nature of the intermittency in eye movement control which is modeled by the Young-Stark sampled data control model is unknown from a physiological point of view. It is becoming increasingly apparent that although the sensory system takes in information continuously and the motor system is capable of producing a continuous output signal, as in smooth pursuit and vergence movements, the controller residing within the central nervous system, possibly at the level of the frontal cortex for eye movements (area 8a), is the site of the intermittency or refractory period of the sampled data movement (Stark, Kupfer and Young, 1965). The following experiments were

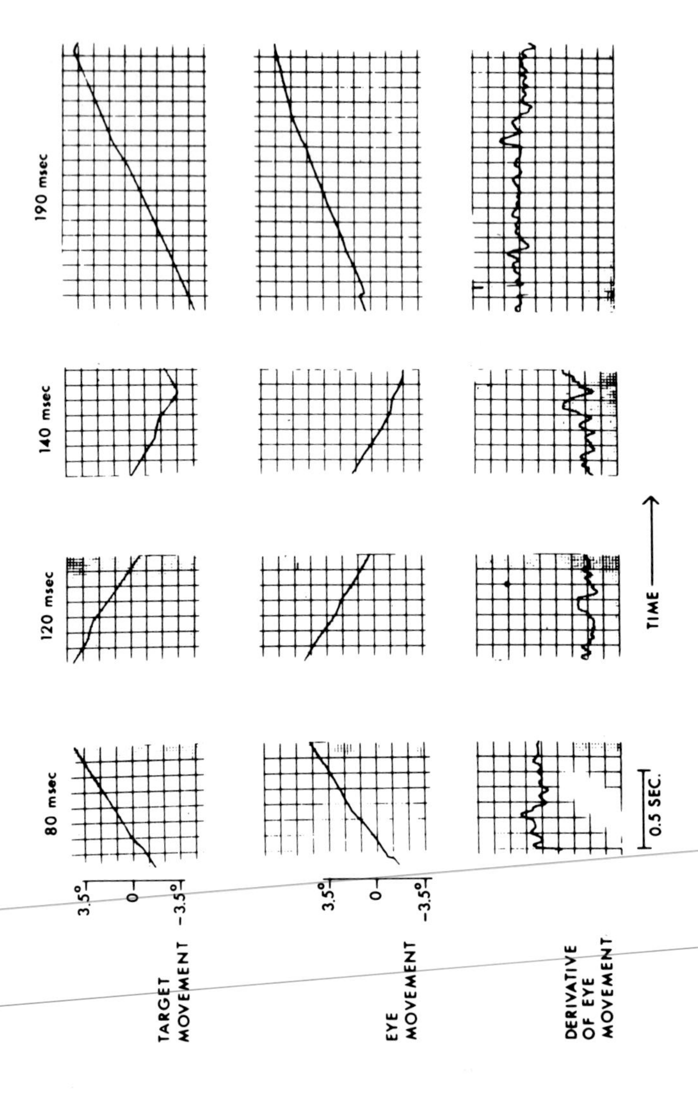

Fig. 19. Crucial pulse experiment. Responses of eye velocity to pulses of change in target velocity. Note absence of a refractory period for smooth pursuit system. Top is target angle; middle, eye angle; bottom, eye velocity. (*Brodkey and Stark*, 1968).

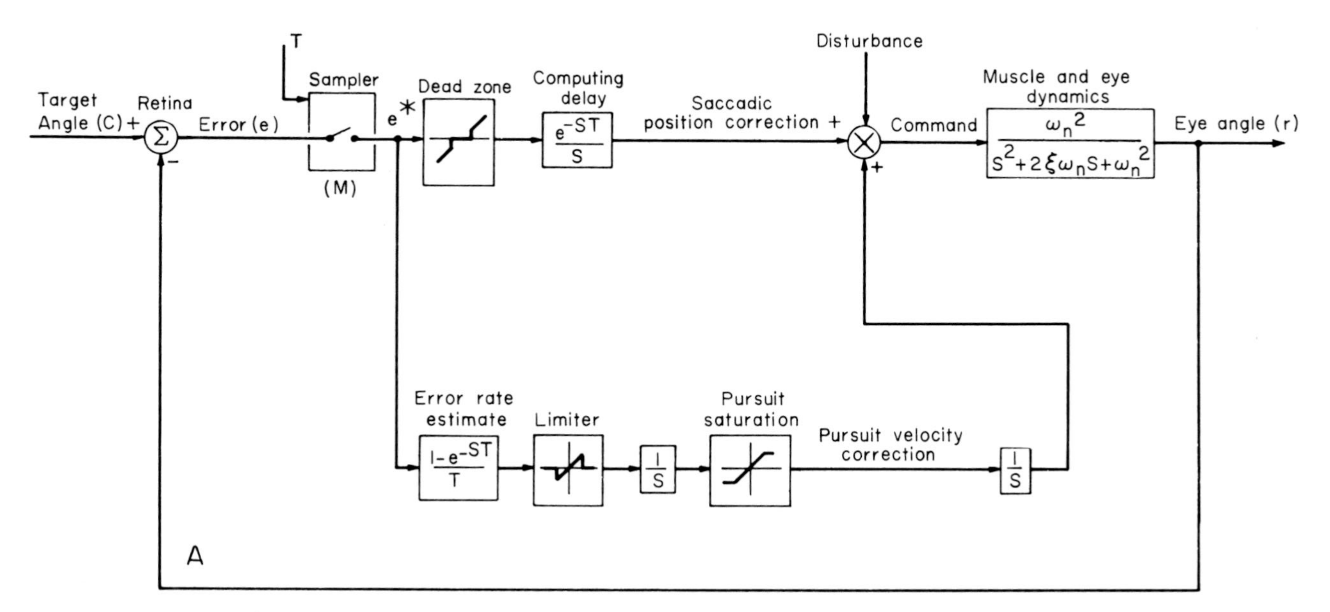

Fig. 20. Dual mode sampled data models. (A) Original Young-Stark sampled data model put forward in 1963 contrasted with two proposed models; (B) by Murthy and Deekshatulu; and (C) by Foster which modify and make continuous the smooth pursuit control path. (*Young and Stark*, 1963 A%B; *Murthy and Deekshatulu*, 1967; *Foster*, 1968).

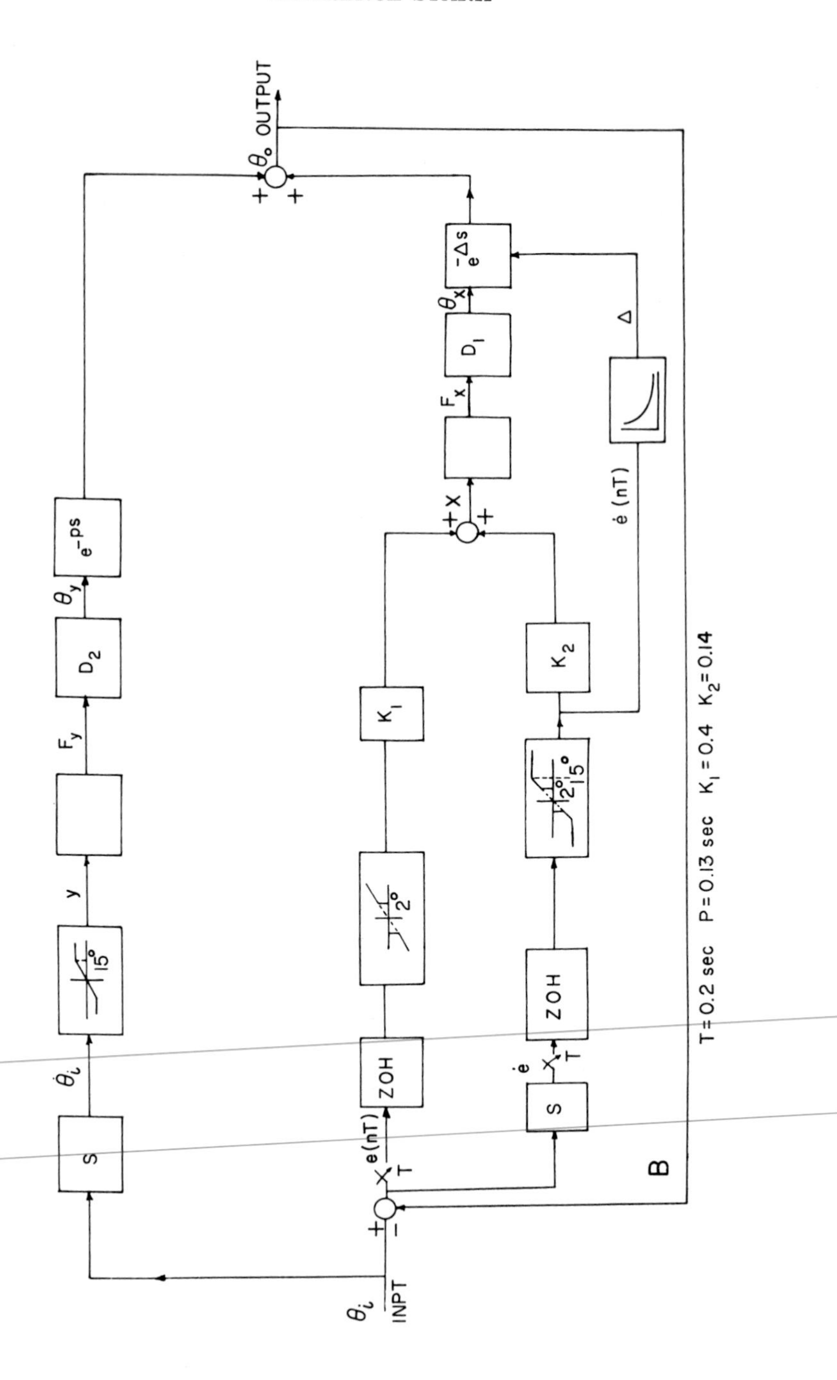

OUTPUT
INPT
ZOH
ZOH
S
S
D₁
D₂
K₁
K₂
B
T = 0.2 sec   P = 0.13 sec   K₁ = 0.4   K₂ = 0.14

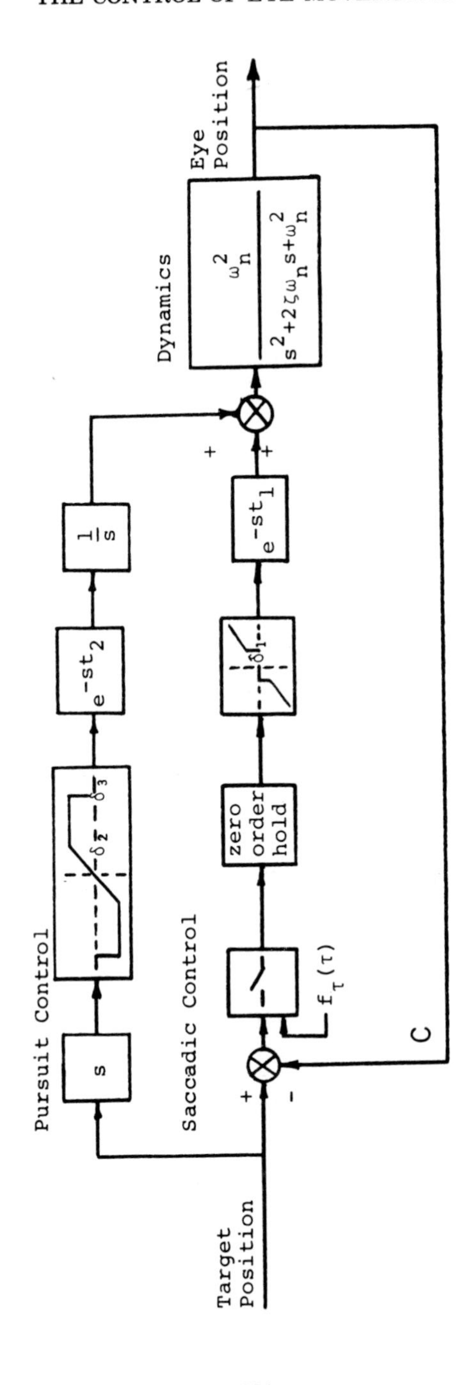
Pursuit Control
Saccadic Control
Dynamics
Target Position
Eye Position
zero order hold
s
1/s
e^-st2
e^-st1
δ1
δ2
δ3
fτ(τ)
C
+
-
ωn^2 / (s^2+2ζωn s+ωn^2)

designed to further define aspects of the intermittent flow of signalling information during the refractory period (Young and Stark, 1962b and Horrocks and Stark, 1964).

It is known that when regular steps of target position are tracked, the subject attempts to predict the occurrence of these target motions and often will anticipate the expected occurrence of a target movement with a saccadic eye movement as shown in Figure 21 (see also below). This distribution of positive and negative delay times is a function of the frequency of the regular target motions as shown by Stark, Vossius and Young (1962). An associated phenomenon, the "error marker", is of importance to indicate the status of information flow under such conditions of variable response times. When eye movement follows target motion with a normal delay of approximately 200 milliseconds, the error in eye movement amplitude is quite small, ranging from one to three percent. When eye movement anticipates the target and estimates amplitude from memory the error is large, as shown in Figure 21, ranging from 10 to 20 percent. Thus we have an indicator, the "error marker", as to whether or not signal information was able to arrive at the controller for precise control of the eye movement. Figure 21 also shows a plot of error as a function of delay time which shows this association of "error marker" with response time, the amplitude of error having a high value for predictive saccades, and a low value for saccades made after a normal delay time and thus after the arrival of visual information.

An even more interesting use of the "error marker" is for those movements wherein the target actually moved to the new position before the eye movement started so that the sensory system was actually in possession of visual information which could have led to low error values. However, in these cases the eye movement occurred so quickly, that is within 80 milliseconds after target motion, that the command signals and the "saccadic anticipatory signal" had most likely already been computed and fixed. Thus these very short positive response times for small delay between target motion and eye movement represent a response related to the prediction response wherein the visual information was not functionally available for precise control of the movement. Under these circumstances, as shown in Figure 22, the error in amplitude of response was large.

As will be discussed below in section IV, the sequences of delay times, anticipatory predictions, and overpredictions show a rather complex behavior which can be modelled as a random process with certain conditional probability restraints. One result of this conditional probability behavior is that it is experimentally rather difficult to find responses occurring with very short delays. Figure 23 is a distribution function showing frequency of occurrence as a function of response time; the marked dip at 0 to 100 milliseconds represents the paucity of responses having short delay times.

How can we interpret this? Experimental results such as shown in Figure 22 suggest that if an eye movement has been decided upon by the controller predicting an anticipated target motion, and if the actual target motion occurs within this short 80 millisecond period preceding the saccade,

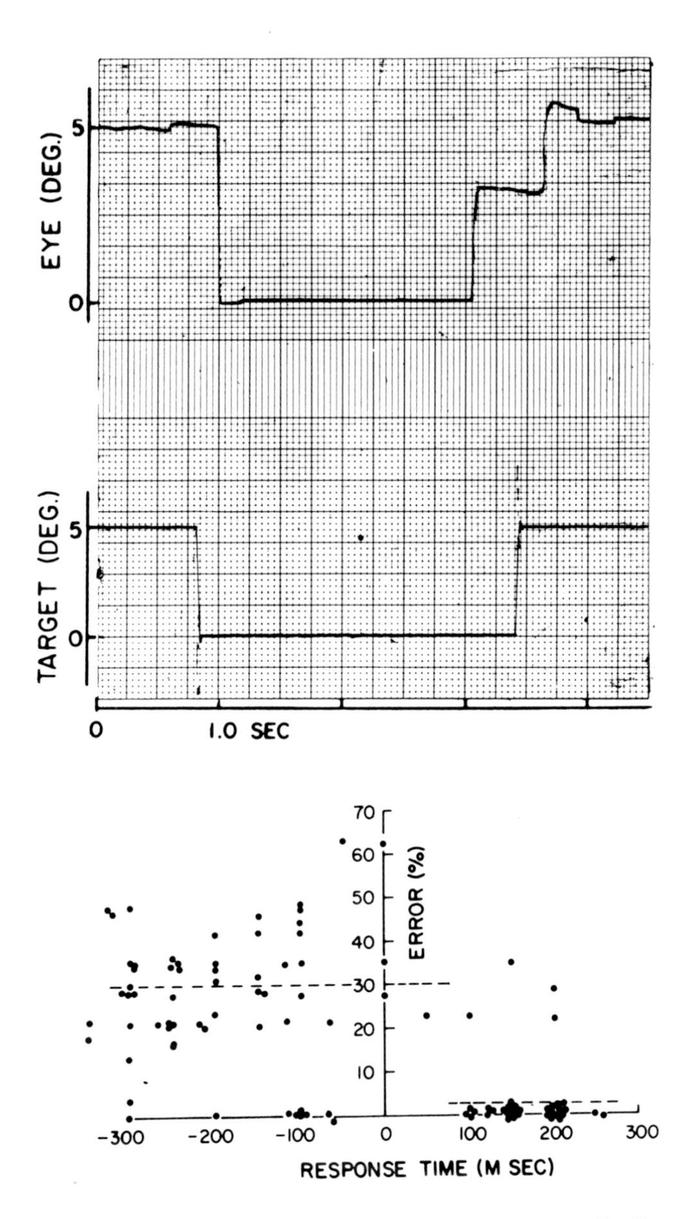

Fig. 21. "Error marker" for predictive responses. Responses to predictable square wave target movement showing both delays and predictions occurring. Plot shows percentage error for various response times. *(Young and Stark,* 1962B; *Stark and Horrocks,* 1964).

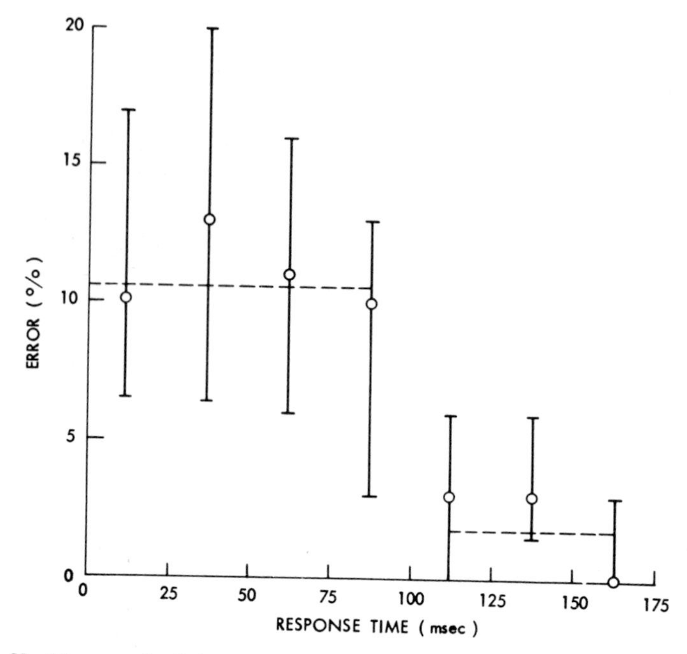

Fig. 22. "Error marker" for predictive responses. Median and interquartile range of prediction error as a function of response time; only delayed responses are shown. Target movement consisted of square waves at 0.4 and 0.5 Hz. Note inability to utilize visual information presented 80 to 100 milliseconds before a saccade. *(Horrocks and Stark,* 1964).

then the functional flow of signal information is blocked. That is, that a possible new and precise error signal from the seen target does not get past the 'opened' saccadic control path, as predicted by the sampled data control model of this intermittent biological system with its neurological 'computing' refractory period. However, the occurrence of the target motion, although incapable of making precise the response motion, does, in a high percentage of cases, cause inhibitory processes to occur which *cancel* the anticipated saccadic movement. Thus we might interpret the experimental data of Figure 23 to indicate that although "first level" error path is open-circuited, secondary "higher level" cancellation paths remain operative.

Saccadic anticipatory signal

The problem of the origin of the control signal for saccadic eye movements has not been solved from a neurological point of view (Stark, Kupfer and Young, 1965) and we had been motivated to study "saccadic suppression" in order to approach this indirectly. Saccadic suppression, a momentary elevation of the visual threshold that occurs in conjunction with all saccadic eye

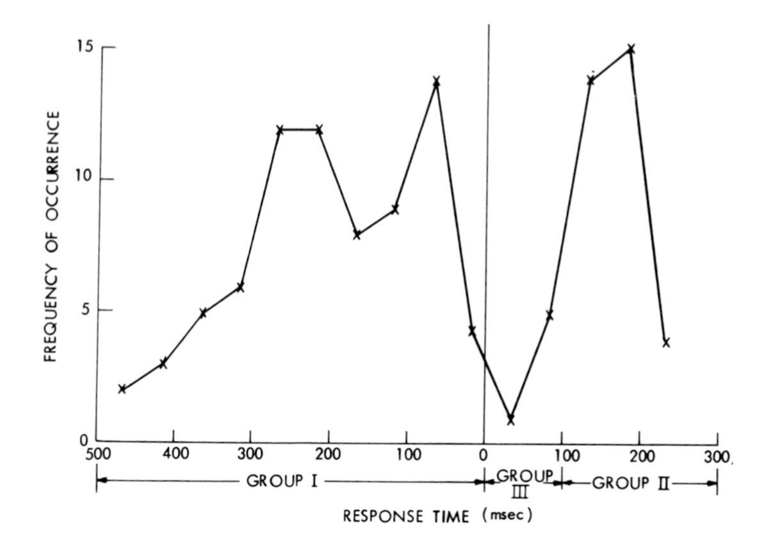

Fig. 23. Cancellation phenomenon. Distribution function of frequency of occurrence of responses having various response times while tracking a predictable target. Note Group I are anticipated or 'negative delay' responses; Group II delayed responses. Note especially the paucity of Group III responses having short positive delays between target motion and eye movement, which indicates that a 'cancellation' of responses occurs at delay times which are too brief for error information to be transmitted to make precise the amplitude of the saccade. *(Horrocks and Stark,* 1964).

movements studied (Latour, 1962; Volkmann,1962; Zuber and Stark, 1966), is accompanied by an objectively measured decrease in the amplitude of the pupillary reflex to light (Lorber, Zuber and Stark, 1965; Zuber, Stark and Lorber, 1966) and by alterations in the visually evoked cortical response in man and animals (Zuber, Stark and Lorber, 1966; Michael and Stark, 1966, 1967). These studies have led to suggestions for the origin of the "saccadic anticipatory signal" and for the locus of action of saccadic suppression (Stark, Michael and Zuber, 1969). They have also raised questions concerning the nature of saccadic suppression as a physiologically important phenomenon in its own right, or as a consequence of the overload produced by the complex "frame of reference" computation which accompanies saccadic movements.

We have postulated that suppression is a functionless consequence of the reconstitution of the visual "frame of reference' initiated by a "saccadic anticipatory signal" sent to the visual system by a central controller for saccadic eye movements (Stark, Michael and Zuber, 1969). Recent experiments, as shown in Figure 24, have indicated that visual acuity is modified only to approximately the same extent as visual threshold, thus suggesting that the 'computational grain' of visual information processing is not changed (Hsiao, Copenhagen, Wilson and Stark, unpublished observations).

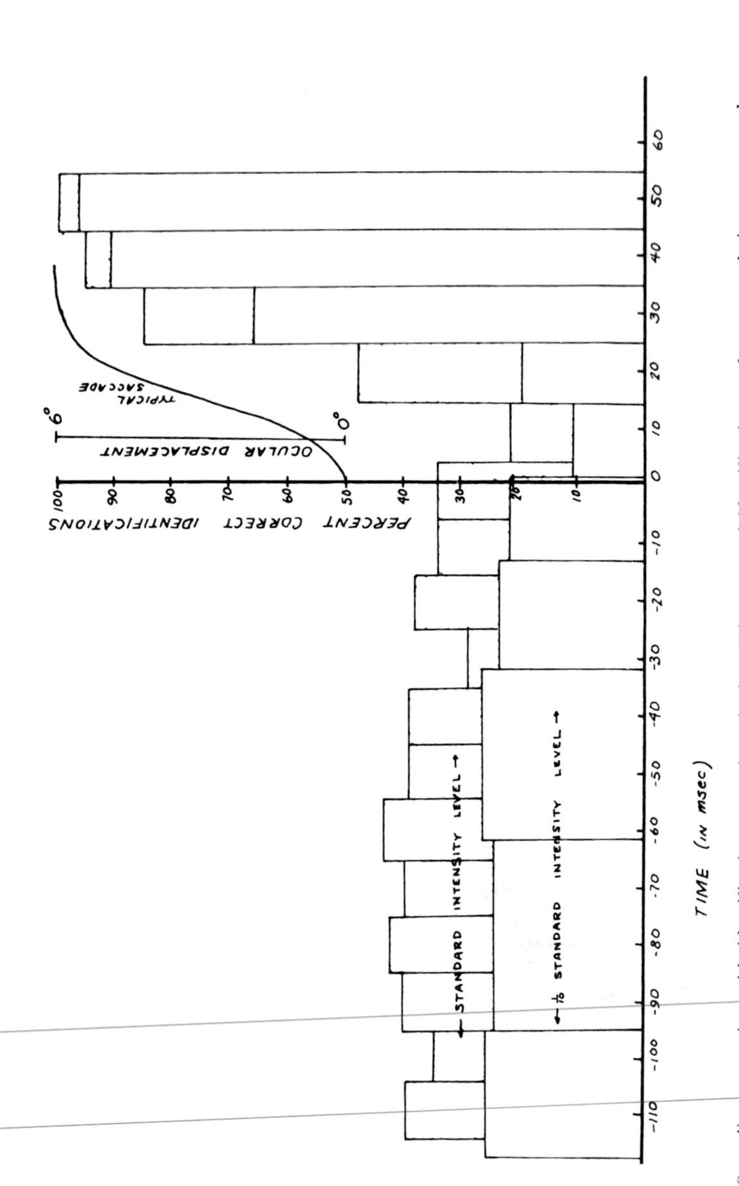

Fig. 24. Saccadic suppression with identification or acuity criterion. Histogram of identification performance relative to temporal occurrence of a 6 degree saccade shows identification of ciphers, or visual acuity, is suppressed approximately one log unit. Time, in msec, from end of stimulus pulse to beginning of saccade. (Unpublished data of *Hsiao, Copenhagen, Wilson and Stark*).

Finally these saccadic suppression studies have suggested a number of neurophysiological studies, now being performed in laboratories throughout the world, which attempt to demonstrate effects concomitant with saccadic suppression, and thus possibly causally related, in various regions of the visual nervous system. Recent studies by Michael and Inchinose (1969) have indicated that receptive field organization in the lateral geniculate body is not changed by rapid eye movements; a result which is consistent with parallel changes in visual acuity and visual threshold during saccadic suppression.

We thus see from the above evidence demonstrating the complexity of mechanisms involved in and available for that feature of eye movement control called "intermittency" and modelled by the Young-Stark sampled data model, that further studies are needed on a broad front, from neurophysiological approaches to modern control theoretic analysis. In this connection recent developments in the general theory of randomly sampled control systems reported by Agnieu and Jury (1969) should be noted. Also according to Starzyk (1969), a pupil of Kulokowsky, a logical pre-condition can be defined for multilevel distribution of control algorithms. If the lower level of control cannot be optimized because of computational limitation, then it is of advantage to accept a suboptimal trajectory and attempt to use higher level control in an adaptive manner. For example, as discussed in the next section (III), the suboptimal saccadic trajectory would be a pre-condition for the predictor feature of eye tracking discussed below in Section IV. The intermittency which can permit "time sharing" (Jury, personal communication), thus may be allocating high level computational facilities among various tasks: trajectory motor control, frame of reference adjustment, 'eigen scan path' pre-programming and visual detection and pattern recognition.

PLANT DYNAMICS TRAJECTORY

Cook-Stark model

For the initial purposes of the Young-Stark sampled data model it was possible to ignore the plant dynamics of the eyeball, orbit, and eye muscles. The dynamics are, of course, of great interest in terms of both the normal physiology of human eye movements and the pathophysiology of various syndromes. When Cook and I turned our attention in this direction, the initial phase of our studies involved a review of the physiology and anatomy of the "plant" so as to obtain a proper topological or logical structure of the elements as well as adequate estimates of the numerical parameters. (Cook and Stark, 1965 a&b; 1966, 1967). We required that the model shown in Figure 25 be homeomorphic in the Bellman sense, that is, that the mathematical elements in the model relate in a one-to-one fashion with the physical, anatomical, and physiological components of the orbit-eyeball-muscle system. The next phase was a careful experimental study of the exact dynamics of the saccadic trajectory for a wide range of initial conditions and amplitudes of movement (Cook, Stark and Zuber, 1966). We were especially concerned to obtain precise

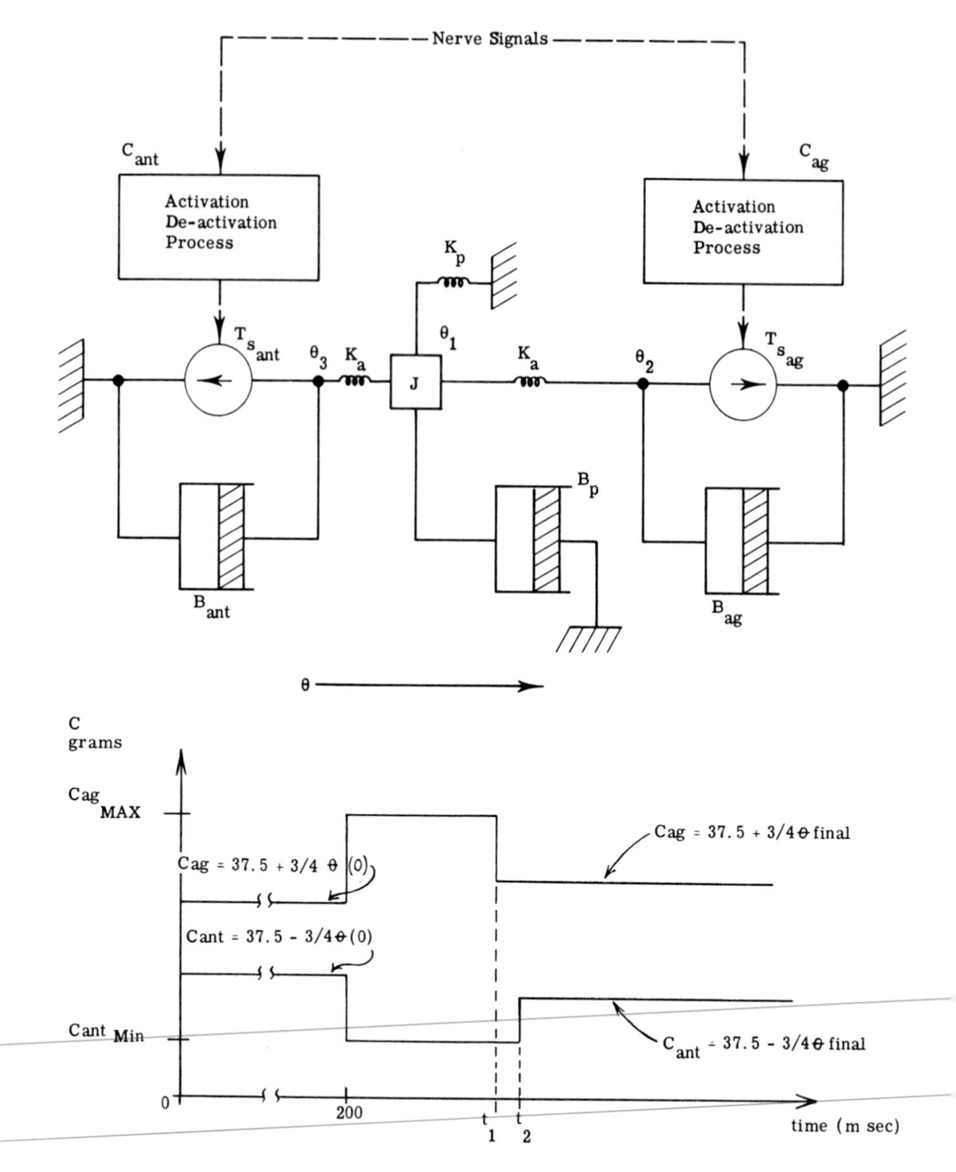

Fig. 25. Cook-Stark model for eye movement mechanism. Above: the activation and deactivation process controls a pair of agonist and antagonist muscle force generators with parallel asymmetrical active "Fenn-effect viscosities" and additional passive elements. Below: Control signals for saccadic eye movements which show the "bang-period" optimal form for a viscous load. *(Cook and Stark,* 1965A, 1967).

velocity profiles so that we could stringently test the behavior of the model in a phase plane analysis. The following phase was to simulate the experimental dynamics with our model, altering and adjusting parameters so that our final representation was made as precise as possible for the particular set of quantitative data (Cook and Stark, 1968b). In the last phase, we explored model behavior in rather abnormal and unusual experiment conditions, both to test the model and to gain insight into such physiological questions as the critical roles of reciprocal innervation and muscle force-velocity asymmetries (Cook and Stark, 1968a).

A brief review of salient features of the model and the controller signals can be made by reference to Figure 25. It now seems clear that there is no true viscosity in the muscle contractile process but rather the "Fenn-effect" (Fenn, 1923) which depends on a limitation in the rate of chemical-to-mechanical energy conversion. Each muscle also has a series elasticity which connects it to the minimal inertia of the eyeball which can be neglected in most treatments. The passive elasticity and viscosity of the orbit also has included in it the passive parallel elasticity of the muscles. The controller signals as shown in Figure 25B are of the form of an optimal controller for a viscous load, that is, "bang-period". This contrasts with the "bang-bang" type of optimal control signal for inertial loads. Electromyographic evidence (Tamler, *et al.,* 1959) supports this form of control signal. Recently, new evidence (Robinson, *et al.,* (1969) has indicated that one of our explicit assumptions concerning the length-tension graph of muscles was not accurate, and we are now carrying out simulations to study how this correction will influence other parameters in the model. The importance of the Blix-Gordon-Huxley length-tension diagram has been re-emphasized recently in conjunction with the sliding filament theory. The main resistive forces in saccadic eye movements are in the asymmetrical force-velocity characteristics, which are functions of activation in our model formulation.

Examples of human eye movement data are shown in Figures 26 and 27; the position and velocity traces of Figure 26 can be replotted to form the family of phase plane trajectories shown in Figure 27. These trajectories have been found to be suboptimal for a controller policy minimizing time to execute a movement; our calculations show that the actual movements take two to four times as long for completion as could be obtained if the system operated with the maximum tension available and attempted a minimum time policy. Such suboptimal trajectories may be a consequence of a system being computationally bound at the first level and requiring multi-level distribution of control algorithms.

Our next procedure was to adjust model parameters to simulate these families of saccadic position and velocity curves occurring with saccades of various amplitudes and initial and final positions. Figure 28 shows the adequacy of our model simulation and is considered positive evidence for the realistic nature of the model structure and the accuracy of its parameters.

We consider that the most important feature of our model is the asymmetrical force-velocity characteristics that define the main viscous load

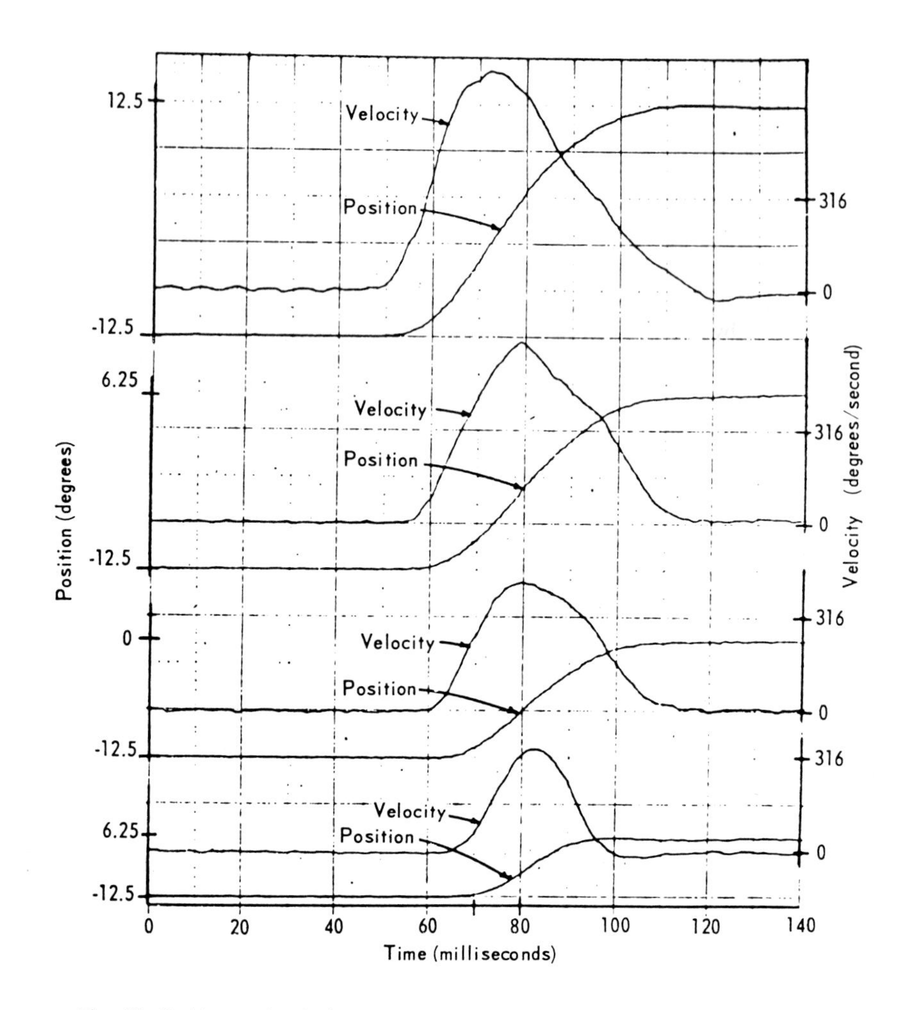

Fig. 26. Position and velocity curves for saccadic movements. Various amplitudes all beginning at —12.5°. Noise in velocity traces are a true rendition of irregularity in muscle control and not an artifact of the measurement technique. Velocity curves are clearly not of the form of a ballistic movement. Ballistic suggestions for eye movements where visco-elastic loads predominate are not tenable. *(Cook, Stark and Zuber,* 1966).

behavior of the movement. These characteristics were first defined as basic to muscle physiology by Fenn and Marsh (1935) and Katz (1939), and are well described by A.V.Hill's equation (Hill, 1938) and perhaps even more accurately by the simplified equations of Carlson (1959). Other previous and current

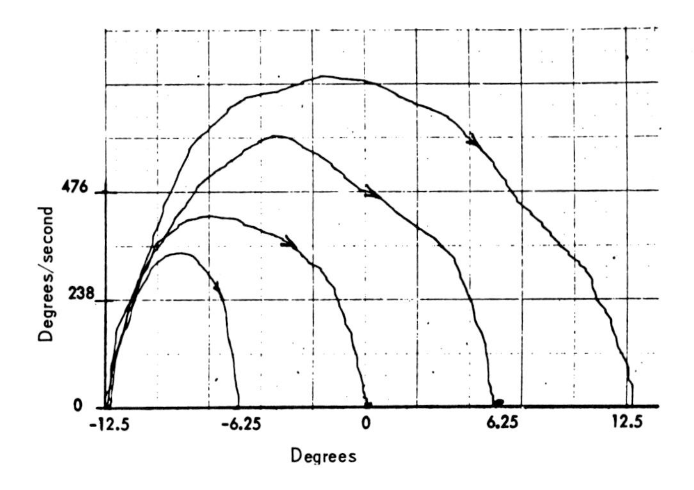

Fig. 27. Phase plane trajectories for saccadic movements. These are same responses shown in Figure 26. *(Cook, Stark and Zuber,* 1966).

models for the eye movement trajectory have ignored this important asymmetrical behavior and have lumped the agonist and antagonist muscles into one force generator-dynamical element, such as the linear second-order differential equation of Westheimer (1954, a&b) and the models of Vossius (1960), Robinson (1964), Childress and Jones (1967) and Thomas (1967). Illustrative of the inadequacies of these models are the results seen in Figure 29, which shows a completely abnormal velocity curve obtained in a simulation by us (Cook and Stark, 1968b) with Robinson's (1964) model.

As a further test of our model, we simulated an important experiment performed by Robinson (1964) wherein the eyeball was held fixed so that an attempted saccade was transformed into an isometric contraction. As shown in Figure 30 our model simulation quite accurately models this abnormal but important experimental behavior. First of all, we use the excellent fit to justify our contention that the topology and logical structure of the model are realistic, and the parameters accurate.

Secondly, we use this prediction of the isometric experiment by the model to assert that during a saccade there is *no* proprioceptive role for receptors in the eye muscles which would tend to provide any kind of feedback control of dynamic form or final position of the saccadic trajectory. Contradicting Vossius (1960), we make this strong assertion because the isometric experiment essentially clamps the system into an open loop configuration with the full target input as the error signal. If, as shown in Figure 30, the model predicts the force program here with the same sequence of controller signals as in making a normal saccadic movement, then clearly no feedback from sensory elements can exist. In addition to this evidence, there is also a minor

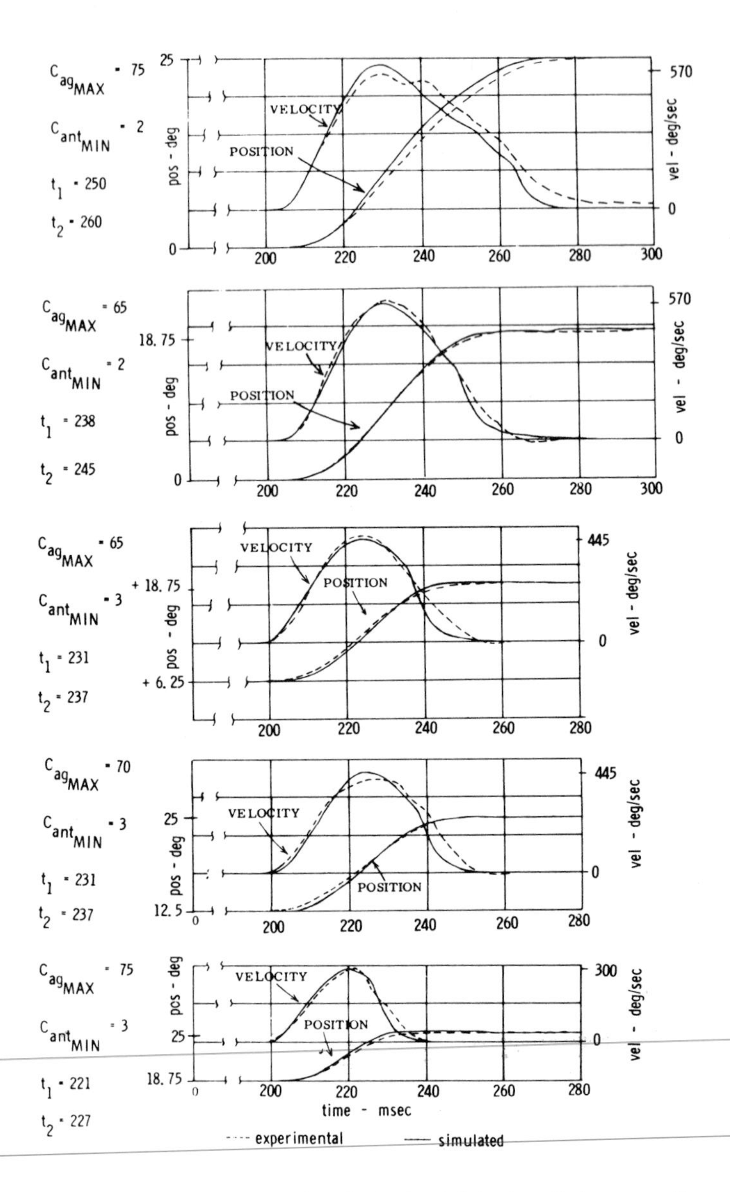

Fig. 28. Comparison of experimental and simulated behavior. Various saccadic eye movements from a different series of experiments. Note amplitude and temporal parameters of controller signals. *(Cook and Stark,* 1965B, 1968B).

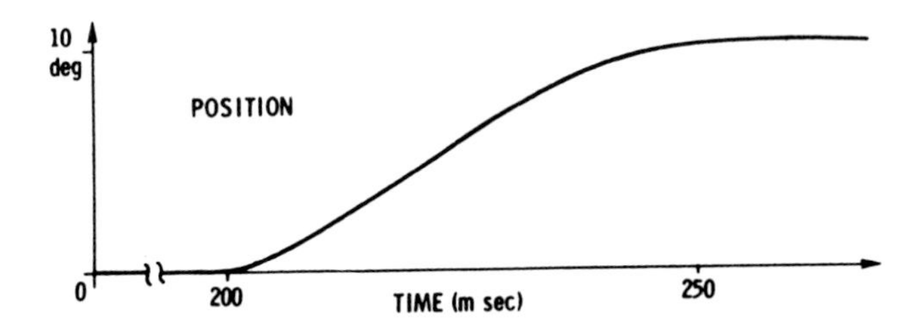

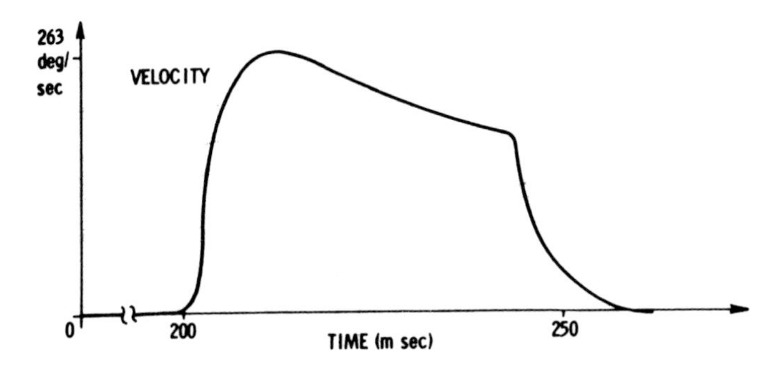

Fig. 29. Abnormal velocity curve in simulations using nonphysiological symmetrical model. This abnormal behavior of an inadequate model reenforces necessity of considering the basic asymmetrical muscle physiology and the important reciprocal innervation characteristics in the modelling of neurological control of saccadic eye movements. *(Cook and Stark,* 1968B)

argument to support the conclusion. The eye movement control system has an elegant and precise sensor, the retina, with which to measure and control versional eye movements. Thus there is no need for a less precise proprioceptor system which, indeed, in competing with the retina, might have adverse influence. Also, consider that the load on the eye muscle system is consistent as opposed to the rapidly changing load configurations for hand or other skeletal movements; the eye is an ideal case to be under open loop control:-the plant is constant and not liable to have disturbing parameter variations. It would be interesting to search under conditions where load does change, as in extreme convergence, and to see whether trajectories alter or whether peripheral compensating mechanisms occur. Further, there are old clinical neurological observations that even with paralysis of an eye muscle and resulting erratic eye movements, the preset frame-of-reference computation corresponding to the preset efferent controlling signal, both driven by the

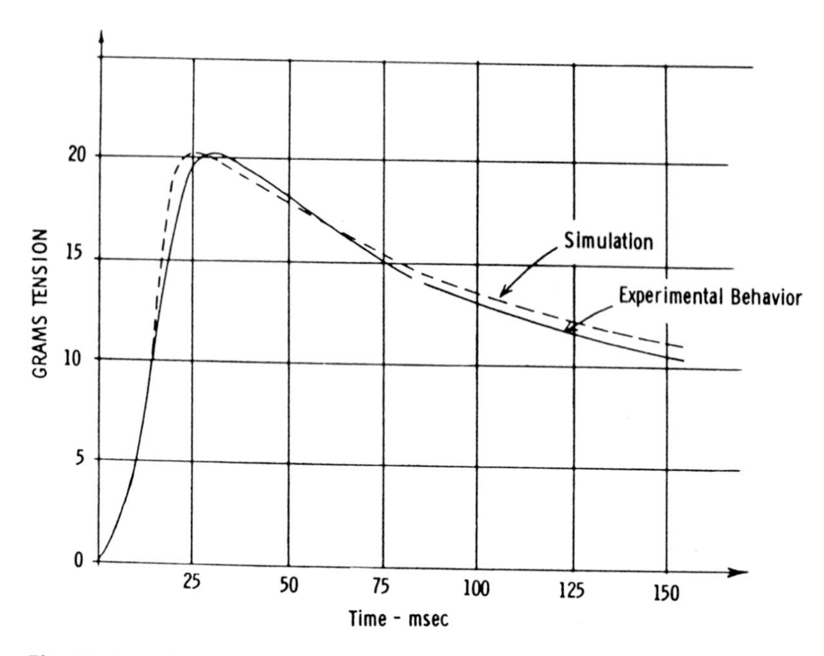

Fig. 30. Isometric eye saccade. Note excellent agreement of simulation to experimental behavior. Function measured in a spring, K=13.5 grams/degree, when eye attempted to execute the saccade from 0 degrees to 6.25 degrees, but was inhibited by the external spring. Experimental curve is based on Robinson. *(Robinson,* 1964; *Cook and Stark,* 1968B).

"saccadic anticipatory signal", continues and, far from being modified by the paralytic process, the world jumps in the opposite direction. Clearly this is an uncompensated-for open loop control malfunction.

What then might be the role of the known proprioceptive sensors? The recent demonstration that they do not act to provide conscious sensation of eye movement is really a straw-man argument since even muscle proprioceptors do not have this function in skeletal movement. It is known, however, that in addition to the ninety percent "local sign" anatomical return of the monosynaptic stretch reflex in skeletal muscle there is a component directed to muscles serving the next-but-one joint (Eccles and Lundberg, 1957). This anatomically provides for coordination of ankle and hip flexes on a primitive "hard-wired" neurological basis. Perhaps the eye muscle proprioceptors so serve head and eye movements, which are important cooperating elements in any visual target tracking task or searching task.

We have noted that these head and eye movements, as shown in Figure 31, are the normal response to wide angle visual target jumps, and although

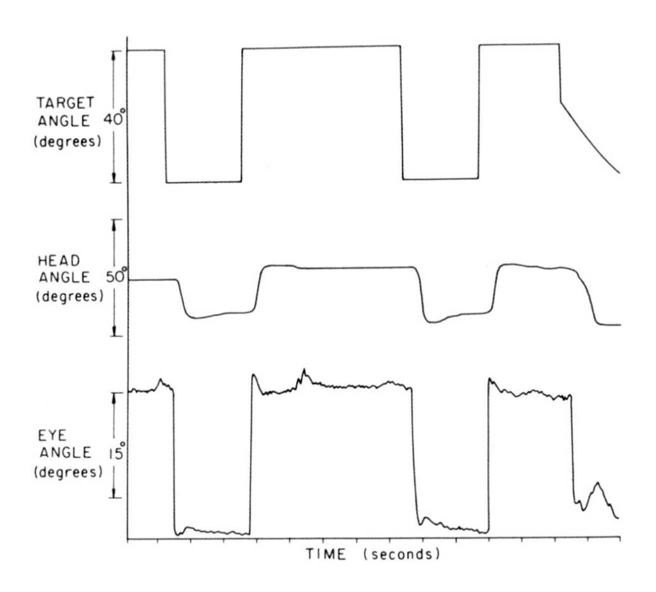

Fig. 31. Head and eye movement. Typical response to a 40° step in target position showing a rapid saccadic eye movement, as well as a concomitant saccadic head angle movement. *(Masek and Stark,* 1963).

the fractional amplitude of either the eye or the head is variable in these movements, their total movement is quite precise. In this way it is possible that the proprioceptive system in eye muscles might help coordinate head movement in a manner similar to the hip-and-ankle reflex coordination. From this point of view, it is interesting that Professor Granit reports that the neck muscles have an extremely high sensory supply of receptors such as spindles. Another possible, but not proven, role of the eye proprioceptors might be in long-term tonic readjustments relating to the head, neck, body and vestibular influences. However, it is clear that on the basis of our model studies of normal saccadic trajectories and the abnormal isometric experiment *no* proprioceptive influence is acting during a saccadic trajectory back onto the controller for eye movement.

Although there are many different types of saccades---fixation micro-saccades only minutes of arc in amplitude, some corrective saccades and staring OKN saccades of the order of one degree, tracking or voluntary saccades ranging up to 30 - 40 degrees---a single pattern of control exists: our model predicts this extremely wide range of open loop movements. Figure 32 shows the non-linear relationship between maximum saccadic velocity and amplitude; all of these widely varying amplitudes fall on the same curve.

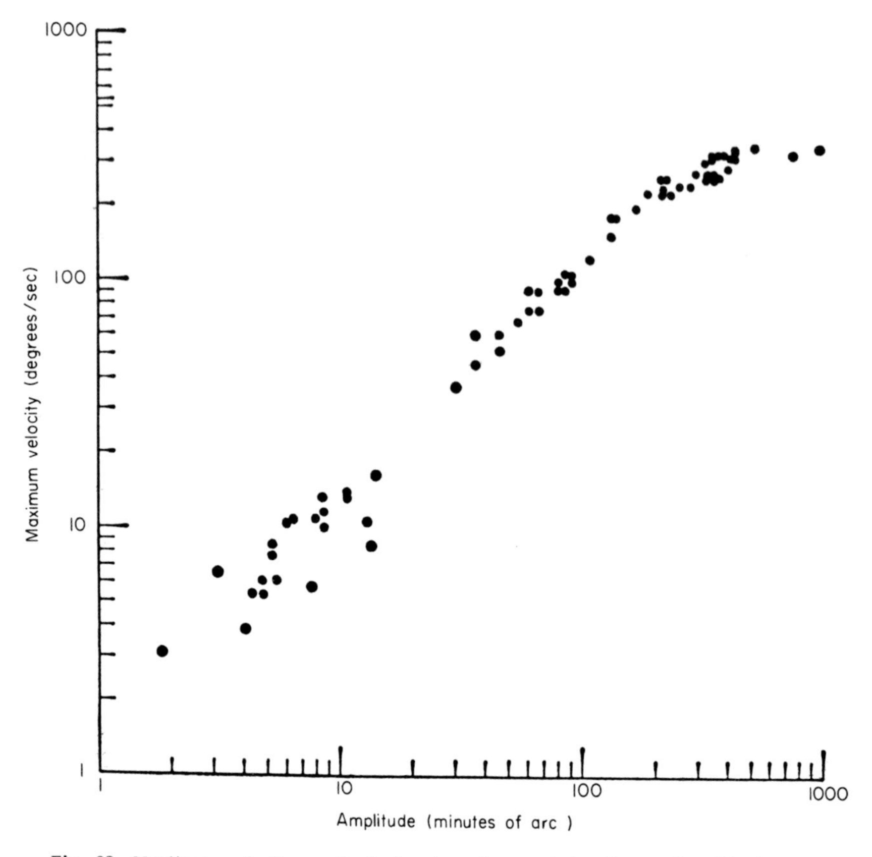

Fig. 32. Nonlinear velocity-amplitude-duration characteristic of saccades. Maximum velocity correlation with amplitude for micro-saccades, corrective saccades, and voluntary saccades over a nearly 1,000 to 1 dynamic range. Duration similarly correlates with amplitude. *(Zuber, Stark and Cook,* 1965).

Animal experiments

During the past few years, Reinhardt and Zuber (1968), Zuber (1968, a&b), Robinson and Fuchs (1969), Collins and his associates and Gauthier and myself have been quantitatively studying the dynamics of eye movements in animals produced by stimulation of appropriate regions in the central nervous system. Although it is agreed that artificial electrical stimulation is unphysiological, still these studies give one an indication of the types of transfer properties between different points in the nervous system and the accompanying plant behavior. Such an experiment (Gauthier and Stark, unpublished) is shown in Figure 33 where both the sixth and the third nerve nuclei are stimulated in the brain stem separately, and also in a special reciprocal stimulation mode, i.e., in coordinated fashion, similar to reciprocal innervation.

Although these studies are in progress, it now seems likely that with careful analysis we will be able to confirm most of the details of the dynamical plant model discussed above. Examples of such quantitative analysis are shown in Figure 34, wherein computer averaged responses as well as Fourier analysis of these time data can be studied.

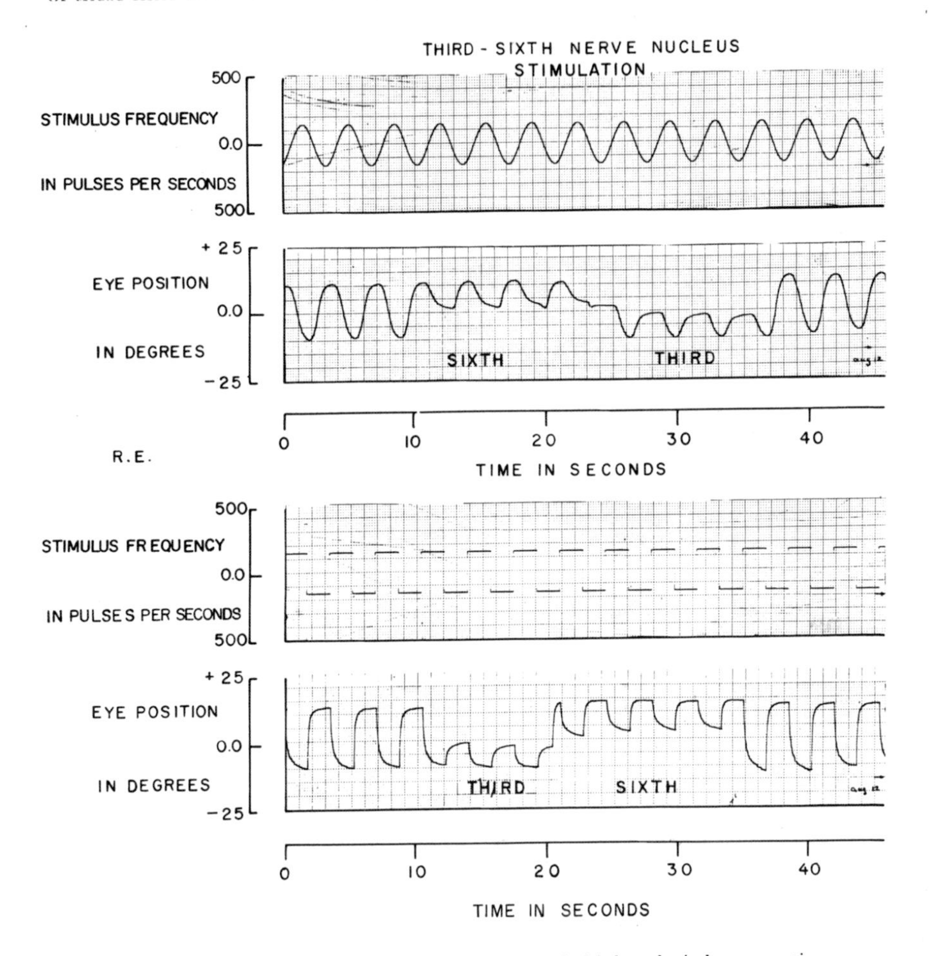

Fig. 33. Dynamic responses of the plant. Example of third and sixth nerve stimulation in anesthetized cat. These time function data indicate importance of "reciprocal stimulation" in obtaining full range of movement, rather smooth sinusoidal form, and linearized responses; shown especially in upper traces. *(Gauthier and Stark,* unpublished experiment).

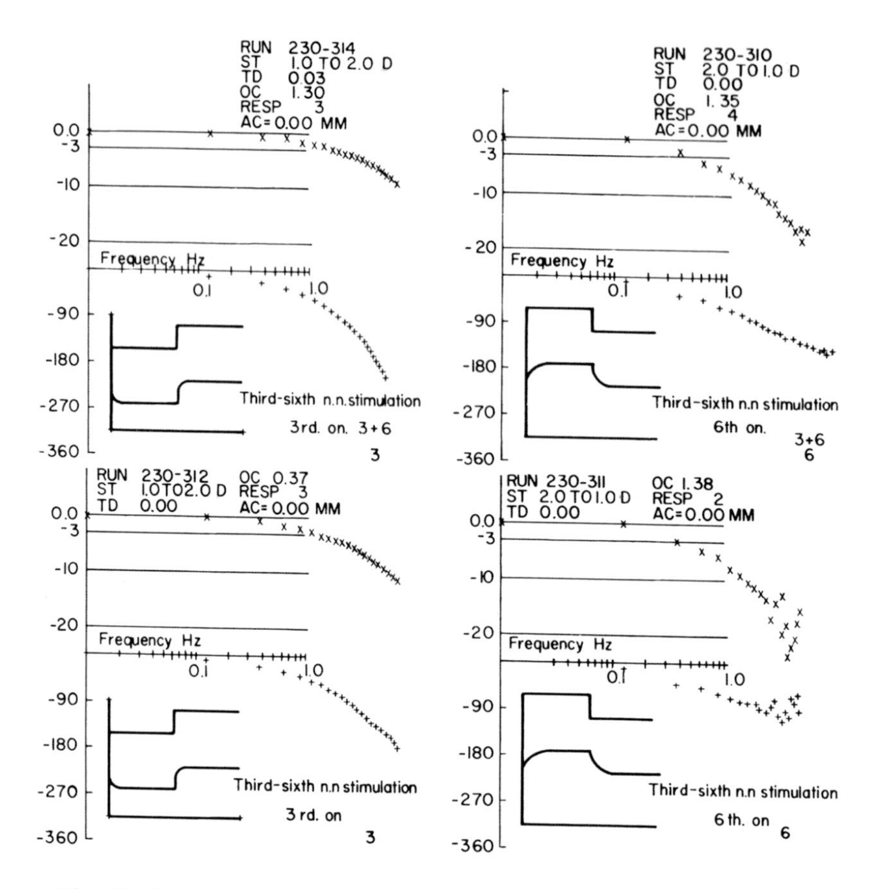

Fig. 34. Frequency responses of the plant. Four averaged time responses for different types of electrically stimulated eye movements in cat. The insets in each figure show the average step response; the full diagrams show the gain and phase functions from the Fourier analysis. Different conditions of stimulation, including amplitude, initial conditions and the reciprocal stimulation mode have their part in changing time constants, attenuation slopes, and phase characteristics of frequency response diagrams. Upper two show reciprocal stimulation, 3rd on -6th off and 6th on -3rd off, respectively; lower two show only agonist stimulation with antagonist unstimulated, 3rd on and 6th on, respectively. *(Gauthier and Stark,* unpublished).

From analysis of these frequency diagrams, it is possible to deduce approximate transfer functions for the linear portions of these movements and, as well, nonlinear changes in parameters as a function of initial conditions, amplitude of movement, and organizational changes of stimulation; by this latter we mean whether or not the stimulus pattern is in the form of "reciprocal stimulation." Although spontaneous tonic activity exists in these preparations, more quantitative interactions of antagonist on agonist dynamics can be produced by artificially stimulated tonic and phasic antagonistic activity. These data can be compared to the detailed piecewise linear approximation to saccadic movements recently reported by us (Zuber, Semmlow and Stark, 1968).

Just as shown in the pupillary system (Smith *et al.*, 1968) recording of single units with respect to eye movement gives additional information, not as troubled by the unphysiological nature of electrical stimulation (Schaefer, 1965; Bizzi, 1968; Wurtz, 1968). Of course, single unit analysis has corresponding difficulties in that the actual sampled neuron may not be representative of the population of neurons driving a particular movement. However, we are pursuing these unit studies in eye movement control which should contribute additional valuable information.

PREDICTION

Eye-hand prediction

The eye movement system has an important adaptive or learning feature, the "prediction operator". This operator was proposed and experimentally defined for the eye by Stark, Vossius and Young (1962) and Dallos and Jones (1963), and similarly for the hand by Stark, Iida and Willis (1961). In these studies prediction was demonstrated in essentially two ways. The first was the increased gain and decreased phase lag found in tracking of single sinusoids, which could be predicted, as compared and contrasted with sequences of superimposed nonharmonically related sinusoids, the pattern of which was too complex to be predicted (even though deterministic and analytical in the mathematical sense). The second was by altered distribution functions of latencies when tracking step changes in target position. These latency distribution histograms were found to depend on whether or not the sequences of step changes in target position were predictable. When the sequences were not predictable, histograms of response times were all positive delays; this delay time can be modelled as a transport delay element in transfer function descriptions of the eye movement system. When the sequences of step changes of target position were regular in time, the eye could predict this time of occurrence of the target step. Thus, these histograms contain both positive and negative response times; further, the distributions were functions of the period of the regular cyclic sequences of target jumps.

Hand movement latencies were found to show similar dependencies of response times and distribution functions of response times on predictable *versus* cyclic regularity of target time (Stark, 1968). The actual latency times are similar, and one question often raised is, how linked are the delayer "computation" times for hand and eye tracking? In experiments wherein simultaneous recordings are made of hand and eye tracking, it is indicated that independent random shifts in latency can occur as well as correlated shifts (Okabe, *et al.*, 1962). Figure 35 is such an experimental analysis which shows how the response times occasionally shift together and occasionally shift in opposite directions when hand and eye movements are simultaneously recorded in a tracking task.

In another experiment shown in Figure 36, either the hand was held steady so that only eye tracking occurred or the eye motion was stopped by slight pressure of a finger on the side of the eyeball. Under these circumstances, hand tracking continued to be quite accurate without eye tracking, thus suggesting that extra-foveal retinal information was sufficient, at least with this set of operating conditions. On the other hand, without hand tracking, eye movement response is much less consistent and accurate; when hand movement starts, rather regular sequences of saccadic eye movements re-occur.

It seems from the above studies (Okabe, *et al.*, 1962; Stark, 1968) that there is an interaction between hand and eye movement which has been exposed but not defined. In any case, it is clear that an important component of the eye-hand tracking system is the behavioral modification produced by the "prediction operator".

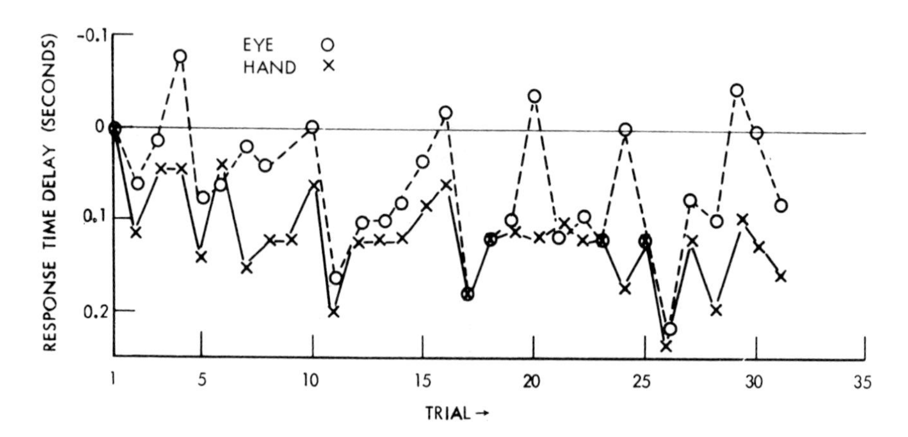

Fig. 35. Hand-eye interaction. Response time-delays for both eye and hand recorded simultaneously; target input square waves of 0.5 cycle/sec. Note both correlations and lack of correlations as a function of sequential order. (*Okabe et al.*, 1962; *Stark*, 1966; *Stark*, 1968).

Pupil and accommodation systems

It is of some interest to note that the pupillary system shows no such prediction operator (Stark, 1968), and for some time it was debatable as to wherein the lens focusing or accommodative system showed such responses (Stark, Takahashi and Zames, 1965). Recently Vandenbrekel, Polse and Stark (unpublished) have obtained data on accommodation and Figure 37 shows changes in distribution of response times which compare with those observed

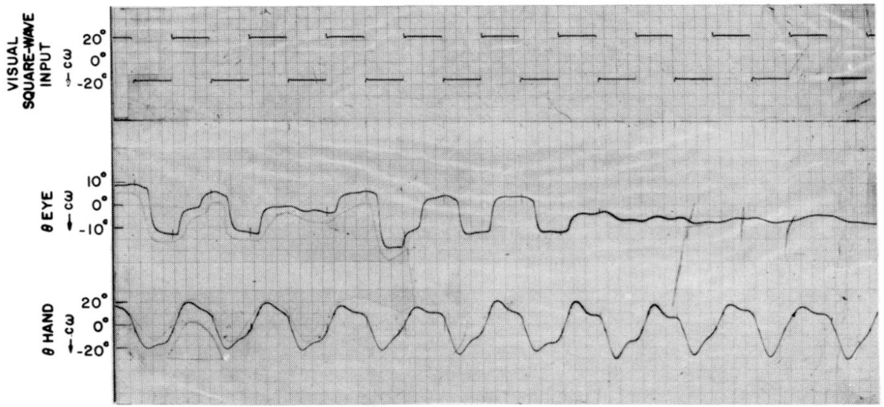

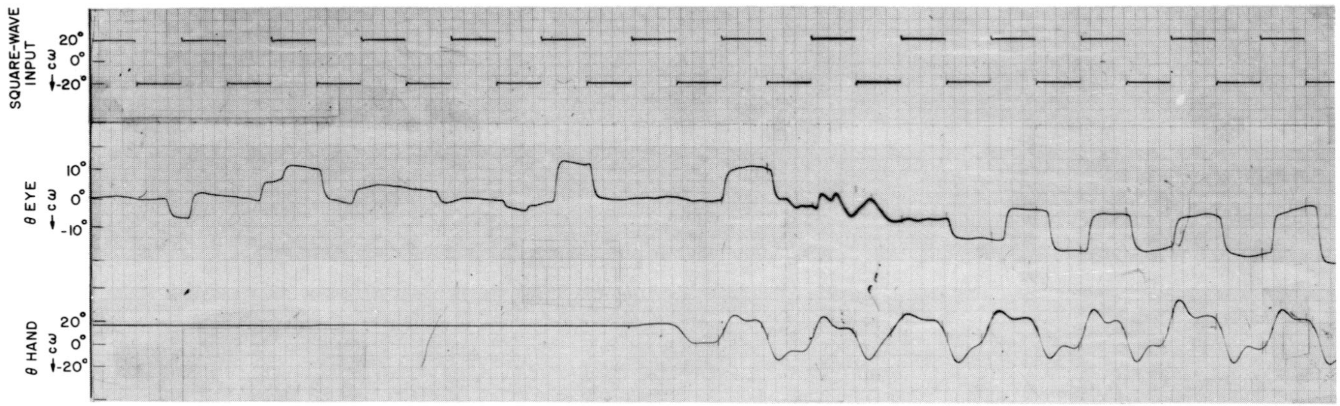

VISUAL SQUARE-WAVE INPUT
cω 20° 0° -20°
θ EYE
cω 10° 0° -10°
θ HAND
cω 20° 0° -20°

SQUARE-WAVE INPUT
cω 20° 0° -20°
θ EYE
cω 10° 0° -10°
θ HAND
cω 20° 0° -20°

Fig. 36. Hand-eye interaction. Time functions of target, eye and hand positions. Above shows eye tracking movement sequences spontaneously halting with no apparent effect on hand tracking; below shows poor or absent eye tracking when hand is still, and market improvement of eye tracking association with hand tracking. (*Okabe et al.*, 1962; *Stark*, 1966; *Stark*, 1968).

in the eye movement versional tracking system. Predictable sequences of step changes in target position (in this case, distance from the subject under monocular viewing conditions) result in a histogram of predictive response times with a mode close to zero delay.

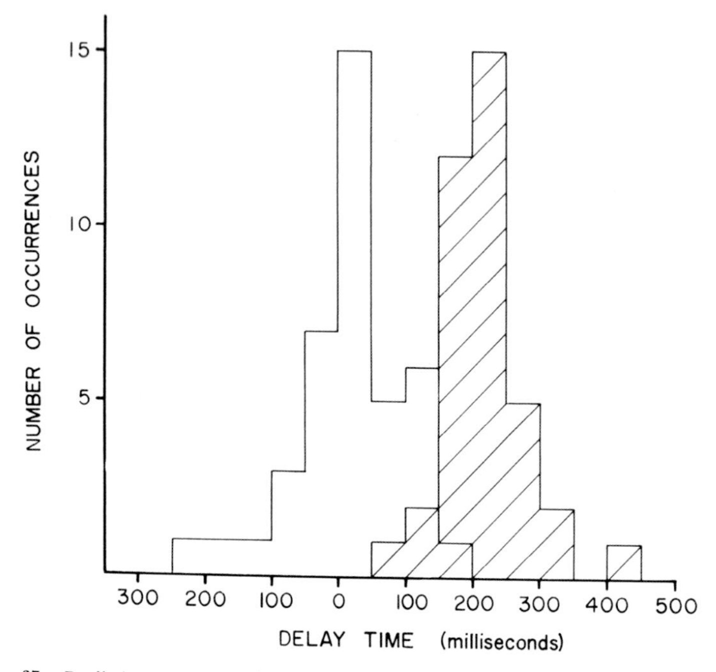

Fig. 37. Prediction operator in accommodation. Two histograms of response time distributions for accommodative human lens system. Note decrease in average delay time and the occurrence of negative delay times indicating anticipatory predictions of regular target movements. *(Vandenbrekel, Polse and Stark,* unpublished data).

Billheimer-Stark conditional probability model

In 1962, Billheimer and I proposed a probabilistic model in the form of a partitioned matrix that could account for the memory dependent pattern in the learning of a periodic predictable wave form. The model can be understood by referring to Figure 38 which defines first the classification of "states" as reaction times which show either no prediction (state A), slight prediction (state B), accurate prediction (state C), slight overprediction (state D), or underprediction. What we seek to have the model do is predict, at least on a statistical basis, the occurrence of these states through a sequence of "stages".

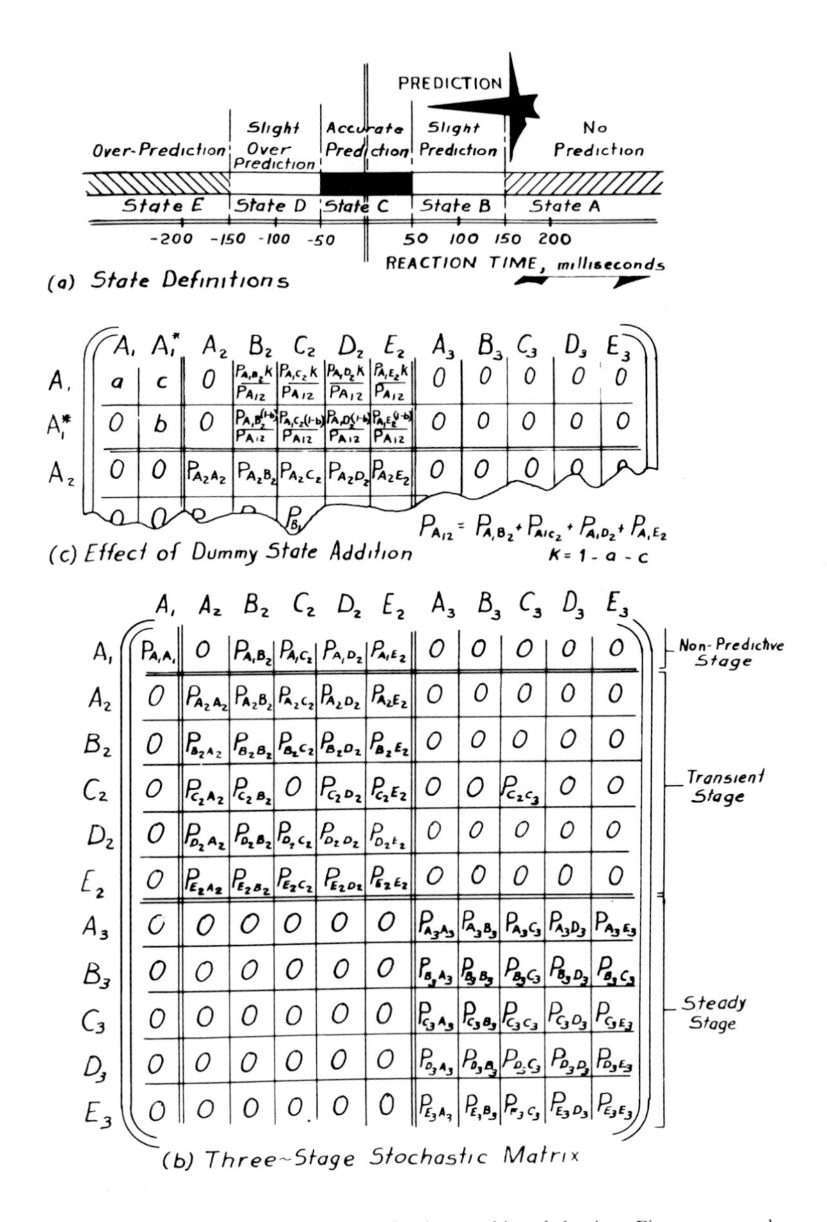

Fig. 38. Markov partitioned model for adaptive tracking behavior. Five states and three stages defined in text. Dummy states are also used to increase variance in accord with experimental findings. (*Billheimer,* unpublished).

These stages are: first, the nonpredictive stage, then a transient stage during which learning is taking place, and finally a steady stage wherein the target motion is being tracked in a predictive fashion. We may define these stages arbitrarily. For example, the transition from stage one to stage two occurs when the empirical data shows the first accurate prediction, $P_{A_1C_2}$. Similarly, stage three, the steady stage, is attained only after two successive accurate predictions, $P_{C_3C_3}$. A further complication of the model was the introduction of dummy or holding states within existing states; this additional degree of freedom enabled the model to predict passage times and also to generate correct variance predictions, which without dummy state transition properties were empirically inaccurate.

An example of the transient tracking behavior of the human hand to regular square waves of target movement is shown in Figure 39. In the upper trace is seen the number of state A responses, with no prediction, in the total sequence of responses studied experimentally. It is seen that the probability of "no prediction" falls rapidly to a very small value. The partitioned and final model responses similarly decrease. In contrast, in the next to bottom trace, state D responses, slight overpredictions, started out with a low probability and finally increased to approximately 0.5 probability of occurrence. These dynamical curves are functions of the frequency of the regular target motion, of the particular subject and his experience, and of the system being studied.

We may compare the eye movement system with hand movement prediction characteristics generated for the same frequency of target input, shown in Figures 40 and 41 respectively. For example, if we look at the upper trace in each figure, the dynamics of the probability of state A or no-prediction responses, we see that the probability only reduces to 0.5 for eye movements, whereas it reduces to 0.2 for hand movements. Another important point of difference is the peaks in slight prediction and slight overprediction found early in the hand movement, Figure 41, but not seen at all in eye movements, Figure 40.

The series of experiments done by Billheimer and Stark (unpublished) on the hand, and by Masek and Stark (1964) on the eye and the hand, support the ability of the partitioning techniques in Markov conditional probability models to provide a mathematical framework capable of supporting the analysis of such adaptive behavioral traits as the prediction operator. These are, of course, black box models: the intricate mechanisms of the neural networks underlying these phenomena will possibly be an exciting field of experimental and theoretical endeavor in the, hopefully, not too distant future. A different and independently developed black box model for similar purposes is now being studied by Professor Fender at Cal Tech and it may be that comparison of these different models will lead to new experimental studies which will further develop the field. Of interest in this connection is the reported absence of predicted eye movements in monkeys in the elegant work of Professor Fuchs (1967, a and b), now at the University of Washington in Seattle. Are monkeys less able to utilize their brains to develop prediction operators, or are they somehow less motivated than are human subjects striving for their doctoral degrees!?

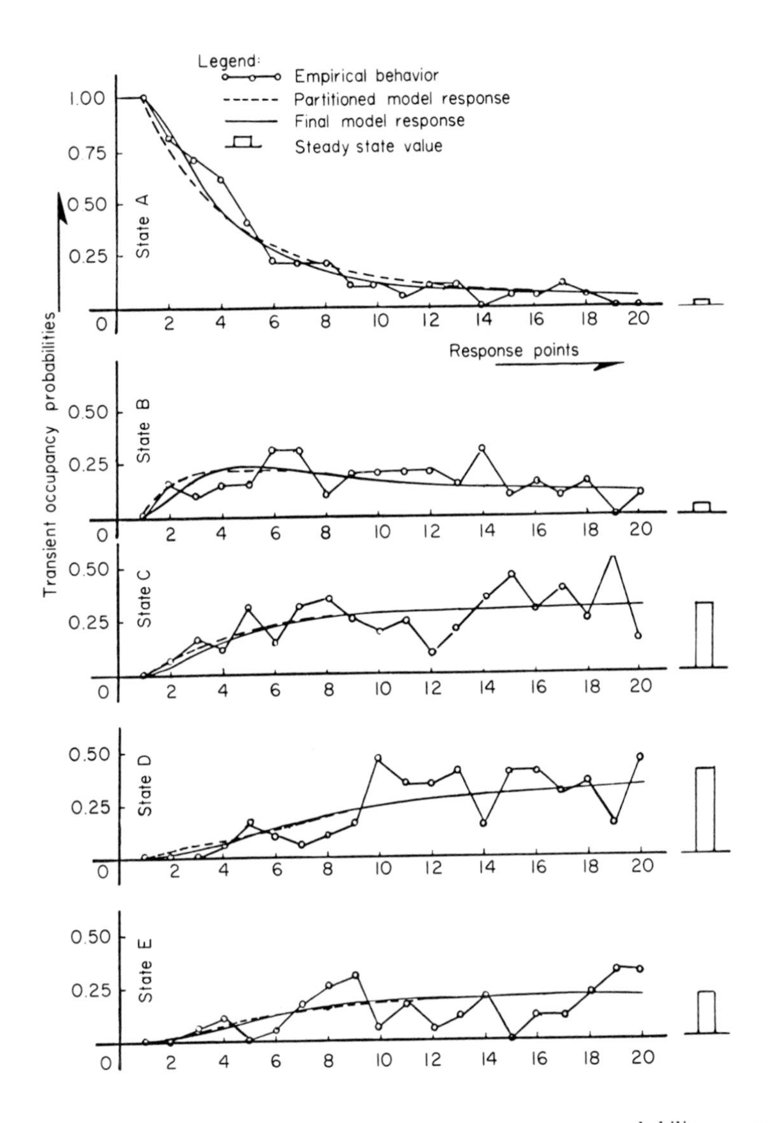

Fig. 39. Adaptive tracking behavior. Shows transient occupancy probability curves for each of five response-time states for empirical behavior, and as calculated from partioned-matrix Markov model; steady-state, or third stage, values shown on right; square wave target at 0.6 Hz. *(Billheimer,* unpublished).

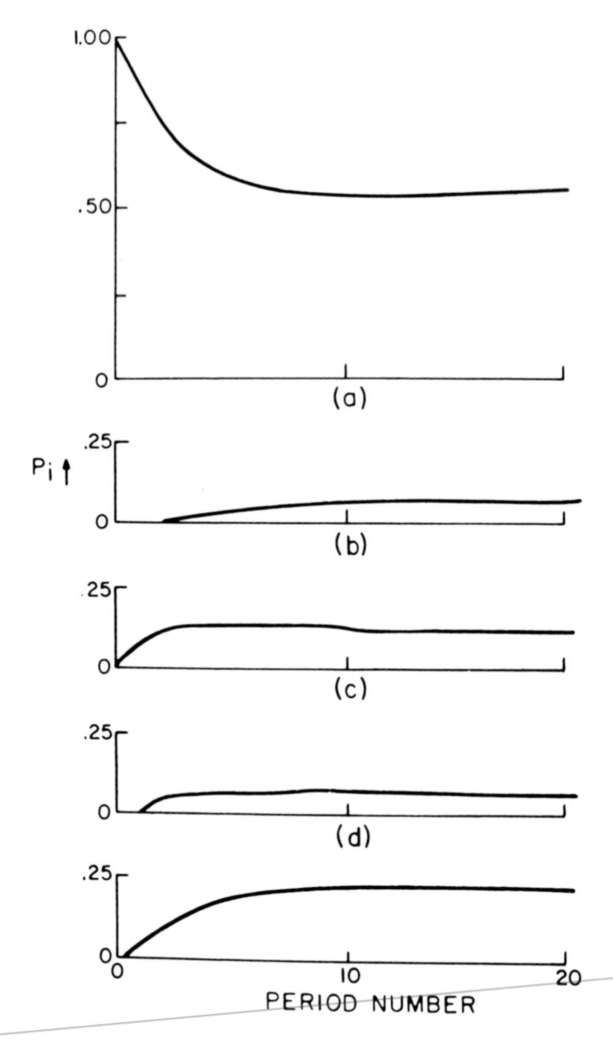

Fig. 40. Adaptive tracking behavior. Eye tracking 0.5 Hz square waves. Computer derived transient state-occupancy probability curves from empirical data and partitioned matrix model. (*Masek and Stark*, 1964).

Pattern recognition of pictures—the "eigen scan path"

With the ability to measure both horizontal and vertical eye movements, discussed in an earlier section, David Noton and I have embarked upon a study of eye movements which occur during normal viewing, such as looking at pictures. A number of artificial conditions have been adhered to in order to

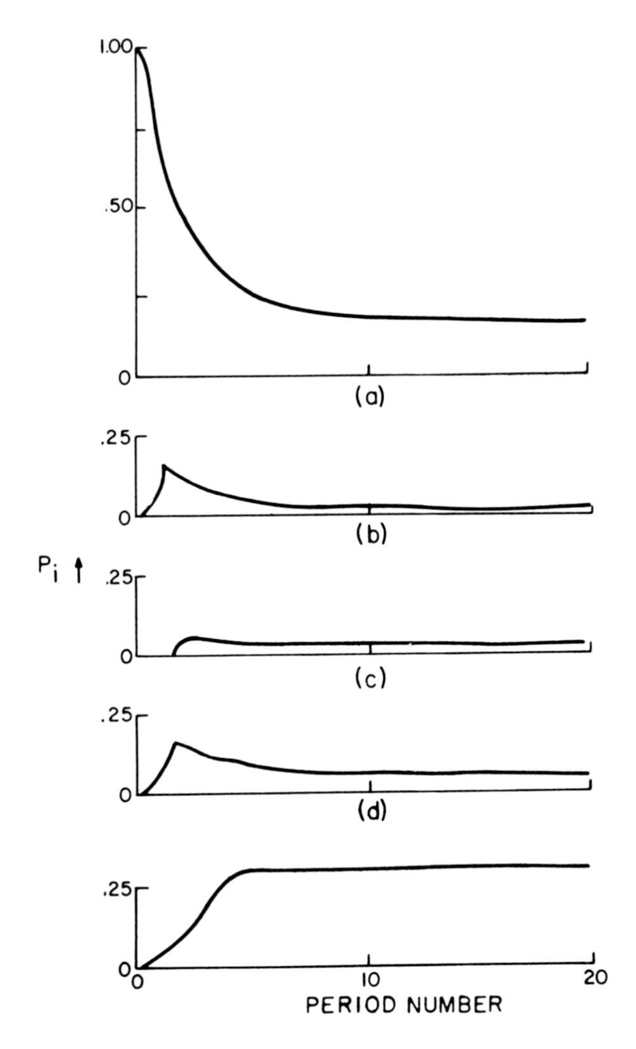

Fig. 41. Adaptive tracking behavior. Hand tracking 0.5 Hz square waves. Computer derived transient state-occupancy probability curve. (*Masek and Stark*, 1964).

provoke a rich experimental situation. The outline figures cover a wide visual field and are drawn with fixed density outlines. A random sequencing slide projector aids us in conveniently presenting the subject with a wide variety of such pictures. The illuminating light is so reduced that eye movements are required to position the fovea over this wide visual field in order to search, identify and recognize the picture. The recordings of the subject's eye

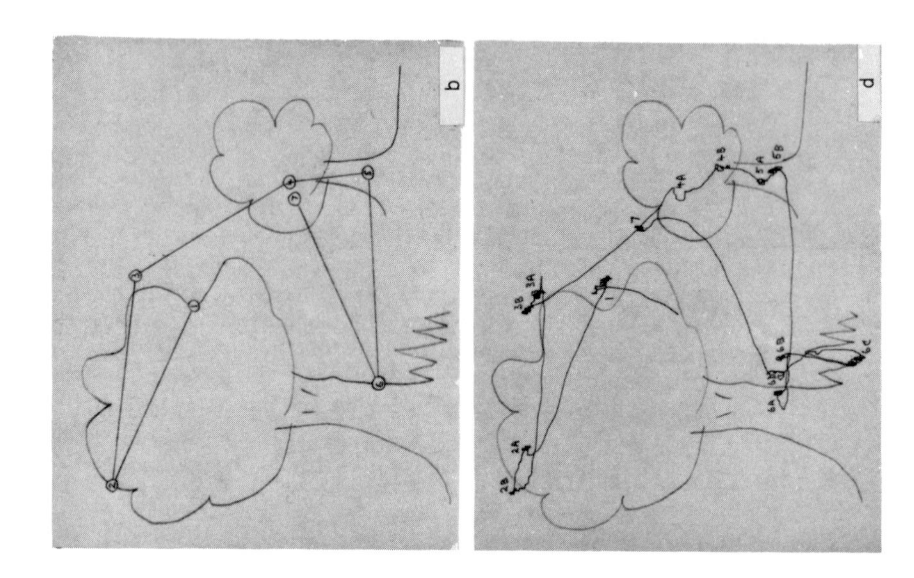
b
d

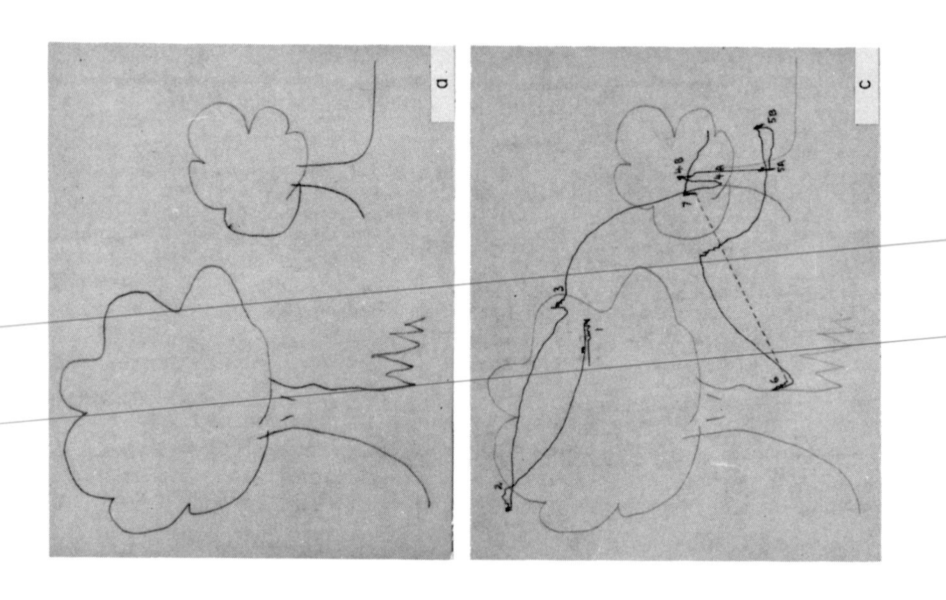
a
c

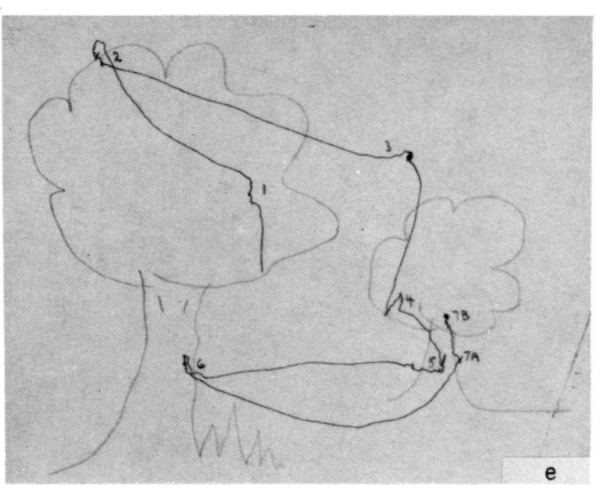

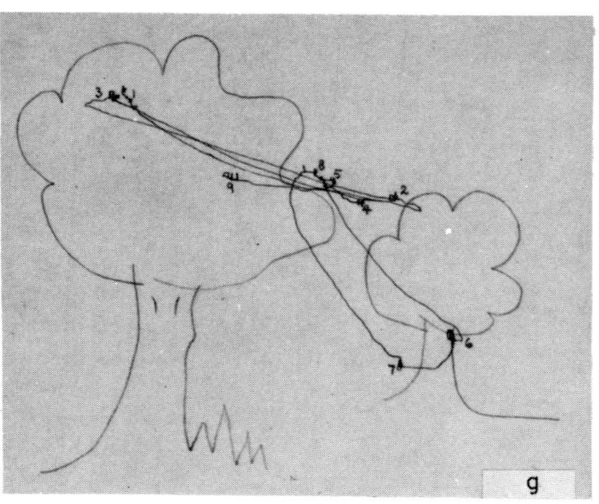

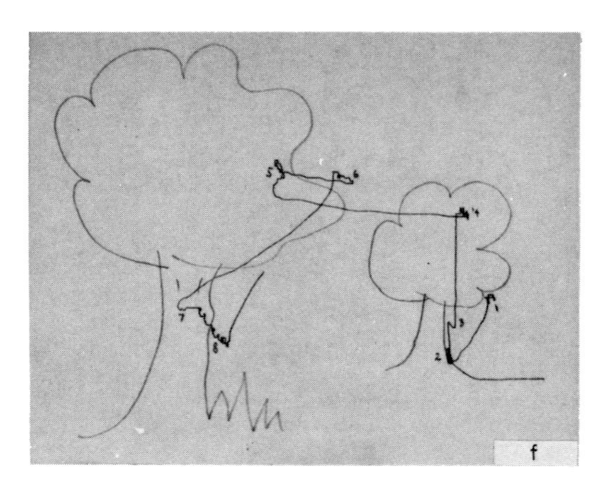

Fig. 42. Eye movement "eigen scan paths". (A) Original line drawing picture shown to the subject for 75 seconds; (B) idealized model "eigen scan path"; (C, D, & E) three of the five occurrences of "eigen scan path" showing minor modifications and deviations from mode. (F & G) are two examples of highly variable and non-characteristic paths which occur approximately seventy percent of viewing time. Note in (C) dashed line represents a hypothetical saccadic trajectory which was obscured by an eye blink measurement artifact. Note also curvilinear nature of saccadic trajectories which indicate that the eyeball is rotated by non-synchronous eye muscle contractions. *(Noton and Stark,* unpublished).

movements are stored on an on-line digital computer, played back in slow motion, and plotted on reproductions of the pattern which he viewed. In this way the pattern of successive objects of regard is explicitly available for study.

What has been discovered is that a characteristic path of sequential saccadic movements occurs for a repetitively significant percentage of the viewing time. This "eigen scan path" is fixed for a particular subject and a particular picture, though it is certainly a function of many operating conditions we have not yet explored. As can be seen in Figure 42, the sequential "eigen scan path" occurs frequently enough and characteristically enough to be identifiable although, of course, minor modifications produce a random distribution about the modal path. In addition to the three examples of the "eigen scan path" shown in the figure, we have also illustrated for the reader's convenience the picture and the idealized "eigen scan path" for the particular subject. In addition, the two bottom figures illustrate sequences of saccadic movements which do not fall into the characteristic scan path pattern; these occur approximately 75% of the viewing time so that they are clearly not inconsequential or insignificant aspects.

The earlier work of Yarbus (1967) showing patterns of saccadic eye movement while viewing pictures demonstrated consistency for a given subject, and explored variations produced by instructions to the subject. These support Yarbus' contention that eye movements reflect aspects of thought processes. Noton's study extends the work of Yarbus by attending to the *temporal* characteristic of the saccadic eye movement sequences; Noton's theory relates these "eigen scan paths" to a sequential theory of pattern recognition which has as its model a computer algorithm for searching, identifying and recognizing patterns or pictures (Noton, 1969 and 1970).

DISCUSSION

The versional eye system has many appealing characteristics: the rapid saccadic trajectory, operating over a dynamic range of 1,000 to 1, which suggests some sophisticated control driving the plant; the intermittent saccadic system showing clearly that computational delays are the limiting dynamic feature in sequential movement; the interactions between the position and velocity in the dual-control mode; and the prediction phenomena and other tactical aspects of the system, such as the "eigen scan paths" found when searching pictures and extracting information. In order to approach these aspects of the control of versional eye movements, we have put forth the Young-Stark sampled data model, the Cook-Stark dynamical model for the saccadic trajectory, and applied the Billheimer-Stark predictive matrix to sequences generated by the prediction operator during adaptive tracking.

The discussion will turn briefly to other neurological control systems and then discourse on modelling in general. Versional eye movements, as presented in this review lead to a need for neuronal models such as the McCulloch-Pitts neural network.

Neurological control systems

Neurological control systems fall into two major groups:

(i) The regulators, of which the pupil is a classical example, are generally continuous and without prediction operators. Many of their essential design characteristics lie in their nonlinear features, such as strong scale-compressions or saturations, and important asymmetries not eliminated by small signal approaches. They are often multi-input systems, present high levels of noise, and "biological" adaptation is commonly found.

(ii) The eye/hand tracking systems have intermittent or refractory period characteristics enabling them to be represented by discrete or sampled-data models. They show prediction operators giving them input adaptive properties, and are otherwise fairly linear with low noise levels.

Just as in the engineering analysis of the eye-movement system, we have put forth a number of model and quantitative descriptions for various members of these two classes, starting with the linear pupil model in 1957 (Stark and Sherman, 1957) which was shortly followed by a nonlinear (Stark, 1959) and a nonlinear stochastic model (Stanten and Stark, 1966, and Sandberg and Stark, 1965). Very similar were the nonlinear models for accommodation (Stark, Takahashi and Zames, 1965); and accommodative vergence (Brodkey and Stark, 1967); and quantitative frequency responses for fusional vergence (Zuber and Stark, 1968).

Hand tracking developed in a somewhat different direction with a quantitative frequency response description (Stark, Iida, and Willis, 1961); a linear model of the proprioceptive response in man with Houk, Atwood and Willis (Stark, 1966, 1968); a sampled-data model in 1963 (Navas and Stark, 1963, 1968); and a Markov partitioned model for predictive sequences and their adaptation (Billheimer, 1962; Masek and Stark, 1964).

It is clear, in my opinion, that the development of a model is a crucial feature in the scientific approach to any system and in particular to these complex biological control systems.

Modelling

Models are simplifications and can never be, nor are desired to be, complete matches for the richness of the experimental phenomena. As McCulloch has explained, the McCulloch-Pitts formal neuron was "poverty stricken" when compared to the richness of neuronal features as seen in the brain; but in this very characteristic of simplicity lies its power.

Models are helpful in many ways. They make *explicit* our assumptions regarding the characterization of a system; they unify and summarize much experimental data, both of the black box behaviorist type and of the anatomical-physiological reductionist type. Often this latter aspect generates a logical structure or topology of the model, which is a most essential and critical feature.

Simulation enables us to become familiar with many aspects of the model behavior. It *tests* mutual consistency of observations and enables us to unify our concepts as to common underlying mechanisms of diverse behaviors. With a model and its active simulation, we can make predictions and suggest new experiments. Then, with this new observational data that the model has helped us generate, we can be led to a new model that is either closer to this increased body of knowledge or is more economical and concise in its formulation.

Models are tools and in one sense can be readily used up and discarded. In another sense, they are "more real" than the observational data or sensory experience of the so-called real world.

Models are hard to develop. Both in the past at MIT and at the University of Illinois at Chicago Circle and at the present time at Berkeley, many experimental studies have been performed and are in progress, which in part supported the previous formulation of a model and in part exposed weaknesses of a model, especially by revealing areas of behavior not covered. This interaction between experiment and modelling is perhaps characteristic of the present day style of scientific research.

Kuhn in his "Structure of Scientific Revolutions" (1962) has described scientific activity on a large scale; what is lacking in his treatment is any attempt to portray the intellectual activity of the scientist on the small scale of year-to-year. Are not,on the one hand, the *formulation* of a new model (here read law or hypothesis as equivalent to model) and, on the other hand, the performance of *experiments* (i) to enrich the detailed confirmation of the model, (ii) to reveal nonpredicted areas of behavior, or (iii) to accumulate clearly unsatisfactory aspects of a model related to his radical emergence of *scientific theory as revolutions* and to his conduct of *normal science,* respectively?

The difference is one of scale. A new model requires a change of paradigm experiments, a change of attributed priorities of underlying mechanisms, a change in vocabulary with which one talks about behavior. It then sets the stage for effective and fruitful experimentation into old and new areas. This very productivity, at first, supports the acceptance of the new model, and later, in the more mature or even senescent phase of the model, enables the accumulation of relationships unsatisfactorily ordered or treated by the model. This then in turn provokes renewed efforts to generate a revolutionary (on a small scale) new model formulation.

Versional Eye Movements

In this brief review of mainly versional eye movements, I have tried to show how the ideas of modern control theory have enabled us to develop behavioral models which treat different aspects of the eye-movement control system. These are, of course, both inter-related and non-unique.

The *dual mode controller* for position and velocity was shown to be present over a variety of types of eye movements and to contain variations and interactions which provide many clues to further experiments. Next the discrete or sampled-data operator raises important questions concerning the basic elements underlying these control mechanisms, in particular, the nature and location of *intermittency* in neurological terms, and the relationship of this computational refractory period to the flow of information, to the saccadic anticipatory signal, and to saccadic suppression. The considerations of the *trajectory* of saccadic movement led us to a model dependent upon certain fundamental characteristics of the contractile mechanism of muscle; and also into considerations of the suboptimal trajectory as an indication of a 'computationally bound' (Stark, 1968) system, requiring multi-level distribution of control algorithms, such as the prediction operator discussed later. The trajectory also was studied by means of neurophysiological experiments, which again points us in the direction of dissecting into the black box and defining the neurophysiological elements. Lastly, the *prediction* operator and the characteristic scan path in pattern recognition brought us well beyond the present state of modern control theory in that we were able to demonstrate and define phenomena for which we have inadequate mathematical tools, or alternatively, where our mathematical tools are merely descriptive and whet our appetitie for more fundamental knowledge.

Neuronal model of McCulloch and Pitts

Finally, I would like to present as a last figure, Figure 43, a synaptic and neuronal model for the control of versional eye movements proposed by Pitts and McCulloch in 1947.

McCulloch was a great pioneer in neurophysiology, the first to look at the central nervous system as an information processing machine, as in the article "How we know universals: the perception of auditory and visual forms" from whence this figure comes. He was interested in proving that neuronal mechanisms of a simple sort, the Pitts-McMulloch formal neurons, when combined in networks, again simpler than brain networks, were able to compute universals for pattern recognition or for controller signals for eye movements. In many ways we must go back to Descartes whose "systems" concepts of the reflex and of reciprocal innervation in a way began the physiology of the central nervous system. It is fitting to note, in this conference, that Descartes used the same horizontal versional eye movement system illustrated in McCulloch's figure and which we have been discussing in our conference today as his exemplary system with which to demonstrate the operation of reciprocal innervation.

In any case, this figure of Pitts and McCulloch is a clear arrow for students of eye movements to follow. While we continue to describe behavior, we must also focus our attention on the neurophysiological mechanisms underlying the various control functions that modern engineering control theory enables us to define.

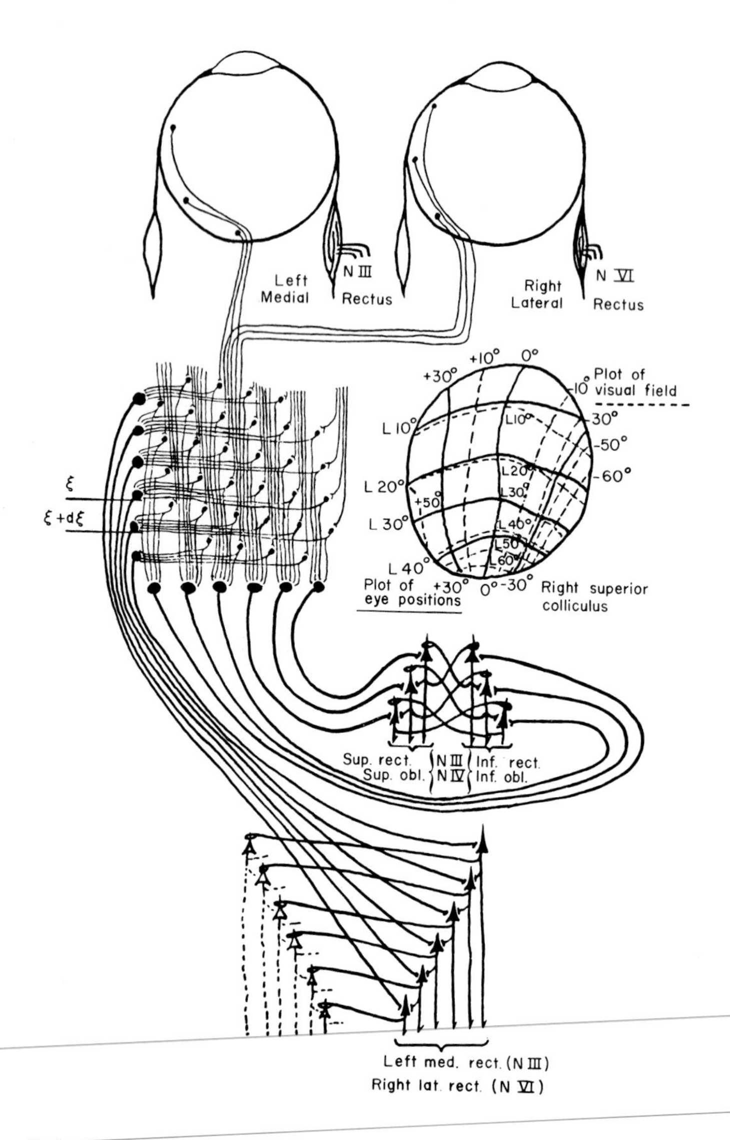

Fig. 43. Early neural model for eye movement control. Diagram showing flow of visual information from retina, through superior colliculus and final common pathway neurons in brain stem, and thence to horizontal eye muscles. Neurons are McCulloch-Pitts formal neurons which, when in proper networks, are capable of computing logical control functions and also of recognizing universals. *(Pitts and McCulloch,* 1947).

CONCLUSION

The Young-Stark model for dual-mode intermittent control, and the Cook-Stark model for reciprocal innervation control of plant dynamics, still represent a considerable compression of the available observational data. The principle new experimental evidence not included by them are continuous features of the pursuit system and the human length-tension characteristics, respectively.

Definitive mathematical modelling has not yet been applied to higher level phenomena of prediction nor to the saccadic anticipatory signal with its frame-of-reference computation and suppression, nor to tactics of saccadic scanning for picture viewing. These and other interactions of versions with visual processes and with eye and hand motor systems are clearly sufficiently complex that satisfactory resolution of important problems may require the development of neuronal level models or new control theoretic insights, or both.

REFERENCES

AGNIEL, R.G., and JURY, E.I. (1969). Stability of nonlinear randomly sampled systems. Presented at Allerton Conference, University of Illinois.

BILLHEIMER, J.W. (1962). *A Markov Analysis of Adaptive Tracking Behavior.* EE Thesis, Mass. Inst. Tech.

BIZZI, E. (1968). Discharge of frontal eye field neurons during saccades and following eye movements in unanesthetized monkeys. *Exptl. Brain Res.* **6,** 69-80.

BRODKEY, J. and STARK, L. (1967). Accommodative convergence: an adaptive nonlinear control system. *IEEE Transactions on Systems Science and Cybernetics,* **SSC-3,** 121-133.

BRODKEY, J.S., and STARK, L. (1968). New direct evidence against intermittency or sampling in human smooth pursuit eye movements. *Nature* **218,** 273-275.

CARLSON, F.D. (1959). Kinematic studies on mechanical properties. **In:** *Tissue Elasticity,* J.W. Remington, ed., Washington, D.C., *Am. Physiol. Soc.,* pp. 55-72.

CHILDRESS, D.S. and JONES, R.W. (1967). Mechanics of horizontal movement of the human eye. *J. Physiol.* (Lond.). **188,**273-284.

COOK, G. and STARK, L. (1965a). Dynamics of human horizontal eye-movement mechanism. *Quart. Prog. Rept., Res. Lab. Electr.* M.I.T. **76,** 343-352.

COOK, G. and STARK, L. (1965b). Human horizontal eye-movement mechanism. *Quart. Prog. Rept., Res. Lab. Electr.,* M.I.T. **77,** 402-412.

COOK, G. and STARK, L. (1966). Dynamics of the saccadic eye movement mechanism. *Proc. Symposium on Biomedical Engineering* **1,** 356-359, Milwaukee.

COOK, G. and STARK, L. (1967). Derivation of a model for the human eye-positioning mechanism. *Bull. Math. Biophys.* **29,** 153-174.

COOK, G., and STARK, L. (1968a). Dynamic behavior of human eye-positioning mechanism. *Communications in Behavioral Biology* **1,** 197,204.

COOK, G. and STARK, L. (1968b). The human eye-movement mechanism: experiments, modeling and model testing. *A.M.A. Arch. Ophthal.* **79,** 428-436.

COOK, G., STARK, L., and ZUBER, B.B. (1966). Horizontal eye movements studied with the on-line computer. *A.M.A. Arch. Ophthal.* **76,** 589-595.

Cornsweet, T.N. (1958). Determination of the stimuli for involuntary drifts and saccadic eye movements. *J. Opt. Soc. Am.* **48,** 808.

Dallos, P.J. and Jones, R.W. (1963). Learning behavior of the eye fixation control system. *IEEE Trans. Automatic Control* **AC-8,** 218-227.

Dodge, R. and Cline, T.S. (1901). The angle velocity of eye movements. *Psychol. Rev.* **8,** 145-157.

Eccles, J.C., Eccles, R.M. and Lundberg, A. (1957). Convergence of monosynaptic excitatory afferents onto many different species of alpha motoneurons. *J. Physiol.* (Lond.), **137,** 22-50.

Fenn, W.O. (1923). A quantitative comparison between the energy liberated and the work performed by the isolated sartorius muscle of the frog. *J. Physiol.* (Lond.). **58,** 173-203.

Fenn, W.W., and Marsh, B.S. (1935). Muscular force at different speeds of shortening. *J. Physiol.* **85,** 277.

Foster, J.D. (1968). A stochastic revised sampled data model for eye tracking. *Man Vehicle Control Laboratory Report,* M.V.T.-68-2, pp. 1-133, Mass. Inst. Tech.

Fuchs, A.F. (1967a). Saccadic and smooth pursuit eye movements in the monkey. *J. Physiol.* (Lond.) **191,** 609-631.

Fuchs, A.F. (1967b). Periodic eye tracking in the monkey. *J. Physiol.* (Lond.). **193,** 161-171.

Hill, A.V. (1938). The heat of shortening and the dynamic constants of muscle. *Proc. Roy. Soc.* (Lond). **B126,** 136.

Horrocks, A., and Stark, L. (1964). Experiments on error as a function of response time in horizontal eye movements. *Quart. Prog. Rept., Research Laboratory of Electronics,* M.I.T. **72,** 267-269.

Katz, B. (1939). The relation between force and speed in muscular contraction. *J. Physiol.* (Lond). **96,** 45.

Kuhn, T.S. (1962). *The Structure of Scientific Revolutions.* University of Chicago Press. Chicago.

Latour, P.L. (1962). Visual thresholds during eye movements. *Vision Research* **2,** 261-262.

Lorber, M., Zuber, B.L. and Stark, L. (1965). Suppression of the pupillary light reflex in binocular rivalry and saccadic suppression. *Nature* **208,** 558-560.

Masek, G. and Stark, L. (1963). Head movements. *Quart. Prog. Rept., Res. Lab. Electr.* M.I.T. **70,** 348-351.

Masek, G. and Stark, L. (1964). Markov modelling technique for predictable visual-motor tracking. *Quart. Prog. Rept., Res. Lab. Electr.* M.I.T. **75,** 180-190.

Merrill, E.G., and Stark, L. (1963a). Optokinetic nystagmus: double stripe experiment. *Quart. Prog. Rept., Res. Lab. Electr.* M.I.T. **70,** 357-359.

Merrill, E.G., and Stark, L. (1963b). Smooth phase of optokinetic nystagmus in man. *Quart. Prog. Rept., Res. Lab. Electr. M.I.T.* **71,** 286-291.

Merrill, E.G., and Stark, L. (1964). Optokinetic nystagmus in man: the step experiment. *Quart. Prog. Rept., Res. Lab. Electr,* M.I.T. **72,** 269-272.

Michael, J. and Ichinose, L. (1969). Effects of organization activity upon visual data processing in the LGB. *Proc. Third Internat. Biophysics Congress,* Cambridge, Mass. p. 258.

Michael, J.A. and Stark, L. (1966). Interactions between eye movements and visually evoked responses in cat, *E.E.G. Clin. Neurophysiol.* **21,** 487-488.

Michael, J.A. and Stark, L. (1967). Electrophysiological correlates of saccadic suppression. *Exptl. Neurol.* **17,** 233-246.

Murthy, D.N.P. and Deekshatulu, B.L. (1967). A new model for the control mechanism of the human eye. *Internat. J. Control* **6,** 263-274.

Nachmias, J. (1959). Two-dimensional motion of the retinal image during monocular fixation. *J. Opt. Soc. Am.* **49,** 901-908.

Navas. F. and Stark, L. (1963). Experiments on discrete control of hand movement. *Quart. Prog. Rept., Res. Lab. Electr.* M.I.T. **69,** 256-259.

NAVAS, F. and STARK, L. (1968). Sampling of intermittency in the hand control system. *Biophys. J.* **8,** 252-302.

NELSON, G.P. and STARK, L. (1962). Optokinetic nystagmus in man. *Quart. Prog. Rept., Res. Lab. Electr.* M.I.T. **66,** 366-369.

NOTON, D. (1969). A proposal for serial, archetype-directed pattern recognition. Record of the 1969 IEEE Systems Science and Cybernetics Conference, Philadelphia.

NOTON, D. (1970). A theory of visual pattern perception. Submitted to *IEEE Trans. on SS&C.*

OKABE, Y., RHODES, H.E., STARK, L. and WILLIS, P.A. (1962). Simultaneous eye and hand tracking. *Quart. Prog. Rept., Res. Lab. Electr.* M.I.T. **66,** 395-401.

PITTS, W. and MCCULLOCH, W. (1947). How we know universals: the perception of auditory and visual forms. *Bull. Math. Biophysics.* **7,** 127-147

RASHBASS, C. (1961). The relationship between saccadic and smooth tracking eye movements. *J. Physiol.* (Lond). **159,** 326-338.

REINHARDT, R. and ZUBER, B.L. (1968). Control of eye position by the lateral rectus muscle in the cat. 21st Ann. Conf. on Engineering in Med. & Biol., Houston, Texas.

ROBINSON, D.A. (1964). The mechanics of human saccadic eye movement. *J. Physiol.* (Lond). **174,** 245-264.

Robinson, D.A. (1965). The mechanics of human smooth pursuit eye movement. *J. Physiol.* (Lond). **180,** 569-591.

ROBINSON, D. and FUCHS, A. (1969). Eye movements evoked by stimulation of frontal eye fields. *J. Neurophysiol.* **32,** 637-649.

ROBINSON, D.A., O'MEARA, D.M., SCOTT, A.B., and COLLINS, C.C. (1969). Mechanical components of human eye movements. *J. Applied Physiology,* **26,** 1-6.

ST. CYR, G. and FENDER, D. (1969). Interplay of drifts and flicks in binocular fixation. *Vision Research* **9,** 245-265.

SANDBERG, A. and STARK, L. (1968). Wiener G-function analysis as an approach to non-linear characteristics of human pupil light reflex. *Brain Research* **11,** 194-211.

SCHAEFER, K. (1965). Die Erregungsmuster einzelner Neurone des Abducenskernes beim Kaninchen. *Pflug. Arch.* **284,** 31-52.

SMITH, J.D., ICHINOSE, L.Y., MASEK, G.A., WATANABE, T. and STARK,L. (1968). Midbrain single units correlating with pupil response to light. *Science* **162,** 1302-1303.

STANTEN, S.F. and STARK, L. (1966). A statistical analysis of pupil noise. *IEEE Trans. on Biomedical Engineering.* **BME-13,** 140-152.

STARK, L. (1959). Stability, oscillations and noise in the human pupil servomechanism. *Proc. Inst. Radio Engineers,* **IRE 47,** 1925-1939.

STARK, L. (1966). Neurological feedback control systems. **In:** *Advances in Bioengineering and Instrumentation,* Ch. 4. Ed Fred Alt, Plenum Press, New York, p. 289-385.

STARK, L. (1968). *Neurological Control Systems: Studies in Bioengineering.* Plenum Press, New York.

STARK, L., IIDA, M. and WILLIS, P.A. (1961). Dynamic characteristics of the motor co-ordination system in man. *Biophys. J.* **1,** 279-300.

STARK, L., KUPFER, C. and YOUNG, L.R. (1965;. Physiology of the visual control system. *NASA Contractor Report* **CR-238,** 1-88.

STARK, L., MICHAEL, J. and ZUBER, B.L. (1969). Saccadic suppression: a product of the saccadic anticipatory signal. Proc. Carnegie Conf. on *The Concept of Attention in Neurophysiology,* Butterworths, London, pp. 281-391.

STARK, L. and SHERMAN P.M. (1957). A servoanalytic study of consensual pupil reflex to light. *J. Neurophysiol.* **20,** 17-26.

STARK, L. TAKAHASHI, Y. and ZAMES, G. (1965). Nonlinear servoanalysis of human lens accommodation. *IEEE Transactions on Systems Science and Cybernetics,* **SSC-1,** 75-83.

STARK, L., VOSSIUS., and YOUNG, L.R. (1962). Predictive control of eye tracking movements. *Institute of Radio Engineers Transactions on Human Factors in Electronics,* **HFE-3,** 52-57.

STRASZAK, A. (1969). On the synthesis of multi-level large scale control systems. *IFAC,* Warsaw, **28,** 48-58.

TAMLER, E., MARG, E., JAMPOLSKY, A. and NAWRATZKI, I. (1959). Electromyography of human saccadic eye movements. *A.M.A. Arch. Ophthalmol.* **62,** 657-661.

TELFORD, C.O. (1931). The refractory phase of voluntary and associative responses. *Exptl. Psychol.* **14,** 1.

THOMAS, J.G. (1967). The torque-angle transfer function of the human eye. *Kybernetik,* **3,** 254-263.

VOLKMANN, F.C. (1962). Vision during voluntary saccadic eye movements. *J. Opt. Soc. Am.* **52,** 571-578.

VOSSIUS, G. (1960). Das System der Augenbewegung (I). *Z. Biol.* **112,** 27-57.

VOSSIUS, G. (1961). Die Regelbewegung des Auges. **In:** *Aufnahme und Verarbeitung von Nachrichten durch Organismen.* Editor VDE, Stuttgart, 149-157.

WESTHEIMER, G. (1954a). Mechanism of saccadic eye movements. *A.M.A. Arch. Ophthal.* **52,** 710-724.

WESTHEIMER, G. (1954b). Eye movement responses to a horizontally moving visual stimulus. *A.M.A. Arch. Ophthal.* **52,** 932-941.

WURTZ, R. (1968). Visual cortex neurons: response to stimuli during rapid eye movements. *Science,* **162,** 1148-1150.

YARBUS, A.L. (1967). *Eye Movements and Vision.* Plenum Press: New York.

YOUNG, L.R., and STARK, L. (1962a). A sampled data model for eye tracking movements. *Quart. Prog. Rept., Research Laboratory for Electronics,* **M.I.T. 66,** 370-383.

YOUNG, L.R. and STARK, L. (1962b). Dependence of accuracy of eye movements on prediction. *Quart. Prog. Rept., Res. Lab. Electr.* **M.I.T. 67,** 212-214.

YOUNG, L.R. and STARK, L. (1963a). A discrete model for eye tracking movements. *IEEE Transactions on Military Electronics* **MIL-7,** 113-115.

YOUNG, L.R. and STARK, L. (1963b). Variable feedback experiments testing a sampled data model for eye tracking movements. *IEEE Transactions for Human Factors in Electronics* **HFE-4,** 38-51.

ZUBER, B.L. (1968). Sinusoidal eye movements from brain stem stimulation in the cat. *Vision Research,* **8,** 1073-1079.

ZUBER, B.L. (1968). Eye movement dynamics in cat: the final motor pathway. *Expt. Neurol.* **20,** 255-260.

ZUBER, B.L., SEMMLOW, J.L. and STARK, L. (1968). Frequency characteristics of the saccadic eye movement. *Biophys. J.* **8,** 1288-1298.

ZUBER, B.L. and STARK, L. (1966). Saccadic suppression: elevation of visual threshold associated with saccadic eye movements. *Exptl. Neurol.* **16,** 65-79.

ZUBER, B.L. and STARK, L. (1968). Dynamical characteristics of the fusional vergence eye-movement system. *IEEE Transactions Systems Science and Cybernetics,* **SSC-4,** 72-79.

ZUBER, B.L., STARK, L. and COOK, M. (1965). Microsaccades and the velocity-amplitude relationship for saccadic eye movement. *Science* **150,** 1459-1460.

ZUBER, B.L., STARK, L., LORBER, M. (1966). Saccadic suppression of the pupillary light reflex. *Exptl. Neurol.* **14,** 351-370.

PURSUIT EYE TRACKING MOVEMENTS

LAURENCE R. YOUNG

A simplistic view of the human eye tracking system recognizes two major modes of tracking: rapid saccadic eye movements and smooth pursuit movements, and assigns complementary functions to them. The saccadic eye movement system supposedly acts to maintain the image of the object of interest on the fovea by a sequence of discrete high velocity jumps. The smooth pursuit system has been assigned the role of stabilization of retinal images, or more particularly matching the angular velocity of the eye to the velocity of the object. This view has led to the development of models by several groups, including the author and his colleagues, which treat the saccadic system as a velocity servomechanism (Fender and Nye, 1961; Young, 1962; Dallos and Jones, 1963). These models have been useful in predicting the response of the eye movement system to a variety of target patterns in a general manner. They have further stimulated experiments which show their shortcomings in detail in a number of ways. This paper deals not with models but with features of the pursuit eye movement system which are known at present and especially with those characteristics which are still uncertain. It will be seen that the pursuit system is not a simple, linear velocity servo based on retinal error velocity.

INPUTS TO THE EYE MOVEMENT SYSTEM

Eye movement records have been examined for tracking a variety of slowly moving targets, including ramps, step ramps, parabolas and pseudo random motion (Rashbass, 1961; Young, 1962; Robinson, 1965). Pursuit eye movements clearly tend to rotate the eye at a velocity approximating that of the target, up to eye velocities of approximately 25 to 30 deg/sec. Since target velocity is a signal which is not directly available, it can only be recreated by the eye movement system on the basis of the sum of eye velocity and retinal slip velocity. At target speeds below 10 deg/sec there appears to be no measurable average steady state difference between target velocity and eye velocity.

Supported by Grants NGL 22-009-025 and NGR 22-009-156 from the National Aeronautics and Space Administration, and by Air Force Contract F33615-69-C-1425.

This precludes the notion of a "type zero" velocity servo system unless it had extraordinarily high gain from retinal slip velocity to change in eye velocity. However, because of the presence of a large pursuit delay, this high gain is not possible for reasons of loop stability.

Avoiding the vexing question of how the velocity error signal is developed and processed, we must ask the next question, what visual signal is being nulled or controlled by the pursuit system? For the laboratory experiments upon which almost all of the models for eye movement have been developed, the target is usually a single, simple, small, discrete object moving against a homogeneous background. There is no question as to what the target is or what the target velocity represents. In a more natural setting, however, and presumably one for which the pursuit eye movement system has evolved, we view moving targets against a rich visual background.

When pursuit eye movements enable the eye to follow an animal running across a field, the image of the animal is relatively stationary on the fovea, whereas the rich image of the background is moving on the retina in both fovea and periphery at a velocity equal and opposite to eye velocity. Why does this visual error rate not produce pursuit eye movements of its own? Similarly, in the case of optokinetic nystagmus, in which pursuit-like smooth eye movements are produced in tracking elements of the background, it is known that a single stationary fixation point is sufficient to greatly diminish or perhaps eliminate this nystagmus. What then is the portion of the visual field which must be stabilized, and how does volition enter the pursuit eye movement input selection?

The size of the moving visual field, as well as its velocity, influences the smooth eye movement response. For visual angles less than about forty degrees the optokinetic nystagmus velocity is reduced, with constant field speed, as the visual angle is reduced (Byford, 1969). Once again, the matter of selectivity and differing requirements for image stabilization on different portions of the retina is raised.

A further complication in specifying the input to the pursuit eye movement system arises in the case of eye movements occurring with free head movements (Sanders, 1963). It is well known that smooth compensatory eye movements can be initiated by vestibular stimulation when the head is turned. These eye movements appear to have the same characteristics as pursuit eye movements in general (not including their reaction time). They tend to stabilize the retinal image of a target which is fixed in the external visual field (Young, 1969). Similarly, smooth compensatory eye movements are generated by neck torsion, especially at low frequencies, presumably through the action of proprioceptors in the neck. Meiry deals separately with these kinds of eye movements resulting from vestibular and proprioceptive stimuli (Meiry, 1969). It is clear that they all form part of a complex multiple-input, single-output command to the smooth eye movement system.

Yet another input to the smooth eye movement system is the little known phenomenon of self-generated smooth eye movements, in the absence of a continuous moving visual signal. Westheimer and Conover (1954) and more recently Steinbach (1968) have demonstrated that some subjects can move their eyes smoothly without a smooth moving target. Such observations suggest that the eye movement system may receive input from a function generator internal to the brain, as well as responding to externally generated signals. Supporting this possibility are experiments by Steinbach and Held (1968). They show that pursuit eye movements can be produced with greatly reduced phase lag and fewer saccades when a subject attempts to follow the active motion of his own hand, in comparison with pure visual tracking of a passively moved arm. The effects of temporal and dynamic as well as spatial transformations on this phenomenon are currently being investigated.

The popularly held view of the pursuit eye movement system being concerned only with velocity information is open to question. At least two kinds of observations indicate that the smooth eye movement system is influenced by the position of the moving target on the retina as well as its velocity. Johnson (1963), and later Robinson (1965) show that in a number of cases targets moving roughly 20 deg/sec are tracked utilizing position error correction that seems to be accomplished entirely by the pursuit system rather than through small saccades. Typically, when the eye is following a constant velocity target and lagging behind it, it will be seen to begin moving at a higher velocity than the target in order to close the positional error gap, and then resume the appropriate constant velocity. The other evidence for consideration of the error as well as the error rate inputs to the smooth pursuit system comes from examination of the corrective nature of slow drifts. It may be argued that slow drifts, falling into the category known as "miniature eye movements," are not properly part of the smooth pursuit mechanism. However, there is no clear dividing line in terms of eye velocity between slow pursuit movements and drift. Yarbus (1967) analyzed his records of fixation drift speed and reported that it varied from zero to approximately 30 minutes of arc/sec, with a mean drift velocity of approximately 6 minutes of arc/sec. However, he also showed a clear example of smooth pursuit interspersed with saccadic correction when tracking an object moving horizontally at a speed of only 5 minutes of arc/sec. Thus, although drift may be considered as "noise" in the smooth pursuit system, it does not appear easily distinguishable from pursuit as a separate mechanism. Most investigators found that for fixation eye movements the drift in the two eyes is essentially independent and random, with microsaccades or flicks performing the role of recentering the image on the fovea. However, recent careful measurements by St. Cyr and Fender (1969a) show that drifts are also corrective in nature, and thus this part of the smooth pursuit system, if it is to be considered, is also responsive to positional error. Furthermore, in cases of ocular motor apraxia, the patient uses smooth pursuit movements to augment inadequate saccades in shifting fixation between stationary points (Cogan, 1952; Young, 1962).

Finally, in considering input to the smooth pursuit eye movement system, one must recognize the strong influence of predictability of object motion. Stark, Vossius and Young (1962) and Dallos and Jones (1963) showed the clear difference between total eye movement tracking of smooth sinusoids and sinusoids which were a component of a pseudo-random motion. The predictability of the signal apparently permits both the pursuit and saccadic systems to reduce the phase lag attributable to their inherent reaction time. It was later shown by Michael and Jones (1966) that there is a continuum of predictability of signals and the effect on eye movement phase lag depends upon the degree of predictability, or the narrowness of the bandwidth of the input spectrum, with wide-band signals and single sinusoids representing the two extremes. Thus it is no surprise that St. Cyr and Fender (1969 b, 1970) observe different frequency response characteristics for the eye movement system depending upon the center frequency and bandwidth of the test spectrum used. Our close examination of tracking records reveals an apparent attempt by the pursuit eye movement system to predict future motion of the target, at least over a period of 100 to 300 milli-seconds ahead. This future motion may be a prediction of many different kinds. Our early model assumed that it was merely a first order extrapolation (assumed target velocity) on the one hand or full pattern prediction, as in the case of phase locked tracking of a sine wave (Young, 1962). Even with a relatively predictable signal, however, the pursuit eye movement system seems to show characteristics of extrapolation which use a variety of information available visually as well as other cues available about future target velocity. This kind of information may of course be increased by other modalities such as vestibular, proprioceptive, or efferent command associated with body movements.

One general pattern of input predictability is for the oculomotor system to track a single sinusoid or narrow-band signal with higher gain than for the same frequency in a wide-band signal. There is also a tendency to track the higher frequency portions of a narrow-band signal with higher gain, a phenomenon explored by St. Cyr and Fender (1969b) and by Watanabe and Yoshida (1969). This lack of stationarity, in which the frequency response is dependent upon the input signal, clearly shows that a single linear model for the system is inadequate. However, the notion of an input-adaptive system has been successfully used in describing other biological systems, and seems applicable to the oculomotor system. The input-adaptive characteristics of the pursuit system are only known in very general terms, i.e. decreased phase lag and high frequency emphasis. Further exploration of the characteristics of an object's motion which lead to predictive tracking seems warranted. Interestingly enough, Fuchs showed that these predictive characteristics are absent in the eye movement system of the monkey which otherwise closely resembles the human system. Care must be taken not to confuse the effects of the well known system nonlinearities (saccadic foveal-dead-zone and pursuit saturation) with true input adaptation. This is especially true when dealing with small motions (less than 1 degree) and high velocity signals, exceeding 30 deg/sec.

Childress (1967) demonstrated that retinal slip of a target is, in itself, not a sufficient stimulus for pursuit tracking. By mechanically releasing the eye from a deviated position, a fixation point image moved slowly across the retina, without inducing correcting pursuit movement.

To summarize the matter of inputs to the pursuit eye movement system, it would appear that pursuit movements result from a single command that integrates information from many sources in order to move the eye at an angular velocity which will minimize the retinal slip and reduce the offset of the image of an interesting object. It must be able to achieve this command either when the eye is stationary and the retinal slip is large or when the eye is moving and retinal slip is small or possibly nil.

PURSUIT EYE MOVEMENT CONTROL CHARACTERISTICS

It is difficult at best to describe quantitatively how a control system works when, as discussed above, it is not known what the system is trying to do. Nevertheless, some characteristics of the pursuit eye movement system in tracking relatively non-predictable simple targets in a homogeneous field with fixed head position have been elucidated and are reviewed in this section.

The first of these characteristics is a delay time in the pursuit loop between the beginning of smooth motion of a visual target and the initiation of a smooth eye tracking movement. This latency has a mean value estimated by Robinson (1965) as 125 milliseconds and by Young, Forster and Van Houtte (1968) as 134 milliseconds. In the absence of a facilitating saccade, to be discussed below, the pursuit eye movement accelerates slowly to its final eye position. Robinson estimates the duration of movement for a 10 deg/sec smooth pursuit response as 133 milliseconds. Young, Forster and Van Houtte account for the smooth changes in pursuit velocity with two dynamic elements in their model for pursuit movements (see Appendix 2).

Variable feedback experiments have been useful in assessing the validity of models developed to describe closed loop behavior. Some portion of the eye movement is added to the target motion to vary the feedback from its normal value of unity. The response of the saccadic eye movement system under variable feedback experiments has been explored at length (Fender and Nye, 1961; Young and Stark, 1963; Robinson, 1965; Fuchs, 1967a,b). The stability of a pursuit system having the dynamic characteristics for normal closed loop tracking mentioned above, can be explored for positive feedback and for increased negative feedback. Clearly the positive feedback system (external feedback greater than unity) will diverge exponentially. One interesting test is the prediction of the lowest frequency of oscillation of a system subjected to increased negative feedback. For the 134 msec delay and the dynamics of the Young *et al.* model, discussed in Appendix 2, the open loop phase lag reaches 180° at 17 rad/sec (2.7 Hz). This is in close agreement with Robinson's (1965) experimental finding that the smooth pursuit system oscillates under excess negative feedback of 3 at a mean frequency of 2.89 Hz. Obviously, as the loop gain is increased further, the frequency of oscillation would be expected to increase. Thus, as Robinson increased the additional external gain to 7 to insure pursuit oscillations, the frequency increased to 3.3 Hz. The value of total negative feedback required for this simple model to oscillate (assuming a geometric feedback of unity normally) is only 2.2. Robinson finds that negative feedback of eight is required to insure sustained pursuit oscillations. However, he points out that total feedback gains of two, four, or six produce oscillations which wax and wane. This is entirely consistent with the notion of a feedback system which breaks into oscillation, detects the periodic oscillations by the prediction capability of the smooth pursuit system, and in turn decreases the effective time delay and causes these oscillations to damp out. Watanabe and Yoshida's (1969) findings support this argument. At a frequency of 3 Hz, pursuit tracking of a single sinusoid lags the input by only 60-80 degrees.

An important characteristic of any biological control system is its forward loop gain - in this case the ratio of pursuit eye velocity to error velocity sensed at the retina. Retinal slip velocity is usually not explicitly measured in the tracking experiments. A plot of eye velocity vs. the difference between target velocity and eye velocity at each test frequency would yield a forward loop frequency response, but it would be very inaccurate as a result of the computation involving small differences between large numbers.

Two techniques have been applied to determining the forward loop gain characteristics of the eye movement control system: opening the loop optically with a normal mobile eye, and using a moving stimulus to an immobilized eye. Young (1962) measured a number of forward loop responses of the pursuit system using an external feedback gain of +1 to cancel the inherent negative feedback. Low frequency estimates of pursuit forward loop gain were obtained from the ratio of eye pursuit velocity to error velocity for input ramps of 5 deg/sec, and for single sinusoids of different frequencies and a complex sum of sinusoids. Examples of typical responses to single sinusoids under these "open loop" conditions are shown in Figure 1 and the frequency responses for variable feedback tracking of pseudo-random signals at different values of total loop gain are shown in Figure 2. All these estimates indicate a low frequency forward loop gain of 2-4 (at frequencies in the vicinity of 0.4 Hz), and a marked drop in gain with frequency, decreasing at slightly more than 6 decibels per octave.

The second method uses a moving target or moving stripe pattern to an immobilized eye (so that the error velocity sensed on the retina is precisely the target velocity) and measures the angular velocity of the other (mobile) eye, which has no vision. The ratio of mobile eye velocity to stripe velocity yields forward loop pursuit gain and avoids the nonlinearity associated with large eye movements, as well as the methodological problems of the earlier technique. Collewijn (1969) thus found an effective forward loop gain of 100. Robinson (1969) points out how this high gain could be made compatible with the Young *et al.* (1968) model via an internal high gain loop cancelling the external feedback, but the modeling concept is on weak ground. The situation concerning foward loop gain may be considerably different for humans, however. Feldman, Atkin and Bender (1969) measured induced mobile eye velocity when vision was through the immobile eye of patients. They found induced slow phase velocities of 20-70 deg/sec for stripe velocities of 10-40 deg/sec. These ratios are considerably closer to the low frequency forward loop gains determined by Young.

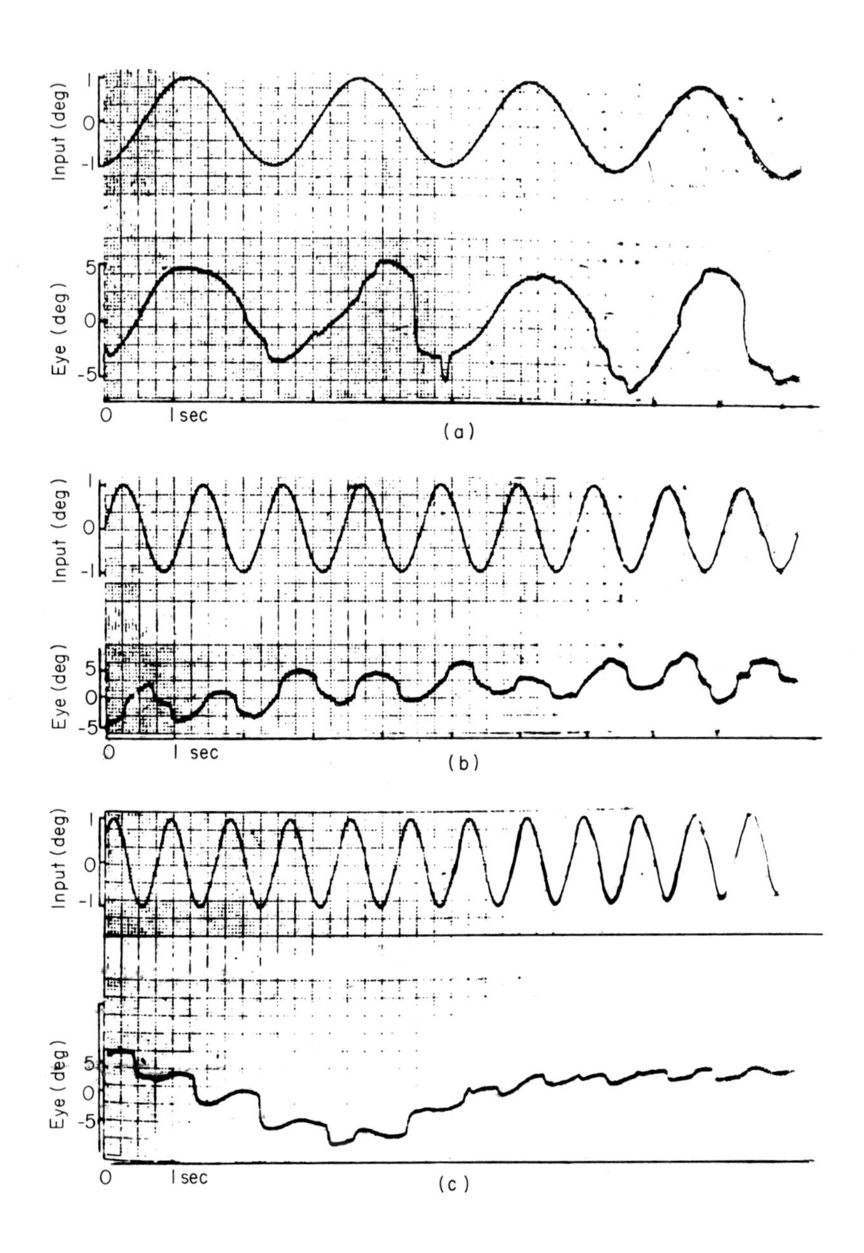

Fig. 1. Open loop sinusoidal tracking (a) 0.4 Hz, (b) 0.8 Hz, (c) 1.2 Hz.

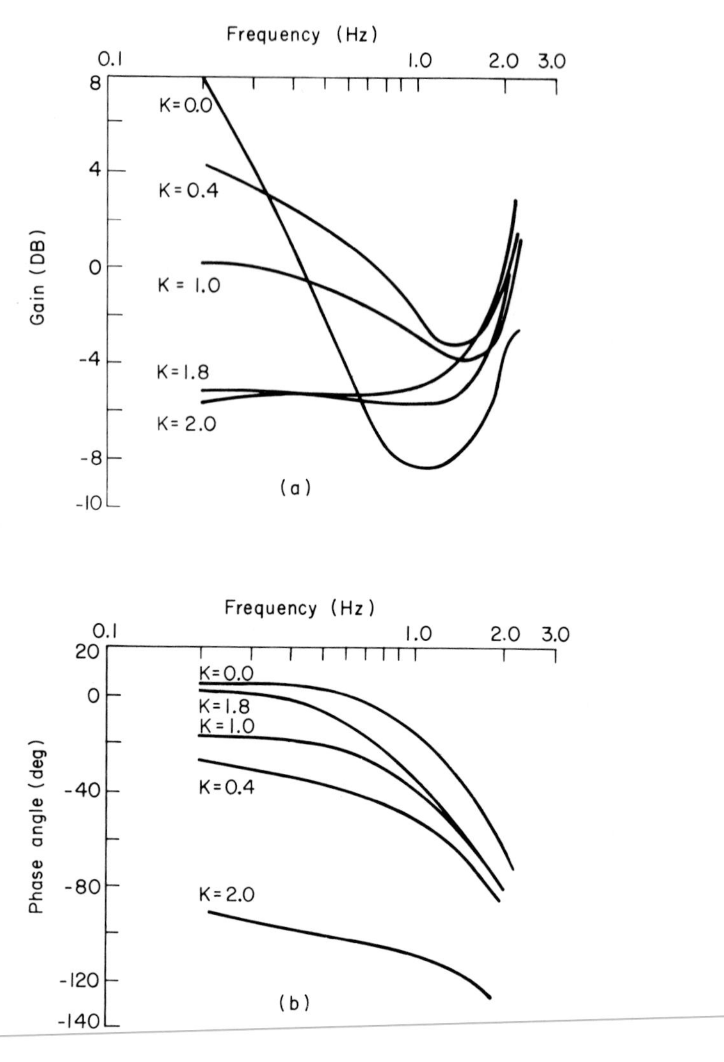

Fig. 2. Frequency responses — variable feedback nonpredictive tracking. (a) Gain, (b) Phase. (K values represent one plus feedback gain.)

An apparent acceleration limitation in the pursuit system is seen in the commonly observed phenomenon in which the failure of the pursuit system to change velocity rapidly results in a buildup of position error, usually corrected by a saccade. This acceleration limitation appears more obvious when reversing directions than when continuing acceleration in the same direction. If such is the case, it could be attributed to a "backlash phenomenon" in which the acceleration is limited by the time required to reverse roles of agonist and antagonist between the sets of extraocular muscles controlling the motion.

The nonlinearity most evident in the pursuit eye movement system is a soft saturation. No reliable measurements of a dead zone for pursuit tracking movements are known to the author, although it becomes difficult to separate tracking movements from drift at rates below 5 minutes of arc/sec. Actual pursuit velocity shows considerable variability, which may be attributable to the varying size of the retinal movement receptive fields (Jung and Spillman, 1967; Richards 1969). As the angular velocity of a target increases, the pursuit velocity also increases, keeping the two velocities approximately equal until the target reaches approximately 15 deg/sec. By 30 deg/sec, the eye velocity is typically less than the target velocity, and frequent position correcting saccades are required to reduce the resulting fixation error (Young, 1962). Under normal circumstances, 30 to 40 deg/sec is the maximum velocity reached by the smooth tracking system, regardless of the target velocity. For target velocities above 40 deg/sec the following eye velocity begins to decrease slightly and more of the tracking is done by saccadic steps. Finally, at target velocities of several hundred deg/sec there appears to be no attempt to reduce retinal slip by smooth pursuit movements. This pattern is reproduced in general form for optokinetic nystagmus in which whole field stimulation is used (Hood, 1967). For moving horizontal stripes, slow phase velocity in the eye roughly matches the angular velocity of the target up to only 40-60 deg/sec, or frequently less, depending on field size and other conditions, and then shifts to a saturation and negative slope region.

An asymmetric nonlinearity may be present in the pursuit system but it has not been explored in detail. It would appear from some of our measurements that, just as in the case of saccadic eye movements, the eye is capable of producing faster pursuit eye movements going from secondary to primary gaze than going in the opposite direction. The three curves in Figure 3 show a typical example of this nonlinearity. The middle curve is for optokinetic nystagmus with the target stripes directly in front of the subject, and shows the linear region, saturation near 40 deg/sec and negative slope of tracking velocity at higher stripe speeds. When the entire pattern is displaced in the direction from which the stripes appear, (forcing eye deviation in the direction of fast phase nystagmus) the nystagmus is enhanced and the linear region extended, in accordance with Alexander's law (upper curve). Just the opposite trend is seen when the eye deviation is away from the fast phase direction.

Some mention should be made of the variety of responses involving the smooth pursuit system which are observed to identical input stimuli. For example, in the response of the eye movement system to a simple ramp or to a step-ramp, one may observe various sequences of one or two saccades and pursuit movements. As discussed in detail by Young, Forster and Van Houtte (1968), the variability in responses to a ramp or step-ramp may be attributable entirely to the random synchronization of samples for the saccadic system, which brings about saccadic corrections at various times during each response.

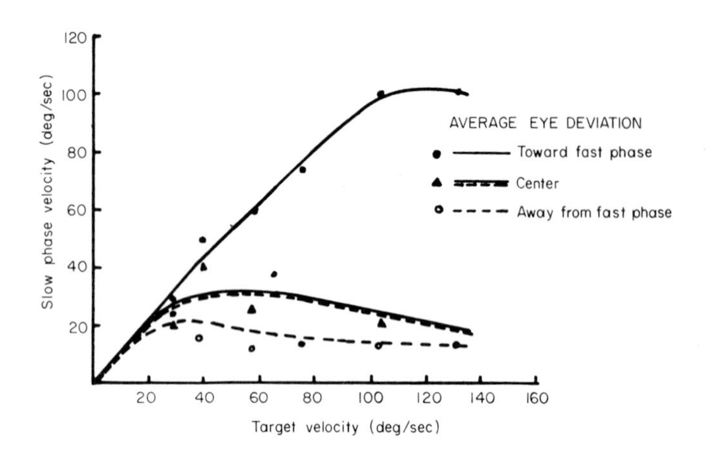

Fig. 3. Optokinetic nystagmus slow phase nonlinearities - (Average values, typical subject).

It is not necessary to assume as wide a variability in the timing of the pursuit responses observed.

Another important characteristic of the pursuit eye movement control system relates to its interaction with saccadic eye movements. It is now clear that although the pursuit eye movement system is capable of changing its angular velocity extremely rapidly, this change only seems to occur simultaneously with a saccadic eye movement in the direction of the velocity change. The exact mechanism for this saccadic facilitation is not known, although it may very well be a phenomenon in the extraocular muscles rather than in the central command to the pursuit system. The saccadic eye movement reaches an angular velocity much greater than that of any subsequent pursuit movement. The muscles need merely decelerate to the level of the required pursuit movement velocity and thus yield a rapid change in pursuit angular velocity. It is clear in the absence of saccades that the slow continuous changes in pursuit velocity referred to previously are readily observable.

APPENDIX 1

THE SACCADIC DEAD ZONE

Some of the data on which the saccadic foveal dead zone is based appears in Figure 4a (Young, 1966). Small targets being fixated were randomly stepped horizontally by angles no greater than one degree, and the time of the corrective saccade, or the lack of response within 800 msec, recorded. The 1962 data was taken with a thin vertical line projected on a screen in a dark room, and the 1965 data used a line on an oscilloscope, with reference grid lines illuminated, in a lighted room. There is no apparent difference in results. The data are replotted in Figure 4b, as the probability of a corrective saccade within *t* seconds, as a function of target step amplitude. A target step of 0.3 degrees elicites a corrective saccade within a nominal reaction time of 0.25 seconds 50 per cent of the time. A foveal dead zone model, which assumes saccades one reaction time after the image appears outside this zone, yields the approximate time given by the dark line.

APPENDIX 2

THE YOUNG-FORSTER-VAN HOUTTE MODEL

The stochastic sampled data model of Young, Forster and Van Houtte (1968), referred to by several participants in this symposium, is not available

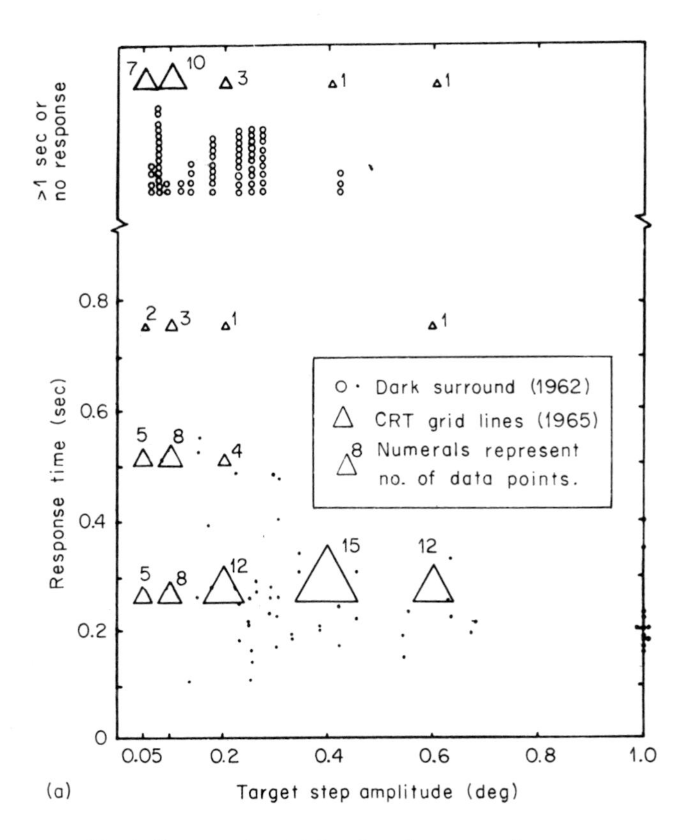

Fig. 4a. Response time as a function of target step size.

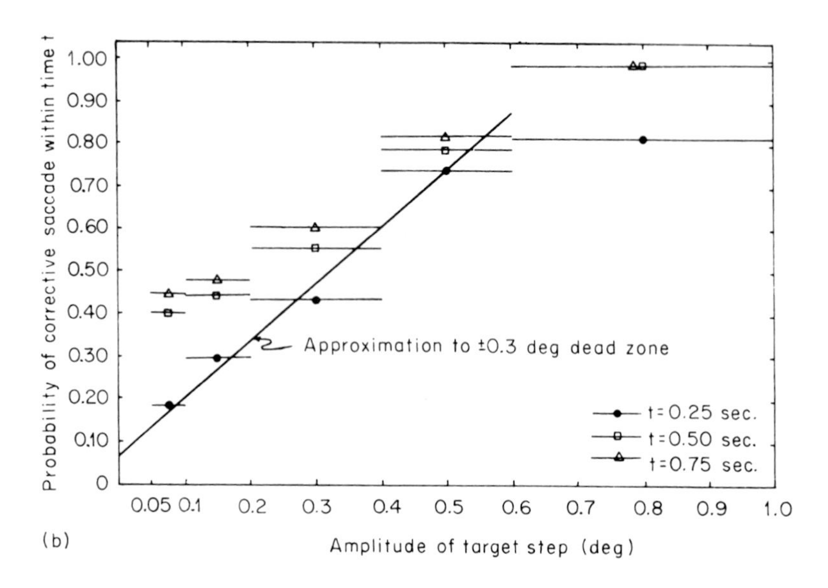

Fig. 4b. Probability of corrective saccade within time *t* versus step amplitude.

in a readily accessible source. It is of limited utility, and merely overcomes some of the detailed shortcomings of the original sampled data model, for example, showing how the uncertainty in sampling instantly leads to a variety of transient responses to identical inputs. The model is reproduced in Figure 5 for reference. The saccadic loop has been altered from the original sampled data model by reducing the delay. The pursuit loop is continuous, acting on target rate (computed from retinal velocity and eye velocity, presumably through some out-flow information). The pursuit loop has a differentiator, nonlinearity and integrator to go from position to velocity and back without exceeding saturation. It also contains a time delay of 134 msec, a first order lag accounting for the 'rounding" of changes in velocity, and a simplified expression for eyeball dynamics which ignores the pre-emphasis and nonlinear aspects that do not affect overall loop performance. It must be noted emphatically that this is merely a non-rational parameter model, which describes some of the average behavior from a black box, input-output point of view. It is useful only in illustrating common characteristics in various types of tracking data. It should not be misapplied as a map or schema for the physiological system, and it does not meet most of the objections to models of this level discussed in the body of this paper.

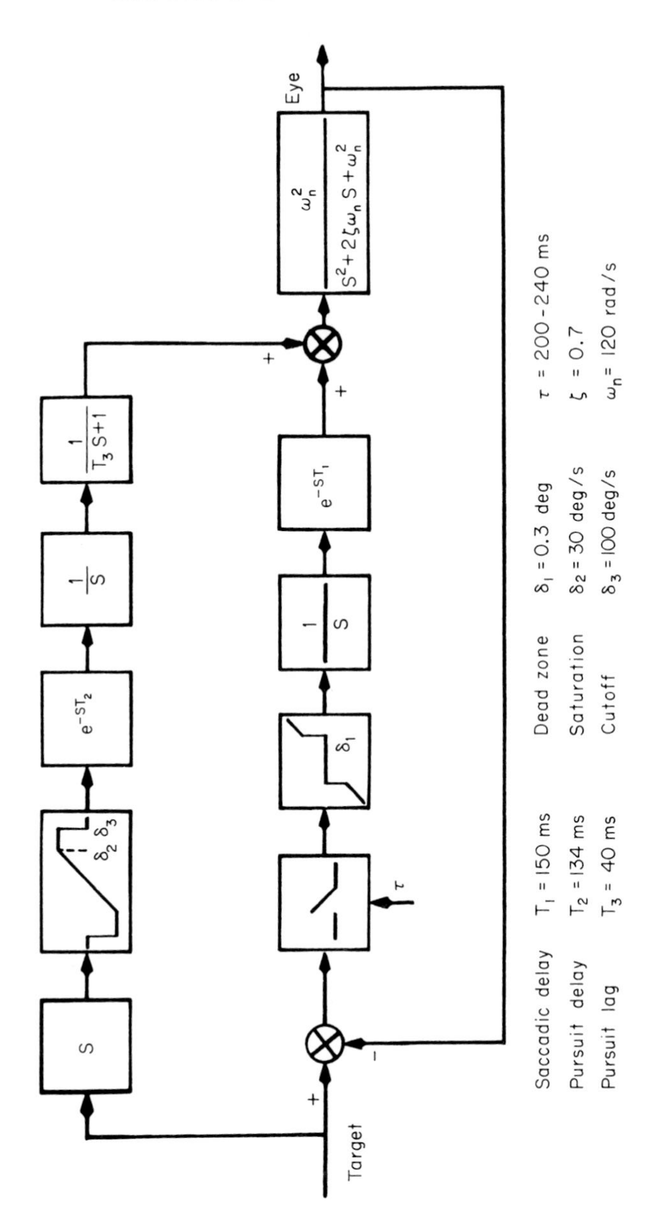

Fig. 5. Eye tracking movement model of Young, Forster and Van Houtte.

ACKNOWLEDGEMENT

The review and comments of Prof. Whitman Richards, Psychology Dept., M.I.T. are gratefully acknowledged.

REFERENCES

Byford, G.H. (1969). Personal communication.

Childress, D.S. (1967). *A Study of the Mechanics of Horizontal Movements of the Human Eye.* Ph.D. Thesis. Northwestern University. Dept. of Electrical Engineering.

Cogan, D.G. (1952). A type of ocular motor apraxia presenting jerky head movements. *Am. Ophth. Oto,* 858.

Collewijn, H. (1969). Optokinetic eye movements in the rabbit: input-output relations. *Vision Res.* **9,** 117-132.

Dallos, P.J. & Jones, R.W. (1963). Learning behaviour of the eye fixation control system. Institute of Electrical and Electronics Engineers, *Trans. on Automatic Control* **AC-8,** 218-227.

Feldman, M, Atkin, A. & Bender, M.B. (1969). Oculomotor responses from visual input to an immobilized eye. Abstract in 4th International Congress of Neurological Surgery, 9th Intl. Congress of Neurology, New York.

Fender, D.H. & Nye, P.W. (1961). An investigation of the mechanics of eye movement control. *Kybernetik.* **1,** 81.

Fuchs, A. (1967a). Periodic eye tracking in the monkey. *J. Phyiol.* **193,** 161-171.

Fuchs, A. (1967b). Saccadic and smooth pursuit eye movements in the monkey. *J. Physiol.* **191,** 609-631.

Hood, J.D. (1967). *Discussion on Myotatic, Kinesthetic and Vestibular Mechanisms,* ed. Aus de Rueck and J. Knight. Little Brown and Co. Boston.

Johnson, L.E., Jr. (1963). Human eye tracking of aperiodic target functions. Report 37-B-63-8. Systems Research Center, Case Institute of Technology, Cleveland, Ohio.

Jung, R. & Spillman, L. (1967). Receptive fields estimation and perceptual integration in human vision. Symposium on Dislexia. Mohawk, New York.

Kris, C. (1960). *Vision: Electrooculography in Medical Physics.* vol. 3, O. Glasser, ed. The Year Book Publishers, Inc. Chicago.

Meiry, J.L. (1969). Vestibular and proprioceptive stabilization of eye movement. Symposium on the Control of Eye Movements, San Francisco, California.

Michael, J.A. & Jones, G.M. (1966). Dependence of visual tracking capability upon stimulus predictability. *Vision Res.* **6,** 707-716.

Rashbass, C. (1961). The relationship between saccadic and smooth tracking eye movements. *J. Physiol.* **159,** 326-338.

Richards, W. (1969). Sensitivity fields for movement. *J. Opt. Soc. Am.* **59,** 1543.

Robinson, D.A. (1965). The mechanics of human smooth pursuit eye movement. *J. Physiol.* **180,** 569-591.

Robinson, D.A. (1969). Models of oculomotor neural organization. Symposium on the Control of Eye Movements, San Francisco Calif.

St. Cyr, G.S. & Fender, D.H. (1969a). The interplay of drifts and flicks in binocular fixation. *Vision Res.* **9,** 245-265.

St. Cyr, G.S. & Fender, D.H. (1969b). Nonlinearities of the human oculomotor system: gain. *Vision Res.* **9,** 1235-1246.

St. Cyr, G.S. & Fender, D.H. (1970). Nonlinearities of the human oculomotor system: time delays. *Vision Res.* **9,** 1491-1503.

Sanders, A.F. (1963). *The Selective Process in the Functional Visual Field.* Thesis. Von Gorcum and Co., Amsterdam.

STARK, L., VOSSIUS, G. & YOUNG, L.R. (1962). Predictive control of eye tracking movement. **HFE-3,** No. 2.

STEINBACH, M.J. (1969). Eye tracking of self-moved targets: the role of errerence. *J. of Exper. Psychol.* **vol. 82, No. 2,** 366-376.

STEINBACH, M.J. & HELD, R. (1968). Eye tracking of observer-generated target movement. *Science.* **161,** 187-188.

VOSSIUS, G. (1961). Die Regelbewung des Auges **In:** *Aufnahme und Verarbeitung von Nachrichten durch Organismen.* Editor VDE, Stuttgart, 149-157; also (1965) *Progress in Cybernetics.* Elsevier Publishing Co. New York.

WATANABE, A. & YOSHIDA, T. (1969). Control mechanism of smooth pursuit eye movement. Proceedings of the 8th ICMBE, Chicago.

WESTHEIMER, G. (1954). Eye movement response to a horizontally moving visual stimulus. *A.M.A. Arch Ophthal.* **52,** 932-941.

WESTHEIMER, G. & CONOVER, D.W. (1954). Smooth eye movements in the absence of a moving visual stimulus. *J. Exper. Psychol.* **47,** 283.

YARBUS, A.L. (1967). *Eye Movements and Vision.* Plenum Press, New York.

YOUNG, L.R. (1962). *A Sampled Data Model for Eye Tracking Movements.* Sc.D. Thesis. M.I.T.

YOUNG, L.R. (1966). The dead zone to saccadic eye movements. Symposium on Biomedical Engineering. Marquette University.

YOUNG, L.R., FORSTER, J.D. & VAN HOUTTE, N. (1968). A revised stochastic sampled data model for eye tracking movements. Fourth Annual NASA-University Conference on Manual Control, U. of Michigan, Ann Arbor, Michigan.

YOUNG, L.R. & STARK, L. (1963). Variable feedback experiments testing a sampled data model for eye tracking movements. *IEEE Trans. on Human Factors in Electronics.* **vol. HFE-4, No. 1,** 28-51.

YOUNG, L.R. (1969). The current status of vestibular system models. *Automatica:* **vol. 5,** 369-383.

ZUBER, B. (1965). *Physiological Control of Eye Movements in Humans.* Ph.D. Thesis, M.I.T.

SECOND THOUGHTS ON SMOOTH PURSUIT

CYRIL RASHBASS

Dr. Young's model for the smooth tracking control of the eye contains the usual flow diagram of black boxes but on this occasion he has healthily filled them with question marks. He has raised some of the problems involved in specifying the system and I should like to add a few more unanswered questions.

1. Dr. Young has suggested that the smooth tracking response is a transformation – albeit non-linear and complicated – of target position or velocity. I am not sure that I agree with him that a signal representing target position or velocity plays much part in the generation of smooth tracking but let us assume for the moment that he is right. Then, as he states, there is no direct way in which the visual system can know where the target is or how fast it is moving; but this signal can be recreated by combining eye position or velocity with retinal image position or velocity. Now, this rings a bell. It may be heresy to say it here, but the eye not only moves, it also sees. One of the problems of vision is concerned with the stability of the position of the outside world and for this we postulate a signal derived by combining retinal position and eye position. (I hasten to explain, lest anyone should be misled, that, being good disciples of Helmoltz, eye position is inferred from outflow information – not a sense of position). Now my first question is – *Could vision and smooth tracking be using the same signal? In other words, does the eye track what it sees?* This suggests a field of experimentation in tracking in which the signal representing eye position is falsified by various techniques in the way that has been used to demonstrate the truth of Helmoltz's outflow theory.

2. Given that retinal slip velocity is a major factor in determining smooth tracking movements – *do we believe that retinal velocity detectors, demonstrated by Barlow and his colleagues (Barlow, Hill & Levick (1964)) in rabbits, are the source of this information?*

3. I have been widely quoted as the authority for asserting that saccadic and smooth tracking systems are independent. I plead guilty and feel that this gives me the special right to assert that they are not independent. I would state the paradox that they can only appear to be independent if there is a conspiracy between them to do so. Imagine two drivers of the same car, one trying to keep the speedometer pointing at 30 m.p.h. and one trying to keep the car alongside another also travelling at 30 m.p.h. Unless there is communication between the two drivers it is easy to see that the velocity

man is going to frustrate the efforts of the position man. Changes in velocity due to the saccades must not be corrected by smooth tracking. Saccadic suppression of vision — the position man putting his hand over the speedometer every time he does something could account for this — but then, *isn't this an interaction?*

4. Task predictability seems to me to be a difficult concept to define for the visual system; bandwidth doesn't seem the appropriate idea because square waves have a broad bandwidth but are eminently predictable. The remarkable property of the smooth tracking system is that not only does it predict, i.e., deduce a probable estimate of where the target is going by inference from where it has been, but it modifies the rules for this inference in the light of where the target has been. This must call for a considerable amount of neurological apparatus and might explain the relative susceptibility of the smooth tracking system to drugs.

One prediction that we can make with great certainty is that we shall need to get together again in a few years' time to discuss the answers to some of these problems.

REFERENCE

Barlow, H. B., Hill, R. M. and Levick, W. R. (1964). Retinal ganglion cells responding selectively to direction and speed of image motion in the rabbit. *J. Physiol.* **173**, 377–407.

CONTROL OF VERGENCE EYE MOVEMENTS

BERT L. ZUBER

Vergence, or disjunctive, eye movements provide the binocular organism[1] with a crucial degree of freedom which permits the fixation of points in visual space at various distances from the organism. Given an arbitrary fixation point in space, the fixation of any point closer to the organism would require a convergence movement (increase in angle between the visual axes). Conversely, the fixation of a more distant point would require a divergence movement (decrease in the angle between the visual axes). In vergence movements, with binocular fixation, the eyes necessarily always move in opposite directions, and usually the movements of the two eyes are of equal magnitude. Although various quantitative measures of vergence have been used (Duane, 1933) the most sensible, and the one most generally used is the magnitude of the angle through which the eye turns in making a vergence movement or in arriving at some position of vergence. These angles may be measured with respect to any line perpindicular to the line joining the centers of rotation of the two eyes. Other measures of vergence are the convergence distance and the meter-angle.

The stimuli eliciting vergence movements involve a change in the distance (or apparent distance) between the fixation point and the eyes of the subject. In general such stimuli bring about two types of modifications of the retinal image of the fixation point. One is a change in the blur pattern of the image, the other is a displacement of the image away from the fovea brought about by a change in the real or apparent distance between the fixation target and the subject.

Supported by U.S. Public Health Service (NB-07777).

[1]Vergence movements are probably only found among some mammals, and may be restricted to primates and higher animals.

These two stimulus characteristics have led to the separation of vergence movements into two classes – fusional and accommodative. The change in the image blur pattern supposedly results in accommodative vergence, while the displacement of the retinal images, resulting in diplopia, or non-fused retinal images, supposedly brings about fusional vergence. There are clearly very few real-world situations in which these two stimulus characteristics are separated.

The clinical ramifications of pathology involving vergence eye movements are vast. Perhaps the most common pathological condition is strabismus or squint, in which the visual axes are chronically misaligned in such a way as to make proper fusion impossible. Amblyopia, partial loss of vision in a misaligned eye, is often seen as a secondary complication of strabismus, and is a forceful example of the many interactions between the visual and oculomotor systems. The completely empirical clinical approach to strabismus is a reflection of our lack of understanding of the mechanism of vergence eye movements. Furthermore, it is ironic, in view of the enormous clinical significance of the vergence system, that this system is perhaps the least studied of all the oculomotor subsystems.

SOME BASIC ASPECTS OF THE SYSTEM RESPONSE

Range of Movement

Duane (1933) reported that the maximum convergence angle for 60 per cent of his normal subjects between the ages of 16 and 40 years was between 21 and 27°. He concluded that this value is little affected by age, and that practice was a more important variable. This corresponds to the range of vergence movement and is roughly equivalent to the angle through which the eye moves in changing fixation from optical infinity to the near point of convergence. It is interesting to note that the range of vergence movement is approximately one fourth the range of eye movement when the same eye makes versional movements.

Accuracy of Movement

A number of investigators have reported significant errors in the final position of the eyes resulting from vergence movements (e.g. Westheimer and Mitchell, 1956; Alpern, 1957; for review see Riggs and Niehl, 1960). Vergence movements were recorded by a variety of methods including direct photography, corneal reflection and electro-oculography. The results of a number of these studies indicated that steady state errors, often as large as 2°, were consistently present after vergence movements. Riggs and Niehl (1960) using a sensitive direct-photographic method to measure eye movement observed no systematic steady state errors larger than about two minutes of arc.

Compound Versional and Vergence Movements

Eye movements between any two arbitrary fixation points consist of both versional and vergence components provided the two points do not lie on a line bisecting the angle formed by the two visual axes (bisector). Pure (symmetrical) vergence movements generally occur only along a bisector. In moving between any two points the eyes are usually conjugately moved in such a way that the intersection of the visual axes falls on the bisector containing the desired fixation point. Pure vergence movement then occurs along that bisector until the intersection of the visual axes and the fixation point coincide. These observations were made by Westheimer and Mitchell (1956) for purely fusional stimuli and by Yarbus (1957) for the general case of stimuli involving both fusional and accommodative components, and for fixation points at different distances and in different directions presented in random order. Both investigations indicated that the vergence component of movement began before the versional component and was essentially continuous, indicating that the two components were algebraically added. A typical compound movement is shown in Fig. 1a taken from Yarbus. The movements of the eyes consist of vergence components (oppositely directed) and conjugate saccades. The dashed curves represent the vergence components preceding the saccade but displaced by the amplitude of the saccade. The overall scheme of this type of movement is shown in Fig. 1b for both convergence and divergence between two fixation points A and B. Note that although the vergence component may precede the versional component, the former still occurs along a bisector.

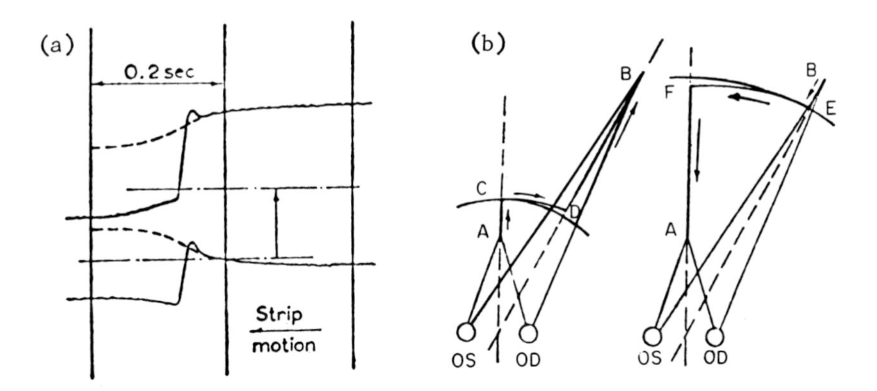

Fig. 1. (a) Typical eye movement resulting from shift in fixation between two arbitrary fixation points. The compound movement consists of both saccadic and vergence components. Dashed curve is presaccadic vergence shifted by amplitude of saccade (Yarbus, 1957).
(b) Schematic representation of eye behavior in type of movement shown in (a). Vergence occurs only along lines bissecting the angle between the two visual axes. Saccadic movement insures that the desired fixation point falls on one of these lines (Yarbus, 1957).

A special class of asymmetrical vergence stimuli has received a considerable amount of attention from investigators. If two fixation points are confined to the visual axis of one eye, then theoretically only movement of the fellow eye is required to shift fixation between the two points. In the nineteenth century Mueller observed that even when the fellow eye was occluded it moved as if to follow the moving target which it could not see (accommodative vergence). This indicated that a purely accommodative stimulus was an effective input to the vergence system. More recent investigations have utilized combinations of accommodative and fusional stimuli (Alpern and Ellen, 1956a, b) as well as purely fusional stimuli (Westheimer and Mitchell, 1956; Alpern, 1957; Zuber, 1967). When the only input is accommodative the resulting accommodative vergence eye movement is uniocular as shown in Fig. 2a. The eye along whose visual axis the target motion occurs stands still. Whenever a fusional stimulus is present (as with binocular viewing, or with purely fusional stimuli), and the target motion has certain temporal characteristics (see below), the pattern of eye movement is binocular. Furthermore, the observed pattern of eye movement is of the same form as that described by Yarbus (1957) for generalized stimulus patterns, consisting of both versional and vergence components. The eye whose visual axis is used for target motion makes a saccade and a vergence movement of the same magnitude but in opposite directions, so that it ends up in the same position it had before moving. An example of this pattern is shown in Fig. 2b. This superfluous eye movement has been cited as evidence for the validity of Hering's Law of equal innervation as applied to vergence movements (Alpern and Ellen, 1956a).

The available electromyographic evidence in this type of experiment is a little confusing. Breinin (1955, 1957) and Tamler, Jampolsky and Marg (1958) recorded electromyographic data that conflicted, but in both studies it was claimed that Hering's Law was verified for this type of eye movement. The interpretation of Hering's Law was at issue: Breinin claimed that equal innervation signals meant for the horizontal recti of the stationary eye were cancelled in the CNS before reaching the muscles; Tamler, *et al* claimed that cancellation occurred in the orbit at the level of the muscles. There has apparently been no rectification of this conflict.

The temporal characteristics of the stimulus in asymmetrical vergence experiments is an additional factor which prevents a clear-cut interpretation and correlation of the results of various studies. The response pattern may be affected by whether the target motion is relatively slow and smooth, or very rapid and stepwise. Furthermore, some investigators have made their observations using the cover test on patients with exo deviations. The consensus seems to indicate that the compound version-vergence response (superfluous movement of the eye whose visual axis is used for target motion) is observed only when the fusional mechanism is operative, and when the target motion is stepwise. On the other hand, when tne stimulus is purely accommodative, the resulting eye movement is uniocular and pure vergence, whether the target motion is smooth or stepwise. This implies a functional separation of these two

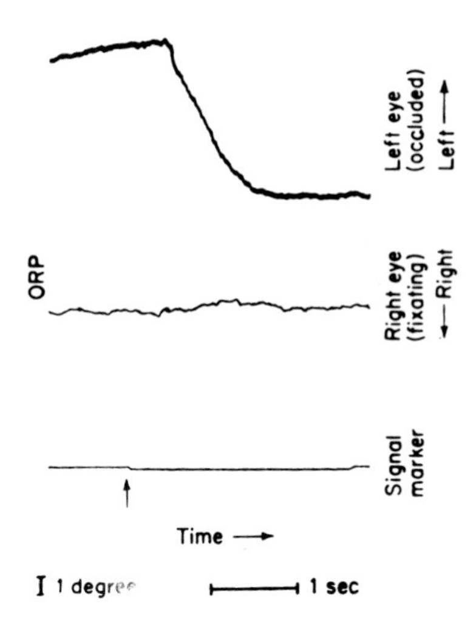

Fig. 2. (a) Accommodative vergence resulting from target motion along visual axis of right eye, left eye occluded (Alpern and Ellen, 1956a).

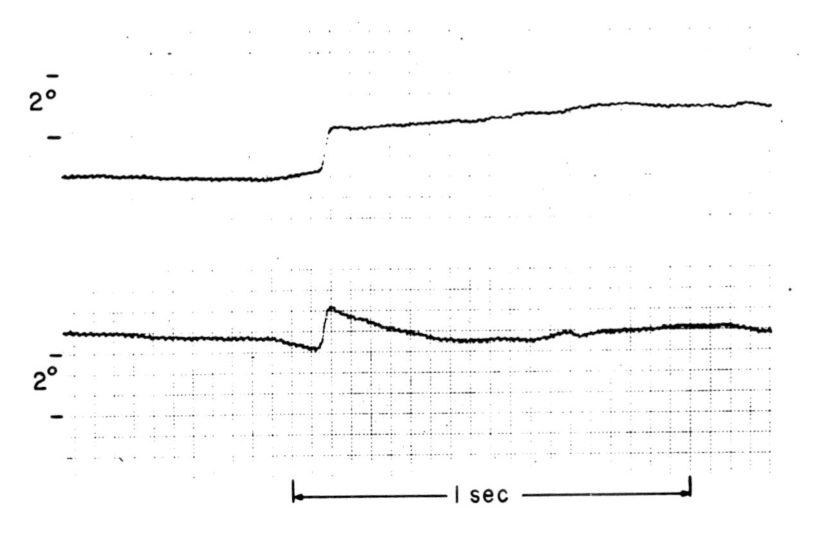

(b) Fusional vergence movements resulting from apparent target movement along the visual axis of one eye, both eyes viewing. Note the similarity between this and Fig. 1a. (Zuber, 1967).

control loops and indicates that the fusional mechanism is responsible for bringing about compound version-vergence eye movement patterns. The relationships between stimulus characteristics and resulting eye movements are summarized in Table 1.

TABLE I

	Target Motion	
Type of Stimulus	Fast	Slow
Pure Fusional or Fusional and accommodative	Binocular, Saccadic and Vergence	Uniocular, Vergence only
Accommodative	Uniocular, Vergence only	Uniocular, Vergence only

The relationship between type of stimulus, target motion and the type of eye movement (gray area) elicited in asymmetrical vergence along the visual axis of one eye. Binocular eye movements, consisting of saccadic and vergence components occur only when a fusional stimulus is present, and when the target motion is fast.

What is needed now is a careful and well conceived study of these two mechanisms wherein stimulus conditions can be carefully controlled. Such a study could reveal the detailed nature of the error signals driving these two control loops. For example, it is only when the fusional mechanism is utilized (e.g., binocular viewing) that a conventional eye movement error signal (lack of coincidence of the target image and the fovea) is generated. The time course of that error signal (target movement) seems to determine the nature of the response. When the target motion is rapid a binocular compound saccadic-vergence response results. If the target motion is relatively slow the response is smooth and uniocular. This is reminiscent of the dichotomy between the stimulus characteristics eliciting saccadic and smooth pursuit eye movements (Dodge, 1903; Westheimer, 1954). It may be that similar mechanisms are brought into play in the case of asymmetrical fusional vergence. For slow target motion it is easy to see that a fusional vergence component and an oppositely-directed versional smooth pursuit component could cancel out in one eye leaving the eye stationary. These are both tracking movements and the innervations causing them would be expected to have roughly similar time courses. This implies, of course, that the movement of the other eye would consist of two smooth components, one fusional vergence and the other smooth pursuit, both moving that eye in the same direction. This remains to be demonstrated. It is also clear that for rapid target motions cancellations could not occur due to the vastly different time courses of innervation causing the saccadic and fusional vergence components of movement. Hence, the binocular compound saccadic-vergence movement.

Independence of Version and Vergence

The preceding discussion indicates that the versional and vergence systems are closely coordinated in the task of fixation of any target in visual space. Another pertinent question is that of the independence of the two components of the coordinated task. Such independence has already been mentioned in reference to the work of Westheimer and Mitchell (1956) and Yarbus (1957) who observed that the versional and vergence components in asymmetrical vergence had different latencies and appeared to be algebraically added. Other investigators have studied the independence of these two systems under different stimulus conditions. Rashbass and Westheimer (1961b) studied eye movements containing both fusional vergence and versional smooth pursuit components. They used both sinusoidal and square wave stimuli, and they were able to independently control and record the vergence and versional components of the stimulus and eye movement. Figure 3, taken from their results, shows the vergence (top) and versional (bottom) components of the eye movement response to sinusoidal target motion in both modalities at 1.0 Hz. The independence of the two responses is clearly seen from this figure. Although the vergence component decreases in amplitude, the versional component continues, and in this example consists of both saccadic and smooth pursuit movements. They concluded that either system independently responded to its own stimulus, regardless of whether the other system was within a latent period, responding or overloaded.

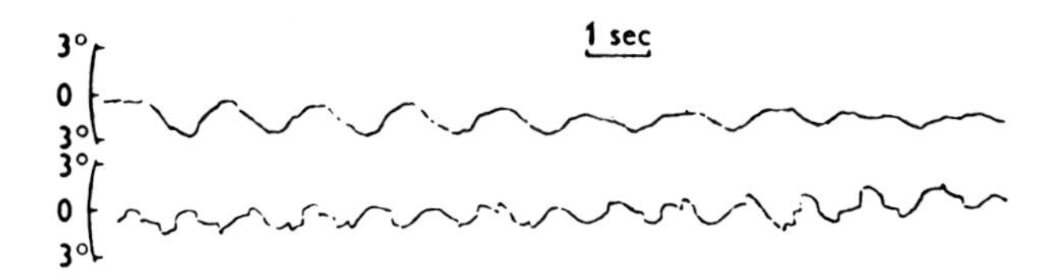

Fig. 3. Vergence (upper trace) and versional (lower trace) components recorded simultaneously during tracking, showing independence (Rashbass and Westheimer, 1961b).

Troelstra and Stark (1963) examined eye movements resulting from stimuli combining both accommodative and versional tracking inputs. Their low frequency sinusoidal target motions were horizontal and were confined to a series of planes parallel to mid-saggital plane. Under such circumstances the movements of an occluded eye were measured, and consisted of accommodative vergence and associated smooth pursuit tracking components. Clearly the inputs for both of these components come from the seeing eye. Given the stimulus configuration, and assuming independence, they were able to calculate the predicted net movement of the occluded eye resulting from accommodative vergence and versional tracking as a function of the position of the saggital plane used for target motion. For one saggital plane position calculations indicated that the vergence and versional components were equal in amplitude but in opposite directions. Therefore, for this plane of target motion it was predicted that there would be no movement of the occluded eye. Their experimental results were in very good agreement with their predictions, leading them to the conclusion that accommodative vergence and versional smooth pursuit movements are independent in that they are algebraically additive. Some of their other data indicated that the accommodative vergence system was much more influenced by fatigue than was the versional tracking system.

Finally, along slightly different lines, Alpern and Wolter (1956) argued that there may be morphological basis for the independence of vergence and saccadic eye movements. Based primarily on the different velocity characteristics of these two types of movements, they proposed two functionally different final common paths histologically distinguished by different nerve fiber diameters and presence or absence of myelin. To date there has been no verification of this hypothesis. Although there are at least two different types of fibers in the extraocular muscles themselves (for Review see Peachey, 1968, and this volume) there has been no clear correlation of muscle fiber type with vergence as opposed to versional movement.

Relations of the Near Triad

A pure accommodative stimulus causes not only a change in the shape of the lens but also associated changes in accommodative vergence and pupil area. The interaction of these three control systems has been referred to as the near triad. Quantification of the static characteristics of these linkages has been the subject of a considerable number of both clinical and non-clinical studies. The voluminous amount of work in this area makes a detailed discussion of these mechanisms impractical at this point. The discussion below is confined to the most basic organizational level, and is primarily based on part of the work of Alpern and his associates (Alpern *et al*, 1961).

These authors used an experimental set up in which steady state accommodation, accommodative vergence and pupil diameter were measured essentially simultaneously as a result of various levels of accommodative stimulation within the range of ±8 diopters. Their data, therefore, represent the static input-output characteristics of the three interacting systems of the near triad. The data for one subject are shown in Fig. 4, where it should be noted that the ordinate for the upper two plots is accommodative response, not accommodative stimulus. They point out that even though the near point of accommodation is exceeded (saturation in the accommodative system, probably due to the mechanical properties of the lens) accommodative vergence continues to increase and pupillary diameter continues to decrease with increasing accommodative stimulation. This was interpreted as indicating that the effective input to both accommodative vergence and the pupillary system is the level of innervation to the ciliary muscle.

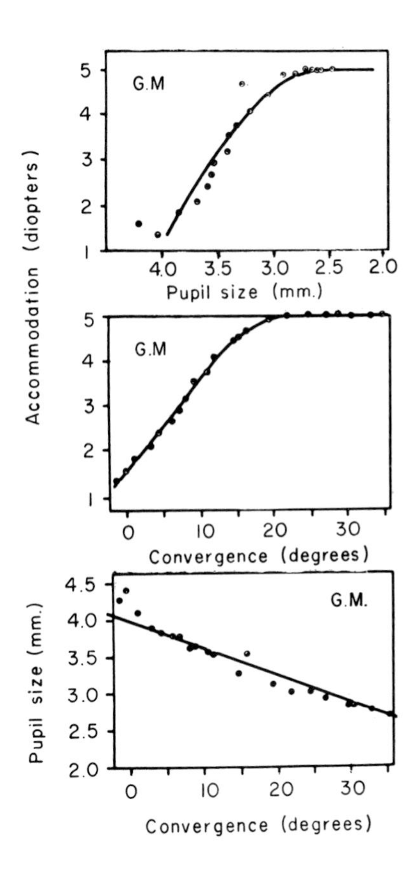

Fig. 4. The static relationship among accommodative response, vergence and pupil size obtained with accommodative stimuli (Alpern, *et al.*, 1961).

One possible interpretation of these observations, consistent with their interpretation, leads to the schematic organizational block diagram shown in Fig. 5. According to this diagram the ultimate input for the three systems in the near triad is the accommodative stimulus. This would be the only readily accessible independent variable; the three otuputs are all dependent variables (see Alpern *et al.* 1959). If the organizational scheme of Fig. 5a is accepted then the presentation of the data in the form shown in Fig. 4 leaves a good deal to be desired, since plotting one dependent variable versus another results in the loss of considerable information. Reconstructed static input-output characteristics of the three systems in the near triad are shown in Fig. 5b. These are based on the data of Alpern *et al.* (1961) and others. For example, Ripps, *et al.* (1962) observed a linear relationship between accommodative response and accommodative stimulus (over a limited range) for the conditions of their experiments. Finally, conceptualizing the near triad in this way raises questions as to

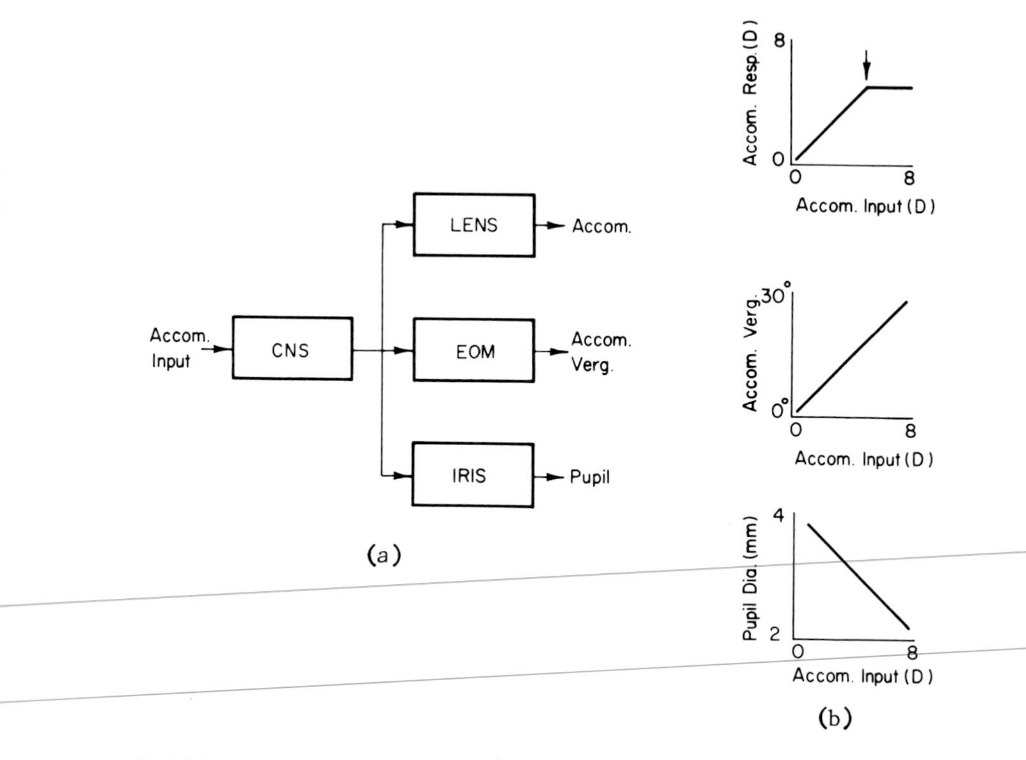

Fig. 5 (a) Block diagram of basic near triad relationships.
(b) Static input-output relationships for the various paths in (a). Ranges derived from existing data. Arrow (top plot) indicates near point of accommodation. Notice in all cases abscissa is independent variable, accommodative input.

the meaningfulness of response measures such as the response accommodative convergence – accommodation ratio (AC/Ar).

The role of fusional vergence movements in the complex interactions of the systems of the near triad is not clear. The question of whether there is a pupillary response associated with fusional movements has not been clearly answered. Part of the reason for this is probably that large purely fusional stimuli may result in changes in level of accommodation (Fry, 1939; Alpern, 1962) which may, in turn, result in associated pupillary responses. Marg and Morgan (1950), after several studies concluded that the pupillary fusion reflex was an artefact, which, when it occurred, probably resulted from inadequate control of accommodative inputs. On the other hand, Backer and Ogle (1964) observed a steady state change in pupillary diameter in response to fusional stimuli (prisms) as well as a transient constriction of the pupil measured either on interposing or removing the prism from the visual axis. In their experiments, Marg and Morgan (1950) intermittently measured both accommodation and pupillary diameter, while Backer and Ogle (1964) continuously measured only pupillary diameter.

CONTROL SYSTEMS STUDIES

A study of the dynamics of vergence eye movements requires that a moving target be presented to the subject and that his eye movements be continuously monitored. All of the most generally used inputs – a variety of transients including pulses, steps, ramps and parabolas, as well as steady state sinusoidal inputs – are useful. Transient inputs may be used to determine the dynamic characteristics of the system if it is linear. However, these inputs are often more useful for clearly demonstrating interesting timing characteristics exhibited by the system, such as the intermittency or refractoriness observed in the versional system (Young and Stark, 1963). Closed loop and open loop frequency response data are usually obtained from steady state sinusoidal responses which are then used to construct the conventional Bode plot or polar plot – graphical representations of the system dynamics.

A stimulus having both symmetrical fusional and accommodative components may be generated using binocular viewing of a target mechanically moved along a line bisecting the angle formed by the two visual axes. Accommodative vergence alone may be studied by restricting target motion to the visual axis of one eye and measuring the resulting movements of the occluded fellow eye. Pure fusional vergence stimuli may be produced by presenting separate identical targets to each eye and varying the separation between the two targets (Westheimer and Mitchell, 1956; Rashbass and Westheimer, 1961a; Zuber and Stark, 1968). Needless to say both targets should be at a fixed distance from the subject and the magnitude of the apparent target motion should be small to prevent accommodative inputs (Fry, 1939). In order to avoid inputs to the versional system the apparent motion of the target should be confined to the midline (symmetrical vergence), which is to say that the error signals for the two eyes should be equal in magnitude and opposite in direction.

Fusional Vergence

Transient Inputs

Pulse Response. Typical fusional convergence pulse responses are shown in Fig. 6. These are computer averages of responses to convergence pulses 2.0° in amplitude with durations of 100 msec and 500 msec. The response to the shorter duration pulse reaches a maximum amplitude of only 0.47° while the response to the longer duration pulse almost matches the amplitude of the stimulus. These responses (Zuber and Stark, 1968) compare favorably with those of Rashbass and Westheimer (1961a) who examined the responses to pulses of constant amplitude and variable duration. These authors were able to record responses to pulses with durations as short as 20 msec, and concluded from their results that vergence movements could be modified as a result of information assimilated during the latent period and during the movement itself. Both Rashbass and Westheimer (1961a) and Zuber and Stark (1968) pointed out the essential difference between this type of pulse response and that observed in the case of saccadic movements. Thus, the vergence system seems to be continuous in contrast to the decidedly refractory nature of the saccadic system.

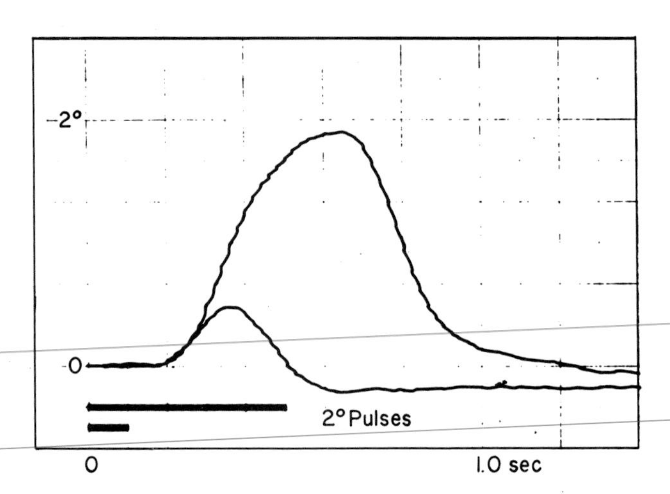

Fig. 6. Computer averages of fusional convergence responses to 2° pulses with 100 and 500 msec durations. Starting position of the eyes (shown as "0") actually represents 6.2° of convergence (Zuber and Stark, 1968).

Step Response. Fig. 7a shows the response to a pulse with a duration of 1.7 sec which is essentially the response to both positive (convergence) and negative (divergence) step stimuli since the eye has time to reach a steady state while the pulse is on. Notice that the asymmetry of the pulse response (Fig. 6) is carried over to the step response – convergence occurs slightly more rapidly than divergence. This asymmetrical nonlinearity can be more clearly observed in Fig. 7b which shows the averages of thirty-five responses to 1.7° step stimuli to both convergence and divergence. Notice that in this case the starting position of the eye is the same in both cases (6.2° of convergence) as opposed to the pulse response of Fig. 7a. Similar asymmetries in vergence responses were noted by Westheimer and Mitchell (1956) although not consistently. The step responses of Rashbass and Westheimer (1961a) also display asymmetries although in some cases these appear to be the opposite of those in Fig. 7, *i.e.*, divergence appears to be the faster component. It is possible that this may be partly attributed to the use of a curvilinear recording system which makes interpretation of symmetry somewhat more difficult.

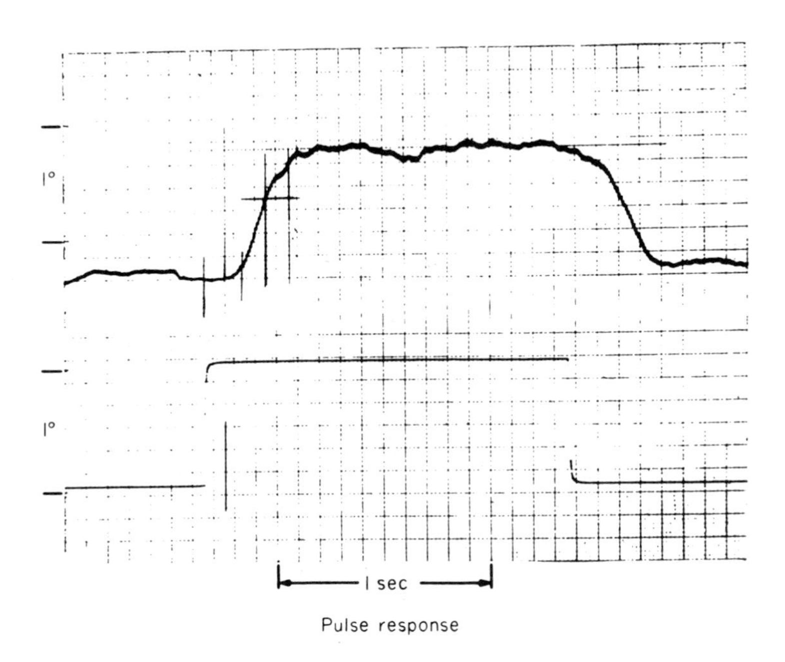

Fig. 7. (a) Single fusional convergence response to a 1° pulse of duration 1.7 sec. Notice asymmetry in response. Starting position as in Fig. 6 (Zuber and Stark, 1968).

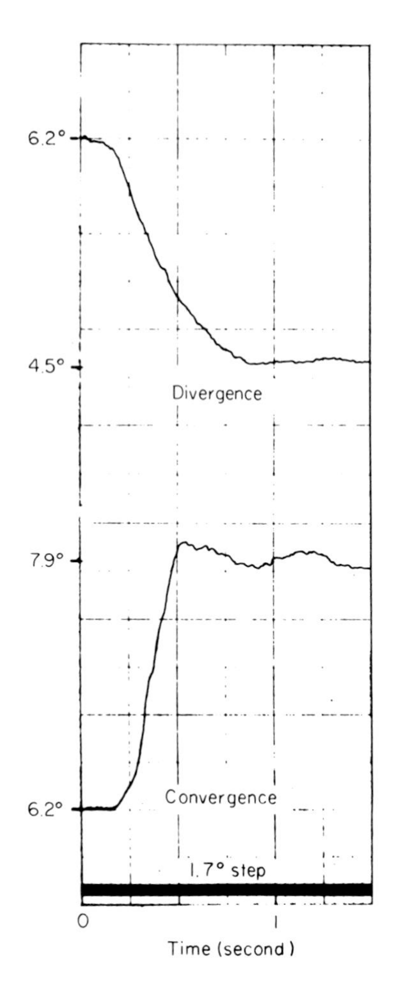

(b) The asymmetrical nonlinearity in the fusional vergence system as exhibited by step responses to convergence and divergence (Zuber and Stark, 1968).

Ramp and Parabola Responses. Single responses to step changes in target velocity *(ramp)* and acceleration *(parabola)* are shown in Fig. 8a and 8b, respectively. Judging from the close similarity of input and output in both cases, the vergence system is apparently capable of performing both constant velocity and constant acceleration movements. Because the system has no effective rapid position correction mechanism similar to the saccadic movement, a position error or offset would be expected during these transient movements, although the rate of change of error magnitude is maintained near zero. Such a position error is incurred because of the latency between stimulus and response. A similar situation is expected in steady state sinusoidal tracking where the position offset would be due both to latency and to the frequency-dependent phase lag introduced by the system dynamics.

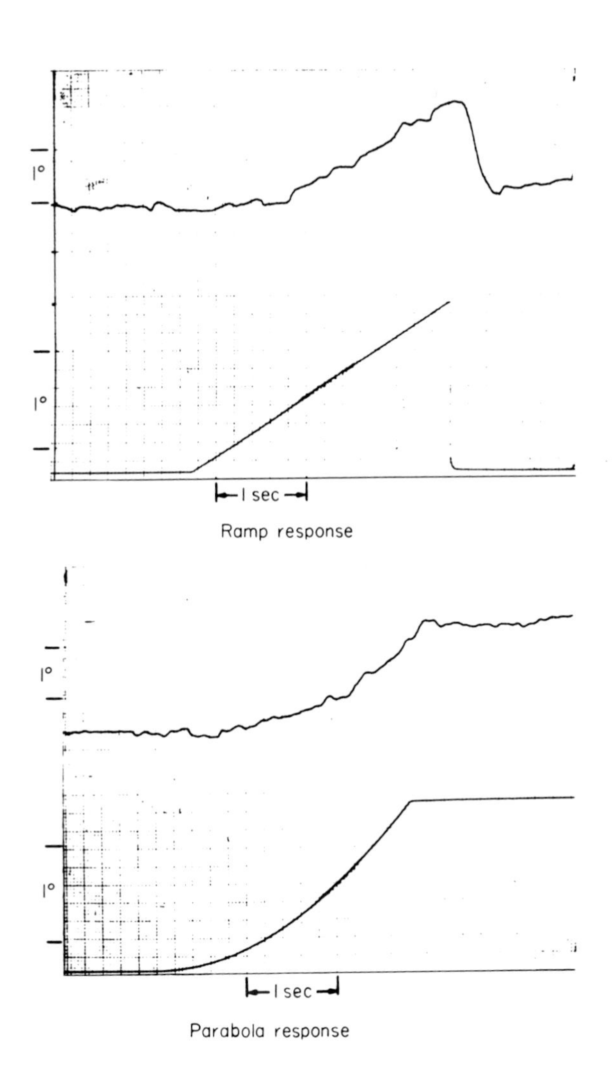

Fig. 8. Ramp (a) and parabola (b) response of fusional vergence. Note the absence of rapid position correction mechanism. Starting position as in Fig. 6 (Zuber and Stark, 1968).

Frequency Response

Closed Loop. Utilizing computer averaging techniques Zuber and Stark (1968) obtained closed loop frequency response data on the fusional vergence mechanism using sinusoidal stimuli in the frequency range of 0.01 to 4.0 Hz. Input amplitudes were 1.7° peak-to-peak or smaller. Although Rashbass and

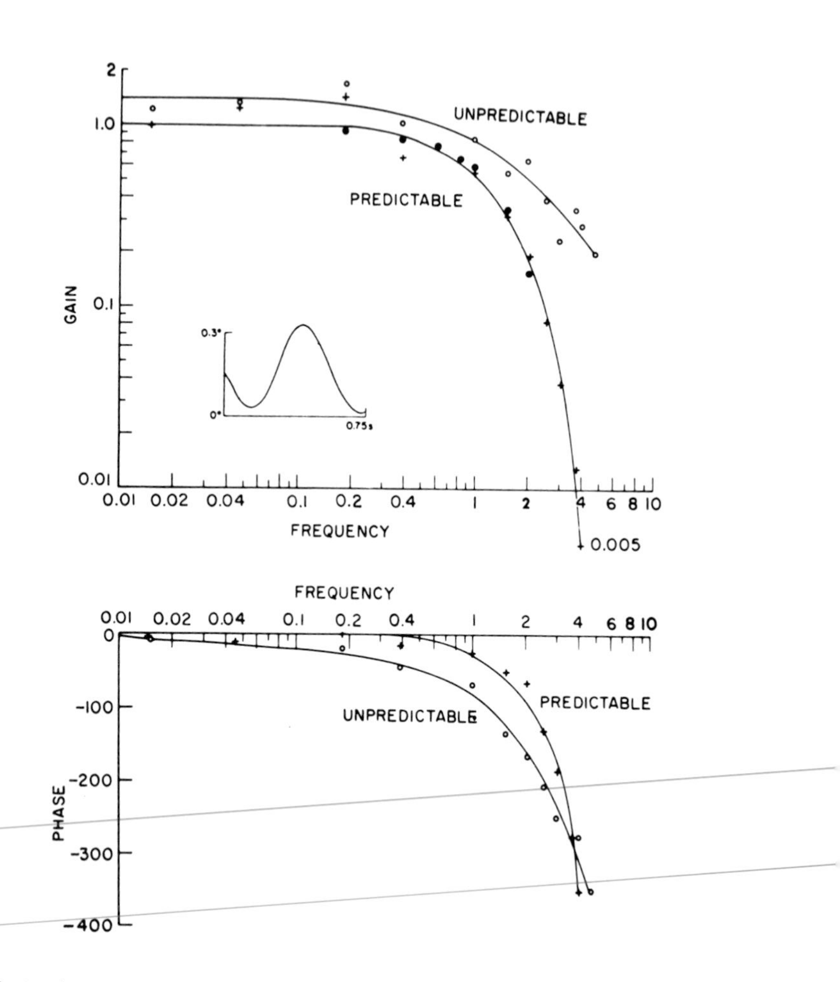

Fig. 9 (a, inset) The average fusional vergence response to a sinusoidal input at 2.0 Hz. with peak-to-peak amplitude of 1.7° about an average convergence level of 6.2°. (Zuber and Stark, 1968).
(b) Predictable and unpredictable closed loop frequency response of fusional vergence from Zuber and Stark, 1968. Closed circles on gain plot are predictable data of Yoshida and Watanabe (1969).

Westheimer (1961b) reported that sinusoidal fusional vergence tracking at 1.0 Hz. died out after the first few cycles of response, Zuber and Stark (1968) observed clear sinusoidal responses in the raw data up to 4.0 Hz. The average response at 2.0 Hz. is shown in Fig. 9a. Yoshida and Watanabe (1969) have also obtained frequency response data up to 2.0 Hz. Closed loop gain and phase data for midline fusional vergence are shown in Fig. 9b. The predictable frequency response was obtained using sinusoidal stimuli at a single frequency, while the unpredictable data were obtained using a mixture of sinusoidal waveforms at different frequencies (Stark, *et al*, 1962). The solid points near the predictable gain curve are the data of Yoshida and Watanabe (1969) for which only gain determinations were made. The difference between the predictable and unpredictable phase curves indicates that for repetitive "monotonous" stimuli the central nervous system is capable of compensating for inherent lags in the system. This is manifested by the consistently smaller phase lag associated with predictable stimuli. A similar phenomenon has been found associated with versional tracking (Stark, et al, 1962).

The difference between the predictable and unpredictable gain curves seems to be the result of an input-amplitude dependent nonlinearity, rather than of prediction. Figure 10 shows predictable frequency response data obtained with three different peak-to-peak amplitude stimuli. The largest amplitude stimulus (1.7°) corresponds to that used in predictable frequency response studies of Fig. 9b, while the smallest amplitude (1.7/3°) is equivalent to the contribution of a single frequency sinusoid to the unpredictable stimulus. These curves are superimposable on their gain curve counterparts in Fig. 9b, indicating that the difference between predictable and unpredictable gain curves resulted from different effective input amplitudes. There is no amplitude-dependent trend in the phase data of Fig. 10. The nonlinearity apparently primarily affects the gain of the system.

Open Loop. The effect of the physiological feedback loop in the fusional vergence system may be cancelled by placing in parallel with it an equivalent artificial *(electronic)* loop such that the effects of the two loops are equal and opposite. One way of doing this is by locking the image of the target onto the retina – practically this means controlling target position with a signal proportional to eye position (Rashbass and Westheimer, 1961a; Zuber and Stark, 1968). Once the loop is opened any error signal *(displacement of target image from fovea)* will result in eye movement, but this movement will not serve to reduce the error. The eye will thus continue to move until it saturates unless the error signal is somehow otherwise reduced. This integrator action of the open loop system is nicely demonstrated in Fig. 11, where it is seen that a small square wave input results in a triangular wave output. The factor of ten difference in the scale of stimulus and response is another reflection of integrator action, specifically a relatively large low frequency gain for the open loop system.

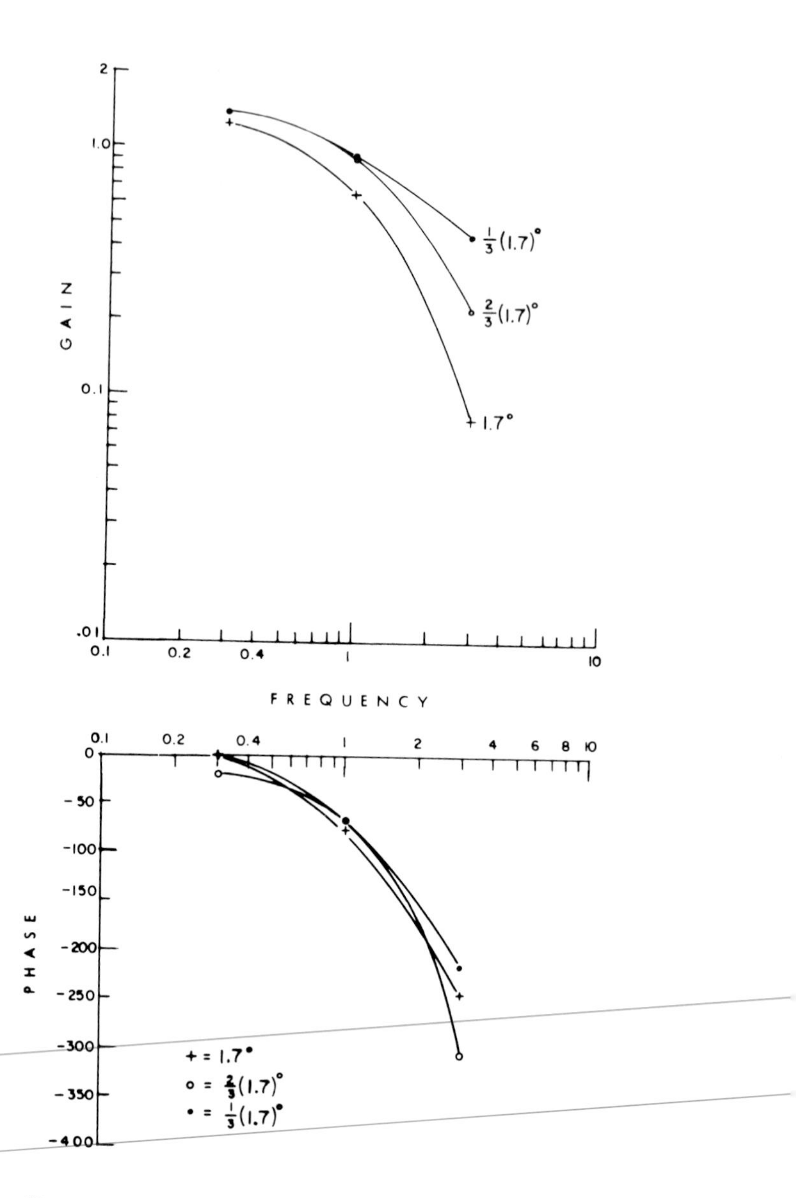

Fig. 10. Effect of input amplitude on fusional vergence closed loop frequency response. An input-amplitude dependent nonlinearity affects primarily the gain of the system and may be used to explain the separation of predictable and unpredictable gain curves in Fig. 9b (Zuber and Stark, 1968).

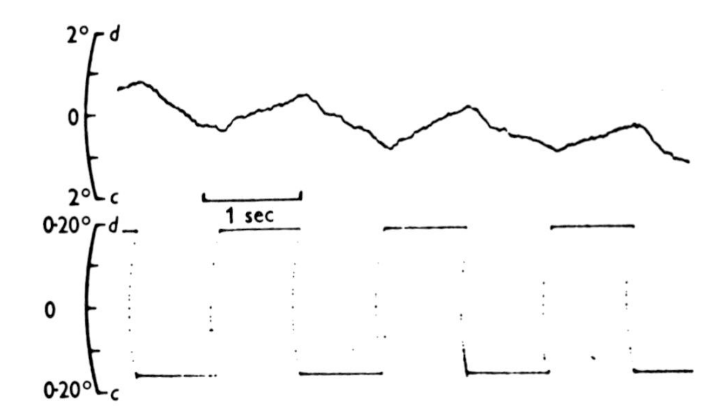

Fig. 11. The integrator action of the open loop fusional vergence system as shown by the triangular wave response to a small square wave input (Rashbass and Westheimer, 1961a).

Open loop frequency response data are shown in Fig. 12. These were obtained using 0.2 to 0.4° peak-to-peak predictable sinusoidal inputs. The straight-line segments of slopes 0, –0.98 and –2.34 were used to approximate the gain data of Zuber and Stark (1968). The open circles represent the data points of Rashbass and Westheimer (1961a). Although their gain measurements were higher, the data points clearly follow the same trend (slope of –1) as the gain data in the corresponding frequency range as measured by Zuber and Stark (1968). The phase data

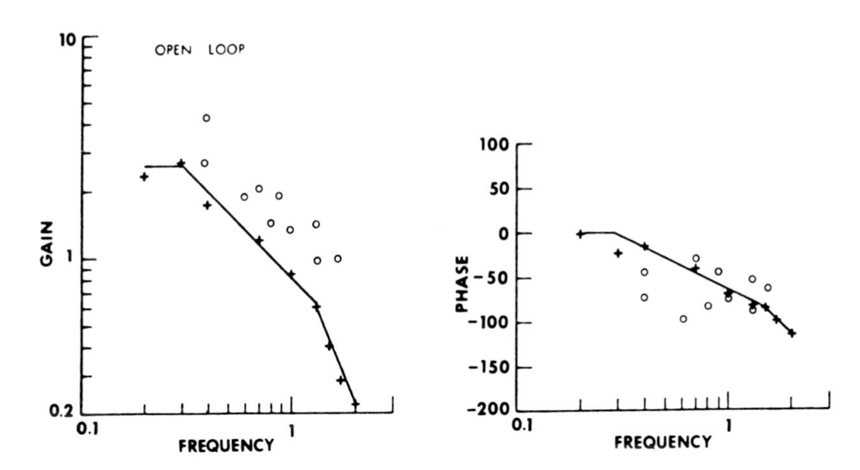

Fig. 12. Open loop frequency response of the fusional vergence system. Straight line approximations are drawn to the data of Zuber and Stark (1968). Open circles are data of Rashbass and Westheimer (1961a).

points from these two studies appear to fall into the same range, although the points of Rashbass and Westheimer (1961a) follow less of a pronounced trend. In both studies it was noted that the open loop system exhibited less than the minimum phase lag predicted from the integrator behavior of the system (–90° at low frequencies). Rashbass and Westheimer (1961a) suggested that prediction might play a role in the reduction of phase lag, but Zuber and Stark (1968) found little difference in the open loop phase characteristics using predictable or unpredictable stimuli.

Finally, the system may be driven into instability oscillations by increasing the loop gain with the electronic feedback path. Theoretically these oscillations should occur at the frequency where the physiologically intact (with no artificial feedback) closed loop system exhibits 180° of phase lag. As shown in Fig. 13, under conditions of artifically increased loop gain the system oscillates smoothly at an average frequency of 2.5 Hz. Figure 9b indicates that the normal closed loop system, with unpredictable stimuli, exhibits 180° of phase lag at approximately 2.3 Hz. Thus, high gain instability oscillations occur at approximately the predicted frequency, providing support for the closed loop frequency response data.

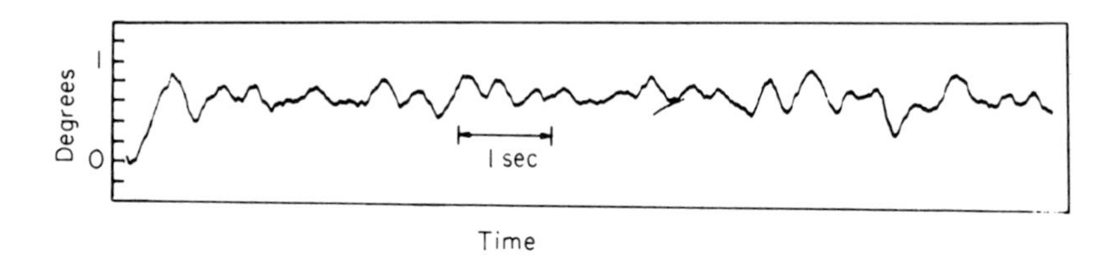

Fig. 13. High gain instability oscillations in fusional vergence caused by artificially elevating the loop gain (Zuber and Stark, 1968).

Accommodative Vergence

There is less available information on the control characteristics of accommodative vergence eye movements than that summarized above for fusional vergence. The reason for this is not clear in view of the fact that an accommodative input is relatively easy to generate as compared to a pure fusional input. A problem of particular interest is the dynamic correspondence between the refractive state of the lens and the position of the fellow eye being driven by the accommodative system. The data on accommodative vergence discussed in previous sections have all been of the static variety.

Transient Inputs

Step Response. Yoshida and Watanabe (1969) measured the response of accommodation and accommodative vergence resulting from a step input to accommodation. The responses to a step input of slightly less than 2 diopters are shown in Fig. 14. There is a remarkable similarity between the details of the two traces, indicating that noise generated in the accommodative system is probably transmitted through the accommodative vergence system, finally appearing superimposed on the oculomotor output.

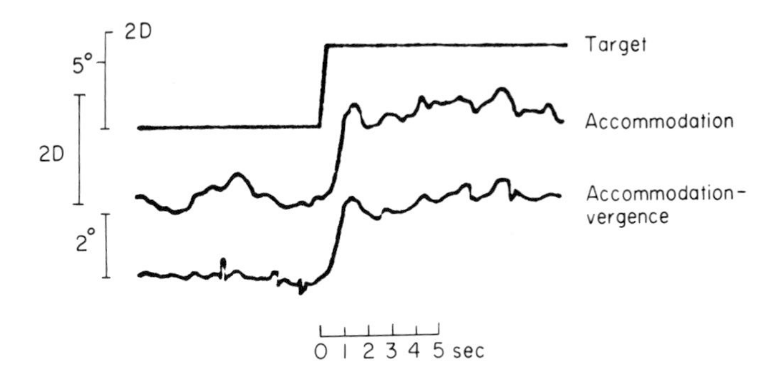

Fig. 14. Accommodative and accommodative vergence response to a step input to accommodation. Notice that much of the noise generated in the accommodative system appears superimposed on the accommodative vergence output (Yoshida and Watanabe, 1969).

Frequency Response

Data from two studies of the closed loop dynamics of accommodative vergence are shown in Fig. 15. The curves are drawn through the data points of Troelstra, et al (1963) while the closed circles represent the data of Yoshida and Watanabe (1969). It is obvious that there are significant differences between these data. Yoshida and Watanabe (1969) measure consistently lower gain and higher phase lag over the entire frequency range. The separation of the gain points from these two studies varies from 10 to 20 db with a distinct trend indicating that the separation increases with increasing frequency. Thus, the difference in the two sets of gain points cannot be reconciled by applying a constant "fudge factor", which might be the case if, for example, different definitions of gain had been used in the two studies. It appears that the two sets of data actually represent different dynamics. The phase data are separated by 20 to 30 degrees of phase lag with no apparent frequency-dependent trend. Considerable variability may also be seen in the accommodative vergence frequency response data obtained by Brodkey and Stark (1967). The reasons for the lack of consistency of data among the few studies of this mechanism is not presently clear.

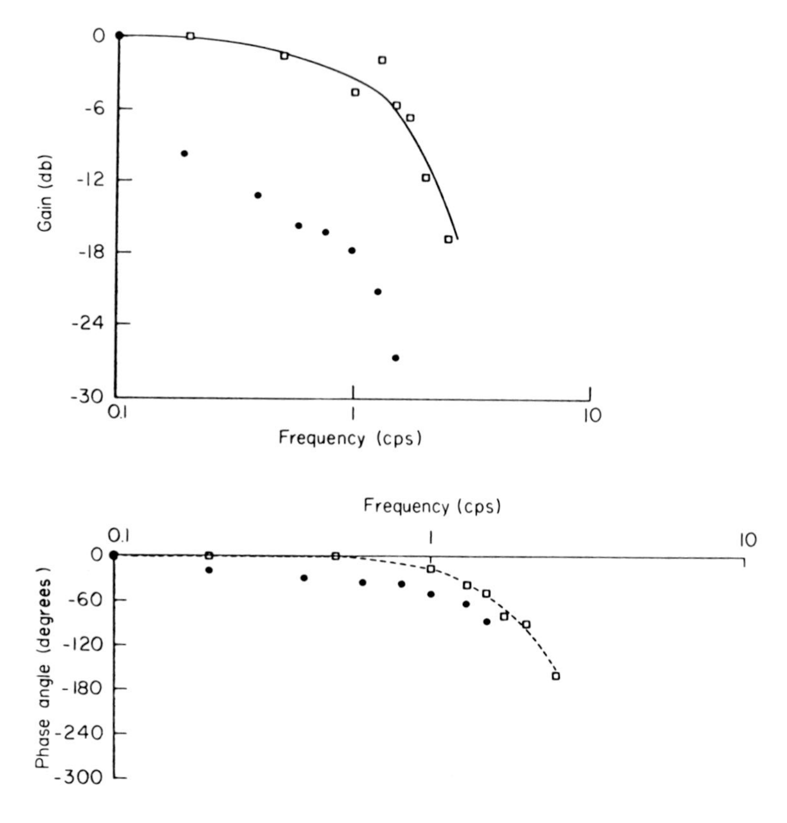

Fig. 15. Closed loop frequency response data for accommodative vergence system. Curves are drawn through the data of Troelstra, *et al.* (1963). Closed circles are data of Yoshida and Watanabe (1969). Lack of consistency in these two sets of data is difficult to explain.

SUMMARY

The vergence system is the stepchild of the oculomotor sub-systems in that it has received considerably less attention from researchers than has the versional system. Complexities are met at the input to the vergence system where either fusional or accommodative stimuli may be used to drive the system. Both of these inputs are difficult to generate compared to relatively simple versional inputs.

When presented with an asymmetrical input the pattern of oculomotor response is determined by the characteristics of target movement, notably target velocity, and by whether or not the fusional mechanism is activated. Under such conditions the eye movement response may be compound, involving the algebraic summation of independent versional and vergence components. In this case a generalized pattern of compound versional-vergence eye movements appears to be followed. Under other conditions vergence movements may be uniocular.

At the output of the vergence system the range of eye movement is about one fourth of the range of versional movements. The system interacts in a complex, and as yet incompletely understood, fashion with the accommodative and pupillary systems as an integral part of the so-called near triad.

Vergence dynamics may be studied by "dissecting" the system through the use of appropriate input formats. Thus, the dynamics of fusional and accommodative vergence movements may be separately studied. The fusional vergence system responds continuously with no apparent refractoriness – movements may be modified by input information coming in during a latent period or during an ongoing movement. During movement the system is apparently satisfied to minimize the rate of change of retinal error, while tolerating a certain *dc* offset resulting either from latency or other inherent lags in the system, or both. This behavior may result from the absence of a rapid position correction mechanism. When responding to periodic or *"monotonus"* inputs a certain amount of prediction may occur, effectively reducing inherent system lags. Two types of nonlinearity are seen in the fusional vergence system. One is an input amplitude dependent nonlinearity which is manifested for inputs as small as a fraction of a degree, and which appears to affect primarily the gain of the system. The second type is an asymmetrical nonlinearity which is manifested in a slightly more rapid convergence response. These nonlinearities make a linear treatment of the fusional vergence system difficult at best.

In the accommodative vergence system recent evidence indicates that noise generated in the accommodative system appears in the oculomotor output. The few available studies of accommodative vergence dynamics are inconsistent and difficult to reconcile. The reason for this is not clear.

It is evident that many gaps remain in our understanding of the vergence eye movement system. When some of these gaps are filled we may begin to understand, for example, how the visual-oculomotor system handles and operates on complex asymmetrical retinal error signals, and what causes the oculomotor imbalance leading to strabismus.

REFERENCES

ALPERN, M. (1957). The position of the eyes during prism vergence. *A.M.A. Arch Ophthal.* **57,** 345-353.

ALPERN, M. (1962). Types of movement. **In,** *The Eye* vol. 3, Davson, H., Ed. Academic Press, Ney York, pp. 63-143.

ALPERN, M. and ELLEN, P. (1956a). A quantitative analysis of the horizontal movements of the eyes in the experiment of Johannes Mueller. I. Methods and results. *Am. J. Ophthal.* **42,** 289-296.

ALPERN, M. and ELLEN, P. (1956b). A quantitative analysis of the horizontal movements of the eyes in the experiment of Johannes Mueller. II. Effect of variation of target separation. *Am. J. Ophthal.*, **42,** 296-302.

ALPERN, M., KINCAID, W.M. and LUBECK, M.J. (1959). Vergence and accommodation III. Proposed definitions of the AC/A ratios. *Am. J. Ophthal.*, **48,** 141-148.

ALPERN, M., MASON, G.L., and JARDINICO, R.E. (1961). Vergence and accommodation. V. Pupil size changes associated with changes in accommodative vergence. *Am. J. Ophthal.* **52,** 762-767.

ALPERN, M. and WOLTER, J.R. (1956). The relation of horizontal saccadic and vergence movements. *A.M.A. Arch. Ophthal.* **56,** 685-690.

BACKER, W.D. and OGLE, K.N. (1964). Pupillary response to fusional eye movements. *Am. J. Ophthal.* **58,** 743-756.

BREININ, G.M. (1955). The nature of vergence revealed by electromyography. *A.M.A. Arch. Ophthal.* **54,** 407-409.

BREININ, G.M. (1957). The nature of vergence revealed by electromyography II. Accommodative and fusional vergence. *A.M.A. Arch. Ophthal.* **58,** 623-631.

BRODKEY, J.S. and STARK, L. (1967). Accommodative convergence--an adaptive nonlinear control system. *IEEE Trans. Sys. Sci. Cyber.* **SSC-3,** 121-133.

DODGE, R. (1903). Five types of eye movements in the horizontal meridian plane of the field of regard. *Am. J. Physiol.* **8,** 307-329.

DUANE, A. (1933). Binocular movements. *Arch. Ophthal.* **9,** 579-607.

FRY, G.A. (1939). Further experiments on the accommodation-convergence relationship. *Am. J. Optom.* **16,** 325-334.

MARG. E. and MORGAN, M.W. (1950). The pupillary fusion reflex. *A.M.A. Arch. Ophthal.* **43,** 871-878.

PEACHEY, L.D. (1968). Muscle. *Ann. Rev. Physiol.* **30,** 401-440.

RASHBASS, C. and WESTHEIMER, G. (1961a). Disjunctive eye movements. *J. Physiol.* **159,** 339-360.

RASHBASS, C. and WESTHEIMER, G. (1961b). Independence of conjugate and disjunctive eye movements. *J. Physiol.*, **159,** 361-364.

RIGGS, L.A. and NIEHL, E.W. (1960). Eye movements recorded during convergence and divergence. *J. Optical Soc. Am.*, **50,** 913-920.

RIPPS, H., CHIN, N.B., SIEGEL, I.M. and BREININ, G.M. (1962). The effect of pupil size on accommodation, convergence and the AC/A ratio. *Invest. Ophthal.* **1,** 127-135.

STARK, L., VOSSIUS, G., and YOUNG, L.R. (1962). Predictive control of eye tracking movements. *IRE Trans. Hum. Fac. Elec.*, **HFE-3,** 52-57.

TAMLER, E., JAMPOLSKY, A., and MARG, E. (1958). An electromyographic study of asymmetric convergence. *Am. J. Ophthal.* **46,** 174-182.

TROELSTRA, A. and STARK, L. (1963). Associated eye movements. Qtrly. Prog. Rept. No. 70, Research Laboratory of Electronics, M.I.T. pp. 342-345.

TROELSTRA, A., ZUBER, B.L., SIMPSON, J.I., and STARK, L. (1963). Pupil variation and disjunctive eye movements as a result of photic and accommodative stimulation. Qtrly. Prog. Rept. No. 69, Research Laboratory of Electronics, M.I.T., pp. 250-253.

WESTHEIMER, G. (1954). Eye movement responses to a horizontally moving visual stimulus. *A.M.A. Arch Ophthal.* **52,** 932-941.

WESTHEIMER, G. and MITCHELL, A.M. (1956). Eye movement responses to convergence stimuli. *A.M.A. Arch. Ophthal.* **55,** 848-856.

YARBUS, A.L. (1957). Motion of the eye on interchanging fixation points at rest in space. *Biofizika.* **2,** 698-702.

YOSHIDA, T. and WANTANABE, A. (1969). Analysis of interaction between accommodation and vergence feedback control systems of human eyes. *Bull. NHK Broadcasting Science Research Lab.* **3,** 72-80.

YOUNG, L.R. and STARK, L. (1963). A discrete model for eye tracking movements. *IEEE Trans. on Military Electron.* **MIL-7,** 113-115.

ZUBER, B.L. (1967). Asymmetrical fusional vergence: Eye movements resulting from target movement along the visual axis of one eye. *Presbyterian-St. Luke's Hosp. Med. Bull.* **6,** 15-20.

ZUBER, B.L. and STARK, L. (1968). Dynamical characteristics of the fusional vergence eye-movement system. *IEEE Trans. Sys. Sci. Cyber.* **SSC-4,** 72-79.

DISCUSSION OF THE CONTROL OF EYE VERGENCE MOVEMENTS

GERALD WESTHEIMER

There are three experiments that I would like to talk about because they tie in Dr. Zuber's presentation with some further aspects of sensory and motor physiology.

The first two relate to the question of how the need for a vergence movement is recognized and its magnitude and direction fixed.

Fig. 1 is a diagram from work done a decade ago by Rashbass and me (Rashbass and Westheimer, 1961) in which the velocity of an open-loop vergence movement is shown against the imposed disparity. Disparity is clearly being measured in the CNS because the vergence velocities shown are achieved immediately (approximately 200 msec) and without feedback. The experiments were done with a single spot in front of each eye in an otherwise dark visual field. Since then, Mitchell and I (Westheimer and Mitchell, 1969) have carried out further experiments to find out what kind of target shapes (one to each eye) will do as well as the two horizontally displaced spots (one to each eye) that were used previously. We originally thought that in this way we could measure the spatial extent of the line units in our cortex which were connected up to produce convergence movements. As it turned out, a large range of target configurations (Fig. 2) will serve equally well to trigger off vergence movements. These movements were specific insofar as target configurations outside the range of the ones illustrated failed to trigger off any movements at all. Also, our vergence movements, when they occurred, were always in the correct direction and never wrong or random. Figure 2 implies that there is a wide range of disparate retinal regions from which non-shape specific stimuli coming in through one eye are compared with just about any stimulus coming in through the other, and the recognition made whether the whole configuration occurred with crossed or uncrossed disparity. This diffuse connection between the uniocular projections contrasted so sharply with the line-specific, usually binocularly-summated projection shown by single unit recordings in the visual cortex (Hubel and Wiesel, 1962), even in the unanesthetized monkey (Wurtz, 1969), that we thought for a while that we might be investigating the bilateral connectivity of a lower projection, say at the level of the superior colliculus. It was, therefore, of particular interest to us to find that one of Sperry and Gazzaniga's subjects, whose

This work was supported in part by the National Institutes of Neurological Diseases and Stroke, U.S. Public Health Service under grant NS-08091.

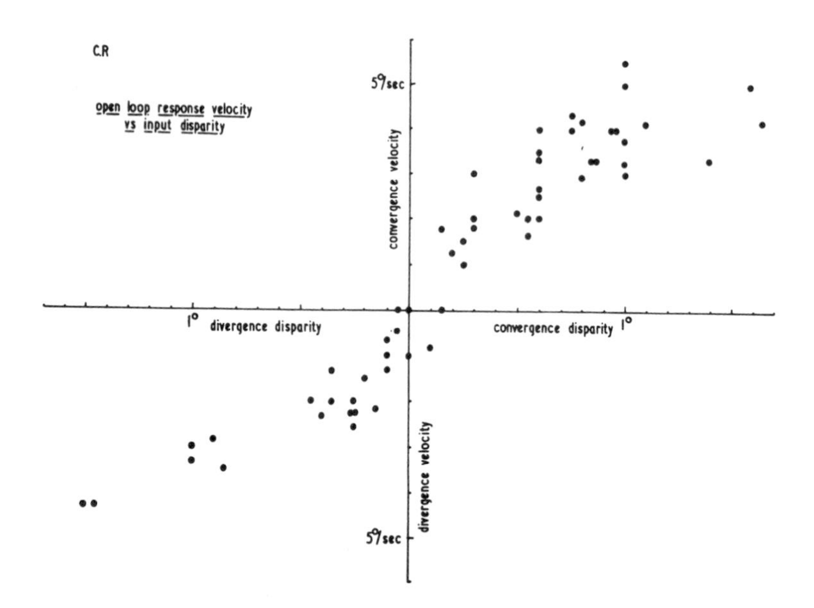

Fig. 1. Experiment on open-loop vergence responses. A spot was seen by each eye. By means of an electro-optical system each spot was moved horizontally so that the pair of spots maintained a fixed binocular disparity during the presentation. This always resulted in a constant velocity vergence movement. This graph gives the relationship between the imposed disparity and the velocity of the resulting eye vergence movements. From *Rashbass, C. and G. Westheimer,* 1961).

corpus callosum had been surgically sectioned, did not evidence vergence movements when the disparate stimulation was such that the eyes and hemispheres were always kept separated. When both eyes' stimulation reached the same hemisphere, this subject made normal vergence movements.

We draw the conclusion that in man there is a cortical projection which keeps the information intact as to which eye received the stimulation but that this information can be pooled over a relatively large area and then compared with that coming in through the other eye for the decision to be reached whether convergence or divergence is needed.

This experiment may be contrasted with the results of a whole series of electrophysiological studies in the cat visual cortex. This series was initiated by Pettigrew (1965) and has since had satisfactory confirmation (Barlow, Blakemore and Pettigrew, 1967; Nikara, Bishop and Pettigrew, 1968; Burns and Pritchard, 1968). Single units were isolated in the visual cortex and their receptive fields measured as seen through each eye. The units were most sensitive to lines of a given direction and could be driven by either eye. However, when a series of such units was checked, it was found that their binocular fields did not coincide (Fig. 3). The phenomenon is independent of eye

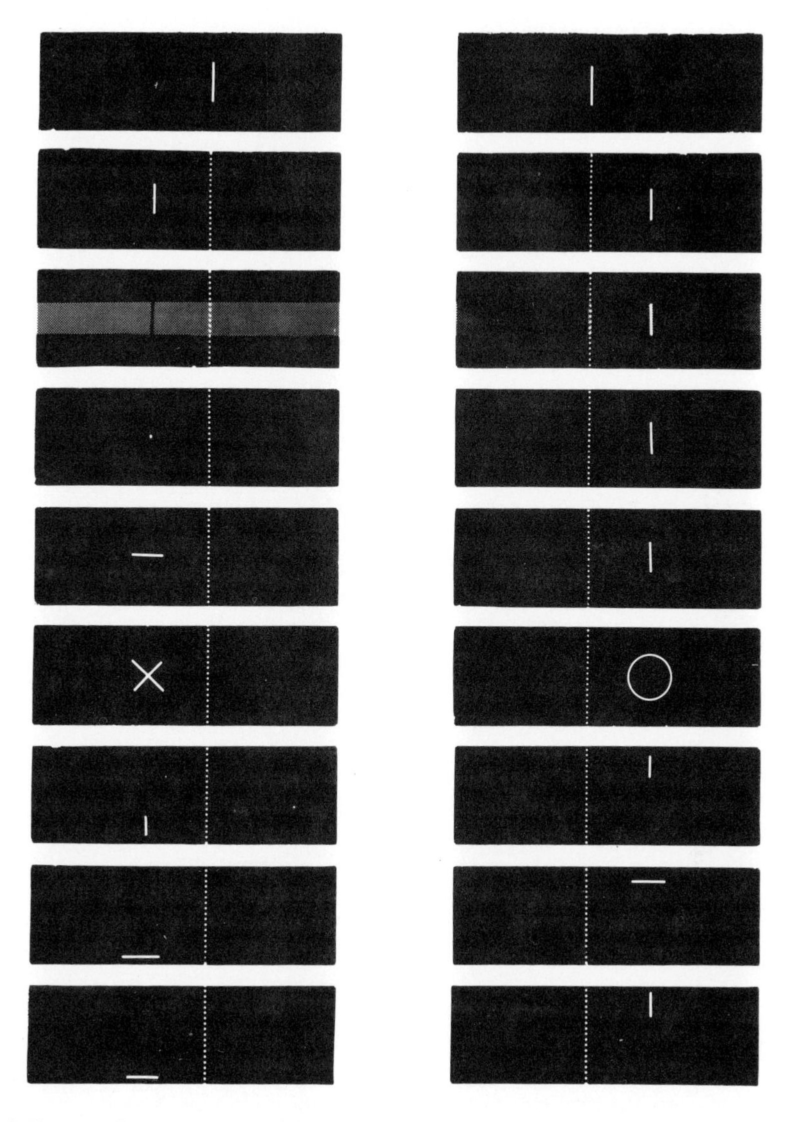

Fig. 2. Target configurations which are all equally effective in initiating a vergence movement. Initially both eyes fixed a vertical line binocularly (top row). This was briefly replaced by one of the presentations shown in each subsequent row. All these disparate targets succeeded in eliciting a vergence movement. The study by Westheimer and Mitchell (1969) contains further details of the spatial and temporal characteristics of disparate configurations that can initiate vergence movements.

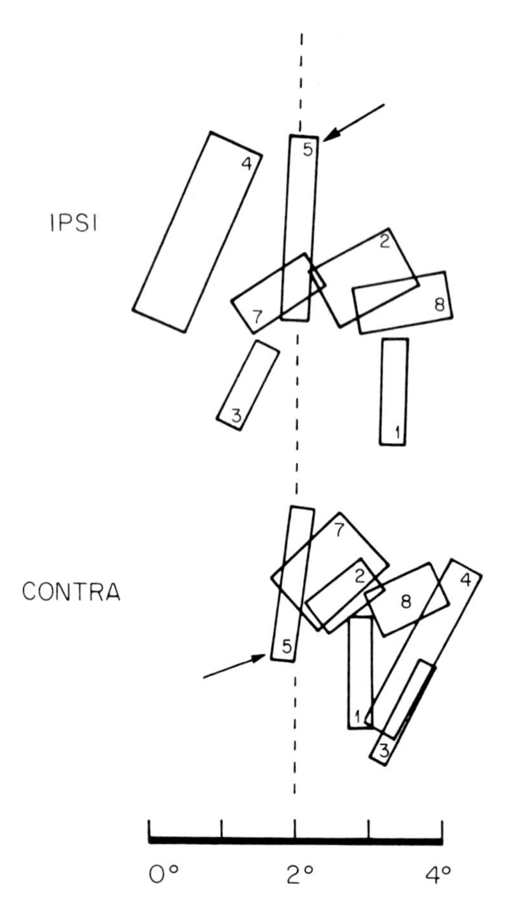

Fig. 3. Receptive field disparities of single units in visual cortex of cat. The contralateral receptive field plots have been positioned beneath those from the ipsilateral eye so that pair 5 are vertically in line. Reprinted by permission from *Nikara, Bishop and Pettigrew* (1968).

movements or any error in the absolute measurement of disparity. It now seems clear that a certain range of disparity is represented in a population of simple (line) cortical units in the primary cortical visual projection. There is no more scatter in the horizontal direction than in the vertical direction (Fig. 4) though there is greater need and capability for handling horizontal disparities. There is even an added aspect of these neurophysiological findings that must appeal to the clinician. The response of these neurons is maximal when a stimulus is presented in the visual field with a certain critical amount of disparity. The response falls off when the stimuli are not presented

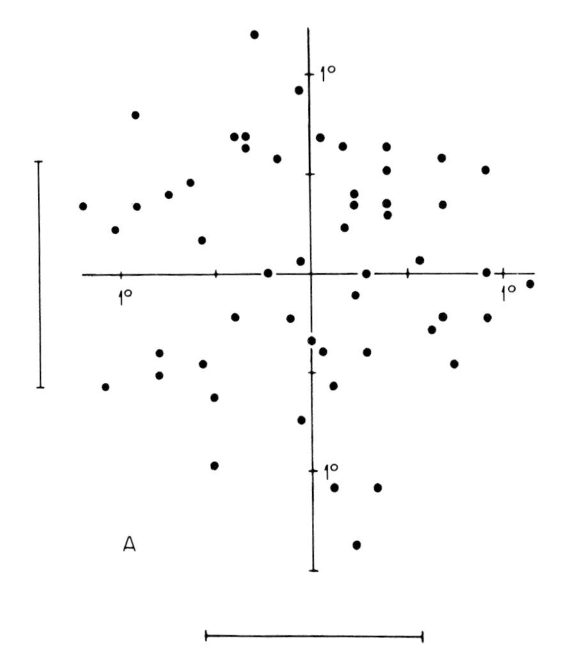

Fig. 4. Horizontal and vertical scatter of receptive field disparities of binocular units in cat visual cortex. Reprinted by permission from *Nikara, Bishop and Pettigrew* (1968).

with this optimal disparity, but in some units there is a clear added reduction of response for a small range of disparities just a little away from the optimum value (Pettigrew, Nikara, and Bishop, 1968). This is certainly reminiscent to the suppression one finds clinically in strabismus.

It is too early to put these findings together into a coherent story about the neural representation of the third spatial dimension. It was first thought that the disparity-specific cortical neurons might subserve the kind of convergence responses specified by Rashbass and Westheimer (1961). But the later findings by Westheimer and Mitchell (1969) suggest that the sensory stimulus to the vergence system is too diffuse to have been funnelled through binocularly responding line elements. It has also been suggested that the spread of disparity of these cortical neurons is the basis of stereopsis. A great number of these units is required to represent in such a manner in the cortex the whole range of target positions, orientations and disparities (perhaps even colors, too) that can be distinguished. I would not be surprised if the neural representation of the third dimension in the cortex is other than by simply duplicating all other functional classifications in a whole new dimension. The separateness and superimposed character of the stereoptic sense of depth makes me suspect that it is something abstracted, perhaps by a system of collaterals organized along this dimension. Clearly this is a problem of considerable conceptual magnitude in which new developments are eagerly awaited.

Now I would like to turn to the motor component of eye vergence movements and review an interesting drug effect. Barbiturates have long been known to interfere with some eye movements. The pursuit movements, in particular, are known to be especially sensitive to barbiturates (Rashbass, 1961). This fact forms a helpful tool in the separation of saccadic and smooth pursuit aspects of a visual tracking task because saccadic movements are highly refractory to barbiturate intoxication. It is significant, therefore, that even a moderate sedative dose of amobarbital can almost totally knock out a normal convergence response (Fig. 5). Since saccadic and vestibular eye movements are perfectly normal when the patient is in this state, the peripheral motor apparatus cannot be involved. And, because the patient's accommodation and pupil responses to a close-up target are normal, his perceptual faculties cannot be impaired to the extent that the need for a vergence movement does not go through to his motor system.

In Fig. 6 we have a detailed set of static measurement of the whole vergence system taken over the course of a single session involving a sedative dose of a barbiturate. The major changes all are seen to follow about the same time course of intoxication and recovery lasting several hours. There is a conspicuous effect on breadth of range of prism vergence (it is reduced), distance heterophoria (it moves towards eso), near phoria (it moves towards exo), near point of convergence (it recedes). Accommodation remains normal throughout so that the ACA is quite markedly lowered.

The synkinesis of accommodation and convergence and the meaning of the influence of barbiturates on the vergence response can best be illustrated with the aid of the schematic diagram of Fig. 7. Each half of the diagram represents the feedback system for one of the two functions. In each case the motor output is compared with the sensory input and an error signal sent centrally. A central processor sends out a signal to the peripheral motor effector. For the case of convergence, the error signal is the target disparity which is the difference between the eyes' vergence position and the target vergence position. In the normal way of operation, a given disparity will lead to a vergence eye movement to bring the eye vergence error to zero, but if the eyes are in a phoria measuring situation, as with a Maddox rod in front of one eye, there is no disparity signal in the usual sense and the system is now open loop. In this state, the influence of extraneous inflows can be measured because any effect they exert will not lead to a correctional eye vergence movement and hence will show up quite openly. Accommodation is such an influence on convergence. When the eyes are made to accommodate and fusion is disrupted, the influence of accommodation on convergence, or clinically, the ACA, or in servo-theory, the cross-talk between the two systems, can be measured. We can view the findings shown in Figs. 5 and 6 in this frame work. The peripheral eye motor system works satisfactorily under

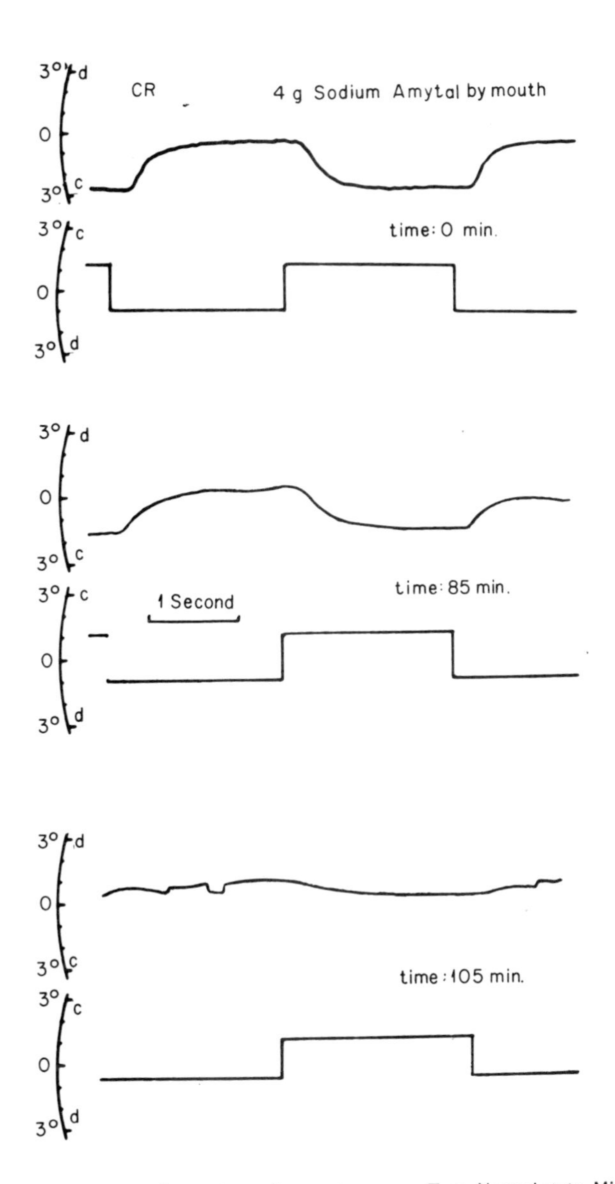

Fig. 5. Eye vergence response to 2° step change in target vergence. Top: Normal state. Middle: 85 min. after ingestion of 260 mgm of amytal sodium. Bottom: 105 min. after ingestion of 260 mgm amytal sodium. From *Westheimer and Rashbass* (1961).

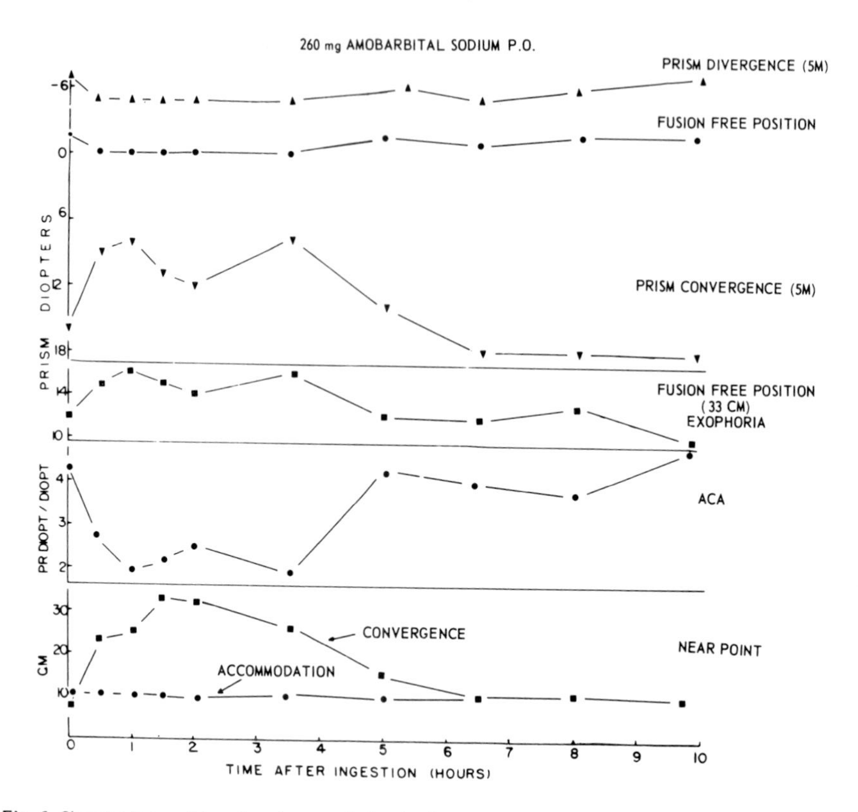

Fig. 6. Changes in a variety of ocular tests following ingestion of 260 mgm amobarbital sodium. Reprinted by permission from *Westheimer* (1963).

barbiturate intoxication because saccadic and vestibular eye movements are normal. Not only have normally triggered vergence movements failed, but also those produced by cross-talk from accommodation, while the accommodational responses themselves seem unaffected. It follows that there is a central (probably midbrain) site for convergence responses that is affected by barbiturates. We can also conclude that the cross-talk signals from accommodation feed into the vergence system at this level or central to it.

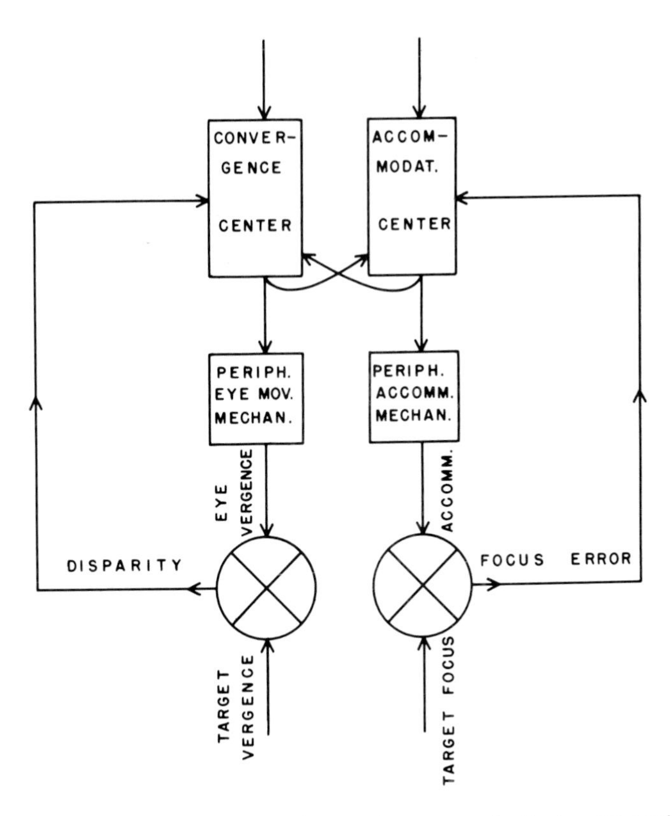

Fig. 7. Schematic diagram depicting accommodation and convergence feedback systems and their interrelationship. Arrow leading from box labeled "Accommodation Center" to box labeled "Convergence Center" is the schematic representation of the accommodation-convergence synkinesis here studied. Reprinted by permission from *Westheimer* (1963).

REFERENCES

BARLOW, H.B., BLAKEMORE, C. & PETTIGREW, J.D. (1967). The neural mechanism of binocular depth discrimination. *J. Physiol.* **193,** 327-342.

BURNS, B.D. & PRITCHARD, R.M. (1968). Cortical conditions for fused binocular vision. *J. Physiol.* **197,** 149-171.

HUBEL, D.H. & WIESEL, T.N. (1962). Receptive fields, binocular interaction and functional architecture in the cat's visual cortex. *J. Physiol.* **160,** 106-154.

NIKARA, T., BISHOP, P.O. & PETTIGREW J.D. (1968). Analysis of retinal correspondence by studying receptive fields of binocular single units in cat striate cortex. *Exper. Brain Res.* **6,** 353-372.

PETTIGREW, J.D. (1965). *Binocular Interaction on Single Units of the Striate Cortex of the Cat.* Thesis submitted for the degree B.Sc. (med) in the Department of Physiology, University of Sydney.

PETTIGREW, J.D., NIKARA. T., & BISHOP, P.O. (1968). Binocular interaction on single units in cat striate cortex: simultaneous stimulation by single moving slits with receptive field in correspondence. *Experim. Brain Research.* **6,** 391-410.

RASHBASS, C. (1961). The relationship between saccadic and smooth tracking eye movements. *J. Physiol.* **159,** 326-338.

RASHBASS, C. & WESTHEIMER, G. (1961). Disjunctive eye movements. *J. Physiol.* **159,** 339-360.

WESTHEIMER, G. (1963). Amphetamine barbiturates, and accommodation-convergence. *Archives of Ophthal. N.Y.* **70,** 830-836.

WESTHEIMER, G. & RASHBASS, C. (1961). Bartiburates and eye vergence. *Nature, Lond.* **191,** 833-834.

WESTHEIMER, G. & MITCHELL, D.E. (1969). The sensory stimulus for disjunctive eye movements. *Vision Res.* **9,** 749-755.

WURTZ, R.H. (1969). Visual receptive fields of striate cortex neurons in awake monkeys. *J. Neurophysiol.* **32,** 727-742.

VESTIBULAR AND PROPRIOCEPTIVE STABILIZATION OF EYE MOVEMENTS

JACOB L. MEIRY

The *eye* perceives body orientation with respect to the environment. This information is of high resolution and is referred to objects observed in the immediate surroundings. In addition, the human can exercise voluntary control of eye movements in searching for a reference to which he relates his orientation. These capabilities of the visual system render the eye as an orientation sensor of prime importance to man. However, the ocular mechanism is by itself a multi-input *servo-control system* with inputs fed to it by other orientation sensors, by the eye itself, and by the voluntary tracking intentions of humans. Therefore, the image of the outside world the eye will provide depends upon the visual and motion conditions in the man-environment system, and the dynamic characteristics of the sensors involved in sensing spatial orientation.

The eye movement control system rotates the eye in order to maintain the image of an object of fixation upon the retina. A displacement of this image is caused by the motion of the visual target and by rotations of the head on the body. The eye movement control system will respond to these motions with two different modes of eye movements: tracking and compensatory movements. Compensatory eye movements rotate the eye in a direction opposite to the rotation of the human body.

The eye has rotational freedom with respect to the skull and the skull as a whole may rotate with respect to the trunk with the neck as a pivot. Accordingly, the eyeball may be considered as mounted on two gimbals with limited freedom of motion with respect to the trunk.

Rotation and translation of the whole gimbal system or relative rotation between the head and the trunk will cause compensatory eye movements. Body motion stimulates the *vestibular system* and rotation of the head upon the trunk excites receptors in the neck. Clearly, the eye, the vestibular system and the receptors in the neck are the motion sensors involved in the eye movement control system.

The schematic diagram in Figure 1 shows the multi-input feature of the eye movement control system. The *semicircular canals* of the vestibular system and the relative *rotation* sensitive, neck receptors are the sensors which provide information about skull rotation in space. Since any rotation of the head, if not compensated by an opposite eye movement, will result in image displacement on the retina, the motion information does not need any processing and is fed directly into the motor end of the eye control servomechanism to initiate immediate compensatory eye movements. The tracking movements branch of the control loop responds to an error between the actual image of a fixation point on the retina and its desired location.

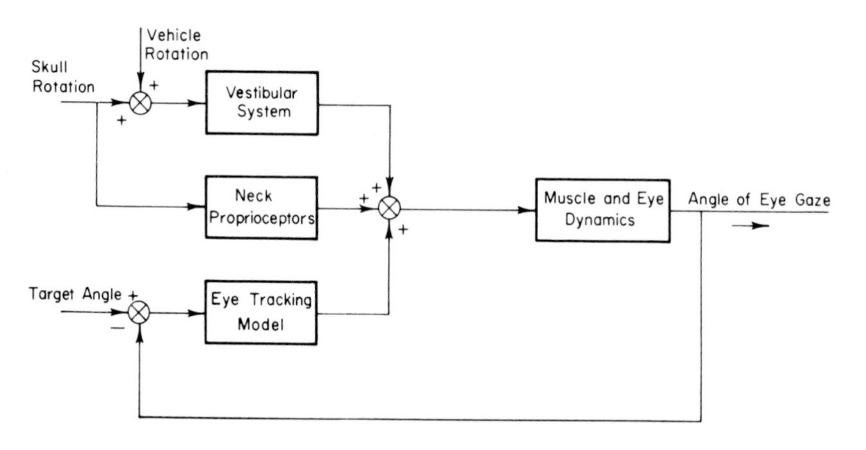

Fig. 1. Block Diagram of the Eye Movement Control System.

ANATOMICAL ASPECTS

The Vestibular System*

The human inner ear is divided into two parts: *1. the cochlea serving auditory function, and 2. a non-auditory portion, the vestibular system.* This structure, also called the labyrinth, lodges the sensors associated with maintenance of balance and orientation in three-dimensional space. One distinguishes between the bony labyrinth and the membranous labyrinth. The bony labyrinth is a cavity tunnelled in the temporal bone of the skull. Its structure forms three

*(Gray's *Anatomy;* Groen (1956-57)).

ducts, the semicircular canals, and the vestibule. This elaborate canal system contains in its cavities the membranous labyrinth suspended in perilymph. The suspension system of the membranous labyrinth does not allow it to move relative to the skull. Thus the accelerations acting on the membranous labyrinth are those applied to the head. The bony semicircular canals lodge the three semicircular canals, while the vestibule contains the utricle and the saccule (Figure 2). The membranous labyrinth contains fluid called endolymph.

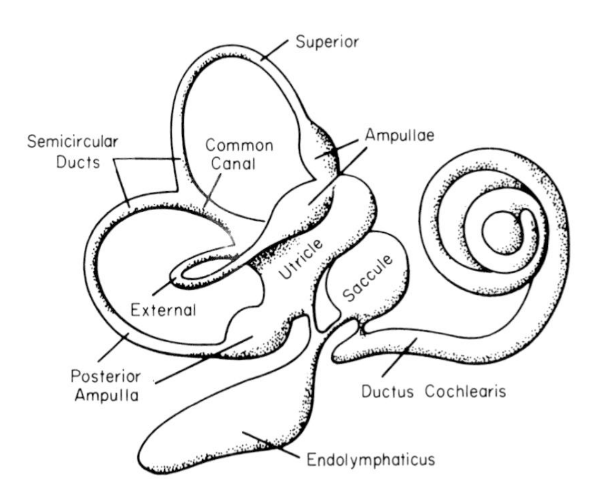

Fig. 2. The Membranous Inner Ear (Barnhill, 1940).

The utricle is the large, oblong sac occupying the vestibule. Its lower part forms a pouch where it thickens over an area of about $6mm^2$ (2mm x 3mm), and is known as the macula. The otolith, a gelatinous substance with calcium carbonate grains in it, and of specific density of around 2.95, is supported over the macula by strands allowing a limited sliding travel of about 0.1mm. The macula is the receptor end of this otolithic organ, providing the bed for the utricular branch of the vestibular nerve. The two utricles (one from each inner ear) are located in the same plane.

The utricle is a multi-dimensional linear accelerometer with the otolith being the moving mass. The plane, associated with the sensor, is relevant in determining the input accelerations to it.

The saccule is an organ with histological structure identical to that of the utricle. The plane of the saccular macula is perpendicular to that of the utricle.

The three semicircular canals are above and behind the vestibule. Their structure is planar, lying in planes which are roughly orthogonal to each other. The horizontal (lateral) canal is in a plane elevated about 25° to 30° from the horizontal plane. The other two canals, the posterior and the superior vertical, are in approximately vertical planes (See Figure 2). Note that the horizontal canals of the two ears lie in the same plane, while the superior canal of the left ear is coplanar with the posterior one of the right ear and vice versa.

The semicircular canals are heavily damped, angular accelerometers. Their arrangement in three perpendicular planes provides a way to sense components of angular acceleration along three axes which are amenable to easy vertorial manipulation.

Anatomy of the Neck – Rotation *

Rotation of the head with respect to the trunk is a coordinated effort of a number of joints and muscles. The head rotates about a vertical axis on a pivot joint. The dens of the axis vertebrae are a pivot around which the atlas rotates. These are the atlanto-axial joints which form a sealed capsule containing a viscous fluid called synovia. The atlanto-axial joints are three: 1. the two lateral atlanto-axial joints together with the ligamentum florum in back and part of the longitudinal ligament in front, form the joint cavity which encloses the space between the atlas and the axis vertebrae; 2. the median atlanto-axial joint is the pivot joint between the dens of the axis and the ring in the atlas.

Simultaneous movement of all the three atlanto-axial joints must occur to allow the rotation of the atlas and the skull with it upon the axis. The angular travel of the head is limited to about 150°. The muscles which produce these movements are the Obliquus capitus inferior, the Rectus capitus posterior major and the Splenius capitus of one side, acting with the Sternocleidomastoid of the other side. Note that rotational motion of the head is induced by three muscles running along the back of the neck counterbalanced by the Sternocleidomastoid muscle which contours the side of the neck. The nerves activating the muscles involved in rotation of the head branch from the cervical plexus, and are believed to be for proprioception.

CONTROL OF LATERAL EYE MOVEMENTS

Compensatory Eye Movements – Vestibular Stimulation

Horizontal eye movements are measured in the presence of relative rotation between the human and the environment about the vertical axes. With body rotation only and in the absence of a visual fixation, these are compensatory eye movements.

The existence of compensatory eye movements accompanying periods of stimulation of the vestibular sensors has been documented extensively (Collins, 1961; Groen, 1956-57; Guedry, 1960; Meiry, 1965). Specifically, compensatory eye movements are considered as an objective measurement of the dynamic

*(Gray's *Anatomy*).

response of the semicircular canals. Rotations of the body around a vertical earth-fixed axis do not involve stimulation of the otoliths which exceeds the threshold level. The compensatory eye movements during such rotations are considered to be controlled by the semicircular canals.

The phenomenon of compensatory eye movements maintained by stimulation of the vestibular sensors is known as vestibular nystagmus. This motion of the eye is characterized by a slow rotation opposite to the direction of rotation of the skull called the "slow phase" and fast return in phase with the rotation, the "fast phase". While the slow phase is clearly for image stabilization purposes, the sharp flick of the fast phase has been explained as a return to a new fixation point after a limit of travel off the center position of the eye was reached or as a process controlled by the central nervous system (Fluur, 1962).

The term cumulative eye position (Meiry, 1965) is used to describe the total compensatory travel, relative to the skull, of the eye from a center position. The cumulative eye position is then the sum of all the segments of slow phase motion put end to end by eliminating the effects of several fixation points introduced through flicks of the fast phase.

A typical vestibular nystagmus record obtained by photoelectric measurement of eye position is presented in Figure 3. The transfer function from input

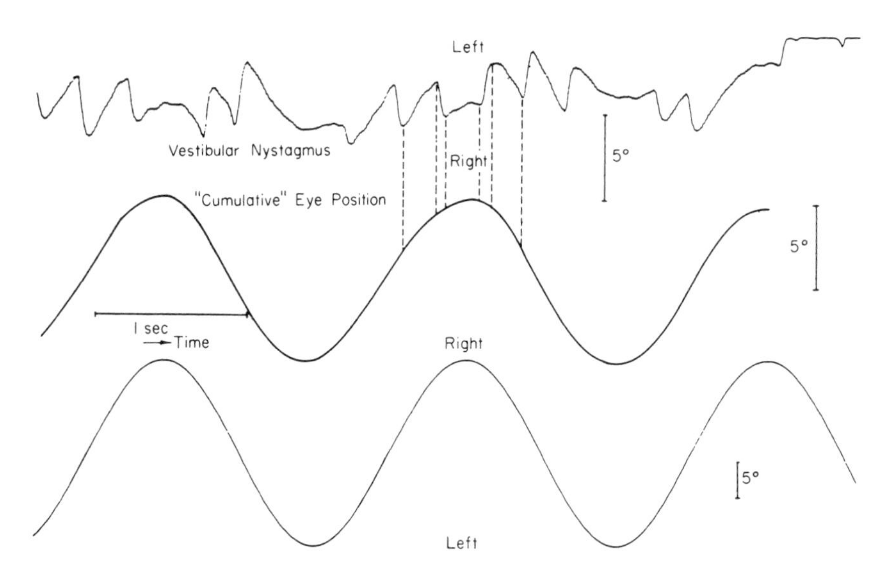

Fig. 3. Vestibular Nystagmus and "Cumulative" Eye Position, f = 0.5 Hz (Note the correspondence of Slow Phase Vestibular Nystagmus and "Cumulative" Eye Position) (Meiry, 1965).

angular velocity to the compensatory eye velocity is approximated as:

$$\frac{\text{eye velocity (s)}}{\text{input angular velocity (s)}} = \frac{-3.2s}{(8s + 1)\,(0.04s + 1)}$$

The frequency response of the system (See Figure 4) indicates a wide range of frequencies with eye movements approximately 180° out of phase with the input motion. However, since the eye movement velocity is only about 40 per cent of the angular velocity of the skull (Jones, 1964) the image upon the retina is not stationary but moves in the direction of rotation. Accordingly, one has to conclude that the vestibular system alone, or more specifically, the semicircular canals cannot achieve space stabilization of the eye when the skull, together with the body, undergoes passive rotations.

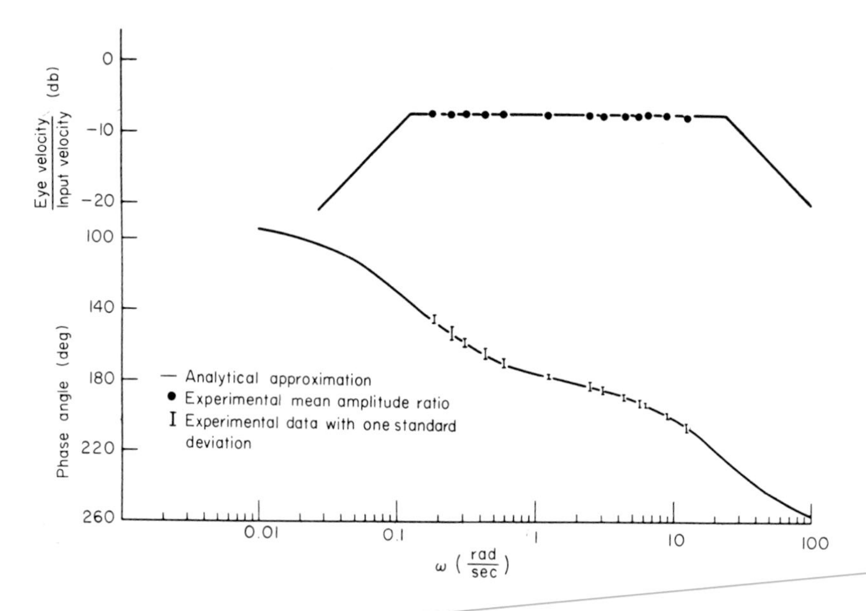

Fig. 4. Bode Plot of Vestibular Compensatory Eye Movements (Slow Phase), (Meiry, 1965).

Environmental Fixation

Rotation of the body and the skull in the presence of a visible fixation point rotating with the subject is referred to as environmental fixation. The situation corresponds to the common condition of travel in a manuevering vehicle whose interior is fully illuminated and the view of the external world is obscured. The fixation point is stationary with respect to the traveller. However, its image upon the retina will move due to the compensatory eye movements initiated by the stimulated semicircular canals. The resulting eye movements exhibit a saw tooth pattern, where the eye is deviated from its mean position by the vestibular branch and returned to it by visual tracking. Consequently, the image of the rotating environment is kept approximately stationary on the retina, the eye remaining within $\pm 0.5°$ of its mean position for inputs up to 2 cps.

Earth-Fixed Fixation Point

If an object in the non-moving surroundings is fixated upon, the control system of the eye will maintain its image on the retina, provided the limits of angular travel of the eye were not exceeded. Physically, the description applies to a human in a rotating vehicle, attempting to look at a given spot outside it. The vestibular compensatory eye movements and the tracking path of the control system are in phase for these conditions. Therefore, they are combining to keep the fixation point image stationary. The frequency response of the eye movement control system with earth-fixed fixation point is presented in Figure 5. Perfect compensation of amplitude is achieved over the range of two decades of frequencies approximately, with the phase lag, however, increasing rapidly beyond 0.5 cps. These results point out the capacity of the control mechanism to maintain a stationary reference for the visual system in the presence of disturbances in the form of vehicle rotations.

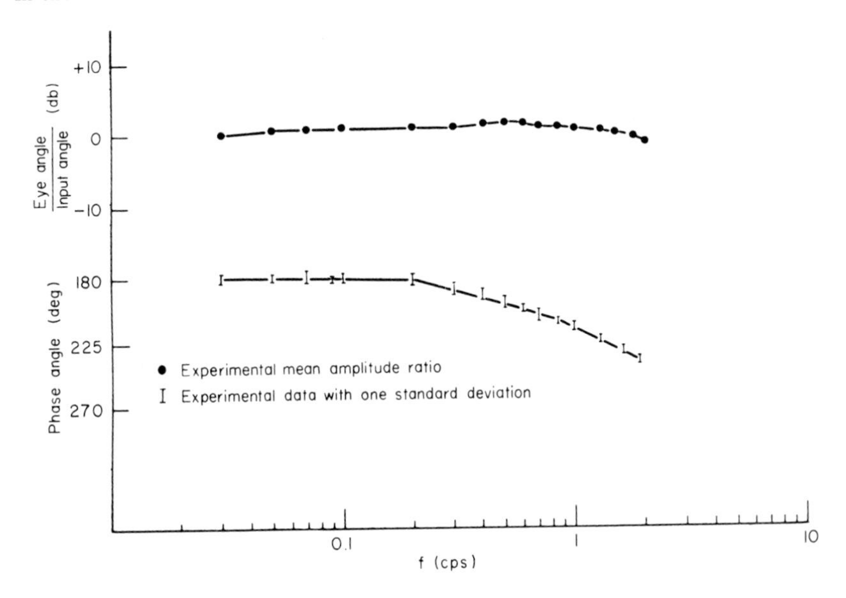

Fig. 5. Bode Plot of Compensatory Eye Movements (Vestibular Stimulation with Earth-Fixation Point) (Meiry, 1965).

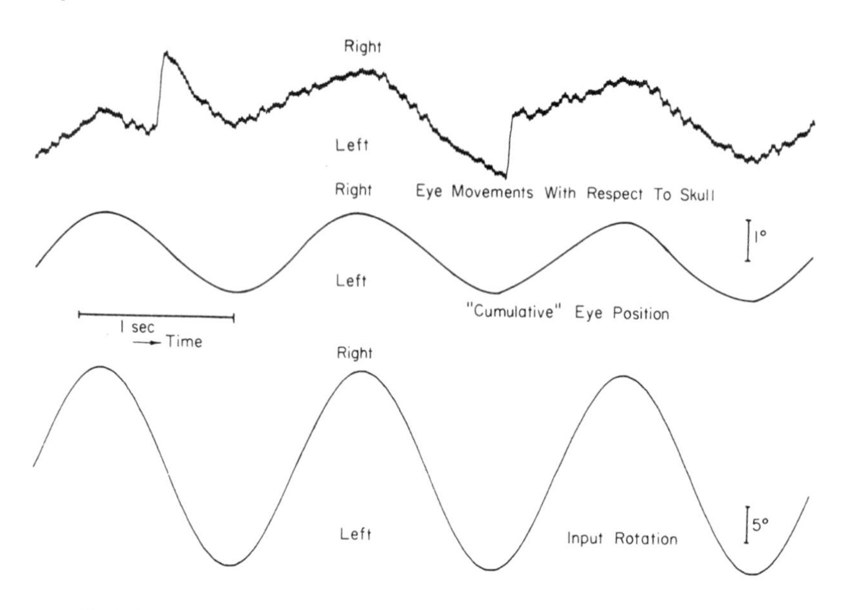

Fig. 6. Compensatory Eye Movements by Neck Receptors, f = 0.6 Hz, (Meiry, 1965).

Compensatory Eye Movements – Neck Proprioceptors

The role of neck receptors as a source of compensatory eye movements has been suggested by physiologists in early literature. As seen in Figure 6, distinct compensatory eye movements are recorded for sinusoidal rotation of the trunk with stationary skull (Meiry, 1965). Examination of the recording emphasizes two characteristic features of the eye motion: *1. eye movements resemble vestibular nystagmus with slow and fast phases; 2. the eye ball is driven in phase with the motion of the trunk.* The latter observation is indeed in agreement with expected compensation for normal head on body rotations. Rotation of the trunk to the left with head fixed corresponds to rotation of the head to the right, while the trunk is stationary. For these relative angular rotations, the compensatory motion of the slow phase should be to the left as is the case at hand.

The frequency response of the experimental data from input angular velocity to compensatory eye velocity is shown in Figure 7. A theoretical fit to the data, in the form of a lag-lead network is given by:

$$\frac{\text{eye velocity (s)}}{\text{input angular velocity}} = \frac{0.325\ (1 + 0.43s)}{(1 + 1.74s)}$$

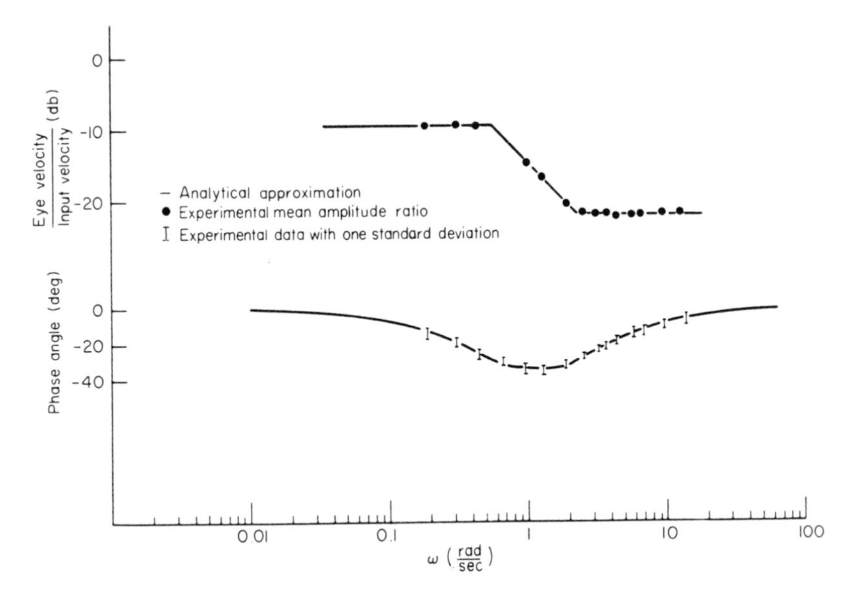

Fig. 7. Bode Plot of Compensatory Eye Movements by Neck Proprioception (Meiry, 1965).

Compensatory Eye Movements – Vestibular and Neck Proprioceptors Stimulation

Frequent movements of the human involve rotation of the head while the eye is fixated upon a given object in the visual field. During these rotating motions, the vestibular system and the neck proprioceptors are stimulated. Therefore, the accompanying eye movements are due to all three of the motion sensors, the eye, the semicircular canals and the neck proprioceptors. The compensation achieved for these circumstances is a measure of the maximum capability of the eye movement control system to preserve a stationary reference on the eye.

The frequency response of the compensatory eye movements measured for these stimuli is presented in Figure 8. The model prediction is the sum of the vestibular and proprioceptive responses as:

$$\frac{\text{eye velocity (s)}}{\text{input angular velocity (s)}} = \frac{-0.325\,(19.2s + 1)\,(1.12s + 1)\,(0.0067s + 1)}{(8s + 1)\,(1.74s + 1)\,(0.04s + 1)}$$

The conclusion one can reach is that the eye movement system is linear over a range of frequencies extending to 2 cps. Obviously then, the compensatory eye movements for combined stimulation of the three motion sensors is

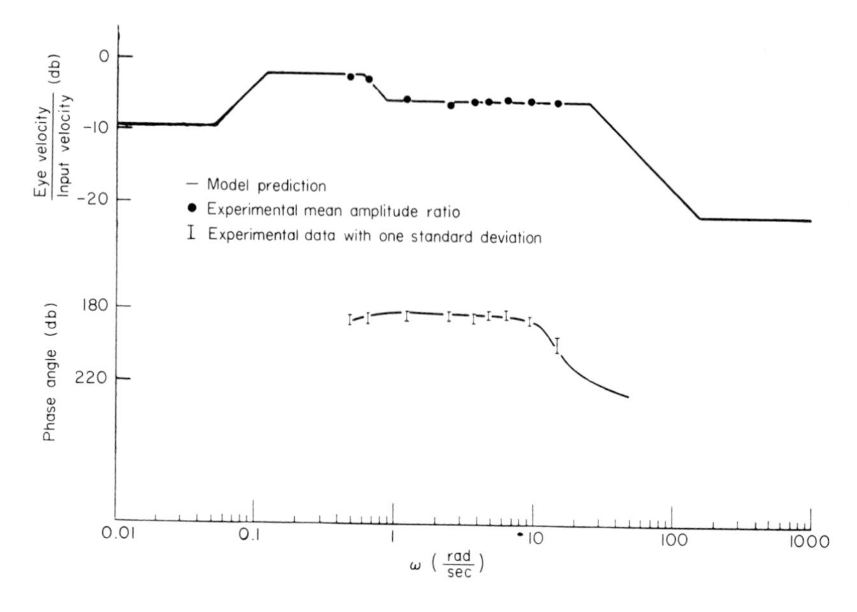

Fig. 8. Bode Plot of Compensatory Eye Movements (Vestibular and Neck Proprioception), (Meiry, 1965).

the vectorial sum of the individual contributions by the semicircular canals, the neck proprioceptors, and visual tracking. The importance of the concept of linearity of the control system is far reaching. By virtue of it, compensatory eye movements are predictable just on the basis of the data on the environmental conditions and a mathematical model of the control system.

In summary, the presence of fixation points, rotation of the skull with respect to the body or rotations of the body as a whole, tend to displace the stationary picture observed by the eye. The degree to which lateral eye movements are stabilized is summarized in Table 1.

ROTATION ABOUT A HORIZONTAL AXIS

Compensatory eye movements for rotations about the sagittal (roll) and the lateral (pitch) axes of the head are readily measured. Jones (1964) reports vestibular nystagmus about the axis of rotation with dynamic response similar in form to the response about the vertical (yaw) axis although with shorter time constants. Experiments by Meiry (1965) to determine the dynamics of the semicircular canals when stimulated in roll confirm the shorter time constant. Since the semicircular canals are arranged in three roughly perpendicular planes one would expect rotation about an intermediate axis to elicit compensatory eye

TABLE I

LATERAL SPACE STABILIZATION OF THE EYE

	No Fixation Point	Environmental Fixation	Earth-fixed Fixation
Vestibular	Partial Compensation of Rotational Rate over Frequencies from 0.02 cps to 4.0 cps	Maintain Eye Angle within $\pm 0.5^{\circ}$ up to 2 cps	Full Compensation up to 2 cps
Neck Proprioceptors	Partial Compensation of Rotational Rate below 0.15 cps	Poor Compensation above 1 cps	Maintain Eye Angle within $\pm 0.5^{\circ}$ up to 2 cps
Vestibular and Neck Proprioceptors	Partial Compensation of Rotational Rate up to 4.0 cps	Maintain Eye Angle within $\pm 0.5^{\circ}$ up to 2 cps	Full Compensation up to 2 cps

movements about that axis. Jones (1964) demonstrated this vectorial summation, however, the difference in time constants mentioned above tends to cause a drift towards the axis with the longest time constant.

Another mode of eye movement response to rotation about the roll axis is counterrolling. This is a rotation of the eyes about the roll axis when the entire body is being rotated about the roll axis of the skull at a constant angular velocity. Since the semicircular canals are heavily damped angular accelerometers they will not respond to this stimulus. Thus dynamic counterrolling is attributed to the stimulation of the utricle as indicated in Figure 9. This figure presents the dynamic counterrolling data of Kellog (1967) superimposed on the frequency plot of the dynamic otolith model of Meiry (1965) and Young and Meiry (1968).

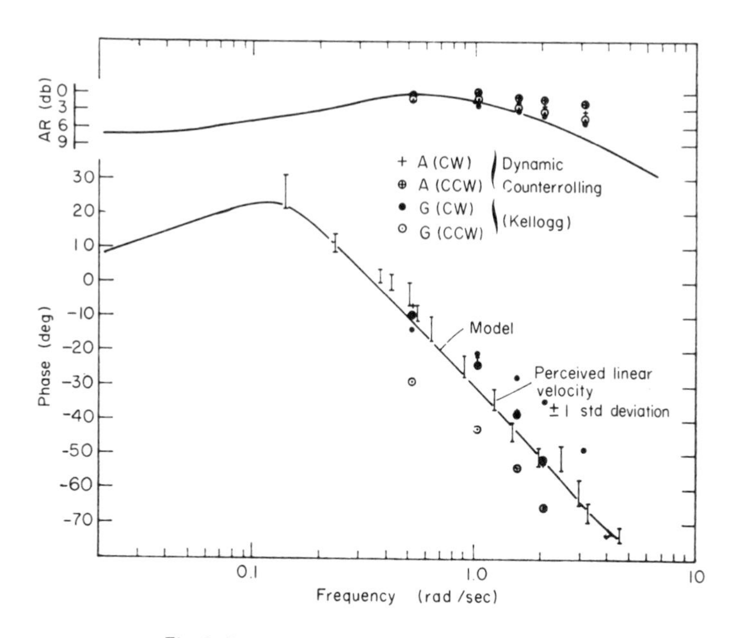

Fig. 9. Perceived Velocity Frequency Response.

LINEAR ACCELERATION NYSTAGMUS

Efforts to elicit horizontal nystagmus by stimulation of the linear motion sensors of the vestibular system have produced rather random results in the past. Recently, Niven *et al* (1965) using sinusoidal linear acceleration applied along the lateral head axis measured consistent nystagmus with slow phase velocity of approximately 9.3°/sec for 18.6 ft/sec² peak acceleration. Their efforts to observe vertical nystagmus for input accelerations along the vertical axis failed. Similarly one can logically reason that linear acceleration along the sagittal axis will not produce any compensatory eye movement mode.

REFERENCES

BARNHILL, J.H. (1940). *Surgical Anatomy of the Head and Neck.* The Williams and Wilkins Co., Baltimore.

CLARK, B., GRAYBIEL, A. and MACCORQUODALE, (1948). The illusory perception of movement caused by angular acceleration and by centrifugal force during flight. II. Visually perceived motion and displacement of a fixed target during turns. *J. Exp. Psychol.*, **38,** 298-309.

COHEN, L.A. (1964). Human spatial orientation and its critical role in space travel. *Aerospace Med.* **35.**

COLLINS, W.E. (1960). Further studies of the effects of mental set upon vestibular nystagmus. US Army Med. Res. Lab., Fort Knox, Ky., Report No. 443.

COLLINS, W.E., CRAMPTON, C.H. and POSNER, J.B. (1960). The effect of mental set upon vestibular nystagmus and the electroencephalogram. US Army Med. Res. Lab., Fort Knox, Ky., Report No. 439.

COLLINS, W.E. and GUEDRY, F.E., Jr. (1961). Arousal effects and nystagmus during prolonged constant angular acceleration. US Army Med. Res. Lab., Fort Knox, Ky., Report No. 500.

CRAMER, R.L., DOWD, P.J., and HELMS, D.B. (1963). Vestibular responses to oscillation about the yaw axis. *Aerospace Med.* **34,** 1031-1034.

FLUUR, E. (1962). The mechanism of nystagmus. *Acta Otolaryng.*, **54,** 181-188.

Gray's Anatomy. (1962). Thirty-third edition. Longmans, Green and Company.

GROEN, J.J. (1956-57). The semicircular canal system of the organs of equilibrium I and II. *Physics in Medicine and Biology.* **1.**

GUEDRY, F.E., Jr., COLLINS, W.E., and SHEFFEY, P.L. (1961). Perceptual and oculomotor reactions to interacting visual and vestibular stimulation. US Army Med. Res. Lab., Fort Knox, Ky., Report No. 463.

GUEDRY, F.E., Jr., and LAUVER, L.S. (1960). The oculomotor and subjective aspect of the vestibular reaction during prolonged constant angular acceleration. US Army Med. Res. Lab., Fort Knox, Ky., Report No. 438.

GUEDRY, F.E., Jr., PEACOCK, L.J., and CRAMER, R.L. (1957). Nystagmic eye movements during interacting vestibular stimuli. US Army Med. Res. Lab., Fort Knox, Ky., Report No. 275.

HIXSON, W.C. and NIVEN, J.I. (1961). Application of the system transfer function concept to a mathematical description of the labyrinth: I. Steady-state nystagmus response to semicircular canal stimulation by angular acceleration. Bureau of Med. and Surg., Project MR005. 13-6001, Subtask 1, Report No. 57.

JONES, G.M. (1964). Predominance of anti-compensatory oculomotor response during rapid head rotation. *Aerospace Med.*, **35**
965-968.

JONES, G.M., BARRY, W., and KOWALSKY, N. (1964). Dynamics of the semicircular canals compared in yaw, pitch and roll. *Aerospace Med.*, **35,** 984-989.

JONES, G.M., and MILSUM, J.H., (1965). Spatial and dynamic aspects of visual fixation. *IEEE Trans. Bio-Medical Engineering,* **BME-2 (2),** 54-62.

KELLOG, R (1967). A mathematical model of the counterolling of the human eye. Third Symposium on the role of the vestibular organs in spact exploration, Pensacola, Fla.

MEIRY, J.L. (1965). The vestibular system and human dynamic space orientation. Sc.D. Thesis, MIT.

MILLER, E.F. (1962). Counterrolling of the human eyes produced by head tilt with respect to gravity. *Acta Otolaryng.*, **54,** 479-501.

NIVEN, J.L. and HIXSON, W.C. Frequency response of the human semicircular canals: steady-state ocular nystagmus response to high-level sinusoidal angular rotations. Bureau Med. and Surg., Project MR005. 13-6001, Subtask 1, Report No. 58.

NIVEN, J.I., HIXSON, W.C., and CORREIA, M.J. (1965). Ellicitation of horizontal nystagmus by periodical linear acceleration. NAMI-953, Naval Aerospace Med. Inst., Pensacola, Fla.

YOUNG, L.R. (1962). *A sampled Data Model for Eye Tracking Movements.* Doctoral Thesis, MIT.

YOUNG, L.R. (1967). A model for linear acceleration effects on the vestibular nystagmus. Third Symposium on the Role of the Vestibular Organs in Space Exploration.

YOUNG, L.R. and MEIRY, J.L. (1968). A revised dynamic otolith model. *Aerospace Med.* **39, No. 6.**

ORGANIZATION OF NEURAL CONTROL IN THE VESTIBULO-OCULAR REFLEX ARC

G. MELVILL JONES

In the preceding chapter, Meiry has considered some of the input/output characteristics of the vestibulo-ocular reflex arc and associated neck proprioceptive mechanisms in the generation of a stabilized visual image during head and body movement. The present chapter examines some of the features which characterise components of the internal organization which brings about those input/output relations. The article draws largely upon the results of experiments conducted by the author in collaboration with various colleagues whose contributions are acknowledged in the text and references.

RESPONSE CHARACTERISTICS OF THE SEMICIRCULAR CANALS

Fig. 1 represents an idealized semicircular canal which essentially comprises a very thin, roughly circular tube (the endolymphatic duct) containing a fluid (endolymph) having mechanical properties which are probably rather similar to those of water. In man, the internal diameter of the thin part of the tube is about 1/3 mm. As a result, during angular acceleration in the plane of the canal the relative fluid flow induced by the fluid's inertia becomes very heavily damped by viscosity, the effects of which are relatively very large compared to those of inertia in a system of such small Reynold's number. An important consequence of this is that in the absence of any obstruction round the canal circuit, the hydrodynamics of the system performs one accurate integration upon

This research was supported by Canadian Defense Research Board Grants in Aid of Research Nos. 9910-37 and 931092.

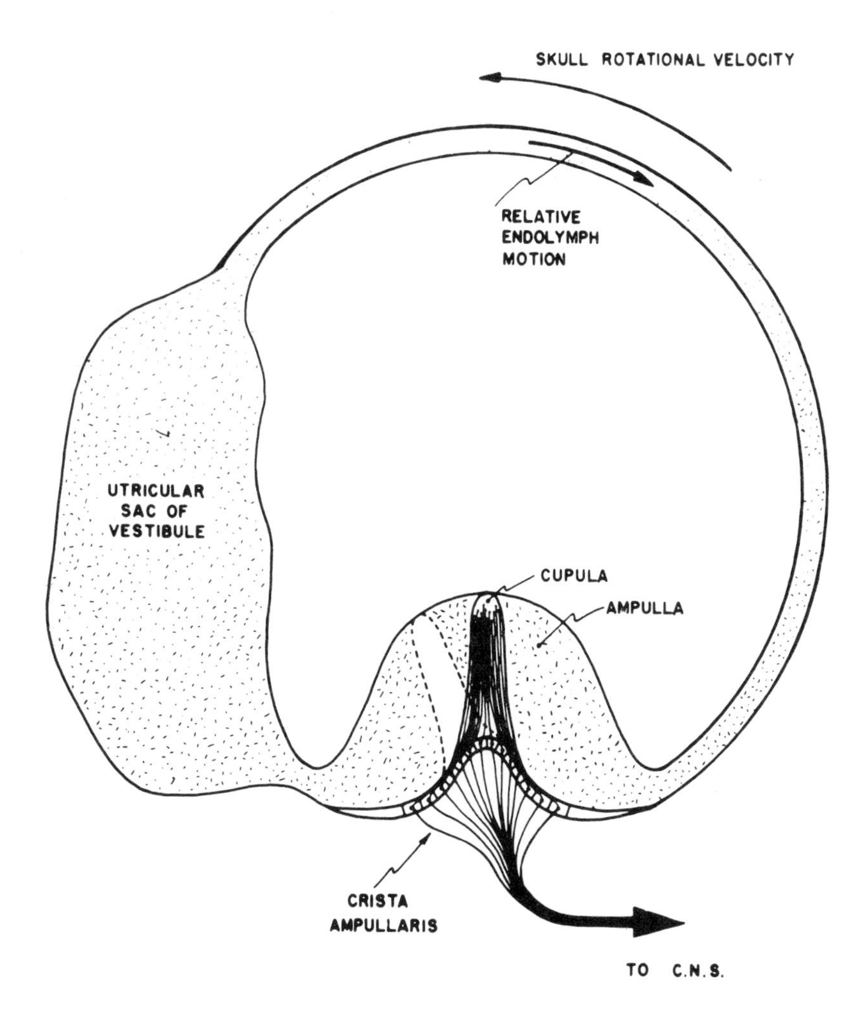

Fig. 1. Diagram of the main functional components of the endolymphatic semicircular canal (From *Melvill Jones & Milsum*, 1965).

the angular acceleration to which the whole system is exposed. Thus the imposed acceleration generates a proportionate relative velocity of fluid flow, and hence the fluid displacement at any instant provides an accurate measure of instantaneous angular velocity. It is important to note that the hydrodynamic response in such a system, being dependent upon the ratio of inertial to viscus terms in the system, is a very rapid one, and therefore for practical purposes the response can be considered instantaneous (Gaede, 1922; Schmaltz, 1925, & 1931).

Of course, in practice as indicated in Fig. 1, the fluid circuit is not free of obstruction. The cupula, in the expanded ampulla, acts like a water-tight spring door which hinges at the base of the cupula and thus deflects through an angle proportional to fluid displacement around the circuit. Hence in the absence of significant effect due to the spring characteristic of the swing door (cupular restoring force) the angle of cupular deflection provides a measure of instantaneous angular velocity in the plane of a canal. This seems to be the normal system response in the canal since natural head movements are usually of too short duration for the cupular restoring force to enter significantly into the response (Steinhausen, 1933; van Egmond, Groen & Jonkees, 1949; Mayne, 1950; Melvill Jones & Milsum, 1965a). However, in order to understand the subsequent account of experimental results, it must be appreciated that when turning movements are prolonged the cupular restoring force substantially modifies the response from that which would be obtained from an unimpeded circular canal.

Functional characteristics of the canal hydrodynamic response may be conveniently summarized in terms of a frequency response diagram as in Fig. 2 (Mayne, 1950; Melvill Jones & Milsum, 1965a). This gives the amplitude and phase data assessed over a wide frequency range of sinusoidal rotational stimuli from mixed experimental and theoretical data. Note particularly that response characteristics are here related to the angular velocity of rotational stimulation, in view of the velocity transducing characteristic implied above. In Fig. 2, it can be seen that over the frequency range 0.1 - 5.0 cps, the response would always be closely in phase with the *angular velocity* of stimulus, with the additional feature of a flat response (amplitude ratio) throughout the range. Over this range, therefore, the system would continue to act as a good angular velocity transducer despite the presence of the elastic cupula. At frequencies below about 0.1 cps, the response of such a system would progressively attenuate with the additional characteristic feature that it would become progressively phase advanced relative to the angular velocity of stimulus.

It could, of course be a chance phenomen that the dimensions of the human canal yield a response such as that in Fig. 2. However, Jones & Spells (1963) and Melvill Jones (1969a) have shown that over a wide range of species, dimensional changes in the canal are just such as to shift the angular velocity transducing range to match the likely change in frequency of head movement due to change in animal size, assessed on the basis of dimensional analysis. It is important to note in this connection that the required changes in canal size are very far from proportionate to changes in animal size. According to the dimensional analysis of Jones & Spells the radius of curvature of the canal and the square of the internal radius of the thin tube should both increase approximately as about the one tenth power of animal body weight. That this is indeed the case is evidenced in Fig. 3 which plots on a log-log basis the measured relationships between animal weight and (a) canal radius of curvature (R) and (b) square of internal tube radius (r^2) for 51 specimens from mammalian species.

Thus it seems probable that the evolutionary process has selected an end-organ which is appropriate specifically for the acquisition of a message having

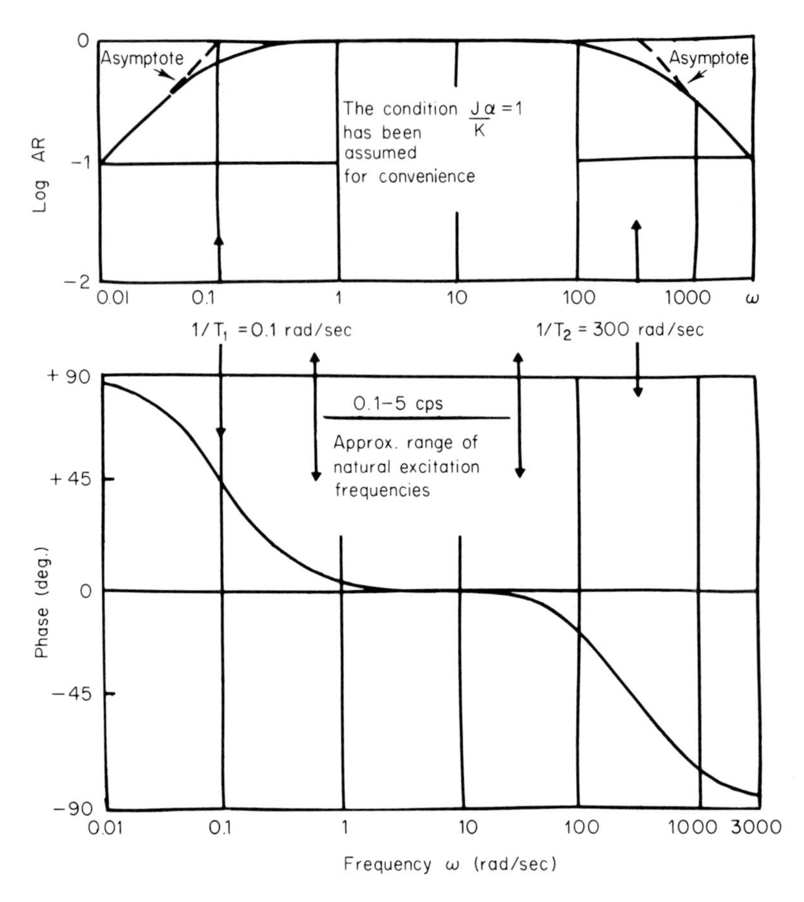

Fig. 2. Frequency response of the human canal. The amplitude ratio (AR) is expressed as the ratio of cupular angle to head angular velocity. Note the working range of frequencies is presumed to lie between 0.1-5.0 Hz (From *Melvill Jones & Milsum,* 1965).

the meaningful content of angular velocity, at least during patterns of head movement encountered in the evolutionary experience. This theme is supported by the further analytical development of Mayne (1965).

THE AFFERENT NEURAL SIGNAL

In view of this special characteristic of the message "collected" by the end-organ, it is of interest to examine the extent to which this message is held intact in the afferent neural communication pathway. For this, experiments have

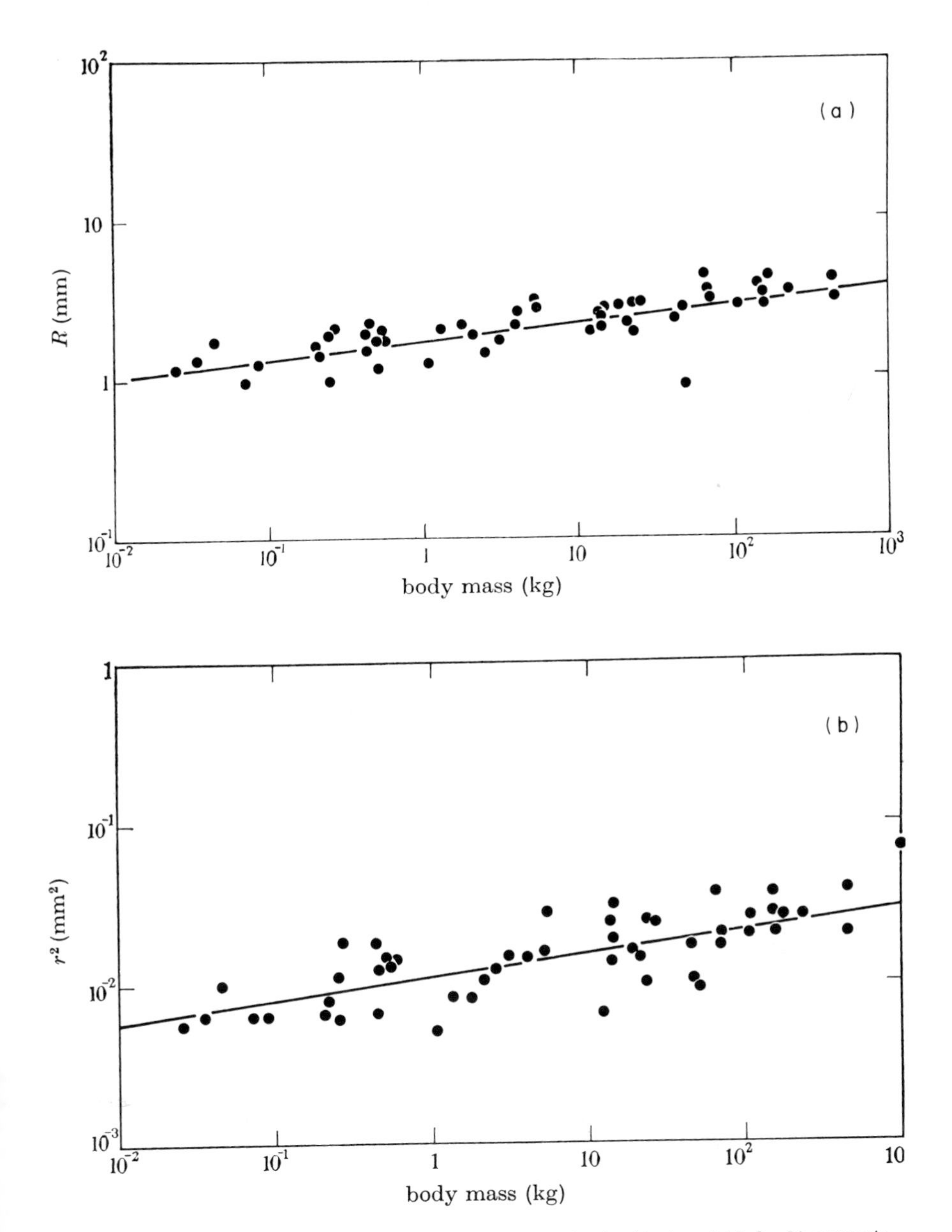

Fig. 3a and b. Relations between critical canal dimensions and animal body weight, for 51 mammals. R = canal radius of curvature; r = internal radius of endolymphatic canal. Calculated regression lines are shown. (From *Jones & Spells*, 1963).

been conducted using the apparatus illustrated in Fig. 4. Essentially, this comprises a stereotaxic platform suspended from four parallel spring cables over a coaxial servo-controlled turntable onto which the platform can be lowered after specifically semicircular canal-dependent neural units have been located in the

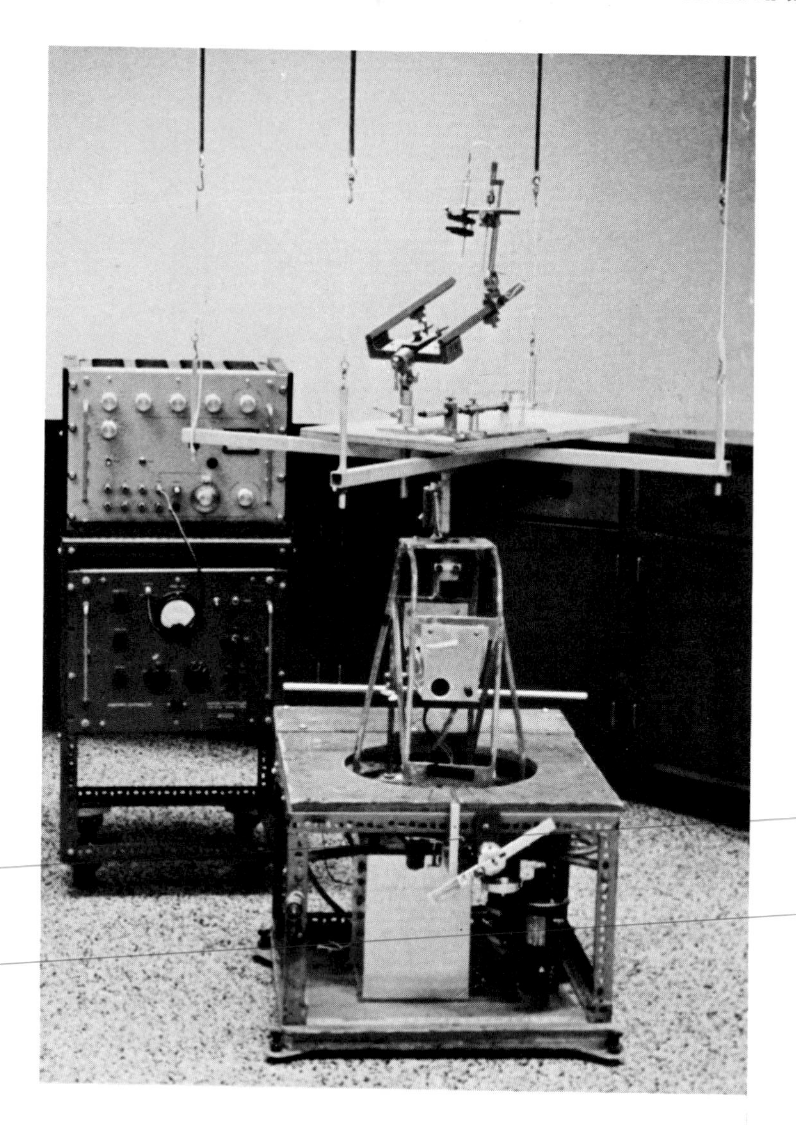

Fig. 4. The slung stereotaxic platform turntable and low frequency wave form generator.

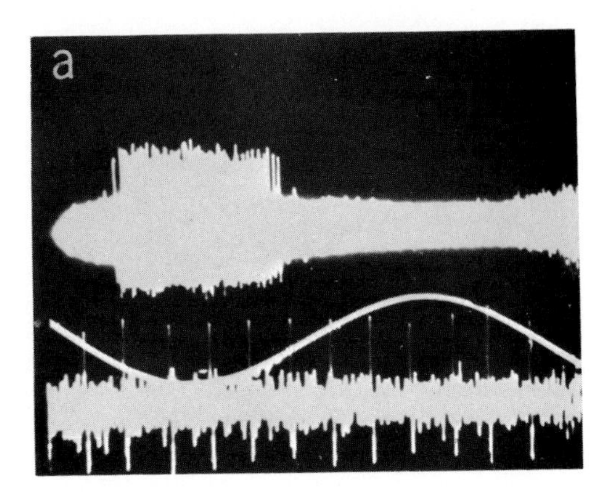

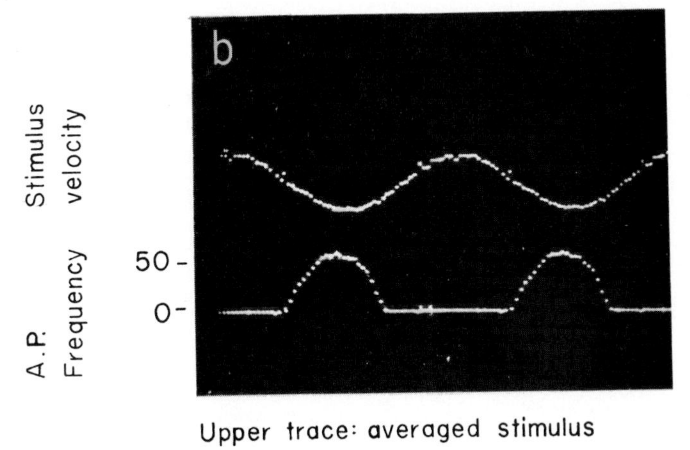

Fig. 5. Response of a lateral canal-dependent neural unit in the left vestibular nucleus to sinusoidal rotation in the plane of the canal. **(a)** Original records of action potentials, stimulus angular velocity and fast sweep of action potential trace, from above down; **(b)** Averaged relation between stimulus angular velocity (upper) and action potential frequency. The averaged records are written out twice to aid visual interpretation, (From *Melvill Jones*, 1969b).

brain stem. In the experiments to be described extracellular steel micro-electrodes were placed in the vestibular nuclei of cats with intact cerebellum, which were decerebrate at the intercollicular level. Fig. 5 illustrates the kind of response obtained from a single specifically horizontal canal-dependent neural unit in the medial vestibular nucleus. The middle trace of the upper photograph gives the *angular velocity* of one sine wave of stimulation. The upper trace gives the corresponding sequence of action potentials in one cycle. The lower trace is a fast sweep recorded to illustrate the unitary characteristic of the recording. Evidently this unit was excited during angular velocity in one direction and inhibited below the threshold of firing during angular velocity in the other direction.

The lower photograph shows the computer-averaged relationships between stimulus angular velocity (upper trace) and action potential frequency (lower trace). The particular feature to notice here is the close phase relationship between the firing frequency of this unit and the stimulus angular velocity (Melvill Jones & Milsum, 1965b).

The top left response in Fig. 6 shows a similar phase dependence upon angular velocity of stimulus in another unit. However, as indicated above (Fig. 2) the phase of response would be expected to advance progressively relative to stimulus angular velocity as the periodic time of sinusoidal stimulus increased. This feature is clearly illustrated in the bottom left record of Fig. 6, which was obtained from the same cell at a periodic time of approximately one *minute*.

Fig. 7 plots the phase characteristics obtained from 21 different neural units. These results may be compared with the expected phase characteristics of the end-organ response drawn at the left-hand end of the bottom curve in Fig. 2. The similarity between theoretical end-organ response and its reflection in the neural message at the cell station represented by the medial vestibular nucleus is rather close (Melvill Jones & Milsum, 1969a).

The closeness with which such neural units may follow the mechanical response of the end-organ is further illustrated in the two right-hand sets of records in Fig. 6. The lower records give the averaged response of the same neurone as illustrated in the left-hand side of the figure, to a step change in angular velocity. The response was a burst of neural activity, initially registering correctly the change of stimulus angular velocity, followed by an exponential decay presumably associated with subsequent elastic restoration of the cupula during maintained steady rotation. The upper right-hand curves show the response to a step change of angular acceleration (triangular trace gives angular velocity), when the response of the end-organ would be expected to rise exponentially to a plateau which would then be held constant at a point determined by the balance between inertial force due to angular acceleration and the elastic restoring force due to cupular deflection. Again this unit responded closely in accordance with such a mechanical response in the end-organ, holding its firing frequency nearly constant for just over one minute (half the periodic time of the triangular wave form of stimulus angular velocity). Similar unpublished results of Melvill Jones & Milsum show a plateau response which is held virtually

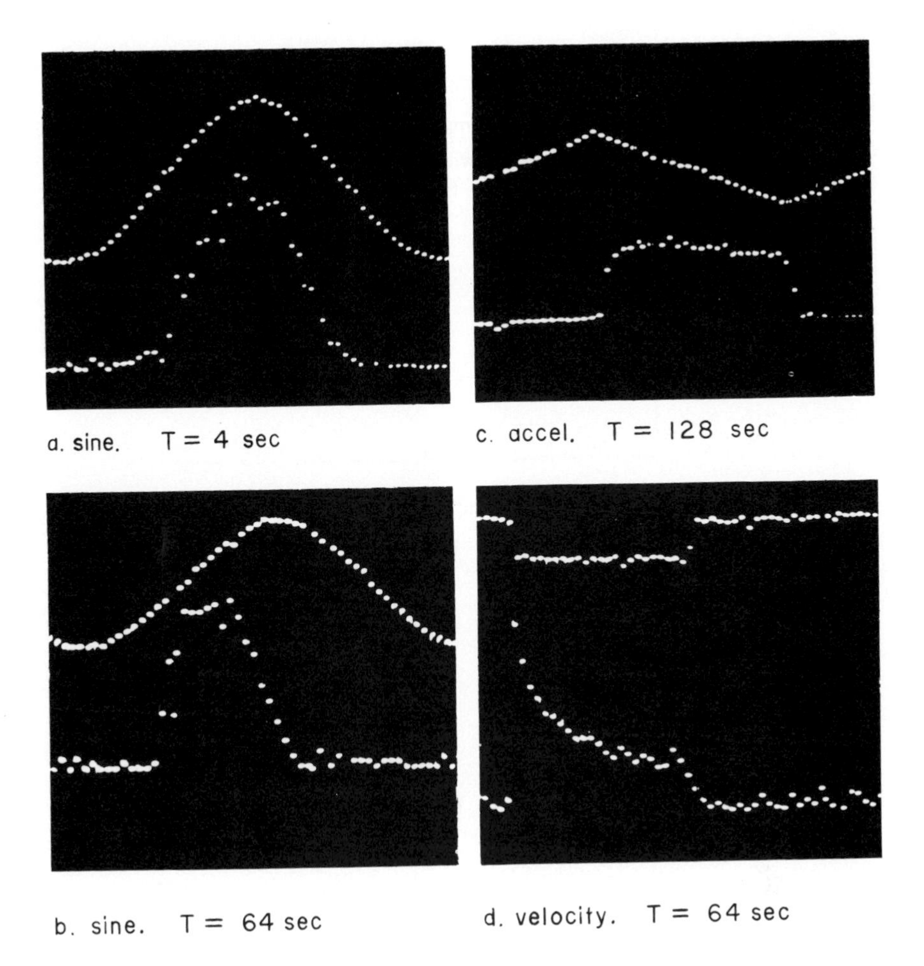

Fig. 6. Averaged stimulus-response relationships obtained from a unit similar to that in Fig. 5. Upper trace of each figure gives stimulus angular velocity profile. Lower trace gives action potential frequency. This cell was taken below its threshold of firing during the "*inhibitory*" half of each cycle. (*Melvill Jones & Milsum*, 1967).

constant for over four minutes continuous unidirectional angular acceleration.

These observations conform with those of earlier investigators (Ross, 1936; Adrian, 1943; Gernandt, 1949; Groen, Lowenstein & Vendrik, 1952). More recently Goldberg & Fernandez (1969) have demonstrated similar relations between stimulus and frequency response of primary afferent vestibular neurones in monkey, and Shimazu & Precht (1965) have clearly defined plateau patterns of response to rotational acceleration in cat vestibular nuclei. It is noteworthy that

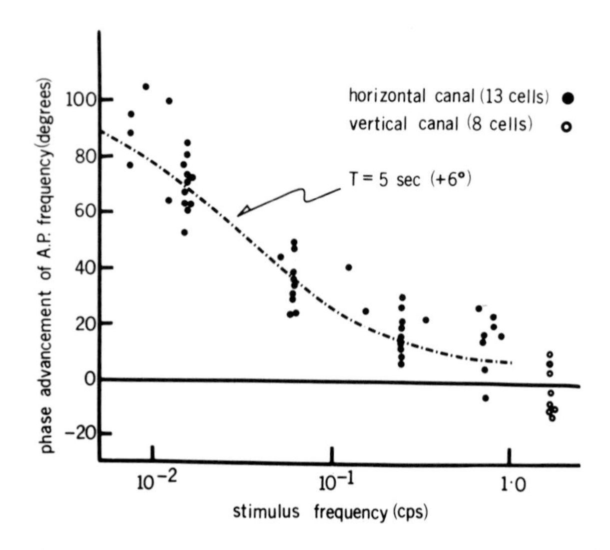

Fig. 7. Phase plot of action potential frequency against the frequency of the sine wave of rotational stimulation. The intermittent line gives the curve to be expected from a cupular restoration time constant of 5 sec with the added feature that the whole curve has been phase advanced by 6° to account for an effect due to dynamic asymmetry in the responses of units taken below threshold during part of the cycle. (From *Melvill Jones & Milsum*, 1967).

the latter authors described stimulated activity of spontaneously silent cells which did not appear to respond in the same way as those which were spontaneously active.

Thus, it seems that at least some neural units carry the mechanical response of the end-organ with good fidelity into the brain stem. The neural message in these cells would in these circumstances continue to carry the meaning of angular velocity of head rotation, at least within the range of angular velocity transduction at the end-organ. The next question arises, how is this message carried forward in the vestibulo-ocular reflex arc to motoneurones in the oculomotor nerves.

THE OCULOMOTOR NEURAL SIGNAL

The shortest pathway from peripheral end-organ to oculomotor nucleus comprises the primary and secondary vestibular neurones with a single relay between them in the vestibular nuclei (Lorente de Nó, 1933; Szentágothai, 1950). The secondary neurones synapse directly with the motoneurones of the IIIrd, IVth and VIth cranial nerves in the corresponding brain stem nuclei (McMasters, Weiss & Carpenter, 1966). It must however be appreciated that in addition to this elementary pathway, which is rapid and excitatory, reciprocal pathways are also involved, generating a differential drive to any particular motor nucleus. For example, the left abducens (VIth) nucleus is excited by direct neurones from the right vestibular nucleus, but it is also influenced by polysynaptic inhibitory pathways from the left nucleus (Richter & Precht, 1968). Probably multi-synaptic influences reach the nuclei via the reticular formation (Lorente de Nó, 1933). Certainly Precht & Shimazu (1965) have shown that primary vestibular nerve stimulation leads to dependent potentials in the bulbo-pontine reticular formation. Presumably, the long-latency responses in motoneurones demonstrated by Horcholle and Tyč-Dumont (1968) (up to about 6 msec as compared with short latency responses of about 2 msec.) are mediated through such reticular pathways.

It seems clear, however, that the final outcome of the differential vestibular drive upon identified motoneurones is always such as to bring about excitation during contraction, and inhibition during relaxation, of the innervated muscle (Tarlo & Melvill Jones, 1968; Precht, Richter & Grippo, 1969). It may appear naive to state this conclusion. But it is emphasised here in order to clarify the point that unidentified unit neural responses in the oculomotor nucleus by no means always conform with this rule. Thus, Melvill Jones & Sugie (1965b), recording from unidentified neurones shown to be located in the abducens nucleus of cat (Prussian blue location of steel electrode tip) detected not only agonistic and antagonistic responses, but also a variety of bi-directional ones. Fig. 8a illustrates a section from the record of an antagonistically acting unit, which fired with a high frequency burst during saccadic *relaxation* of the corresponding lateral rectus, but was completely silent during a saccade in the direction associated with ipsi-lateral rectus contraction. In Fig. 8b, a single electrode tip simultaneously detected single agonistically and antagonistically acting units, indicating that these need not necessarily be located differently in the nucleus. Fig. 9 shows two bi-directional cell responses. In Fig. 9a, the cell fired very fast (up to 500 AP/sec) during saccades in the agonistic direction, and also, but at a much slower speed (70-80 AP/sec) during saccades in the antagonistic direction. In Fig. 9b, the bi-directional response of a spontaneously firing unit is illustrated, in which the characteristic feature was sudden, complete silence during saccades in *both* directions. Precht, Richter & Grippo (1969) found antagonistically acting unit responses in the VIth nucleus which could not be excited antidromically, but did not report bi-directional ones. Possibly the absence of bi-directional ones was due to their preparation being decerebrate and decerebellate, leading to few saccades during vestibular stimulation; whilst the preparation of Melvill Jones & Sugie was intact and under light ether anaesthesia, when an almost normal vestibulo-ocular response can, with care, be obtained.

It is not the purpose of this article to elaborate on these multivariant patterns of activity, and they are only mentioned here to emphasise the importance of motoneurone identification before proceeding to investigate response characteristics in the final neurone pathway innervating extraocular muscles. In

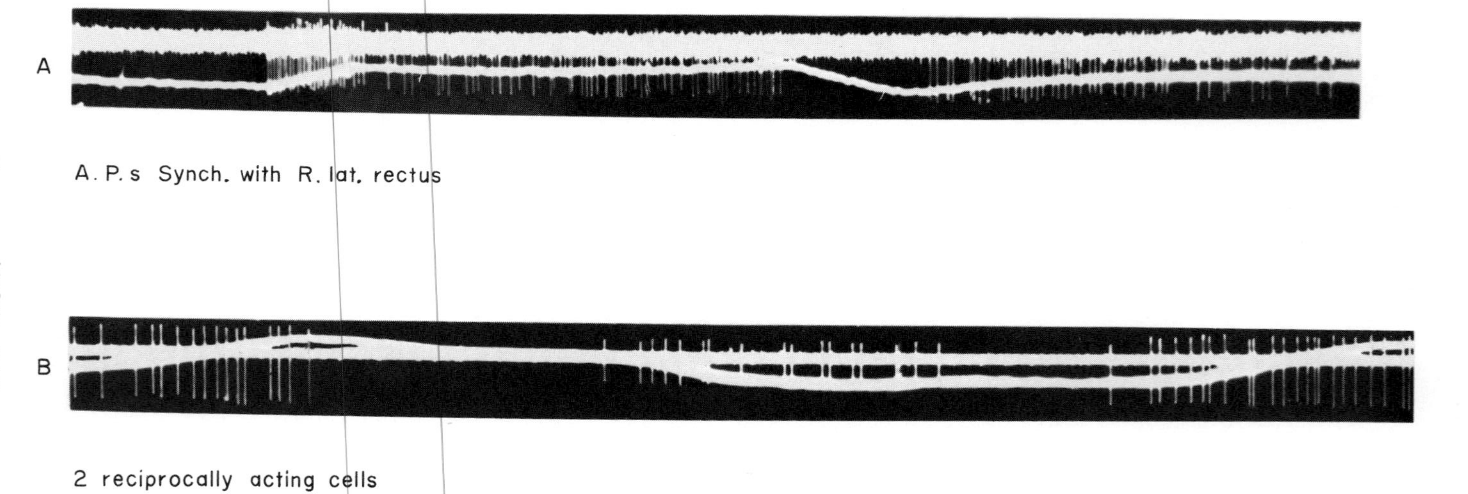

Fig. 8. Records obtained from cells in the left abducens nucleus during sinusoidal rotational stimulation of the semicircular canals in cats under light ether anaesthesia. Curved lines give uncalibrated eye angle (**a**) antagonistic unit, actively firing during relaxation of ipsilateral rectus muscle. (**b**) simultaneous records of two differentially acting units obtained from the same electrode tip. Although located in the region of the abducens nucleus, these cells were not identified as motoneurones.

A
Fast firing synch. with L. lat. rectus
EYE RIGHT
B
A.P.s inhibited in both directions
1 sec

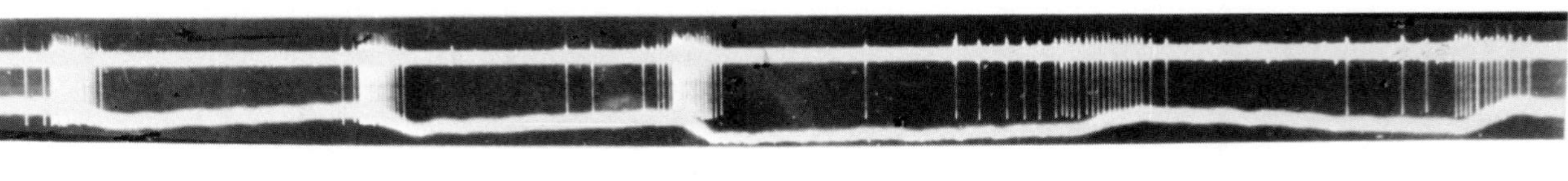

Fig. 9. Records from bidirectional units in the region of the left abducens nucleus but not identified as motoneurones.

this laboratory two approaches have been adopted, using, on the one hand Bach-y-Rita's (1964) approach to the motoneurone trunk in its subpontine course, and on the other hand antidromic identification of unit action potentials in the abducens nucleus. The responses of identified VIth nerve motoneurones were examined during adequate rotational stimulation of the semicircular canals, applied in the same way as in the investigation of vestibular unit responses (Milsum & Melvill Jones, 1969; Melvill Jones & Milsum, 1969a).

Fig. 10 shows tracings obtained by Mergler & Melvill Jones (1969) from records such as those in Figs. 5 & 6 when saccades had been temporarily eliminated by light ether anaesthia. The upper trace gives the stimulus angular velocity whilst the lower three traces give the firing frequency profile observed in this single unit during sinusoidal rotational stimuli of periodic times 1.2, 4.0 and 64.0 sec. So long as the frequency of oscillatory stimulus was sufficiently high to approximate the frequency range of angular velocity transduction in the semicircular canal, the phase of the neural signal in the oculomotor neurone remained closely tied to the angular velocity of stimulus. In these circumstances, it seems that at least in some neurones, the neural message is similar to that contained in vestibular neurones (Figs. 5 & 6), which in turn reflect the angular velocity message transduced in hydrodynamic components of the canal end-organ. Furthermore, as the periodic time for rotational stimulus increased beyond the lower cut-off frequency of the canal (Fig. 2), so the phase of the neural response in the oculomotor neurone became advanced, by approximately 90°, as would be expected from the mechanical characteristics of the end-organ (Fig. 7). At the time of writing, insufficient data have been collected to warrant a definitive statement. But it seems from results obtained to date, both from motor neurones in the nerve trunk and from antidromically identified cell bodies in the nucleus itself, that the neural message transduced by the mechanical components of the canal end-organ is carried in an essentially unchanged form through the vestibular nucleus to the extra-ocular motor neurone system.

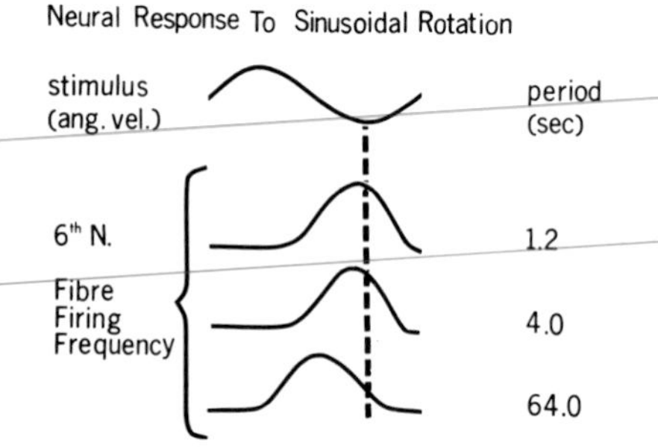

Fig. 10. Tracings of averaged responses obtained from a "teased" mononeurone in the left VIth nerve, to illustrate similar stimulus-response relationships to those found in the vestibular nuclei (Fig. 5 and 6). (From *Mergler and Melvill Jones*, 1968).

The recent results of Precht, Richter & Grippo (1969) add weight to this conclusion. They recorded responses of identified motoneurones in the abducens nucleus of cat during rotational acceleration of the whole animal, and found patterns of change in firing frequency which were almost indistinguishable from those of neural units in the vestibular nuclei (Shimazu & Precht, 1965). For example, during acceleration in an ''excitatory'' direction a spontaneously firing motoneurone would exponentially increase its firing frequency towards a plateau, as in the top right-hand response of the vestibular unit in Fig. 6. Furthermore, the measured time constants of these exponential rises were similar for vestibular and motor neurones (in the range 5-10 sec).

THE OCULAR COMPONENT OF RESPONSE

An important inference from these observations is that, during normal patterns of head movement, the firing frequency of oculomotor neurons tends to be tied specifically to the angular velocity of head rotation. If further results support this conclusion it would seem unlikely that the neural stage of integration required for converting an angular velocity input signal into an angular eye position takes place in the central nervous system, as has been suggested might be the case by Robinson (1968). Presumably, then, we would expect to find the necessary transformation in the peripheral oculomotor system and it therefore becomes of particular interest to examine the relationship between the firing frequency of motor neurones and corresponding eye angle (extraocular muscle length) during the normal patterns of rotational head stimulation. The attempt is therefore currently being made to obtain synchronous records of rotational head velocity motor neurone firing frequency, and eye angle relative to the skull during sinusoidal head rotation. Of course, such a procedure requires a functionally intact oculomotor system and as before the objective is to obtain records in a condition of light ether anaesthesia, sufficient just to suppress the saccadic component of response. Fig. 11 shows records from a single nerve fiber in the VIth trunk together with simultaneous records of stimulus angular velocity, and resulting eye angle.

This motor unit was silent in the unstimulated state and only fired during a portion of the cycle close to peak excitation. However, it can be seen that the center of each period of active firing corresponds closely with maximum compensatory eye angular velocity (i.e. maximum slope of the eye angle record). Current results suggest this finding represents a general feature of neuromuscular transduction in the oculomotor system of the cat, which in turn suggests that the second integration required by Robinson (1968) must occur at this level in the system rather than in the central nervous system. Of course, how this may be achieved is a matter for speculation. Perhaps the ocular torque induced by a given firing frequency in motor neurones would be expected to induce a rate-dependent eye movement on account of high viscus damping in the orbit (Robinson, 1964). Alternatively, or in addition, the possibility that rate dependent negative

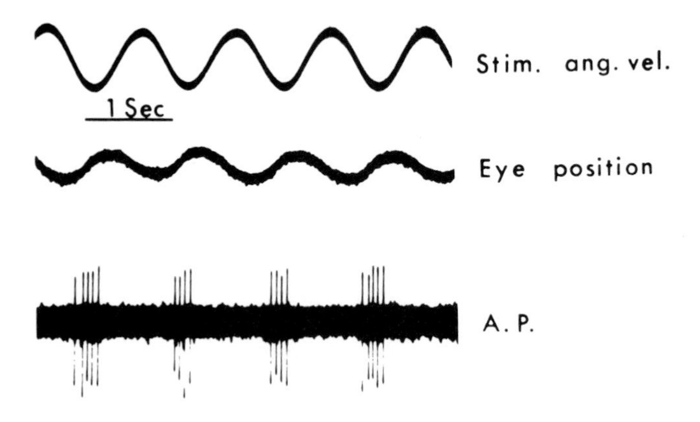

Fig. 11. Relations between rotational stimulus angular velocity, eye position in the skull and action potentials of a single motoneurone in the left VIth nerve. Left-going stimulus angular velocity and eye movement both registered upwards. (From *Mergler & Melvill Jones*, 1968).

feedback (dynamic stretch reflex) obtained from rate dependent stretch receptor information, could theoretically lead to the same event.

THE INFLUENCE OF SACCADES UPON DYNAMIC RESPONSE OF THE OCULOMOTOR SYSTEM

A further feature of Fig. 11 is that compensatory eye angular velocity is some 25-30° phase advanced with respect to the corresponding stimulus angular velocity (note that the eye response is here inferred to be in phase with stimulus angular velocity when the response is in the properly organised compensatory direction). Melvill Jones & Sugie (1965a) and Sugie & Melvill Jones (1966 & 1969) have shown that this is a consistent phenomenon in the cat, but that with the introduction of saccadic eye movements such phase advancement tends to disappear, and the compensatory response then becomes closely in phase with stimulus angular velocity.

Fig. 12 is a short section of record from an experiment in which an intact animal was ether anaesthestized just to the point of saccade disappearance. The anaesthetic was then removed and continuous recording of stimulus and response maintained throughout the period of recovery. At some time during the recovery sequence saccades would intermittently occur during some cycles as indicated in the figure. Over an appropriate portion of the record it was possible to obtain equal numbers of cycles with and without a contained saccade. Without exception the presence of a single saccade just preceding maximum eye deviation restored the phase relationship between stimulus and response. Note that in Fig. 12 the stimulus record is of head angle, not head angular velocity.

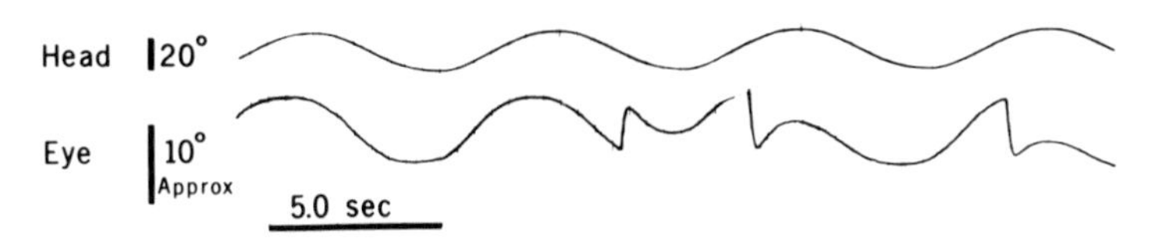

Fig. 12. Influence of saccades upon phase relation between stimulus (head angle, upper trace) and eye angle relative to the skull. Head displacement left = up; eye displacement left = down.

It was concluded from this that in addition to canal dynamics we must include a term equivalent to a first order lag system having time constant in the region of 0.5 - 1.0 sec. Such a system would lead to phase advancement in the undisturbed smooth response and would also account for the restoration of phase after a saccade occurring in a direction opposite to the prevailing compensatory eye movement. In effect this conclusion supposes that whenever the eye is deviated from its central position an angular velocity towards the central position, and proportional to the instantaneous deviation from it, must be algebraically added to the eye angular velocity induced by the reflex drive.

It is interesting to note the pattern of eye movement to be expected from such a system in response to a step change of head angular velocity in the absence of saccades. Fig. 13 illustrates responses obtained to right and left in an intact cat, again under just sufficient ether anaesthesia to remove saccades.

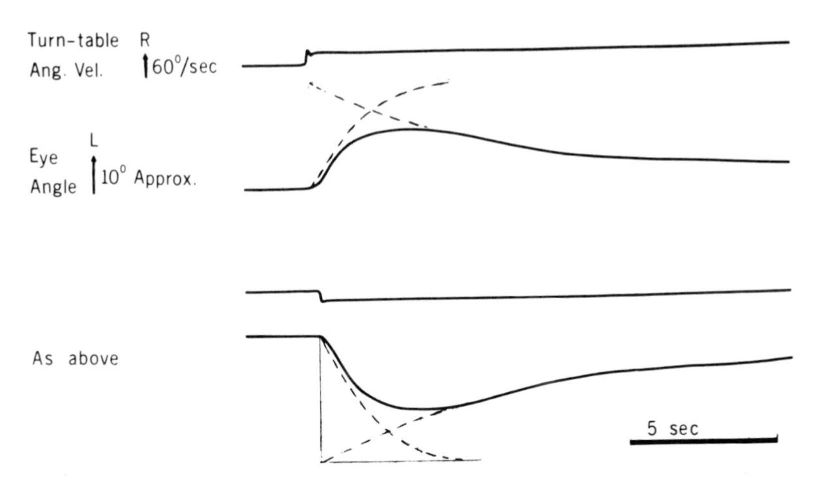

Fig. 13. Ocular responses to step changes in canal angular velocity in the absence of saccades. (From *Sugie & Melvill Jones*, 1966).

The step changes in head angular velocity were chosen to have magnitude unlikely to cause saturation of eye rotation. A relatively fast rise to peak angular displacement of the eye followed by a relatively slow exponential return towards the zero position was regularly observed under these conditions. This pattern is indeed in conformity with the results observed in Fig. 12, with the special features that (a) the initial rise towards peak would be dominated by the time constant of the supposed first order lag system, whilst the subsequent exponential return would be dominated by the long time-constant of the canal. Fig. 14 which is reproduced from Fig. 13 of Sugie and Melvill Jones (1966) provides further evidence that such a system is at play. The upper two traces give the stimulus head angular position and corresponding compensatory nystagmoid trace of eye movement, from a record chosen for the special feature that it contained one saccade per half cycle. The third trace gives the simulated "primary" component which would be associated with a response such as the smooth one in Fig. 11 and the non-saccadic part of Fig. 12. The lowest curve shows that the "secondary" component turns out to be a series of exponential decays induced by the saccadic displacement of the eye first in one direction and then in the other. It seems then as though we have to consider the actual response, at least in the cat, as being the sum of two components, named above as the primary and secondary ones.

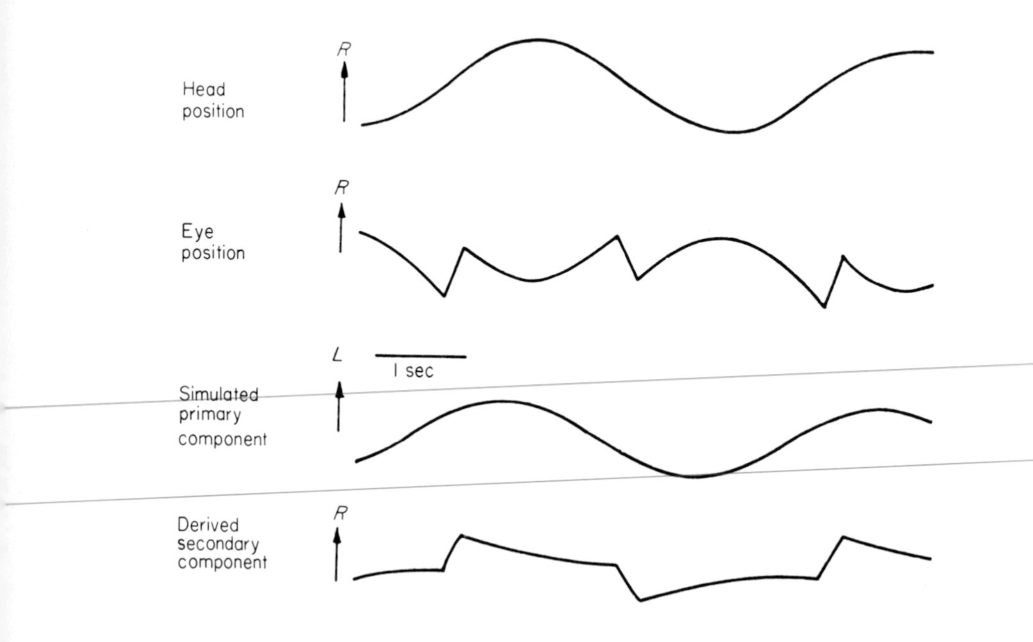

Fig. 14. Demonstration of primary and secondary components of response in the vestibulo-ocular reflex, as described in the text. (From *Sugie & Melvill Jones,* 1966).

For simplicity, these authors assumed a system in which there was always a constant interval between saccades, but the magnitude of each saccade was a function of the canal-induced input. Fig. 15 was proposed as the simple model of cat's vestibulo-ocular reflex system. The input of head position is fed into the canal dynamics which then passes through a primary pathway direct to the oculomotor system and operates on eye position through the oculomotor dynamics proposed as the first order lag system. During nystagmus, however, the output of the canal dynamics is fed through a parallel sampled pathway in which a sampling interval say of 0.3 sec may be assumed, with the particular feature that the magnitude of each triggered response in this pathway (secondary or saccadic pathway) was proportional to the sampled canal signal. The triggered output would be fed through a suitable gain control to sum negatively with the primary pathway, so that in the real event the summed effect would be fed through oculomotor dynamics to generate eye position. The first order lag oculomotor dynamics proposed here does not seem to be out of line with either the results of Zuber (1968) who examined the oculomotor response to sinusoidal modulation of VIth nerve stimulation, or Robinson (1965) who proposed a series of voigt elements in the oculomotor plant. The time-constant represented in Fig. 15 would presumably correspond approximately to the longest time-constant of Robinson's voigt elements. It is true that in man, the latter seems to be considerably shorter than in the cat. But as shown by Sugie & Jones (1966) and in more detail by Outerbridge (1969) the introduction of intermittent saccades can, to a remarkable degree, offset the consequence of a short time constant.

REVIEW OF THE OVERALL SYSTEM

Thus, reviewing the vestibulo-ocular reflex arc, it is suggested from the above findings and inferences that, at least during natural movements, the hydrodynamic response of the semicircular canal leads to the generation of an afferent neural signal containing the essential meaning of head angular velocity. This signal is then fed forward through subsequent neural relays to the oculomotor nuclei in a form which is largely unchanged and hence retains the angular velocity message. This then generates a "primary" oculomotor response after passing through a first order lag system, with the special added feature that a "secondary", saccadically generated, signal, also operating through the subsequent first order lag system, tends to restore correct phase (and presumably amplitude) relations between the response and the original stimulus head movement.

The nicety of such an arrangement is emphasized by the fact that the canal response is essentially dependent upon the inertia of the canal's contained endolymph. Hence, the canal response generates an output dependent upon movement of the head relative to inertial space. With this output carrying the message of head angular velocity relative to space, it seems entirely appropriate that the subsequent carriage of the message through the neural reflex arc in a

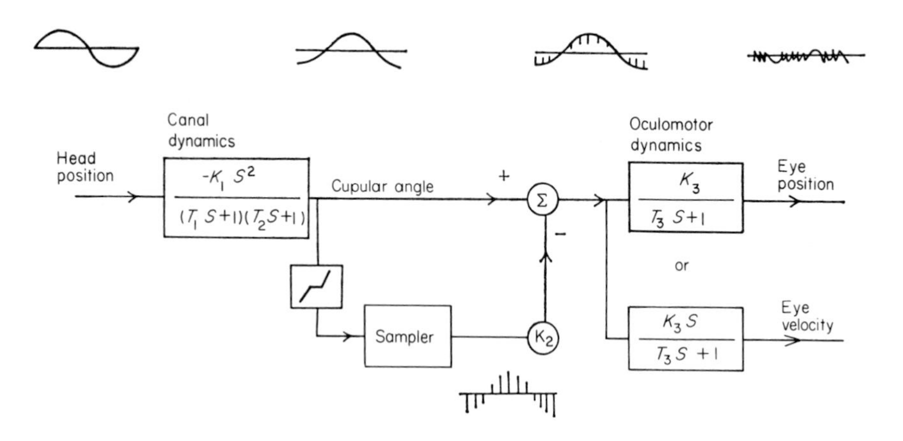

Fig. 15. A simple model of the vestibulo-ocular reflex arc proposed by Sugie and Melvill Jones (1966), incorporating the saccadic influence upon slow-phase nystagmoid response as evidenced in Figs. 12, 13 and 14.

virtually unchanged form leads in the end to a drive which generates corresponding eye angular velocity relative to the head. Due to the anatomical pathways described or referred to by Carpenter (reference earlier chapter in this book) the eye response operates in a compensatory direction. The eye thus becomes stabilised relative to inertial space and hence visual fixation upon the stationary world is automatically established during head rotation.

ACKNOWLEDGEMENT

The author wishes to acknowledge with appreciation the technical assistance of Mr. W. Ferch (Electronics), Mr. F. Lewertoff (Mechanics) and Mrs. T. Lewertoff (Histology).

REFERENCES

Adrian, E. D. (1943). Orientation discharges from vestibular receptors in the cat. *J. Physiol.* **101**, 389–407.

Bach-y-Rita, P. and Murata, K. (1964). Extraocular proprioceptive responses in the VI nerve of the cat. *Quart. J. Exp. Physiol.* **49**, 409–417.

Gaede, W. (1922). Uber die Bewegunge der Flussigkeit in einem rotierenden Hohlring. *Arch. Ohr.-, Nas.-, und Kehlkheilk,* **110**, 6.

Gernandt, B. (1949). Response of mammalian vestibular neurones to horizontal rotation and caloric stimulation. *J. Neurophysiol.* **12**, 173–184.

Goldberg, J. M. and Fernández, C. (1969). Responses of first-order vestibular afferents of the squirrel monkey to angular acceleration. *Symposium on Systems Analysis in Neurophysiology, Brainerd, Minn.,* pp. 176–191.

Groen, J. J., Lowenstein, O. and Vendrik, A. J. H. (1952). The mechanical analysis of the responses from the end-organs of the horizontal semicircular canal in the isolated elasmobranch labyrinth. *J. Physiol.* **117**, 329–346.

Horcholle, G. and Tyč-Dumont. (1968). Activitiés unitaires des neurones vestibulaires et oculomoteurs au cours du nystagmus. *Exp. Brain. Res.* **5**, 16–31.

Jones, G. M. and Spells, K. E. (1963). A theoretical and comparative study of the functional dependence of the semicircular canal upon its physical dimensions. *Proc. R. Soc. B.* **157**, 403–419.

Lorente de Nó, R. (1933). Vestibulo-ocular reflex arc. *Arch. Neur. Psychiat.* Chicago. **30**. 245–291.

Mayne, R. (1950). The dynamic characteristics of the semicircular canals. *J. Comp. Physiol. Psychol.* **43**, 309–321.

Mayne, R. (1965). The functional parameters of the semicircular canals. Tech. Report GERA-1056, Goodyear Aerospace Corpn., Arizona. Also in report under NASA contract No. NAS9-4460.

McMasters, R. E., Weiss, A. M., and Carpenter, M. B. (1966). Vestibular projections to the nuclei of the extra-ocular muscles. Degeneration resulting from discrete partial lesions of the vestibular nuclei in the monkey. *Amer. J. Anat.* **118**, 163–194.

Melvill Jones, G. (1969a). The function significance of semicircular canal size. In: *Handbook of Sensory Physiology,* Berlin: Springer–Verlag. (In press).

Melvill Jones, G. (1969b). Dynamic cross-coupling in the semicircular canals: A non–mathematical appraisal. *Proceedings of the 18th International Congress of Aerospace Medicine,* September 1969, Amsterdam, Netherlands. Editor: D. E. Busby. (In Press).

Melvill Jones, G. and Milsum, J. H. (1965a). Spatial and dynamic aspects of visual fixation. *IEEE Trans. Biomed. Eng.,* **BME-12**, 54–62.

Melvill Jones, G. and Milsum, J. H. (1965b). Neural dynamics of vestibular transduction. *Proc. 18th Ann. Conf. on Eng. in Med. & Biol.* **7**, 38–39.

Melvill Jones, G. and Milsum, J. H. (1967). Relations between neural and mechanical responses of the semicircular canal. *Proc. 38th Ann. Sci. Meeting, Aerospace Med. Assoc.* pp. 252–253.

Melvill Jones, G. and Milsum, J. H. (1969a). Characteristics of neural transmission from the semicircular canal to units in the vestibular nuclei of cats. *J. Physiol.* (In Press).

Melvill Jones, G. and Sugie, N. (1965a). Evidence for a new component of response in the oculomotor system. *Proc. 23rd Internat. Congress of Physiol. Sci.* p. 419.

Melvill Jones, G. and Sugie, N. (1965b). Patterns of neuronal response in the region of the VIth nerve nucleus during controlled rotational stimulation of the semicircular canals. *Proc. Canad. Fed. Biol. Socs.* **8**, 14.

Mergler, D. and Melvill Jones, G. (1969). Relation between neural drive and clinical response in the oculomotor system. *Proc. Aerospace. Med. Ann. Sci. Meeting,* pp. 160–161, San Francisco.

Milsum, J. H. and Melvill Jones, G. (1969). Dynamic asymmetry in neural components of the vestibular system. *Ann. N. Y. Acad. Sci.* **156**, 851–871.

Outerbridge, J. (1969). *Experimental and Theoretical Investigation of Vestibularly Driven Head and Eye Movements.* Ph.D. Thesis, Dept. of Physiology McGill University, Canada.

Precht, W. and Shimazu, H. (1965). Functional connections of tonic and kinetic vestibular neurones with primary vestibular afferents. *J. Neurophysiol.* **28**, 1014–1027.

Precht, W., Richter, A., and Grippo, J. (1969). Responses of neurones in cat's abducens nuclei to horizontal angular acceleration. *Pflügers Arch.* **309**, 285–309.

Richter, A. and Precht, W. (1968). Inhibition of abducens motoneurones by vestibular nerve stimulation. *Brain. Res.* **11**, 701–705.

Robinson, D. A. (1964). The mechanics of human saccadic eye movement. *J. Physiol.* **174**, 245–264.

Robinson, D. A. (1965). The mechanics of human smooth pursuit eye movement. *J. Physiol.* **180**, 569–591.
Robinson, D. A. (1968). The oculomotor control system: A review. *Proc. IEEE*, **56**, 1032–1049.
Ross, D. A. (1936). Electrical studies on the frog's labyrinth. *J. Physiol.* **86**, 117–146.
Schmaltz, G. (1925). Versuche zu einer Theorie des Erregungs-vorganges im Ohrlabyrinth. *Pflüg. Arch. ges. Physiol.* **207**, 125–128.
Schmaltz, G. (1931). The physical phenomena occurring in the semicircular canals during rotatory and thermic stimulation. *Proc. Roy. Soc. Med.* **25**, 359–381.
Shimazu, H. and Precht, W. (1965). Tonic and kinetic responses of cat's vestibular neurons to horizontal angular acceleration. *J. Neurophysiol.* **28**, 991–1013.
Steinhausen, W. (1933). Uber die Funktion der Cupula in den Bogengangsampullen des Labyrinths. *A. Hals.-, Nas.-, Ohren-heilk.* **34**, 201–211.
Sugie, N. and Melvill Jones, G. (1966). Eye movements elicited by head rotation. *Bull. Electrotech. Lab. Japan.* **30**, 598–606.
Sugie, N. and Melvill Jones, G. (1969). Eye movements induced by head rotation. *IEEE Trans. on SSC.* (In Press).
Szentágothai, J. (1950). The elementary vestibulo-ocular reflex arc. *J. Neurophysiol.* **13**, 395–407.
Tarlo, D. and Melvill Jones, G. (1968). Unit activity in cat abducens nerve fibers during vestibularly driven eye movements. *Proc. Canad. Fed. Biol. Socs.* **11**, 125.
van Egmond, A. A. J., Groen, J. J., and Jongkees, L. B. W. (1949). The mechanics of the semicircular canals. *J. Physiol.* **110**, 1–17.
Zuber, B. L. (1968). Sinusoidal eye movements from brain stem stimulation in the cat. *Vision Res.* **8**, 1073–1079.

MODELS OF OCULOMOTOR NEURAL ORGANIZATION

DAVID A. ROBINSON

Block diagrams of oculomotor organization serve as a compact description of system behavior but seldom have much bearing on the way in which the real system, composed of nerve and muscle, actually operates. The models thus do not contribute much to the neurophysiology (or neurology) of eye movements and incur the danger of suggesting that there actually are segregated portions of the nervous system which perform the differentiation, integration and other operations indicated in the boxes of the diagrams. An increasing number of results are emerging from stimulation, ablation and unit recording in oculomotor pathways, especially that important region between the superior colliculi and the vestibular nuclei, and this information will one day allow us to replace black boxes with neural networks. The following speculations are an exercise in this effort. They offer little in the way of conclusions and mostly indicate the difficulties encountered in trying to fill in a few of the black boxes with some sort of neural arrangement that is compatible with known structure and function. These hypothetical schemes attempt to anticipate what must eventually be discovered by neurophysiological experimentation and are offered here in the hope of provoking debate and further investigation.

The vestibular-ocular reflex

It is appropriate to start with this system since it is phylogenetically old and is generally thought to form a substrate overlaid by the more complicated

This investigation was supported by Public Health Service Research Grant NB08633-01, from the National Institute of Neurological Diseases and Stroke.

visually mediated eye movement systems. The shortness of the path and our knowledge of semicircular canal and oculomotor muscle function helps a great deal in specifying what the interposed neural elements must do and so, perhaps, how they may do it. The three neuron arc described by Szentágothai (1950), shown in Fig. 1 for horizontal eye movements, forms a skeleton for the reflex. Szentágothai described only excitatory connections but recently Richter & Precht(1968)have shown that the vestibular nuclei directly inhibit the ipsilateral abducens nuclei. It would be most unusual if the vestibular nuclei did not then also inhibit the contralateral medial recti. These connections are also shown in Fig. 1 making it a slight extension of the basic three neuron arc described by Szentágothai.

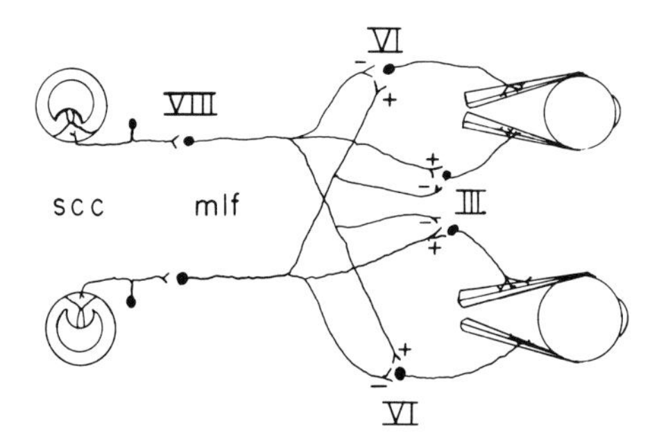

Fig. 1. Szentagothai's three neuron arc for horizontal gaze. Semicircular canal (scc) afferents pass through the vestibular nuclei (VIII) and ascend in the medial longitudinal fasciculus (mlf) to excite (+) the oculomotor (III) and abducens (VI) nuclei. Inhibitory fibers (–) inferred from the work of Richter & Precht (1968) are included.

One might be tempted to utilize the tonic activity of the semicircular canals to account for the 15g of tone (Robinson *et al.*, 1969) observed in extraocular muscles in the primary position. The simple arc in Fig. 1 could account for such tone if the inhibitory connections were left out but their inclusion means that each canal by itself, reciprocally innervates the musculature and the opposing influences may cancel out at the motor nuclei. The fact that drowsiness and depressants knock out muscle tone before interfering with vestibular afferent signals also implies that vestibular tonic activity is not the cause of motor tone and its source probably arises from a more general activation process.

The function of the vestibulo-ocular reflex is to stabilize the visual axes in space by changing the position of the eyes in the orbit an amount equal and opposite to a change of position of the head in space. The scheme in Fig. 1 cannot accomplish this. Since the canals are stimulated by head acceleration, a double integration must occur between canal excitation and eye position. The first integration occurs mechanically in the cupula of the canal over the range .017 Hz to 17 Hz (Jones & Milsum, 1965) and in this range the afferent discharge is proportional to head velocity. An additional integration must therefore occur in the brain stem. It probably occurs in polyneuronal chains in the reticular formation.

Fig. 2 shows a hypothetical network to accomplish this integration. The integrator must not be directly connected to either source of vestibular afferents since each contains a constant level of activity. It is necessary that the difference in activity between the two canals be integrated as shown in Fig. 2. These decussating fibers are similar to those described by Shimazu and Precht (1966). There are many ways to construct a nerve net so that it performs integration over a given bandwidth. A fairly simple one is to utilize re-excitation; that is, cells excite their neighbors and are re-excited by them. A nerve net, randomly connected in this way with the proper synaptic weightings will, if briefly excited, tend to retain its activity regeneratively. The activity will decay slowly and the network will appear to have the transfer function $1/(s+\alpha)$. Lorente de Nó (1933) has described such a system of reverberating collaterals but this choice for the integrating nerve net must remain a speculation until microelectrode recording in the reticular formation and medial longitudinal fasciculus can shed more light on the matter.

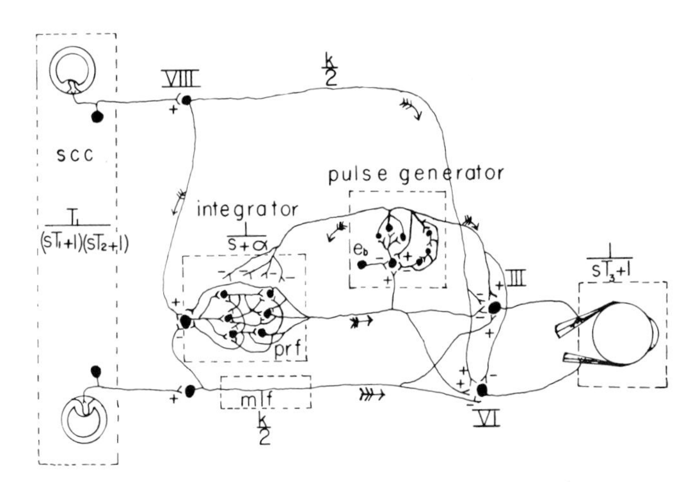

Fig. 2. An extension of the simple three neuron arc of Fig. 1 by the addition of an integrator and pulse generator in the pontine reticular formation (prf). The neural integrator converts the head velocity information flowing in from the semicircular canals (scc) to position information for use by the extraocular muscles. The pulse generator circuit executes the fast phase of vestibular nystagmus. Excitation is indicated by +, inhibition by -.

Since an integration is required in the brain stem path, the direct connections of the three neuron arc might seem to interfere with the accomplishment of this purpose. However this is not so as shown by the following analysis. The transfer function of the semicircular canals (afferent discharge rate divided by head acceleration) is

$$\frac{T_1}{(sT_1 + 1)(sT_2 + 1)}$$

where T_1 and T_2 are about 10 sec and 10 msec respectively. Within the spectral range where the canals integrate $[(1/T_1) < s < (1/T_2)]$, the transfer function is approximately $1/s$. The neural integrator with a transfer function of $1/(s+a)$ is in parallel with the direct three neuron arc. If the transmission of the latter is k (the sum of the transmissions of $k/2$ from each canal), the total brain stem transmission is

$$k + \frac{1}{s+a} = \frac{k(s+a)+1}{s+a}.$$

In the frequency range $s > a$ (in which the nerve net behaves like an integrator) this simplifies to $(ks + 1)/s$. The zero (numerator) in this transfer function occurs because rate information is being passed directly to the motor nuclei along the medial longitudinal fasciculus. It is proposed that its function is to overcome the lag inherent in the final common path. Although the torque-angle transfer function of the eyeball, muscles and supporting tissue is at least fourth order (Robinson, 1964), contains a small resonant peak (Thomas, 1967), and non-linear elements (Cook, 1968), it is dominated by viscoelasticity and, for many purposes, such as the simple considerations here, may be approximated by a simple lag of the form $1/(sT_3 + 1)$. (For the eye of the awake fixating human, T_3 is about 115 msec (Robinson, 1964)).

Therefore the approximate transfer function from head acceleration to eye position is,

$$\left(\frac{1}{s}\right)\left(\frac{sk+1}{s}\right)\left(\frac{1}{sT_3+1}\right) = \frac{1}{s^2}\frac{(sk+1)}{(sT_3+1)} = \frac{1}{s^2}, \text{ if } k = T_3.$$

Thus, if k has the right value (namely about 0.115), a simple double integration as required by the function of the reflex, is achieved. Looked at another way, the direct path k feeds high frequency velocity information directly to the final common path and the final integration is performed mechanically by the sluggish elements of the orbit. The low frequency components, which the globe could follow, are integrated by the nerve net in the pontine reticular formation. Fig. 3 shows pictorially how the two brain stem pathways cooperate to produce accurate compensatory eye movements during a quick movement of the head. Gernant has estimated k at about 0.25 (Gernant, 1968) but it is a bit early to attempt numerical correlation between brain stem physiology and nerve net models.

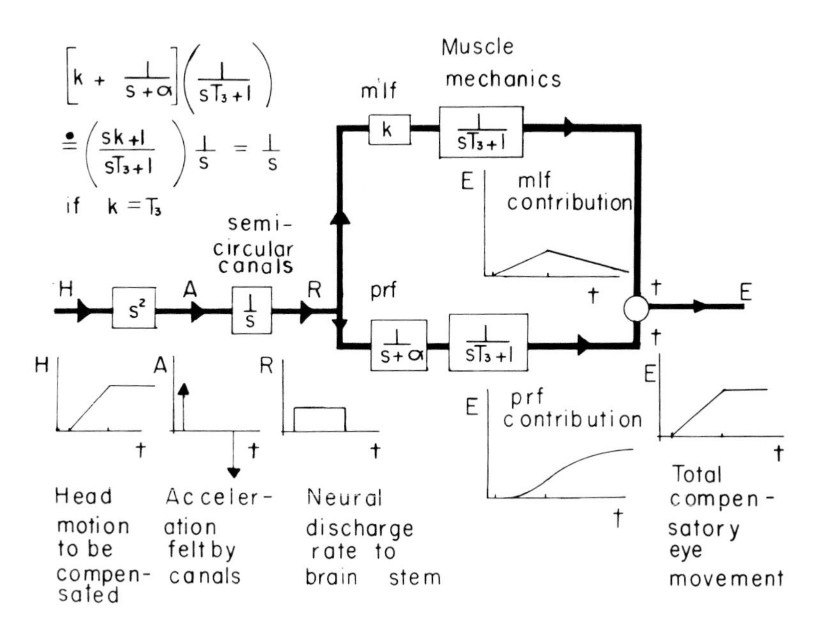

Fig. 3. The signals created by a sudden turn of the head (H). The canals are excited by head acceleration (A) and produce a neural afferent whose rate (R) is proportional to head velocity. This is processed in turn by two paths, the medial longitudinal fasciculus (mlf) and muscle mechanics which integrates high frequency components and the pontine reticular formation (prf) which integrates low frequency components. The sum of the two paths produces an eye movement (E) equal (and opposite) to the head movement stimulus.

The system shown in Fig. 2 is for one eye and only one direction of slow phase eye movement. To complete the picture one must imagine connections being made to the yoke muscles of the other eye and then the whole diagram overlaid by the mirror image of itself to create movements in the opposite direction. The picture is further complicated if one considers that all three pairs of canals must be properly connected to all three antagonistic muscle pairs of each eye. The experimenter, recording single units in the brain stem of a behaving animal, is painfully aware of the complexity created by these three degrees of freedom.

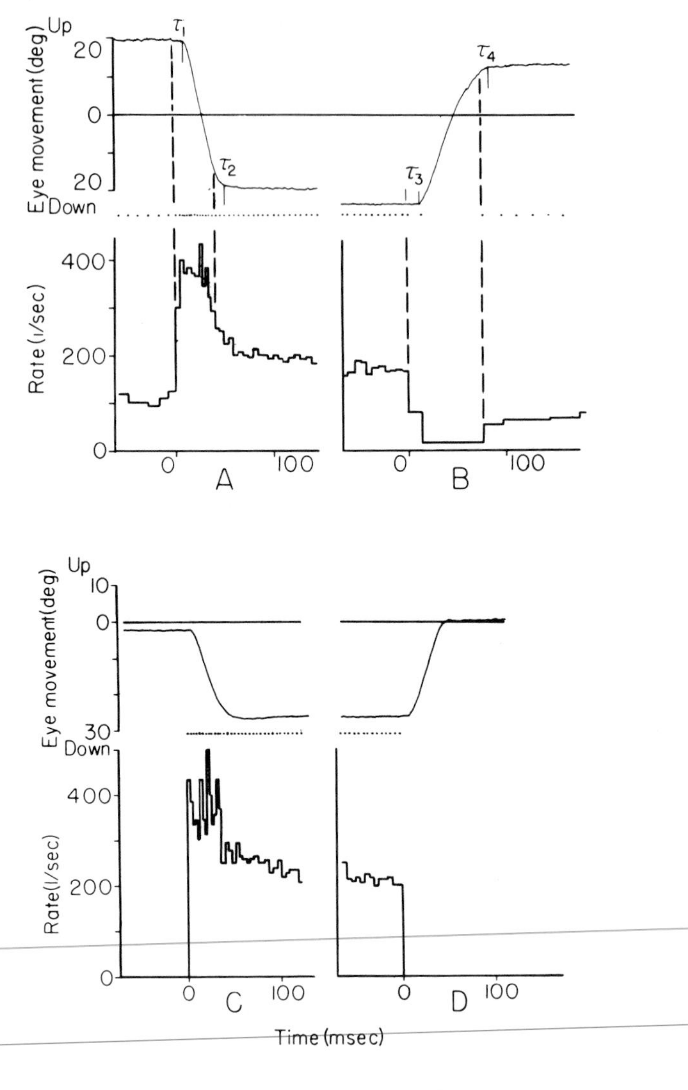

Fig. 4. The time course of single unit activity in the oculomotor nucleus of the awake intact monkey during spontaneous saccadic eye movements. During on saccades (into the field of action of the muscle) the units burst at high discharge rates (A and C) and during off saccades are inhibited (B and D). The unit in C and D has a high threshold and only fires when the eye looks sufficiently into the on field. The row of dots incidate the occurrences of spikes and the instantaneous frequency is plotted below.

The system so far described stabilizes the visual axes in space over a certain frequency range for head excursions too small to trigger the fast phase of vestibular nystagmus. If the head turns too far, a fast phase, or saccade occurs since, from a survival standpoint, it is better to stabilize about a new axis in space than to loose stabilization altogether and visual acuity with it. Many experiments have shown that the fast phase is triggered centrally and not peripherally (McCouch, 1932). Often, when a man is suddenly rotated from rest, the first eye movement he makes may be a fast phase although his eyes started in the primary position (Jones, 1964). Since the amplitude of the fast phase and the eye position at which it occurs is quite variable for a constant vestibular excitation it would appear that the fast phase trigger threshold fluctuates considerably and is probably under the influence of the state of alertness and especially the nature of objects seen in the advancing peripheral visual field. Once the threshold is exceeded by the integrator output, an all-or-nothing burst of neural activity drives the eyes in the opposite direction in a fast phase. The pulsatile nature of this saccadic movement has been well established by electromyography (Miller, 1958; Tamler, 1959), by measuring isometric muscle tension in the intact eye (Robinson, 1964) and on single muscles detached from the globe during surgery (Robinson *et al.*, 1969), and by single unit recording in the abducens nucleus (Schaefer, 1965) and nerve (Yamanaka, 1968) of rabbit and cat during vestibular nystagmus. Fig. 4 illustrates results from my own laboratory. It depicts activity typical of single units in the oculomotor nucleus of the intact awake monkey during spontaneous saccadic eye movements. The examples demonstrate that motor units burst at high discharge rates during saccades into the field of action of that muscle and are strongly inhibited during saccades in the opposite direction. Fig. 4 also illustrates that the duration of intense excitation (or inhibition) is equal to the duration of the saccade (and consequently proportional to its amplitude).

The need for this pulsatile activity is clear when one considers the overdamped nature of the globe torque-angle transfer function. If one uses the oversimplified function $1/(sT_3 + 1)$ for the plant, Fig. 5a illustrates how a pulse is used to move the eye rapidly and a step is used to hold it there. Thus saccades are produced by a pulse-step combination of applied force. By similar reasoning, pulse-ramps of force are required to produce nystagmus as shown in Fig. 5b. Consequently, one must add, as shown in Fig. 2, a neural pulse generator network which is triggered into activity when the neural integrator output exceeds a (fluctuating) threshold level (e_b) and which must inhibit one motor nucleus, powerfully activate the opposite nucleus and reset the integrator. Resetting the integrator is an important function of the pulse generator. It will not do to simply over-ride or uncouple the motor nuclei temporarily from the integrator output since, when they are recoupled, the integrators will drive the eye back to the last remembered position which is just what is not wanted. The memory of the integrator must be wiped out so it can start to integrate again from a new level. Fig. 2 indicates one simple way to do this by completely

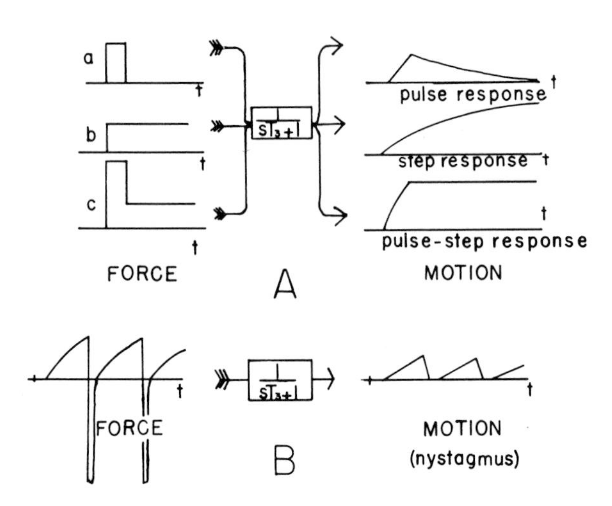

Fig. 5. A simplified illustration of the pulsatile nature of extraocular muscle force to produce saccades or the fast phase of nystagmus. A. If the globe torque-angle transfer function is approximated by a simple lag (T_3), a saccade-like movement (c) can be thought of as the combined response to a pulse (a) and a step (b). B. A combination of alternating ramps and pulses is required of the extraocular muscles to produce nystagmus.

inhibiting all the integrator cells. One cannot, as an alternative, apply the pulse to the integrator input since it cannot integrate negative inputs. It is proposed that as animals developed foveas and created the need for a saccadic system so as to be able to ''look at'' things (that is, place an object's image rapidly onto the fovea) these same fast phase pulse generators were appropriated by the visual system for the purpose of making saccades. For this reason, the specific form chosen for the pulse generator shown in Fig. 2 is deferred for the discussion of the saccadic system.

When the complementory integrator and pulse generator to handle movements in the opposite directions are added to Fig. 2 one has a neural model for the entire vestibulo-ocular reflex in one plane for one eye. The model proposed in Fig. 2 is probably not far from wrong from a functional standpoint. The details of the integrators and pulse generators remain to be elucidated but their existance may be inferred with some certainty. Where in the pontine reticular formation the cells and fibers lie which mediate this activity is one of the goals of oculomotor neurophysiology. I should now like to speculate on how this basic reflex can be overlaid by the more complex visually controlled saccadic and smooth pursuit systems.

The saccadic system

The pulsatile system of Fig. 2 for making saccades is insensitive to absolute eye position. Its responsibility is only to get the eye from one place to another as quickly as possible and not to hold it there. The simplest visual act is steady fixation and in trying to introduce a visually mediated eye positioning system into the primitive arrangement of Fig. 2 one is made more aware of the distinction between these two requirements; to move the eye quickly and then to hold it there. Fig. 2 contains a means to do the former but not the latter. This leads to the question of whether one should consider the existence of a fixation system independent of, and in addition to, the saccadic system or whether both services are performed by a single system. The latter would be better designated as the positioning system rather than the saccadic system as is now the custom. There are several lines of evidence to favor the former distinction. When an animal is lightly depressed by drugs (sodium pentobarbital, phencyclidine hydrochloride (Sernylan, Parke Davis), and diazepam (Valium, Roche), all give the same results with respect to eye movements) the animal is still able to make saccadic eye movements but has lost the ability to make smooth pursuit movements (optokinetic nystagmus driven by a rotating mirror) and also the ability to maintain fixation away from the primary position. A vigorous visual or acoustic stimulus will produce a saccade in the direction of the stimulus followed at once by a slow, more or less exponential drift of eye position back to the primary position. This suggests that although both saccades and fixation are visually initiated optomotor responses, their prenuclear motor organization is sufficiently different that one response can occur without the other. The simultaneous loss of fixation and smooth pursuit movements may not be a coincidence if one considers that fixation is the special case of pursuit when the target velocity is zero. Thus it is a moot question whether the saccadic or the smooth pursuit system (as currently represented in the literature) are responsible for fixation.

Another bit of evidence concerns single unit behavior in the motor nuclei. Their discharge rates increase as both eye position (at zero velocity) or eye velocity (at any given position) increase in the on direction (the direction of action of that muscle). The eye velocity dependence leads directly to the burst in rate during on saccades when the eye velocity is very large. Between different units there can be a 6:1 spread in the sensitivity of rate to eye velocity relative to the sensitivity to eye position. Put another way, two units having the same rate dependency on position can have quite different burst rates during on saccades (e.g. 700/sec vs. 125/sec). This behavior suggests that position and velocity commands cannot reach the nucleus on the same set of presynaptic fibers but arise from different structures, one concerned with position (fixation) the other with movement (saccades).

For these reasons it is proposed that the fixation system be distinguished as a separate system whose function is to hold the eye wherever it is put, and that the function of the saccadic system be contracted to exclude fixation and be concerned only with the rapid movement itself. In this context the foundation for the saccadic system is already contained in Fig. 2. Indirect evidence concerning the dynamics of the neural pulse generators shown there come from the results of stimulating the frontal eye fields (Robinson & Fuchs, 1969). A short pulse train (30 msec) delivered to the frontal eye fields of the awake macaque produces a conjugate contralateral saccade with a latency of about 25 msec. It occurs in an all-or-none fashion at a threshold (typically 0.2 ma) and the amplitude and direction of the saccade depends only on where the cortex is stimulated being independent of stimulus intensity (above threshold), train length, pulse width, pulse rate and initial eye position. No other types of eye movement could be produced by stimulation although smooth movements, centering, nystagmus and vergence movements could all be produced by using anesthesia. As the electrode moved from point to point, saccade size ranged from 1 to 70 deg.

The frontal eye fields project to the ventral layers of the superior colliculi (Kuypers, 1967) and the presumption is that excitation of these fibers provokes a response along optomotor pathways arising in or near the superior colliculi and involving tegmental and pretectal areas. This latter pathway is presumed to be phylogenetically old and must have subserved the first tectally derived optokinetic movements. Frontal eye field stimulation thus eventually arrives in the brain stem and triggers the neural pulse generators which create saccades.

The fact that the saccades occurred in an all-or-none fashion above a fixed threshold suggests the circuit analogue of the one-shot multivibrator. This feature of saccades has long been implied in the use of the term ballistic, indicating a phenomenon which, once started, cannot be stopped or modified until it has run its course. Such systems (the nerve action potential is a well known biological example) generally exhibit refractoriness and when a conditioning stimulus is delivered to the frontal eye fields, a subsequent test stimulus shows that an evoked saccade is followed by a 50 msec absolute refractory period and then another 50 msec relative refractory period. Thus, the neural circuits being excited seem to possess all the classical behavior patterns of the one-shot multivibrator.

I have suggested a specific circuit for the pulse generator of Fig. 2 simply for the sake of argument. The circuit, shown in detail in Fig. 6, is the simplest form possible from a circuit standpoint and one which is easily realized in a nerve net. It consists of a unidirectional saturating amplifier normally kept in an off state by a biasing signal e_b and triggered on by an input signal e_1. Positive feedback e_2 through attenuator λ ($\lambda < 1$) locks the amplifier on in full saturation momentarily. A negative feedback path delayed by a time constant T finally overwhelms the positive feedback, unlocks the amplifier and turns it off. The signal wave forms shown in Fig. 6 indicate how each pulse is followed by a refractory period. It is clear from Fig. 6 how aggregates of cells can accomplish, by excitation and inhibition, the same behavior shown by the circuit diagram. There are of course innumerable alternate possibilities for a neural arrangement, all of them more complicated than the one shown, to accomplish the same purpose. The correct organization must await progress in single unit recording and the tracing of anatomical connections.

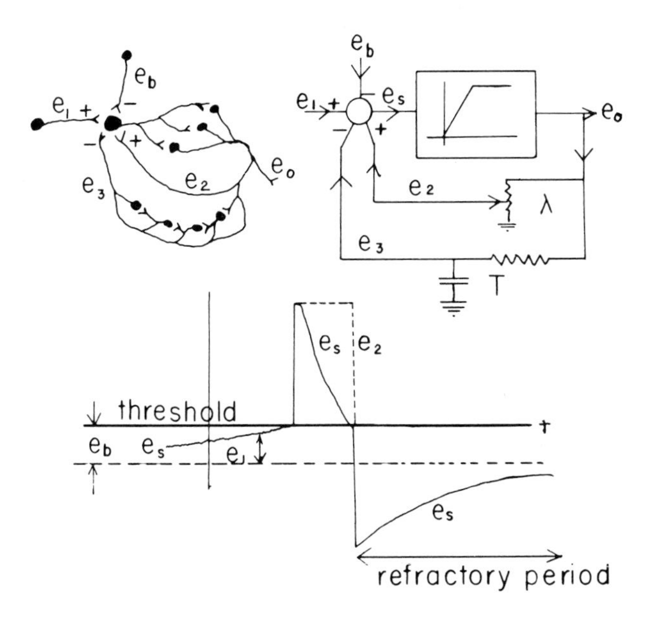

Fig. 6. A very primitive form of one-shot multivibrator circuit with its nerve net analogue similar to the one shown in Fig. 2. The wave forms are shown below during a pulse and subsequent refractory period in voltages or their neural analogue, discharge rate.

When a conditioning stimulus is given to one frontal eye field and the test stimulus to the opposite side, no refractoriness is demonstrable and the two evoked saccades (opposite in direction) may be made to occur back to back. The simplest explanation for this, as suggested in Fig. 2, is that there are two antagonistic pulse generators, one for left, the other for right saccades, each with its own post-pulse refractory period to restimulation from that cortex which excites it. Other interesting properties of these networks emerge when two sites in the frontal eye fields, which evoke saccades of different sizes and directions are stimulated simultaneously. The pulse generators are turned nearly full on during a pulse so that larger saccades are produced by longer pulse durations. Since evoked saccade amplitude depends on where, rather than how, the frontal eye field cortex is stimulated, there must be a network, presumably caudal to the tectum, which translates the somatotopic locality of excitation into pulse duration. In the model of Fig. 6 the usual way of altering pulse duration is changing the time constant (changing the inhibitory transmission time in the neural network). However, there is little point in speculating how the neural networks actually carry out this transformation. When two points on the frontal eye fields are stimulated simultaneously an odd thing happens; a single saccade results but its amplitude may be smoothly varied between the extremes of the two saccades evoked singly by changing the relative strengths of the two stimuli. Fig. 7 is an example (hypothetical for illustrative purposes) of this behavior. Stimulation of the left cortex at a threshold of 0.2 ma produces a right 20° saccade. A 15° left saccade is evoked from the right cortex at a threshold, I_2 of 0.3 ma. As I_1 decreases from threshold and I_2 increases from zero, the right saccade drops in amplitude until, at some pair of current values, the result is complete cancellation. Beyond this the saccade grows in the other direction. This indicates that the network that translates cortex stimulus site into pulse duration must also receive fibers from the cortex contralateral to the frontal eye field which excites it and when conflicting messages reach it along several descending fiber paths, calling for saccades of different amplitudes and directions, it somehow reaches a compromise between them and produces a saccade of intermediate amplitude. It is important to note that when the net saccade in Fig. 7 is very small (e.g. 2 deg) its duration is appropriate to its size. That is, the 2 deg saccade has a duration of 20 msec and consequently cannot be the

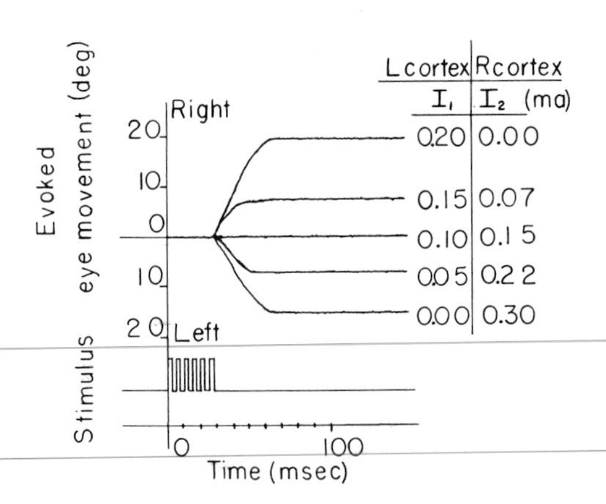

Fig. 7. A constructed example (for illustrative clarity) of saccades evoked by simultaneously stimulating the left frontal eye field of the macaque with a stimulus train of intensity I_1 (ma) and the right frontal eye field with intensity I_2 (ma). As I_1 decreases and I_2 increases, the saccade to the right decreases in amplitude, reverses, and becomes a left saccade in a smooth continuous manner.

leftover result of a struggle at the motor level of the two original saccade commands whose durations were 30 msec. It is also interesting that stimulus I_2 begins to decrease the amplitude of the saccade evoked by I_1, at current values well below threshold.

Fig. 8 summarizes the behavior for horizontal saccades. The left cortex excites the right pulse generator *R* and vice versa through unknown networks *N* (dotted lines) which responds to *which* fibers (not how many) entering it are active and produce pulses of appropriate width to create large or small saccades in either direction. The right pulse generator is placed tentatively on the right side to conform to the observation that below the level of the 3rd nucleus, stimulation creates ipsilateral eye movement (Bender, 1964).

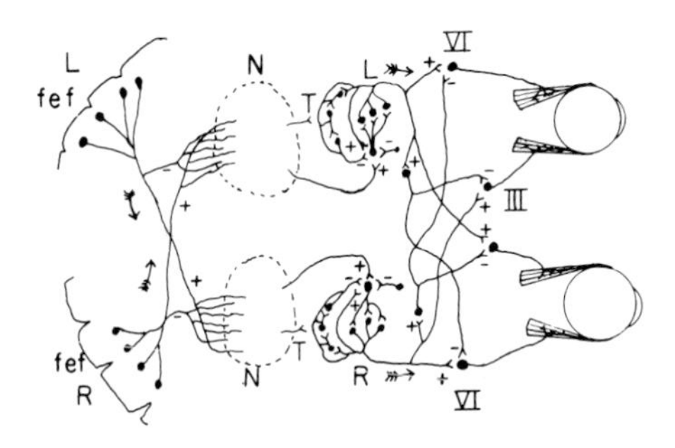

Fig. 8. A scheme suggested by the saccadic eye movements that are produced by frontal eye field (fef) stimulation. Two neural pulse generators R and L create saccades to the right and left respectively. They are connected with reciprocal innervation to yoke muscles. Each pulse generator is post-stimulus refractory to subsequent stimulation of the contralateral cortex but not the ipsilateral cortex. The neural networks N, thought to lie between the tectum and the eye muscle nuclei, trigger the pulse generators and somehow modulate pulse width or saccade size (shown by fibers marked T) according to which (not how many) fibers descending from the cortex are stimulated. When both eye fields are stimulated simultaneously, the pulse width is increased (+) by contralateral corticofugal fibers and decreased (–) by ipsilateral fibers.

In summary, sets of brain stem neural networks are proposed to create saccadic eye movements. They utilize a phylogenetically old organization responsible for maintaining fixation in the new position. Frontal eye field stimulation reveals several interesting properties of the pulsatile networks themselves and focuses attention on pathways arising in the superior colliculi, to which the frontal eye fields project, which play a vital but unknown role in translating visual information into eye movement commands.

The smooth pursuit system

Superficial inspection of the smooth pursuit system in man suggests, at first, the model shown in Fig. 9. The evidence of Rashbass (1961) and Fender (1962) indicate that this system responds only to target velocity and is not responsible for bringing the target to the fovea. This behavior is simulated in Fig. 9 by differentiating the error *e* to get slip velocity $\dot{e}$ and then integrating with some gain G. This permits the system to ignore sudden movements of either eye or target because of the non-linear error velocity cut-out element. Thus, the system tracks motion of the visual field but is indifferent to any absolute position error *e* between any part of the visual field and any special part of the retina. The question arises of whether the pursuit system tracks over a velocity range or whether it can also hold the eye steady when the visual field is stationary, that is, can it track arbitrarily small velocities down to and including zero velocity? The latter situation might be called a relative-position tracking system to indicate that it does respond to zero frequency but is distinct from the absolute-position systems of foveal tracking.

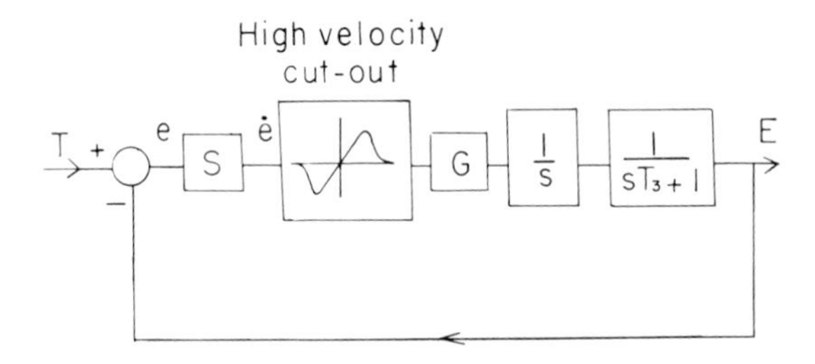

Fig. 9. A simple model of the smooth pursuit system. The scheme tracks target motion, T, but is independent of absolute error, e, between target and eye, E. Rapid jumps in target position are not followed because of the high velocity cut-out element.

Recent experiments by Collewijn (1969) indicate that the optokinetic following system of the rabbit, an afoveate animal, is a relative-position tracking system. The rabbit's eye matches the visual field velocity, with a slip velocity of about 20%, down to a field velocity of 0.003 deg/sec at which point the slip or error velocity is only 0.0006 deg/sec or one revolution a week. This is a remarkably slow movement. When the rabbit's eyes are drawn from their resting position by a drum rotation and the drum is stopped, the eyes remain deviated (Collewijn). Thus, the same system that produces optokinetic following also holds the eye in steady gaze. The implication of this is that the primate smooth pursuit system may also be a relative-position tracking system and it is possible that the saccadic system may get the target to the fovea but the pursuit system keeps it there.

In order to track arbitrarily low velocities, the differentiator and integrator must be assumed to be perfect. That is, if they are approximated by $s/(sT+1)$ and $1/(sT+1)$, then one must have a zero time constant and the other an infinite time constant. This assumption is quite unrealistic from a neurological standpoint and can easily be avoided by the reasonable supposition that relative position information is made available to the oculomotor system. Such a scheme, quite speculative, is shown in Fig. 10. For low target velocities it is a simple position tracking system. It does not follow high target velocities and after slipping, it attempts to resume relative-position tracking around a new retinal location. Relative target error e_r is obtained by subtracting a retinal offset position signal R from the absolute error e_a between target position T and eye position E. So long as the target moves slowly, e_r stays small (less than the threshold level e_{rm}), the G_1/s loop is inoperative and the system, overall, is a simple zero order position tracking system. When the target jumps rapidly so that e_r is large, the G_1/s loop changes the offset R until e_r is once again small. The system then resumes position tracking but about a new retinal position. If the target continues to move so that e_r remains large, the G_1/s loop remains active and is equivalent to the operation $s/(s+G_1)$ in the forward path. Consequently it acts as a differentiator and simulates the behavior of the simpler system in Fig. 9. The integrator in the G_1/s loop is not an analogue integrator but could come about physically by the transfer of the tracking task from an organization of receptive fields at one retinal location to another nearby. In the scheme of Fig. 10 the analogue integrator $1/(s+a)$ could be the same as that utilized by the vestibular system in Fig. 2 and permits the hypothesis that the

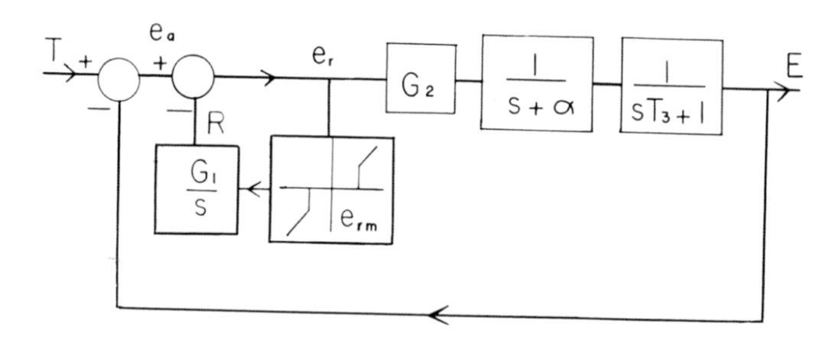

Fig. 10. Another method of achieving relative-position tracking. When relative error e_r is small, the system tracks the target based on position, not velocity information. If the target jumps, e_r is returned to zero by relocating the retinal position R about which subsequent tracking would then take place.

slow phase components of vestibular and optokinetic nystagmus share the same brain stem mechanisms. Fig. 10 is presented not only to show a scheme more neurologically plausible than that in Fig. 9 but to indicate by example that many alternate schemes are possible and modeling of the smooth pursuit system is still in a very primitive stage.

In the above considerations, the roles of the motion sensitive and directionally selective units found in the visual system, especially in the superior colliculi (Michael, 1969; Sterling, 1969), have not appeared explicitly. Clearly these units, as reported in the literature, are not likely to participate in following movements at low velocities such as 0.01 deg/sec. The rabbit's tracking system follows the movement of the majority of images in its visual field. It does not track small objects moved in the field. Thus motion sensitive units can have an important role to play in reporting the motion of elements moving within the visual field without being involved in eye movement. On the other hand they could also play a role in tracking but only when the slip velocity is great enough to excite them (typically 1-20 deg/sec). The actual mechanisms used in detecting small position and velocity errors clearly involve sensitivity to both temporal and spatial changes. The latter aspect is usually ignored in block diagrams which only deal with temporal phenomena at a few discrete points in a lumped model and cannot easily deal with spatial interactions among many parallel transmission paths. For this reason, block diagrams and their transfer functions are quite inadequate to deal with the visual afferent side of optomotor feedback systems.

Collewijn's results also produced another complication in smooth pursuit modeling. He immobilized one eye, stimulated it with moving stripes and measured the nystagmus of the opposite occluded eye. In the range 0.2 to 0.02 deg/sec the open loop gain measured in this way was about 100. Using sinusoidal stripe motion, the phase shift was compatible with a pure delay of 150 msec. Those familiar with control theory may see at once that the gain and delay are badly incompatible with stability. Fig. 11 shows the root locus for the system in Fig. 9 to which has been added a delay $e^{-s\tau}$ where τ is 150 msec. As mentioned earlier, T_3, for man is about 115 msec. The figure shows that instability is reached when the open loop gain is only 1.17. The system is so unstable that large changes in T_3 or the addition of lead or lag transfer functions do not help sufficiently to change the result.

Estimating delay by phase shift is an indirect method although the result is compatible with human smooth pursuit latencies (130 msec) during foveal tracking of small targets. In case movement of the entire visual field should produce a shorter latency, the pursuit latency to full field stimulation was measured in monkey (by the sudden rotation of a mirror) and man (by stripes moving on a tangent screen) and it was found that the latency did not change. Thus, it is unlikely that Collowijn's paradox is due to a mistaken overestimation of the delay. Oddly, when a similar open loop experiment is performed on the goldfish (Easter) the result is quite different; the open loop gain is only slightly larger than 1. It is surprising that two afoveate lateral-eyed vertebrates show such a difference. The difference may lie in the degree of coupling between the two eyes rather than in the characteristics of the optomotor reflex of one eye considered singly.

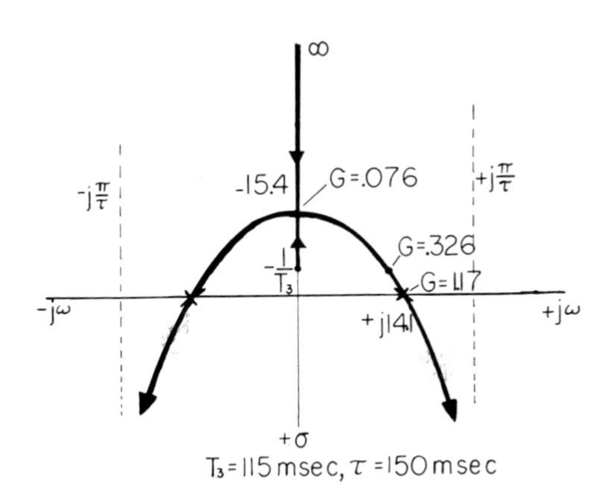

Fig. 11. The root locus plot of the scheme in Fig. 9 if a delay τ of 150 msec is added to the forward path. The system becomes unstable at a gain G of only 1.17 and is badly unstable if the gain is 100 as found by Collewijn in the rabbit.

Young's early model of the pursuit system (Young, 1963) achieved stability by sampling. Subsequent experiments (Robinson, 1965) indicated that the system is probably continuous. Attempts to simulate the system with this restriction quickly led to instability and to avoid this, Young, Forster and Van Houtte (1968) utilized a scheme of efference copy. The revised model was first shown as an open loop, unity gain system shown in Fig. 12a (only elements important to this discussion are shown). Of course target position T (or velocity) in space is not available to the system from retinal information alone and the implication intended in this model is that, as shown explicitly in Fig. 12b, an efference copy signal, *ec*, in this case a neural report of eye velocity $\dot{E}$, is fed back positively and, adding to error velocity $\dot{e}$, centrally reconstructs target velocity $\dot{T}_r$. This scheme is equivalent to Fig. 12a if the transmission along the path 1-2-3 exactly matches that along 1-4-5 so that the outer negative feedback is exactly cancelled by the internal positive feedback. To make the two paths match dynamically, the efference copy signal, taken off before the plant, since there is much evidence that reafferents from muscle proprioceptors are not involved, must pass through a central replica of the plant dynamics. Since it is probable that the pursuit system tracks velocities down to, and including, zero, one might chose to consider the equivalent arrangement of Fig. 12c which invokes position efference copy and eliminates the need for all the differentiators in Fig. 12b. Absolute-position tracking may be converted to relative-position tracking by some scheme similar to that of Fig. 10. Various delays that must occur in the paths have also been made explicit in Fig. 12c.

The valuable feature of this efference copy is that it resolves Collewijn's paradox. Clamping the stimulated eye removes the outer negative feedback loop.

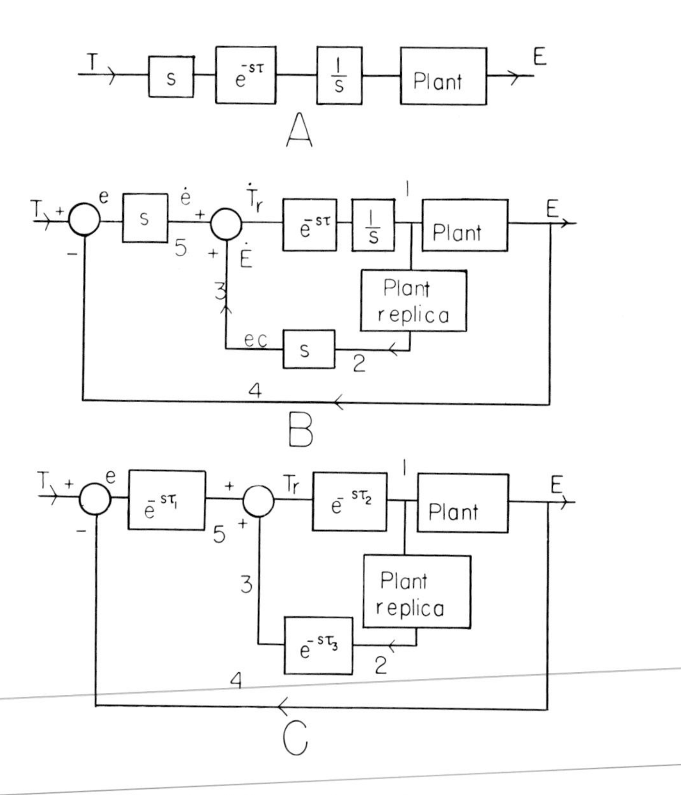

Fig. 12. **A.** The basic elements of the smooth pursuit system proposed by Young et al. (1968). The system contains no feedback because of the instability illustrated in Fig. 11 when feedback is used and the system is not sampled. **B.** An elaboration of A in which the built-in negative feedback is effectively removed by internal positive feedback in the form of efference copy which permits the central reconstruction of absolute target velocity $\dot{T}_r$. This system has a large central latency, a high open loop gain and is stable. **C.** Another version of the same scheme that utilizes position rather than velocity efference copy feedback. The delays in the various pathways are shown explicitly.

The unopposed inner positive feedback loop then creates the appearance of a very high gain. The scheme in Fig. 12 has infinite gain but this can be reduced to finite values by slightly reducing the gain of the efference copy path. On the other hand, the system is stable, closed loop, so long as the two paths 1-2-3 and 1-4-5 have the same transmission. In Fig. 12c this requires that the two delays τ_1 and τ_3 be the same. The closed loop latency $\tau_1 + \tau_2$ can be any desired value without affecting stability. Thus the model permits long latencies and high ''open loop'' gains without causing instability. There remains the technical problem of finding out how much imbalance due to biological sloppiness can be tolerated in the two feedback loops before instability is once again a problem.

The above speculations seem to indicate that when one attempts to assign neurological mechanisms to models of the pursuit system, one discovers that the models so far proposed are so greatly oversimplified that they must be considerably modified not only to make them more compatible with the capabilities of neural networks but simply to make them conform to experimental observations. The studies of optokinetic movements in rabbit (Collewijn, 1969), crab (Horridge, 1968) and goldfish (Easter) indicate that further quantitative and analytical experiments on the comparative physiology of the pursuit system may be of great value in deducing the nature of the organization in primates. No attempt has been made to simulate and test the schemes presented. Their function is only to indicate that of all the visually mediated eye movements, pursuit and fixation are the most elementary and the least understood and they represent a fertile field for investigation by both theoretical and experimental research.

REFERENCES

BENDER, M.B. & SHANZER, S., (1964). Oculomotor pathways defined by electric stimulation and lesions in the brain stem of monkey. **In** *The Oculomotor System*, M.B. Bender, ed., N.Y., Harper and Row.

COLLEWIJN, H., (1969). Optokinetic eye movements in the rabbit: input-output relations. *Vision Res.*, **9**, 117-132.

COLLEWIJN, H., *Personal communication.*

COOK, G. & STARK, L. (1968). Dynamics of the saccadic eye-movement system. *Comm. Behav. Biol.*, **1**, 197-204.

EASTER, S.S., Jr., *Personal communication.*

FENDER, D.H. (1962). The eye movement control system: evolution of a model. **In**, Neural Theory and Modeling, R.F. Reiss, ed., *Proc. Ojai Symp.*, Stanford, Stanford Univ. Press.

GERNANT, B.E., (1968). Interactions between extraocular myotatic and ascending vestibular activities. *Exptl. Neur.*, **20**, 120-134.

HORRIDGE, G.A. & BURROWS, M., (1968). Tonic and phasic systems in parallel in the eyecup responses of the crab *carcinus*. *J. Exp. Biol.*, **49**, 269-284.

JONES, G.M. (1964). Predominance of anti-compensatory oculomotor response during rapid head rotation. *Aerospace Med.*, **35**, 965-968.

JONES, G.M. & MILSUM, J.H. (1965). Spatial and dynamic aspects of visual fixation. *IEEE Trans. Bio-med. Eng.*, **BME-12**, 54-62.

KUYPERS, H.G. & LAWRENCE, D.G. (1967). Cortical projections to the red nucleus and the brain stem in the rhesus monkey. *Brain Res.*, **4**, 151-188.

LORENTE de NÓ, R. (1933). Vestibulo-ocular reflex arc. *Arch. Neurol. and Psychiat.*, **30**, 245-291.

McCOUCH, G.P. & ADLER, F.H. (1932). Extraocular reflexes. *Am. J. Physiol.*, **100**, 78-88.

MICHAEL, C.R. (May, 1969). Retinal processing of visual images. *Sci. Am.*, **220**, 105-114.

MILLER, J.E. (1958). Electromyographic pattern of saccadic eye movements. *Am. J. Ophthal.*, **46**, 183-186.

RASHBASS, C. (1961). The relationship between saccadic and smooth tracking eye movements. *J. Physiol.*, **159**, 326-338.

RICHTER, A. & PRECHT, W. (1968). Inhibition of abducens motoneurones by vestibular nerve stimulation. *Brain Res.*, **11**, 701-705.

ROBINSON, D.A. (1964). The mechanics of human saccadic eye movement. *J. Physiol.*, **174**, 245-264.

ROBINSON, D.A. (1965). The mechanics of human smooth pursuit eye movement. *J. Physiol.*, **180**, 569-591.

ROBINSON, D.A., O'MEARA, D.M., SCOTT, A.B., and COLLINS, C.C. (1969). The mechanical components of human eye movement. *J. Appl. Physiol.*, **26**, 548-553.

ROBINSON, D.A. & FUCHS, A.F. (1969). Eye movements evoked by stimulation of the frontal eye fields. *J. Neurophysiol.*, **32**, 637-649.

SCHAEFER, K.P. (1965). Die Erregungsmuster einzelner Neurone des Abducens-Kernes beim Kaninchen. *Pflüger's Arch.*, **284**, 31-52.

SHIMAZU, H. & PRECHT, W. (1966). Inhibition of central vestibular neurons from the contralateral labyrinth and its mediating pathway. *J. Neurophysiol.*, **29**, 467-492.

STERLING, P. & WICKELGREN, B.G. (1969). Visual receptive fields in the superior colliculus of the cat. *J. Neurophysiol.*, **32**, 1-15.

SZENTÁGOTHAI, J. (1950). The elementary vestibulo-ocular reflex arc. *J. Neurophysiol.*, **13**, 395-407.

TAMLER, E., MARG, E., JAMPOLSKY, A., and NAWRATZKI, I. (1959). Electro-myography of human saccadic eye movements. *A.M.A. Arch. Ophthal.*, **62**, 657-661.

THOMAS, J.G. (1967). The torque-angle transfer function of the human eye. *Kybernetik*, **3**, 254-263.

YAMANAKA, Y. & BACH-Y-RITA, P. (1968). Conduction velocities in the abducens nerve correlated with vestibular nystagmus in cats. *Exptl. Neur.*, **20**, 143-155.

YOUNG, L.R. & STARK, L. (1963). Variable feedback experiments testing a sampled data model for eye tracking movements. *IEEE Trans. of the Professional Tech. Grp. on Human Factors in Electronics*, **HFE-4**, 38-51.

YOUNG, L.R., FORSTER, J.D. and VAN HOUTTE, N. (March, 1968). A revised stochastic sampled data model for eye tracking movements. Fourth Annual NASA-University Conf. on Manual Control, Univ. Mich., Ann Arbor, Mich.

TIME DELAYS IN THE HUMAN EYE-TRACKING SYSTEM

DEREK H. FENDER

This symposium has been memorable for the wealth of new information that has emerged concerning the oculomotor system and for the number of shibboleths which have fallen by the wayside. For example, we have heard that the dichotomy between retinal image displacement and retinal image velocity as stimuli for saccades and for smooth following motions is by no means clear cut; the original ideas of a synchronous sampling mechanism have been softened, and following this lead, the purpose of this paper is to attempt to lay to rest the myth of the predictor mechanism. Most of this work has been carried out in conjunction with Gaetan J. St-Cyr. In two papers (St-Cyr and Fender, 1969a, 1969b) we have examined the response of the human eye tracking system in two-dimensional following tasks. The target motions used for this work ranged from the sum of a small number of sinusoids along each of the horizontal and vertical axes to various bandwidths of Gaussian sequences along each axis. Both monocular and binocular viewing conditions were examined.

The outcome of this work was to point up the nonlinearities of the oculomotor pursuit system. For example, on the average, the response has fairly well behaved low-pass characteristics, but the gain of the system is a function of the class of target motion---the gain at any frequency is reduced as the target motion becomes more complex. However, if the stimulus motion consists of a small number of sinusoids packed into a narrow frequency band, the gain increases with increasing frequency within the band; this is in contrast to the overall low-pass frequency characteristics of the system. Further, if the stimulus motion consists of a small number of sinusoids distributed over the bandwidth of the oculomotor system, there is a preferential response to the component having the highest frequency, power being robbed from lower frequency components if necessary to support the higher frequency enhancement.

Despite these nonlinear modes of behavior, the output of the system does not contain harmonic frequencies or sum-and-difference frequencies if the stimulus motion consists of a small number of sinusoids.

Turning now to the phase of the response of the oculomotor system in tracking tasks, the visual axis lags behind the target motion at all frequencies. This phase lag is relatively well behaved, increasing monotonically with increasing frequency and showing no behavior comparable with the rise of gain in narrow frequency bands. The phase lag does however change with the class of stimulus motion; in general the lag is greater as the target motion becomes more complex.

In many of the previous models of the oculomotor system it has been assumed that a linear representation is adequate, or at least a quasi-linear system with lumped nonlinearities. In general, the linear transfer function is obtained by curve-fitting to the gain of the system. This transfer function carries with it fixed phase characteristics. Unfortunately, when the phase of the real eye movement system is measured, it is found that the phase is generally much less than the model predicts. The normal escape from this impasse is to postulate that the eye-retina-brain complex is an intelligent organism which can analyse the target motion and predict where it will go next. The visual axis can thus be positioned ahead of time and so the phase lags of an unintelligent, minimum-phase system can be avoided.

Although this argument is very persuasive and has held sway for nearly a decade, it turns entirely on the forced linearization of a highly nonlinear system. If the invalidity of this process is accepted, than the whole idea of a predictor fails. Since the system is nonlinear, it cannot be represented by a transfer function, hence there is no theoretical datum of phase with which to compare the real phase of the response. Without this datum, who is to say that the system 'predicts', unless the phase lags are actually reduced to zero or even turned into a phase lead? The experimental evidence, however, is that neither of these two conditions ever occurs.

Having expressed our firm disbelief in what we acknowledge to be a time-honored feature of the oculomotor system, the responsibility of describing a more credible model rests with us.

We believe that the phase-lags which we measure for the oculomotor system, and all similar data derived from the work of other authors, can adequately be represented by simple time delays, but that the value of the delay, obtained by seeking the lag for maximum correlation between input and output of the system, is a function of the class of target motion. Some of these delay times are shown with phase-lag data obtained from the estimated cross power spectra between input and output in Figure 1.

Our concern is to identify the parameter of the tracking task which sets the delay time. If we calculate the rate of information transfer between the target motion and the tracking response of the visual axis, we obtain the results shown in Figure 2. Information transfer rate, R, is reduced as the

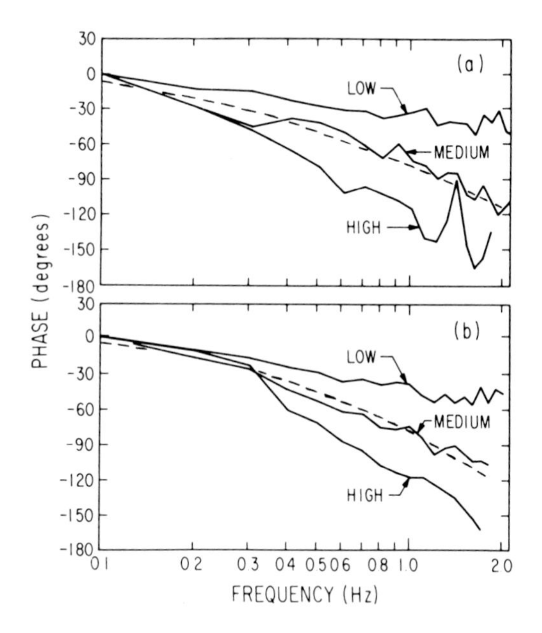

Fig. 1. Phase of left visual axis as a function of frequency when tracking three different band widths (low, medium, and high) of Gaussian sequences. **(a)** Vertical motion. **(b)** Horizontal motion. The appropriate time-delay for the medium band width curve is shown in each case as a dotted line.

delay time increases; the delay time, T, is adequately represented by a linear expression of the form

$$T = T_i + H/R$$

where T_i is the intercept of the line on the time axis. The time T_i can be equated with the transit time for nerve impulses to travel from the retina, through various central structures to the oculomotor nuclei and finally to the extraocular muscles. The value of T_i was found to be close to 65 msec for all subjects; this is not an unreasonable transit time for the neural messages.

The increased loss of information is consistent with the idea that the system subjects the input signal to some form of averaging process which extends over progressively lengthening periods of time as the delay increases. We have examined many models of this effect and believe that some credance can be placed in the process described below.

Let us assume that a finite amount of radiant energy must be absorbed by the retinal photoreceptors in order to produce a primary electrical event,

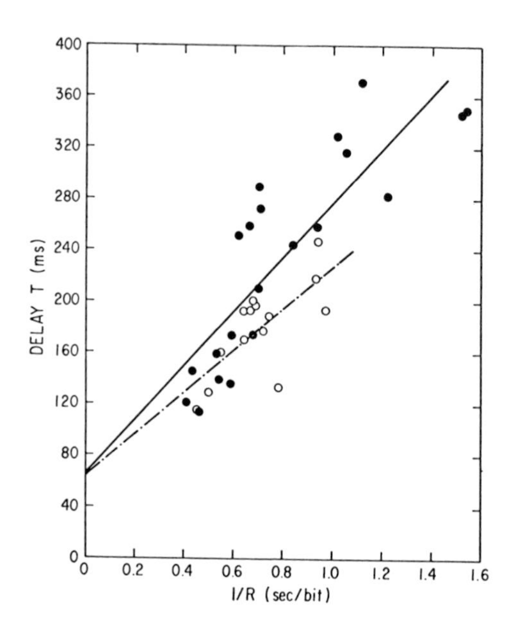

Fig. 2. Average delay of the oculomotor system response to band limited Gaussian sequences versus the reciprocal of the rate of transfer of information from target position to eye position. Data for two subjects.

and that these events must be integrated, both over time and over space, by the neural networks of the optic tract in order to produce the amount of excitation necessary to elicit a corrective eye movement. The time $(T\text{-}T_i)$ can thus be equated with the time required for the retinal image to travel over sufficient receptors to produce threshold excitation for a corrective eye movement.

We have the complete time history of the path of the retinal image; hence we can calculate δt, the mean time which a point image spends on one receptor. Moreover, since we know the time $(T\text{-}T_i)$ for each class of target motion we can also calculate the value of δs, the retinal distance swept by the image during the time $(T\text{-}T_i)$. If our hypothesis is correct, the corresponding values δs and δt should be related by a hyperbolic equation of the form:

$$(\delta s - \delta s_0)(\overline{\delta t} - \delta t_0) = C$$

where δs and δt are threshold values for space and time respectively. Our data is represented by an equation of this form at the p=0.05 level of significance.

From this evidence we conclude that our hypothesis has some validity; the delay time is thus the time required by the retinal image to sweep across enough receptors so that the integrated neural messages can generate the minimum afferent signal necessary to elicit corrective eye movements.

REFERENCES

St-Cyr, G. J. and Fender, D. H. (1969a). Non-linearities of the human oculomotor system: Gain. *Vision Research*, **9**, 1235–1246.

St-Cyr, G. J. and Fender, D. H. (1969b). Non-linearities of the human oculomotor system: Time delays. *Vision Research*, **9**, 1491–1503.

SUBJECT INDEX

SUBJECT INDEX

D

E

SUBJECT INDEX

F

L

M

SUBJECT INDEX

O

T

U

V